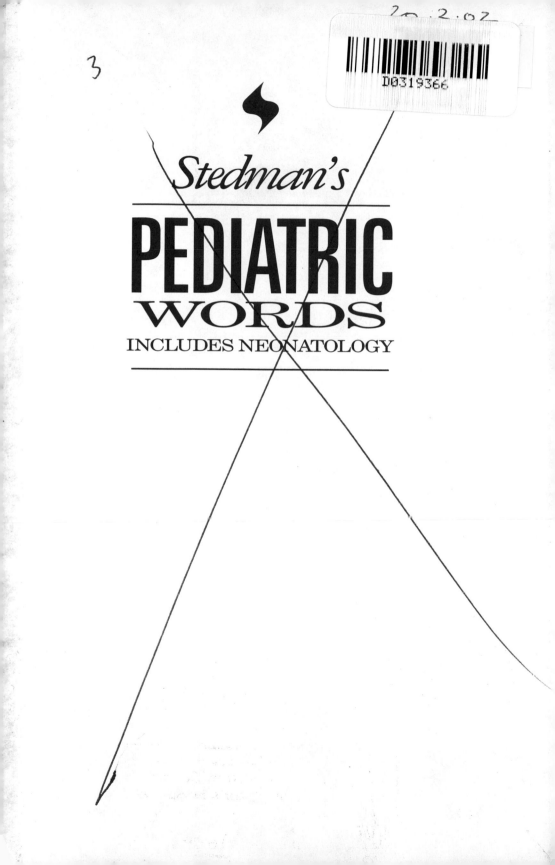

3

20.2.02

D0319366

Stedman's

PEDIATRIC
WORDS

INCLUDES NEONATOLOGY

Stedman's

PEDIATRIC

WORDS

INCLUDES NEONATOLOGY

Reference Collection

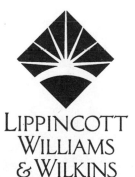

LIPPINCOTT
WILLIAMS
& WILKINS

Series Editor: Beverly J. Wolpert
Associate Managing Editor: Trista A. DiPaula
Associate Managing Editor: William A. Howard
Art Director: Jennifer Clements
Production Manager: Julie K. Stegman
Production Coordinator: Kevin Iarossi
Typesetter: Peirce Graphic Services, Inc.
Printer & Binder: Victor Graphics, Inc.

Printed in the United States of America

2001

Library of Congress Cataloging-in-Publication Data

Stedman's pediatric words includes neonatology
    p. ; cm.
    ISBN 0-7817-3057-0 (alk. paper)
    1. Pediatrics—Terminology. 2. Neonatology—Terminology. I. Title: Pediatric
words includes neonatology. II. Stedman, Thomas Lathrop, 1853–1938.
    [DNLM: 1. Pediatrics—Terminology—English. 2. Neonatology—
Terminology—English.
WS 15 S812 2001]
RJ47 .S74 2001
618.92'0001'4—dc21

2001029177
01
1 2 3 4 5 6 7 8 9 10

Contents

Acknowledgments

An important part of our editorial process is the involvement of medical transcriptionists — as advisors, reviewers, and/or editors.

We extend special thanks to Jeanne Bock, CSR, MT, and Nicole G. Peck for editing the manuscript, helping resolve many difficult questions, and contributing material for the appendix sections. We also extend thanks to Natasha Brown for working on the appendix and to Helen Littrell for performing the final prepublication review.

We are grateful, as well, to our MT Editorial Advisory Board members, including Natasha Brown; Wendy Ryan, RHIT; Jenifer F. Walker, MA; and Sandra Wideburg, CMT, who were instrumental to the development of this reference. They recommended sources and provided valuable judgment, insights, and perspectives.

Others important to this edition include Rose M. Berry; Marty Cantu, CMT; Shemah Fletcher; Elizabeth Willard Gorsline, CMT; Deborah B. Hahn, CMT; Diane Hernandez, CMT; Kathy Hess, CMT; Nancy Hill, MT; Sandy Kovacs, CMT; Robin Koza; Kathryn C. Mason, CMT; P. Michael Murphy, CMT; Beverly S. Oberline, CMT; Anna Parr, CMT; Laura A. Pitts; Diana Rezac, CMT; Cheri Sawyer, CMT; and Diane LeMieux Zook, CMT.

Barb Ferretti played an integral role in the process by reviewing the content files for format, updating the database, and providing a final quality check.

As with all our *Stedman's* word references, this resource incorporates the suggestions and expertise of our many contacts in the medical transcriptionist community. Thanks to all of our advisory board participants, reviewers, and editors; AAMT meeting attendees; and others who have written us with requests and comments — keep talking, and we'll keep listening.

Editor's Preface

It's a miracle of life: two microscopic cells join; then they grow and multiply, forming tissues, membranes, muscles, bones, and organs, until eventually they form a tiny human being, composed of body systems working together to carry out the functions of life. The mother needs care of her own to help nurture and eventually bring this little individual into the world. Once born, this new being has its own specific set of needs requiring specialized care.

Never before have parents had more cause for concern or awe regarding the healthcare of their children. Doctors are now able to perform innovative surgery on a fetus still in its mother's womb, providing opportunities to correct debilitating deformities even before birth. Some of the worst scourges of our time, as well as the commonplace, touch even the smallest lives: AIDS, cancer, herpes, congenital anomalies, genetic defects, maternal addiction with inherent fetal prematurity, withdrawal syndrome, cerebral palsy, cystic fibrosis, mental retardation, fetal alcohol syndrome, syphilis, gonorrhea, and infant and child abuse/neglect, as well as chickenpox, respiratory syncytial virus (RSV), rotavirus, mumps, meningitis, increasingly resistant streptococcal infections, rubella, influenza, and the "common" cold.

The advances in pediatrics are of great interest to us as both parents and medical transcriptionists. We worry: What are the chances my child could develop this illness? What if she has an adverse reaction to her routine immunizations? Will he be born healthy? Our hearts are touched when we transcribe reports of the trials children and their parents go through to attain better health. Unfortunately, these innocent lives can be touched by tragedy through an accident, abuse, society, the environment, or simply genetics. Our goal, while we may not be able to cure these children ourselves, is to provide an accurate medical record so that the physicians can provide the best care possible.

Medical advances, from in vitro fertilization to selective reduction, have created subspecialties within the specialty of pediatrics. The growth of these subspecialties has introduced many new terms into the field of pediatrics, and those terms have now been documented and compiled in this first edition of *Stedman's Pediatric Words*.

We searched for emerging and existing terminology specific to the field of pediatrics with the goal that this book would provide a wide range of specialty terms to make the medical records you transcribe the most accurate possible. We believe we are offering a unique reference book covering terminology that will be heard throughout the field of pediatrics, beginning at the time of birth through adolescence.

We thank all of you who have sent in suggestions that were subsequently incorporated into this first edition of *Stedman's Pediatric Words*. Additional thanks goes to Barb Ferretti for her consistent and ever-present assistance and contributions to the entire Stedman's Word Book Series.

Jeanne Bock, CSR, MT
Nicole G. Peck

Publisher's Preface

Stedman's Pediatric Words offers an authoritative assurance of quality and exactness to the wordsmiths of the healthcare professions—medical transcriptionists, medical editors and copyeditors, health information management personnel, court reporters, and the many other users and producers of medical documentation.

In the specialties of pediatrics, a single, comprehensive collection of terms is difficult to identify. These fields of pediatrics and neonatology encompass a vast array of terms from dermatology to cardiology, ranging from birth to age eighteen. Over the past few years, we have received requests and suggestions from MTs to create a separate pediatric and neonatology wordbook. As the requests increased, we realized that medical language professionals need a single, comprehensive reference for pediatrics and neonatology.

In *Stedman's Pediatric Words,* users will find thousands of words as they relate to immunization, growth, and development, as well as the many subspecialties of pediatrics. Users will also find terms for protocols, diagnostic and therapeutic procedures, new techniques, and lab tests, as well as equipment names and abbreviations with their expansions. The appendix sections provide anatomical illustrations with useful captions and labels, sample reports, and common terms by procedure, as well as normal lab values, Apgar scores, developmental milestones, recommended immunizations, routine immunizations for HIV-infected children, oral rehydration fluids and infant formulas, poisonous plants, and drugs by therapeutic category and key word.

This compilation of more than 100,000 entries, fully cross-indexed for quick access, was built from a base vocabulary of approximately 66,000 medical words, phrases, abbreviations, and acronyms. The extensive A-Z list was developed from manufacturers' literature, scientific reports, books, journals, CDs, and websites (please see list of References on page xvi).

We at Lippincott Williams & Wilkins strive to provide you with the most up-to-date and accurate word references available. Your use of this word-book will prompt new editions, which we will publish as often as updates and revisions justify. We welcome your suggestions for improvements, changes, corrections, and additions—whatever will make this *Stedman's* reference more useful to you. Please complete the postpaid card at the back of this book, and send your recommendations care of "Stedman's" at Lippincott Williams & Wilkins.

Explanatory Notes

Medical transcription is an art as well as a science. Both approaches are needed to correctly interpret the dictation of a physician, whose language is a product of education, training, and experience. This variety in medical language means that there are several acceptable ways to express certain terms, including jargon. *Stedman's Pediatric Words* provides variant spellings and phrasings for many terms. These elements, in addition to complete cross-indexing, make *Stedman's Pediatric Words* a valuable resource for determining the validity of terms as they are encountered.

Alphabetical Organization

Alphabetization of main entries is letter by letter as spelled, ignoring punctuation, spaces, prefixed numbers, or other special characters. For example:

Benylin
Benzac
5-Benzagel
Benzamycin

Terms beginning with Greek letters show the Greek letters spelled out and listed alphabetically. For example:

alpha, α
    a. fetoprotein
    interferon a.
    a. lactalbumin (ALA)

In subentry alphabetization, the abbreviated singular form or the spelled-out plural form of the noun main entry word is ignored.

Format and Style

All main entries are in **boldface** to expedite locating a sought-after term, to enhance distinction between main entries and subentries, and to relieve the textual density of the pages.

Irregular plurals and variant spellings are shown on the same line as the singular or preferred form of the word. For example:

atrium, pl. atria
hypogammaglobulinemia, hypogammaglobinemia

Hyphenation

As a rule of style, multiple eponyms (e.g., Mears-Rubash approach) are hyphenated. Also, hyphens have been added between a manufacturer and one or more eponyms (e.g., Vital-Metzenbaum dissecting scissors). Please note that in many cases, hyphenation is a question of style, not of accuracy, and thus is a matter of choice.

Possessives

Possessive forms have been dropped in this reference for the sake of consistency and conformance with the guidelines of the American Association for Medical Transcription (AAMT) and other groups. Please note, however, that in many cases, retaining the possessive, like hyphenating, is a question of style, not of accuracy, and thus is a matter of choice. To form the possessive of a word, simply add the apostrophe or apostrophe "s" to the end of the word.

Cross-indexing

The word list is in an index-like main entry-subentry format that contains two combined alphabetical listings:

1) A *noun* main entry-subentry organization, which is typical of the A-Z section of medical dictionaries like *Stedman's:*

iris
  i. dilator
  stellate i.

trunk
  t. control
  pulmonary t.

(2) An *adjective* main entry-subentry organization, which lists words and phrases as you hear them. The main entries are the adjectives or modifiers in a multiword term. The subentries are the nouns around which the terms are constructed and to which the adjectives or modifiers pertain:

pancreatic
  p. ring
  p. tumor

vaginal
  v. discharge
  Monistat V.

This format provides the user with more than one way to locate and identify a multiword term. For example:

irregular
  i. cortex

cortex
  irregular c.

fetal
  f. tracheal occlusion

occlusion
  fetal tracheal o.

stage
  s. A infection

infection
  stage A i.

It also allows the user to see together all terms that contain a particular descriptor, as well as all types, kinds, or variations of a noun entity. For example:

acid
  acetic a.
  amoxicillin-clavulanic a.
  a. maltase deficiency (AMD)

dermatitis
  candidal diaper d.
  d. gangrenosa infantum
  juvenile plantar d.

Wherever possible, abbreviations are separately defined and cross-referenced. For example:

NICU
  neonatal intensive care unit

neonatal
  n. intensive care unit (NICU)

unit
  neonatal intensive care u. (NICU)

References

In addition to the manufacturers' literature we gather at various medical meetings, scientific reports from hospitals, and the lists of our MT Editorial Advisory Board members from their daily transcription work, we used the following sources for new terms in *Stedman's Pediatric Words:*

Books

Avery GB, Fletcher MA, MacDonald MG, eds. Neonatology: Pathophysiology and Management of the Newborn. Baltimore: Lippincott Williams & Wilkins, 1999.

Behrman RE, Kliegman RM, Jenson HB, eds. Nelson Textbook of Pediatrics, 16th Edition. Philadelphia: Saunders, 1999.

Betz CL, Snowden LA, eds. Mosby's Pediatric Nursing Reference, 4th Edition. St. Louis: Mosby, 1999.

Coleman JG. The Early Intervention Dictionary: A Multidisciplinary Guide to Terminology. Bethesda, MD: Woodbine House, 1999.

Finberg L, ed. Saunders Manual of Pediatric Practice. Philadelphia: Saunders, 1998.

Fleischer GR, Ludwig S, Henretig FM, Ruddy RM, Silverman BK, eds. Textbook of Pediatric Emergency Medicine, 4th Edition. Baltimore: Lippincott Williams & Wilkins, 1999.

Garson A, Bricker JT, Fisher DJ, Neish SR. The Science and Practice of Pediatric Cardiology, 2nd Edition. Baltimore: Lippincott Williams & Wilkins, 1997.

Gennrich J, ed. Pediatric Drug Reference, Year 2000 Edition. Mission-Viejo, CA: Current Clinical Strategies Publishing, 1999.

Gilbert P, ed. Dictionary of Childhood Health Problems, 2nd Edition. Chicago: Fitzroy Dearborn Publishers, 1999.

Herzog D. Reviews in Child & Adolescent Psychiatry. Baltimore: Lippincott Williams & Wilkins, 1998.

Lance LL. 2000 Quick Look Drug Book. Baltimore: Lippincott Williams & Wilkins, 2000.

Menkes JH, Sarnat HB, eds. Child Neurology, 6th Edition. Baltimore: Lippincott Williams & Wilkins, 2000.

Pyle V. Current Medical Terminology, 8th Edition. Modesto, CA: Health Professions Institute, 2000.

Schwartz WM, Bell LM, Bingham PM, Chung EK, Friedman DF, Mulberg AE, eds. The 5 Minute Pediatric Consult, 2nd Edition. Baltimore: Lippincott Williams & Wilkins, 1999.

Staheli LT. Fundamentals of Pediatric Orthopedics, 2nd Edition. Baltimore: Lippincott Williams & Wilkins, 1998.

Stedman's Medical Dictionary, 27th Edition. Baltimore: Lippincott Williams & Wilkins, 2000.

Taketomo CK, Hodding Hurlburt J, Kraus DM. Pediatric Dosage Handbook, 6th Edition. Hudson, OH: Lexi-Comp, 1999.

Tessier C. The American Association of Medical Transcriptions Book of Style. Modesto, CA: AAMT, 1995.

Wong D. Pediatric Quick Reference, 3rd Edition. St. Louis: Mosby, 2000.

Zeichner SL, Read JS, eds. Handbook of Pediatric HIV Care. Baltimore: Lippincott William & Wilkins, 1999.

Journals

Contemporary Pediatrics. Montvale, NJ: Medical Economics, 1999–2000.

Current Opinion in Pediatrics. Baltimore: Lippincott Williams & Wilkins, 1999–2000.

Journal of the American Academy of Child and Adolescent Psychiatry. Baltimore: Lippincott Williams & Wilkins, 1999–2000.

Journal of Pediatric Gastroenterology and Nutrition. Baltimore: Lippincott Williams & Wilkins, 1998–2000.

The Journal of Pediatrics. St. Louis: Mosby, 1999–2000.

The Latest Word. Philadelphia: Saunders, 1996–2000.

MT Monthly. Gladstone, MO: Computer Systems Management, 1996–2000.

Pediatric Annals. Thorofare, NJ: Slack Incorporated, 1996; 2000.

Pediatric Emergency Care. Baltimore: Lippincott Williams & Wilkins, 1999–2000.

The Pediatric Infectious Disease Journal. Baltimore: Lippincott Williams & Wilkins, 1999–2000.

Pediatric News. Short Hills, NJ: Saunders, 1996.

Pediatric Research. Baltimore: Lippincott Williams & Wilkins, 1999–2000.

Pediatrics. Elk Grove Village, Il.: American Academy of Pediatrics, 1996; 1999–2000.

CDs

McMillan JA, DeAngelis CD, Feigin RD, Warshaw JB, eds. Oski's Pediatrics: Principle and Practice, 3rd Edition on CD-ROM. Baltimore: Lippincott Williams & Wilkins, 1999.

Websites

http://generalpediatrics.com

http://ww2.med.jhu.edu/peds/neonatology

http://www.aacap.org

http://www.aap.org

http://www.hpisum.com

http://www.medscape.com/Home/Topics/pediatrics/pediatrics.html

http://www.mtdesk.com

http://www.pcc.com/lists/pedtalk.archive/

http://www.pedinfo.org

A2
thromboxane A2
a-2
a-2 antiplasmin (a-2AP)
a-2 antiplasmin coagulation
inhibitor
a-2 antitrypsin (a-2AT)
a-2 antitrypsin inhibitor
a-2 macroglobulin (a-2M)
a-2 macroglobulin coagulation
inhibitor
AA
acetabular anteversion
acute appendicitis
atlantoaxial
AA40
Varian Spectra AA40
A-a
alveolar-arterial
A-a gradient
AAA
achalasia-addisonianism-alacrimia
AAA syndrome
AABR, A-ABR
automated auditory brainstem response
AABR hearing screening
AAC
augmentative and alternative
communication
AACAP
American Academy of Child and
Adolescent Psychiatry
AAD
antibiotic-associated diarrhea
AADPPO
alveolar-arterial difference in partial
pressure of oxygen
Aagene syndrome
AAI
axial acetabular index
AAMD
American Association on Mental
Deficiency
AAMR
American Association on Mental
Retardation
A antigen
AAP
American Academy of Pediatrics
a-2AP
a-2 antiplasmin
a-2AP coagulation inhibitor
AAPCC
American Association of Poison Control
Centers

AaPO₂
arterial to alveolar oxygen tension ratio
Aarskog-Scott syndrome
Aarskog syndrome
AASH
adrenal androgen-stimulating hormone
AAST
American Association for the Surgery of
Trauma
AAST Organ Injury Scaling of
vulva, vagina, bladder, urethral,
rectal injury (grade I–V)
AAT
animal-assisted therapy
a-2AT
a-2 antitrypsin
a-2AT coagulation inhibitor
a/b
influenza a/b
ABA
applied behavior analysis
abacavir (ABC)
a. sulfate
Abate
Abbokinase
ABC
abacavir
absolute band count
airway, breathing, circulation
ABCDE
airway, breathing, circulation and control
bleeding, disability, exposure
ABCDE assessment
abdomen
acute a.
bloated a.
distended a.
milk lines of a.
scaphoid a.
tympanitic a.
abdominal
a. ballottement
a. breathing
a. bruit
a. cavity
a. coarctation
a. compartment syndrome (ACS)
a. distention
a. epilepsy
a. heterotaxy
a. incision
a. mass
a. metroplasty
a. migraine
a. muscular deficiency

abdominal *(continued)*
    a. pain
    a. percussion
    a. pregnancy
    a. radiograph
    a. rectopexy
    a. sheath
    a. tenderness
    a. tuberculosis
    a. ultrasound
abdominis
    diastasis recti a.
abdominopelvic
abdominoscrotal hydrocele
abducens
    a. facial paralysis
    a. nerve
    a. palsy
abduct
abduction
    a. cast
    defective eye a.
    forefoot a.
    resisted a.
    a. splint
abductor lurch
Abelcet
aberrancy
aberrant
    a. coronary artery
    a. course
    a. course of testicular descent
    a. regeneration
    a. right subclavian artery (ARSA)
    a. subclavian artery
    a. supraventricular tachycardia
    a. vitamin D metabolism
aberration
    heterosomal a.
    newtonian a.
abetalipoproteinemia
ABG
    arterial blood gas
ability
    cognitive a.
    Illinois Test of
      Psycholinguistic A.'s (IPTA)
    McCarthy Scales of Children's A.'s
    Revised Tests of Cognitive A.
Abiotrophia
    A. defectiva
    A. elegans
ablation
    laser a.
    mucosal intact laser tonsillar a.
    (MILTA)
    percutaneous transluminal coronary
    rotational a. (PTCRA)

    stellate ganglion a.
    transurethral a.
    valve a.
ablative surgery
ablepharon macrostomia syndrome
    (AMS)
ABM
    adult bone marrow
abnormal
    a. aortic valve attachment
    a. cortical visual input
    a. dysfluency
    a. face
    a. facies
    a. glucosylceramide storage
    a. head size
    A. Involuntary Movement Scale
      (AIMS)
    a. laxity of upper airway
    a. mitochondrion
    a. palate
    a. palpebral fissure
    a. penile curvature
    a. phonation
    a. placentation
    a. respiratory pattern
    a. transit
    a. vaginal bleeding
    a. vasculature flow pattern
abnormality
    cardiac a.
    central serotonin a.
    chromosomal a.
    congenital enamel a.
    conotruncal a.
    dermatoglyphic a.
    electrographic background a.
    extracardiac a.
    Fairbank skeletal a.
    fishmouth a.
    gyral a.
    multiple endocrine a.'s (MEA)
    palpable bony a.
    perisylvian a.
    platelet a.
    posterior fossa malformation,
      hemangiomas, arterial anomalies,
      coarctation of aorta and cardiac
      defects, eye a.'s (PHACE)
    regional wall motion a.
    Ribbing skeletal a.
    spinal cord injury without
      radiographic a. (SCIWORA)
    ST-segment a.
    ST-T wave a.
    tuberous breast a.
    T-wave a.

abnormally wide splitting of second heart sound
ABO
> ABO hemolytic disease
> ABO incompatibility

aboral flow
abortion
> induced a.
> spontaneous a.
> therapeutic a. (TA)
> threatened a.

abortive poliomyelitis
abortus
> *Brucella a.*

Aboulker stent
ABP
> ambulatory blood pressure
> arterial blood pressure

ABPA
> allergic bronchopulmonary aspergillosis

ABPM
> ambulatory blood pressure monitoring

ABPN
> American Board of Psychiatry and Neurology

ABR
> auditory brainstem response

abrachia
Abramson classification
abrasion
> basal pleural a.
> basilar pleural a.
> corneal a.

abrogated neonatal alveolization
abruptio
> placenta a.
> a. placentae

abruption
> placental a.

abscess
> amebic hepatic a.
> amebic liver a.
> auricular a.
> Bartholin gland a.
> Bezold a.
> biliary a.
> breast a.
> Brodie a.
> a. cavity
> cold a.
> cranial epidural a.
> crypt a.

> dental-alveolar a.
> embolic a.
> epidural a.
> extradural a.
> intermuscular a.
> intersphincteric a.
> intraabdominal a.
> ischiorectal a.
> metastatic tuberculous a.
> myocardial a.
> neonatal scalp a.
> orbital subperiosteal a.
> otogenic brain a.
> paravertebral a.
> parenchymal a.
> perianal a.
> periappendiceal a.
> perirectal a.
> peritonsillar a.
> psoas a.
> retroesophageal a.
> retropharyngeal a.
> retrotonsillar a.
> spinal epidural a.
> subdural a.
> subperiosteal a.
> subphrenic a.
> supralevator a.
> tuberculous a.
> tuboovarian a.
> visceral a.

abscessus
> *Mycobacterium a.*

absence
> a. attack
> a. of branch pulmonary artery
> congenital a.
> a. epilepsy
> myoclonic a.
> protein-induced vitamin K a. (PIVKA)
> a. of rectal muscles
> a. seizure
> a. status
> a. status epilepticus
> testicular a.

absent
> a. antihelical fold
> a. menses
> a. patella
> a. prostate
> a. pulmonary valve syndrome

NOTES

absent *(continued)*
    a. radius
    a. tears
    a. testis
absolute
    a. band count (ABC)
    a. CD4 count
    a. length gain
    a. lymphocyte count
    a. neutrophil count
    a. nucleated red blood cell (ANRBC)
    a. temperature
    a. weight gain
absorbance
    time-of-flight and a. (TOFA)
absorbed
    rabies vaccine, a. (RVA)
absorbent gelling material (AGM)
Absorbine
    A. Antifungal
    A. Jock Itch
    A. Jr. Antifungal
absorptiometry
    dual-energy x-ray a. (DEXA)
absorption
    coefficient of fat a.
    defective tryptophan a.
    fat a.
    mean fraction a.
    vitamin B_{12} a.
absorptive hypercalciuria
ABSR
    auditory brainstem response
abstinence syndrome
abstract thinking
ABT
    alternating breath test
Abt-Letterer-Siwe syndrome
abuse
    child a. (CA)
    child physical a.
    emotional a.
    mandated reporter (of child a.)
    maternal substance a.
    sexual a.
    a., sexuality, safety assessment
    spousal a.
    substance a.
    verbal a.
abuser
    child of substance a. (COSA)
ABVD
    Adriamycin (doxorubicin), bleomycin, vinblastine, dacarbazine
A-C
    Robitussin A-C

AC
    acromioclavicular
      Guaituss AC
      AC joint
A1c
    hemoglobin A1c
a.c.
    ante cibum (before meals)
A-Caine Rectal
acalculous cholecystitis
Acanthamoeba
    A. castellani
    A. culbertsoni
    A. keratitis
    A. polyphagia
    A. rhysodes
acanthocyte
acanthocytosis
acantholysis bullosa
acanthosis
    a. nigricans
    paraductal a.
acardiac fetus
Acarosan
acatalasemia
acatalasia
accelerate
accelerated
    a. atherosclerosis
    a. hypertension
    a. junctional ectopic tachycardia
    a. rejection
acceleration-deceleration force
acceleration injury
accentuation
    perifollicular a.
acceptance stage
accessory
    a. auricle
    a. chromosome
    a. muscle
    a. muscle retraction
    a. navicular
    a. nipple
    a. protein
    a. soleus
    a. spleen
    a. tragus
accident
    cerebrovascular a. (CVA)
    neonatal vascular a.
accidental ingestion
Accolate
accommodation
    pupils equal, round, reactive to light and a. (PERRLA)
accommodative esotropia

accreditation
>   Commission on Office
>   Laboratory A. (COLA)

accretion
>   mass a.
>   neural tissue a.

ACCS
>   acute change clinical score

Accu-Chek test

AccuLevel

accumbens
>   nucleus a.

accumulation
>   dermatan sulfate a.
>   glycogen a.
>   heparin sulfate a.
>   ketoacid a.
>   lipid a.

Accupep formula

Accurbron Aerolate III

AccuStat Strep A assay

Accutane effect

ACE
>   angiotensin-converting enzyme
>   antegrade continence enema
>   ACE inhibitor

Acel-Imune
>   A.-I. HibTITER
>   A.-I. vaccine

acellular
>   a. pertussis
>   a. pertussis vaccine

acentric chromosome

Acephen

aceruloplasminemia

Aceta

acetabula (*pl. of* acetabulum)

acetabular
>   a. anteversion (AA)
>   a. dysplasia
>   a. index (AI)
>   a. labrum
>   a. roof

acetabuli
>   protrusio a.

acetabuloplasty
>   Pemberton a.

acetabulum, pl. **acetabula**
>   shallow a.

acetamide
>   modafinil a.

acetaminophen
>   hydrocodone and a.
>   oxycodone and a.
>   propoxyphene and a.

acetate
>   aluminum a.
>   Cortone A.
>   depomedroxyprogesterone a.
>   (DMPA)
>   desmopressin a.
>   Florinef A.
>   glatiramer a.
>   histrelin a.
>   leuprorelin a.
>   medroxyprogesterone a. (MPA)
>   megestrol a.
>   methylprednisolone a.
>   octreotide a.
>   sermorelin a.
>   sodium a.

acetazolamide

acetic acid

acetoacetate

acetonide
>   triamcinolone a.

acetonuria

acetylcholine

acetylcholinesterase histochemical stain

acetyl-CoA
>   a.-CoA carboxylase
>   a.-CoA dehydrogenase

acetylcysteine drug

acetylsalicylic acid

ACGME
>   American College of Graduate Medical
>   Education

achalasia
>   familial a.

achalasia-addisonianism-alacrimia (AAA)
>   a.-a.-a. syndrome

Achard syndrome

ache
>   stomach a.

acheiria

Achenbach
>   A. Child Behavior Checklist
>   A. questionnaire

Aches-N-Pain

achievement
>   Kaufman Test of Educational A.
>   (K-TEA)
>   Woodcock-Johnson Tests of A.

NOTES

Achilles
    A. tendon
    A. tendon insertion
    A. tendon lengthening
    A. tendon xanthoma
Achillis
    tendo A.
achlorhydria
acholic stool
achondrogenesis syndrome
achondroplasia
    homozygous a.
    a. syndrome
achondroplastic dwarfism
achromians
    incontinentia pigmenti a.
achromic nevus
Achromobacter xylosoxidans
Achromycin
    A. Ophthalmic
    A. Topical
    A. V Oral
acid
    acetic a.
    acetylsalicylic a.
    all-*trans*-retinoic a.
    alpha-aminoadipic a.
    alpha-ketoadipic a.
    alpha-ketoisocaproic a. (alpha-KIC)
    alpha-linolenic a. (ALA)
    amino a.
    aminocaproic a.
    5-aminosalicylic a.
    amoxicillin-clavulanic a.
    anti-deoxyribonucleic a. (anti-DNA)
    arachidic a.
    arachidonic a.
    argininosuccinic a.
    ascorbic a.
    aspartic a.
    bile a.
    branched-chain amino a.
    branched-chain fatty a. (BCFA)
    branched deoxyribonucleic a. (bDNA)
    a. ceramidase deficiency
    citrate and citric a.
    complementary deoxyribonucleic a. (cDNA)
    conjugated linoleic a. (CLA)
    C-palmitic a.
    deoxyribonucleic a. (DNA)
    dibasic amino a.
    diisopropyl iminodiacetic a. (DISIDA)
    dimercaptosuccinic a.
    docosahexaenoic a. (DHA)
    docosapentaenoic a.

    eicosapentaenoic a.
    elevated bile a.
    epsilon-aminocaproic a.
    erucic a.
    essential amino a.
    essential fatty a. (EFA)
    ethacrynic a.
    ethylenediaminetetraacetic a. (EDTA)
    excitotoxic amino a. (EAA)
    fatty a.
    folic a.
    folinic a.
    formic a.
    formiminoglutamic a. (FIGLU)
    free fatty a.
    gamma-aminobutyric a. (GABA)
    glutamic a.
    gossypol acetic a. (GAA)
    homovanillic a. (HVA)
    hydroxyeicosatetraenoic a.
    hypochlorous a.
    iduronic a.
    imino a.
    isobutyric a.
    isovaleric a.
    kinetoplast deoxyribonucleic a. (kDNA)
    lactic a.
    linoleic a.
    linolenic a.
    a. lipase deficiency disease
    long-chain fatty a.
    long-chain polyunsaturated fatty a. (LCPUFA)
    a. maltase
    a. maltase deficiency (AMD)
    A. Mantle
    medium-chain fatty a. (MCFA)
    mefenamic a.
    messenger ribonucleic a. (mRNA)
    methylmalonic a.
    methylsuccinic a.
    mitochondrial deoxyribonucleic a. (mtDNA)
    mycophenolic a.
    N-acetylaspartic a.
    nalidixic a.
    neuraminic a.
    nicotinic a.
    nonessential amino a.
    omega fatty a.
    omega-3 fatty a.
    orotic a.
    palmitic a.
    pantothenic a.
    paraaminosalicylic a.
    a. peptic disease

phenylacetic a.
phenylpyruvic a.
a. phosphatase
phytanic a.
plasma linoleic a.
plasma very-long-chain fatty a.
polyunsaturated fatty a. (PUFA)
pteroylglutamic a.
pyruvic a.
quinolinic a.
a. reflux
retinoic a.
ribonucleic a. (RNA)
salicylic a.
serum amino a.
serum uric a.
short-chain fatty a. (SCFA)
short-chain polyunsaturated fatty a.
  (SCPUFA)
sulfur and salicylic a.
thioctic a.
ticarcillin/clavulanic a.
tranexamic a.
trans fatty a. (tFA)
trichloroacetic a. (TCA)
umbilical venous plasma amino a.
undecylenic a.
unsaturated linolenic a.
uric a.
urinary orotic a.
urine organic a.
urine vanillylmandelic a.
urocanic a.
ursodeoxycholic a. (UDCA)
valproic a.
vanillylmandelic a. (VMA)
very long chain fatty a. (VLCFA)
xanthurenic a.

acid-base disorder
acidemia
branched-chain amino a.
gamma-aminobutyric a. (GABA)
glutaric a. (type I, II)
hyperpipecolic a.
isovaleric a.
lactic a.
methylmalonic a.
mevalonic a.
organic a.
orotic a.
pipecolic a.
propionic a.

acid-fast
a.-f. bacillus
a.-f. sputum smear
a.-f. stain
acidification
disordered renal a.
acidified serum lysis test
acidity
fecal a.
acidophilus
Lactobacillus a.
acidosis
chronic respiratory a.
congenital lactic a.
cord blood a.
diabetic a.
fetal a.
hyperchloremic metabolic a.
hyperchloremic renal a.
hyperchromic a.
hypokalemic a.
lactic a.
metabolic a.
nonanion gap metabolic a.
organic a.
primary lactic a.
renal tubular a. (RTA)
respiratory a.
acid-Schiff staining
aciduria
alpha-aminoadipic a.
alpha-ketoadipic a.
argininosuccinic a.
beta-aminoisobutyric a.
ethylmalonic-adipic a.
glutaric a. (type I, II)
HMG a.
3-hydroxy-3-methylglutaric a.
isovaleric a.
3-methylglutaconic a.
methylmalonic a. (MMA)
mevalonic a.
organic a.
orotic a.
paradoxical a.
urocanic a.
xanthurenic a.
acinar artery
Acinetobacter
acinic cell carcinoma

NOTES

ACIP
  Advisory Committee on Immunization
  Practices
acitretin
ACL
  anterior cruciate ligament
aclasis
  diaphyseal a.
Aclovate
ACLS
  advanced cardiac life support
acne
  acute febrile ulcerative a.
  a. conglobata
  cosmetic a.
  a. cyst
  drug-induced a.
  a. fulminans
  a. (grade I–IV)
  gram-negative a.
  halogen a.
  neonatal a.
  a. neonatorum
  occupational a.
  a. rosacea
  steroid a.
  toddler-age nodulocystic a.
  truncal a.
  a. vulgaris
acnes
  Propionibacterium a.
acoustic
  a. admittance
  a. blink reflex
  a. meningioma
  a. nerve
  a. neuroma
  a. reflectometry
  a. reflex test
  a. respiratory motion sensor
  (ARMS)
  a. schwannoma
  a. trauma
acquired
  a. abducens palsy
  a. angioedema (type I, II)
  a. antithrombin III deficiency
  a. ascending undescended testis
  a. C1 INH deficiency
  a. cutis laxa
  a. epileptic aphasia
  a. growth hormone deficiency
  a. heart disease
  a. hemophilia
  a. hypogammaglobulinemia
  a. hypothalamic lesion
  a. hypothyroidism

  a. immune deficiency syndrome
  (AIDS)
  a. immunodeficiency
  a. immunodeficiency syndrome
  (AIDS)
  a. inflammatory Brown syndrome
  a. melanocytic nevus (AMN)
  nosocomially a. (NA)
  a. nystagmus
  a. PAP
  a. platelet disorder
  a. pneumonia
  a. protein C, S deficiency
  a. 6th nerve palsy
  a. torticollis
  a. urticaria
acquisita
  epidermolysis bullosa a.
acquisition
  intrauterine a.
  multiple gated a. (MUGA)
acral
  a. cyanosis
  a. keratotic papule
  a. skin lesion
acridine orange stain
acrid odor
acrivastine
acrobrachycephaly
acrocallosal syndrome
acrocephalopolysyndactyly
acrocephalosyndactyly (type I–V)
acrocephaly
acrochordon
acrocyanosis
  peripheral a.
acrodermatitis
  a. chronica atrophicans
  a. enteropathica
  papular a.
  papulovesicular a.
acrodynia
acrodysostosis syndrome
acrofacial
  a. dysostosis
  a. dysostosis (Nager type)
acromegaly
acromelic shortening
acromesomelic dysplasia
acromioclavicular (AC)
  a. joint
  a. ligament
acromion process
acroosteolysis
acropustulosis
  a. of infancy
  infantile a.
acrorenal syndrome

acrorenocular syndrome
acrorenomandibular syndrome
acrylic splint
ACS
    abdominal compartment syndrome
    acute chest syndrome
    anterior cricoid split
ACT
    activated clotting time
act
      Americans with Disabilities A.
       (ADA)
      Child Abuse Prevention and
       Treatment A.
      Education for All Handicapped
       Children A.
      Family Medical Leave A. (FMLA)
      Individuals with Disabilities A.
      Individuals with Disabilities
       Education A. (IDEA)
      self-harming a.
Actagen
ACTG
    AIDS Clinical Trials Group
    ACTG 076, 316 protocol
ACTH
    adrenocorticotropic hormone
    ACTH gel
    ACTH stimulation test
    ACTH unresponsiveness
Acthar gel
ActHIB vaccine
ACTH-stimulated 17-
  hydroxypregnenolone
Acticort Topical
Actidil
Actidose-Aqua
Actidose with Sorbitol
Actifed Allergy Tablet
Actigall
actigraphy
    limb a.
actin
    muscle a.
actinic prurigo
Actinobacillus actinomycetemcomitans
Actinomadura madurae
Actinomyces
    A. *georgiae*
    A. *gerencseriae*
    A. *graevenitzii*
    A. *israelii*

    A. *meyeri*
    A. *naeslundii*
    A. *neuii*
    A. *odontolyticus*
    A. *pyogenes*
    A. *viscosus*
actinomycetemcomitans
    Actinobacillus a.
actinomycin D
actinomycosis
    cervicofacial a.
action
    excessive insulin a.
    muscarinic a.
activate
activated
    a. charcoal
    a. clotting factor X
    a. clotting time (ACT)
    a. partial thromboplastic time
      coagulation test
    a. partial thromboplastin time
      (APTT)
    a. T cell
activation
    polyclonal B cell a.
activator
    gli family zinc-finger
      transcriptional a.'s
active
    a. ignoring
    a. immunization
    a. and intense crying state
    a. learner
    a. sleep (AS)
activity
    antigravity a.
    aspartoacyclase hydrolytic a.
    cause-and-effect a.
    ceramidase a.
    conjugation a.
    a.'s of daily living (ADL)
    epileptiform a.
    high-voltage slow a. (HVSA)
    H and Lewis blood group a.
    low-voltage electrocortical a.
      (LVECoG)
    low-voltage fast a. (LVFA)
    oxidative-reductase a.
    PK a.
    plasma renin a.
    play a.

NOTES

activity *(continued)*
    ristocetin cofactor a.
    vagal a.
actometer
acuity
    baseline visual a.
    VEP a.
    visual a.
Acular Ophthalmic
acuminate
    a. papule
    a. plaque
acuminatum, pl. **acuminata**
    condyloma a.
acupuncture
Acuson 128/XP10 scanner
acuta
    pityriasis lichenoides et
    varioliformis a. (PLEVA)
acute
    a. abdomen
    a. acalculous cholecystitis
    a. acquired neutrophilia
    a. adrenal crisis
    a. angle closure glaucoma
    a. anterior uveitis
    a. appendicitis (AA)
    a. ascending radiculomyelitis
    a. aseptic meningitis syndrome
    a. atrophic candidiasis
    a. bacterial endocarditis
    a. barotitis
    a. biliary disease
    a. bronchiolitis
    a. bronchitis
    a. cerebellar ataxia
    a. cerebellar ataxia of unknown cause
    a. cerebellitis
    a. chagasic encephalitis
    a. change clinical score (ACCS)
    a. chest syndrome (ACS)
    a. childhood ataxia
    a. childhood ITP
    a. circulatory collapse
    a. coalescent mastoiditis
    a. confusional migraine
    a. cystitis
    a. dacryocystitis
    a. disseminated encephalomyelitis (ADEM)
    a. disseminated histiocytosis
    a. epidemic conjunctivitis
    a. epiglottitis
    a. eruptive lichen planus
    a. exudative tonsillitis
    a. fatty liver
    a. fatty liver of pregnancy (AFLP)

    a. febrile neurophilic dermatosis
    a. febrile ulcerative acne
    a. fibrinous pericarditis
    a. flaccid paralysis
    a. follicular tonsillitis
    a. fulminant colitis
    a. fulminant disease
    a. glomerulonephritis
    a. graft-versus-host disease (AGVHD, aGVHD)
    a. headache
    a. hemarthrosis
    a. hemorrhagic conjunctivitis
    a. hemorrhagic edema of infancy (AHEI)
    a. hemorrhagic pancreatitis
    a. hydrocephalus
    a. illness
    a. infantile hemiplegia
    a. infectious colitis
    a. infectious polyneuritis
    a. inflammatory demyelinating polyneuropathy (AIDP)
    a. influenza A encephalitis
    a. injury
    a. insulin response
    a. intermittent porphyria (AIP)
    a. interpersonal loss
    a. interstitial myocarditis
    a. iridocyclitis
    a. iron poisoning
    a. labyrinthitis
    a. life-threatening event (ALTE)
    a. lower respiratory infection (ALRI)
    a. lower respiratory tract infection (ALRTI)
    a. lymphatic leukemia
    a. lymphoblastic leukemia (ALL)
    a. lymphocytic leukemia (ALL)
    a. lymphonodular pharyngitis
    a. mastoid osteitis
    a. megakaryoblastic leukemia
    a. meningoencephalitis syndrome
    a. motor-axonal neuropathy (AMAN)
    a. motor-sensory axonal neuropathy (AMSAN)
    a. MS
    a. myeloblastic leukemia
    a. myelogenous leukemia
    a. myeloid leukemia (AML)
    a. myeloradiculitis
    a. myocardial infarction (AMI)
    a. necrotizing ulcerative gingivitis (ANUG)
    a. neuritis
    a. neuronopathic Gaucher disease

a. nonlymphoblastic leukemia (ANLL)
a. nonlymphocytic leukemia
a. on chronic SCFE
a. osteomyelitis
a. otitis media (AOM)
a. pancarditis
a. parotitis
a. pelvic inflammatory disease
a. pericoronitis
a. perinatal conjunctivitis
A. Physiology and Chronic Health Evaluation (APACHE)
a. pneumonitis
a. postinfectious glomerulonephritis (APGN)
a. postinfectious nephritis
a. poststreptococcal glomerulonephritis (APSGN)
a. pseudomembranous candidiasis
a. purulent conjunctivitis
a. pyelonephritis
a. radiation syndrome
a. recurrent ataxia
a. rejection
a. renal failure (ARF)
a. renal parenchymal inflammation
a. respiratory disease (ARD)
a. respiratory distress syndrome (ARDS)
a. respiratory infection (ARI)
a. retroviral syndrome
a. rheumatic carditis
a. rheumatic fever (ARF)
a. schistosomiasis
a. scombroid intoxication
a. secondary localized peritonitis
a. sera
a. sinusitis
a. spasmodic laryngitis
a. spastic paraparesis
a. splenic sequestration
a. splenic sequestration crisis
a. streptococcal gangrene
a. stress disorder (ASD)
a. subdural hematoma
a. subglottic stenosis
a. suppurative otitis media
a. suppurative thyroiditis
a. surgical mastoiditis
a. syphilitic leptomeningitis
a. torticollis

a. total asphyxia
a. tracheitis
a. transfusion reaction
a. transverse myelitis
a. traumatic compartment syndrome
a. tubular necrosis (ATN)
a. urticaria
acute-phase
a.-p. attrition
a.-p. reactant
Acutrainer
Acutrim Precision Release
acyanotic
a. cardiac anomaly
a. congenital defect
a. congenital heart disease
a. lesion
a. tetralogy of Fallot
acyclovir
acylcarnitine
a. analysis
a. profile
A-D
Imodium A-D
AD
Asperger disorder
autosomal dominant
a.d., AD
auris dextra (right ear)
ADA
adenosine deaminase
American Diabetes Association
Americans with Disabilities Act
ADA diet
adactyly
Adagen
Adair-Dighton syndrome
Adalat CC
adamantinoma
Adamkiewicz
artery of A.
Adam position
Adams forward-bending test
Adams-Oliver syndrome
Adams-Stokes syndrome
adapalene
Adapin Oral
adaptability
a., partnership, growth, affection, resolve (APGAR)
poor a.

NOTES

adaptation
 bowel a.
 immediate extrauterine a.
adapter
 Briggs T-a.
 side-port a.
adaptive
 a. behavior
 a. chair
 a. delay
 a. development
 a. domain
 a. switch
ADB
 anti-DNase B
 ADB antibody
 ADB titer
ADCC
 antibody-dependent cell-mediated
  cytotoxicity
ADD
 attention deficit disorder
add-back therapy
Adderall
Addison disease
addisonian
 a. crisis
 a. syndrome
adducted great toe
adduction
 a. deformity
 eye retraction with a.
 forefoot a.
adductor
 a. angle
 a. interosseous compartment
 a. spasm
adductus
 a. clubfoot
 congenital metatarsus a.
 forefoot a.
 a. of forefoot
 metatarsus a. (MA)
 simple metatarsus a.
adefovir dipivoxil
adeloscentis
 Bifidobacterium a.
ADEM
 acute disseminated encephalomyelitis
  recurrent ADEM
adenine
 a. nucleotide
 a. phosphoribosyltransferase
adenitis
 bacterial cervical a.
 cervical a.
 inguinal a.
 mesenteric a.

 periodic fever, aphthous stomatitis,
  pharyngitis, cervical a. (PFAPA)
 salivary a.
 tuberculous a.
adenocarcinoma
 clear-cell a.
Adenocard
adenohypophysis
adenoid
adenoidal hypertrophy
adenoidectomy
 tonsillectomy and a. (T&A)
adenoiditis
adenoma
 benign hepatic a.
 beta cell a.
 eosinophilic a.
 islet cell a.
 pituitary a.
 a. sebaceum
 thyrotropin-secreting pituitary a.
adenomatoid malformation
adenomatosis
 beta cell a.
 islet cell a.
 multiple endocrine a. (MEA)
adenomatous
 a. colonic polyposis
 a. polyp
adenopathy
 cervical a.
 inguinal a.
 phenytoin-associated a.
 preauricular a.
adenosarcoma
adenosine
 a. deaminase (ADA)
 a. deaminase deficiency
 a. triphosphatase
 a. triphosphate (ATP)
adenosis
adenosylcobalamin
adenosyltransferase
 cobalamin a.
adenotomy
adenotonsillar hypertrophy
adenotonsillectomy
adenotonsillitis
adenoviral
 a. pneumonia
 a. tonsillitis
adenovirus
 a. 7
 enteric a.
 a. infection
 a. type 3
adenylate cyclase

adenylosuccinate
- a. deficiency
- a. lyase deficiency (ASLD)

adequate caliber of anus

ADH
- antidiuretic hormone

adhalin gene

ADHD
- attention deficit hyperactivity disorder

adherens
- fascia a.

adherent pseudomembrane

adhesiolysis

adhesion
- fimbrial a.
- labial a.
- platelet a.
- tongue-lip a.

adhesiotherapy

adhesive
- a. band
- a. otitis
- Testoderm with A.

ADI
- atlantodens interval
- autism diagnostic interview

adiabatic effect

adiadochokinesia

Adie
- A. chronic pupillary syndrome
- A. pupil

adipocyte

adiponecrosis subcutanea neonatorum

adipose tissue

adiposity

adiposogenital syndrome

adipsia

ADI-R
- Autism Diagnostic Interview-Revised

aditus admission antrum

adjusted age

adjustment disorder

adjuvant

ADL
- activities of daily living
- Amsterdam Depression List

ad libitum diet

Adlone Injection

ADMCKD
- autosomal dominant medullary cystic kidney disease

administration
- Food and Drug A. (FDA)
- rectal a.
- RSV immunoglobulin for intravenous a. (RSV-IGIV)
- silver nitrate a.

admittance
- acoustic a.
- peak a.
- static a.

adnexal torsion

adolescence

adolescent
- a. bunion
- Computerized Diagnostic Interview for Children and A.'s (cDICA, C-DICA)
- Functional Impairment Scale for Children and A.'s (FISCA)
- a. idiopathic scoliosis (AIS)
- Interview Schedule for Children and A.'s (ISCA)
- a. obesity
- A. and Pediatric Pain Tool (APPT)
- Pictorial Instrument for Children and A.'s (PICA)
- Scale for Children and A.'s
- a. scoliosis
- a. seborrhea
- Service Assessment for Children and A.'s (SACA)
- a. tibia vara

ADOS
- Autism Diagnostic Observation Schedule

ADPKD
- autosomal dominant polycystic kidney disease

ADR
- adverse drug reaction

adrenal
- a. androgen-stimulating hormone (AASH)
- a. calcification
- a. cortex
- a. cortical carcinoma
- a. crisis
- a. excess
- a. gland
- a. hematoma
- a. hemorrhage
- a. hyperplasia

NOTES

adrenal *(continued)*
    a. insufficiency
    a. medulla
    a. suppression
    a. tumor
adrenalectomy
Adrenalin Chloride
adrenaline
adrenalitis
    necrotizing a.
adrenarche
    premature a.
adrenergic
adrenocortical
    a. hyperplasia
    a. insufficiency
    a. stress
adrenocorticotropic
    a. hormone (ACTH)
    a. hormone insufficiency
adrenogenital syndrome
adrenoleukodystrophy (ALD)
    neonatal a.
    X-linked a.
adrenomedullary
adrenomyeloneuropathy
Adriamycin
    A. (doxorubicin), bleomycin,
      vinblastine, dacarbazine (ABVD)
    A. PFS
    A. RDF
Adrucil Injection
Adsorbocarpine Ophthalmic
Adsorbonac Ophthalmic
adult
    American Association on Mental
      Deficiency Adaptive Behavior
      Scale for Children and A.'s
    a. bone marrow (ABM)
    a. NCL
    a. polycystic disease
    a. progeria
    a. Refsum disease
    a. T-cell leukemia/lymphoma
      (ATLL)
adult-directed instruction
adulthood
adult-onset
    a.-o. hypogammaglobulinemia
    a.-o. polycystic kidney disease
    a.-o. spinocerebellar ataxia
adultorum
    scleredema a.
Advair Diskus
advanced
    a. cardiac life support (ACLS)
    A. Formula Oxy Sensitive Gel
    Imodium A.

    a. life support (ALS)
    a. oxidation protein product
      (AOPP)
    a. pediatric life support (APLS)
    a. trauma life support (ATLS)
Advance formula
advancement
    mandibular a.
    maxillary a.
adventitia
adventitial
    a. pulmonary sound
adventitious
    a. choreiform movement
    a. deafness
Advera formula
adverse
    a. drug reaction (ADR)
    a. food reaction
Advil
    Children's A.
Advisory Committee on Immunization
    Practices (ACIP)
advocacy
    protection and a. (P & A)
advocate
adynamia episodica hereditaria
adynamic ileus
adysplasia
    hereditary renal a.
    hereditary urogenital a.
AEA
    antiendomysium antibody
AED
    antiepileptic drug
Aedes triseriatus
aEEG
    amplitude-integrated
      electroencephalogram
AEP
    auditory evoked potential
AER
    auditory evoked response
aeration
    lung a.
    unequal a.
aeroallergen
aerobic
aerobics
    digital auditory a. (DAA)
AeroBid-M Oral Aerosol Inhaler
AeroBid Oral Aerosol Inhaler
AeroChamber spacer device
Aerolate
    Accurbron A. III
    A. III
    A. JR
    A. SR S

Aeromonas hydrophila
aerophagia
Aeroseb-Dex Topical Aerosol
Aeroseb-HC Topical
aerosol
    Aeroseb-Dex Topical A.
    Breezee Mist A.
    cromolyn sodium inhalation a.
    Decaspray Topical A.
    Dexacort Phosphate Turbinaire
      Intranasal A.
    Isoetharine Bronkometer A.
    Medihaler-ISO Inhalation A.
    a. therapy
    Tilade Inhalation A.
aerosolization
aerosolized
    a. amphotericin B
    a. racemic epinephrine
    a. ribavirin
Aerosporin Injection
aerotitis
aeruginosa
    Pseudomonas a.
aestivale
    hydroa a.
AF
   amniotic fluid
    Lotrimin AF
    SSD AF
AFAFP
   amniotic fluid alpha fetoprotein
AFDC
   Aid to Families with Dependent Children
afebrile
    a. bactcrcmia
    a. convulsion
    a. pneumonia syndrome
    a. seizure
affect
    a. attunement
    Eating Disorders Inventory Score
      for Interoceptive Awareness A.
    flat a.
affective storm
affectivity
    negative a.
afferent vessel
affricate
AFI
   amniotic fluid index
Afipia felis

aflatoxin poisoning
AFLP
   acute fatty liver of pregnancy
AFO
   ankle-foot orthosis
AFP
   alpha fetoprotein
africae
    Rickettsia a.
African
    A. Burkitt lymphoma
    A. tick bite fever
    A. trypanosomiasis
africanum
    Mycobacterium a.
Afrin
    A. Children's Nose Drops
    A. Nasal Solution
    A. Saline Mist
Afrinol
Aftate
afterload
    LV a.
    ventricular a.
afzelii
    Borrelia a.
AGA
   antigliadin antibody
   appropriate for gestational age
   average for gestational age
agalactiae
    Streptococcus a.
agammaglobulinemia
    Bruton a.
    X-linked a. (XLA)
aganglionic
    a. bowel
    a. colon
    a. megacolon
    a. rectum
aganglionosis
    congenital intestinal a.
    long-segment a.
    total colonic a.
    zonal a.
agar
    blood a.
    charcoal a.
    chocolate a.
    a. gel precipitation technique
    Hektoen a.
    a. immunoprecipitin technique

NOTES

agar *(continued)*
    nalidixic acid a.
    NMN biphasic blood a.
    Novy-McNeal-Nicolle biphasic
      blood a.
    a. plate
    Ryan a.
    Thayer-Martin a.
    xylose lysine deaminase a.

age
    adjusted a.
    appropriate for gestational a.
      (AGA)
    average for gestational a. (AGA)
    birth weight for gestational a.
      (BWGA)
    chronological a.
    corrected gestational a.
    delayed bone a.
    developmental a.
    Dubowitz/Ballard Exam for
      Gestational A.
    functional a.
    gestational a. (GA)
    growth-adjusted sonographic a.
      (GASA)
    hand-wrist bone a.
    large for gestational a. (LGA)
    mean a.
    mental a.
    postconceptional a. (PCA)
    postnatal a.
    small for gestational a. (SGA)
    A.'s and Stages Questionnaire
      (ASQ)

agency
    child protective a.
    lead a.
    local education a. (LEA)
    protective service a.

agenesia corticalis

agenesis
    anorectal a.
    callosal a.
    caudal a.
    a. of cerebellar vermis
    cervical a.
    a. of corpus callosum
    corpus callosum a.
    cortical a.
    gonadal a.
    hereditary renal a.
    lumbosacral a.
    a. of lung
    pancreatic a.
    partial a.
    penile a.
    renal a.

    sacral a.
    thyroid and pituitary a.
    unilateral renal a.

agent
    antianxiety a.
    antidysrhythmic a.
    antimicrobial a.
    antiplatelet a.
    antistaphylococcal a.
    anxiolytic a.
    betamimetic a.
    chemotactic a.
    chemotherapeutic a.
    emetic a.
    Hawaii a.
    neuromuscular blocking a.
    nondepolarizing paralyzing a.
    Norwalk a.
    prokinetic a.
    Snow Mountain a.
    TWAR a.
    W-Ditching a.

age-related pharmacodynamic response

age-to-dose pattern

agglomeration schedule

agglutination
    a. assay
    latex a. (LA)
    latex particle a.
    rickettsial a.
    a. test

agglutinin
    cold a.

aggregated mucopolysaccharide

**Aggregate Neurobehavioral Student
  Health & Education Review System**

aggregation
    defective primary platelet a.
    platelet a.

aggression
    inattention-overactivity with a.
      (IOWA)

aggressive
    a. behavior
    a. conduct disorder

aging
    premature a.

agitation

aglossia-adactylia syndrome

AGM
    absorbent gelling material

agminated lentigo

agnogenic myeloid metaplasia (AMM)

agnosia
    auditory a.
    finger a.
    verbal-auditory a. (VAA)

agonist
    beta-2 a.
    beta-adrenergic a.
    inhaled beta-2 a.
    motilin receptor a.
Agoral Plain
agoraphobia
agouti protein
agranulocytosis
    infantile a.
AGVHD, aGVHD
    acute graft-versus-host disease
agyria
agyria-pachygyria cortical dysplasia
AH
    antihyaluronidase
      AH antibody
      AH titer
AHEI
    acute hemorrhagic edema of infancy
AHF
    antihemophilic factor
A-hydroCort Injection
AI
    acetabular index
    anal index
Aicardi-Goutiéres disease
Aicardi syndrome
AID
    artificial insemination by donor
    artificial insemination donor
aid
    communication a.
    Compoz Nighttime Sleep A.
    crawling a.
    electronic communication a.
    A. to Families with Dependent
      Children (AFDC)
    Foille Medicated First A.
    hearing a.
    low-vision a.
    mobility a.
    Swim-Ear water drying a.
    vibrotactile hearing a.
AIDP
    acute inflammatory demyelinating
    polyneuropathy
AIDS
    acquired immune deficiency syndrome
    acquired immunodeficiency syndrome
      AIDS Clinical Trials Group
      (ACTG)

      AIDS Clinical Trials Group
        protocol
      AIDS encephalopathy
      AIDS gastropathy
AIE
    autoimmune enteropathy
AIHA
    autoimmune hemolytic anemia
AIMS
    Abnormal Involuntary Movement Scale
    Alberta Infant Motor Scale
AIN
    autoimmune neutropenia
ainhumlike
    a. constriction
    a. constriction of digit
AIP
    acute intermittent porphyria
air
    a. arthrogram
    a. embolism
    a. embolus
    a. enema
    extrapulmonary extravasation of a.
    free peritoneal a.
    high-efficiency particulate a.
    (HEPA)
    humidified a.
    a. hunger
    a. leak
    a. leak test
    a. pollution
    a. reduction
    reflux of a.
    room a.
    A. Shields incubator
    subdiaphragmatic a.
    a. swallowing
    a. trapping
airbag injury
airborne allergen
air-contrast barium enema
Airet
air-filled heart
airflow
    laminar a.
    turbulent a.
air-fluid level
AirPacks backpack
airplane glue
Airshields jaundice meter
airspace

NOTES

AirTEC model backpack
airway
    abnormal laxity of upper a.
    a. branching
    a., breathing, circulation (ABC)
    a., breathing, circulation and
      control bleeding, disability,
      exposure (ABCDE)
    a. conductance
    double-lumen a.
    a. epithelium
    extrinsic compression of a.
    a. fluoroscopy
    laryngeal mask a. (LMA)
    a. management
    a. obstruction
    a. obstruction syndrome
    a. occlusion
    a. opening pressure (P_{ao})
    a. protection
    reactive a.
    a. reactivity testing
    a. resistance
    reversible obstructive a.
    a. smooth muscle
    a. transmural pressure
AIS
    adolescent idiopathic scoliosis
AIT
    auditory integration thinking
    auditory integration training
AIUM
    American Institute of Ultrasound in
    Medicine
Akaike score
akari
    Rickettsia a.
Akarpine Ophthalmic
akathisia
AK-Beta Ophthalmic
AK-Chlor Ophthalmic
AK-Con Ophthalmic
AK-Dex Ophthalmic
AK-Dilate Ophthalmic Solution
akinetic
    a. mutism
    a. seizure
akiyami
AK-Mycin
AK-NaCl
AK-Nefrin Ophthalmic Solution
Akne-Mycin
AK-Pentolate
AK-Poly-Bac Ophthalmic
AK-Pred Ophthalmic
AK-Spore
    AK-S. H.C. Otic
    AK-S. Ophthalmic Ointment

AK-Sulf
AK-Taine
AKTob Ophthalmic
AK-Tracin Ophthalmic
AK-Trol Ophthalmic
ALA, pl. alae
    alpha lactalbumin
    alpha-linolenic acid
ala
    nasal a.
Ala-Cort Topical
alacrima, achalasia, adrenal insufficiency
Aladdin Infant Flow System
alae (*pl. of* ALA)
alae nasi
Alagille syndrome
Alamast ophthalmic solution
alanine
    a. aminotransferase (ALT)
    a. transaminase (ALT)
alaninuria
alar flaring
Ala-Scalp Topical
Alateen
Alazide
alba
    cutis marmorata a.
    pityriasis a.
    pneumonia a.
Albalon Liquifilm Ophthalmic
albendazole
Albers-Schönberg
    A.-S. disease
    A.-S. syndrome
Alberta Infant Motor Scale (AIMS)
Albert Einstein Neonatal Developmental
    Scale
albicans
    Candida a.
albinism
    cutaneous a.
    generalized a.
    localized a.
    Nettleship-Falls ocular a.
    ocular a. (OA)
    oculocutaneous a. (OCA)
    partial oculocutaneous a.
    tyrosinase-negative
      oculocutaneous a.
    tyrosinase-positive a.
albopapuloid Pasini form of dominant
    dystrophic epidermolysis bullosa
Albright
    A. hereditary osteodystrophy
    A. syndrome
albuginea
    tunica a.
albumin

Albuminar
albumin-bound toxin
albuminocytologic dissociation
albuminuria
Albumisol
Albunex
Albutein
albuterol
    sustained-release a.
Alcaine
Alcaligenes xylosoxidans
alcaptonuria
Alcare formula
alclometasone
alcohol
    benzyl a.
    cetyl a.
    ethyl a. (EtOH)
    isopropyl a.
    a. and other drugs (AOD)
    A. Use Disorders Inventory Test
    (AUDIT)
alcoholic
    child of a. (COA)
    children of a.'s (COA)
    a. tincture
    a. tincture of opium
alcoholism
alcohol-related neurodevelopmental
    disorder (ARND)
alcohol, tobacco, and other drugs
    (ATOD)
Alconefrin Nasal Solution
ALD
    adrenoleukodystrophy
Aldactazide
Aldactone
Aldara
Alden-Senturia collection trap
Alder anomaly
aldolase
    creatinine a.
Aldomet
aldosterone
    a. deficiency
    a. excretion rate
    a. replacement therapy
aldosteronism
    juvenile a.
Aldrich
    hypoganglionic segment of A.
    A. syndrome

ALEC
    artificial lung-expanding compound
alendronate
alert inactivity
alertness
    quiet a.
    a., response to voice, response to
    pain, unresponsive (AVPU)
    state of a.
Alesse
aleukia
    congenital a.
Aleve
Alexander
    A. anomaly
    A. aplasia
    A. disease
    A. operation
alexithymia
alfa
    dornase a.
    epoetin a.
    poractant a.
Alfenta
alfentanil
AL 110 formula
algae
    blue-green a.
algal oil
alginate
    calcium a.
alglucerase
algodystrophy
Algo newborn hearing screener
ALGO 1-plus
algorithm
    Burg a.
Alice in Wonderland syndrome
alignment
    body a.
    ocular a.
    torsional a.
alimentary
alimentation
    parenteral a.
Alimentum formula
aliphatic hydrocarbon
aliquot
Alitra Q formula
Alkaban-AQ
alkalemia
alkalemic

NOTES

alkali
   a. infusion
   a. therapy
alkaline
   a. phosphatase (ALP)
   a. reflux
alkalinization
alkalosis
   cerebral lactic a.
   diet-induced hypochloremic
     metabolic a.
   hypochloremic metabolic a.
   respiratory a.
Alka-Mints
Alka-Seltzer Plus Children's Cold Medicine
Alkeran
ALL
  acute lymphoblastic leukemia
  acute lymphocytic leukemia
Allegra
allele
   papG a.
allele-specific oligonucleotide hybridization
allelic gene
Allemann syndrome
Allen
   A. and Capute neonatal
     neurodevelopmental examination
   A. chart
   A. Kindergarten Picture Cards
   A. picture test
Aller-Chlor Oral
Allercon
Allerest
   A. Children's Tablets
   A. Eye Drops
   A. Headache Strength
   A. 12 Hour Nasal Solution
   A. Maximum Strength
Allerfrin
allergen
   airborne a.
   contact a.
   A. Ear Drops
allergenic
allergen-induced asthma
allergic
   a. bowel disease
   a. bronchopulmonary aspergillosis (ABPA)
   a. colitis
   a. conjunctivitis
   a. contact dermatitis
   a. crease
   a. diaper rash
   a. encephalitis

   a. encephalomyelitis
   a. enterocolitis
   a. eosinophilic gastroenteritis
   a. esophagitis
   a. gape
   a. gastroenteropathy
   a. polyp
   a. rhinitis
   a. rhinitis perennial
   a. rhinoconjunctivitis
   a. salute
   a. shiner
   a. sinusitis
allergy
   barley a.
   cow's milk a. (CMA)
   gluten a.
   milk a.
   milk-protein a.
   milk/soy-protein a.
   non-IgE-mediated food a.
   pollen a.
   a. treatment
   Triaminic A.
AllerMax Oral
Allerphed
Allgrove syndrome
alligator forceps
alloantibody
allocate
allogenic, allogeneic
   a. BMT
   a. bone marrow transplantation
   a. stem cell transplantation
allograft
   composite a.
   cryopreserved valved a.
   dura mater a.
   a. rejection
alloimmune
   a. neonatal neutropenia (ANN)
   a. thrombocytopenia
   a. thrombocytopenic purpura
alloimmunization
Alloiococcus otitidis
alloisoleucine
allopurinol
allowance
   recommended daily a. (RDA)
   recommended dietary a. (RDA)
all-progestin contraceptive
all-terrain vehicle (ATV)
all-*trans*-retinoic acid
Almora
alobar holoprosencephaly
Alocril
Alomide

alopecia
  a. areata
  cicatricial a.
  generalized a.
  marginal a.
  pyoderma a.
  secondary a.
  a. totalis congenita
  toxic a.
  traction a.
  traumatic a.
  a. universalis
  a. universalis totalis
ALP
  alkaline phosphatase
  bone ALP
Alpern-Boll Developmental Profile
Alpers
  A. disease
  A. syndrome
alpha
  a. fetoprotein (AFP)
  interferon a.
  A. Keri soap
  a. knockout
  a. lactalbumin (ALA)
  macrophage inflammatory protein-
    1 a.
  a. proteobacteria
  recombinant human MIP-1 a.
    (MIP-1 alpha)
  a. thalassemia
alpha-1
  a.-1 antitrypsin deficiency
  a.-1 antitrypsin disease
  a.-1 proteinase inhibitor (A1PI)
alpha-2a
  interferon a.-2a
alpha-adrenergic receptor
alpha-aminoadipic
  a.-a. acid
  a.-a. aciduria
alpha-antilysin deficiency
alpha-2b
  interferon a.-2b
alphabet
  manual a.
alpha-chemokine receptor
alpha-glucosidase deficiency
alpha-granule
  giant platelet a.-g.

alpha-ketoadipic
  a.-k. acid
  a.-k. aciduria
alpha-ketoisocaproic acid (alpha-KIC)
alpha-KIC
  alpha-ketoisocaproic acid
alpha-linolenic acid (ALA)
alpha-lipoprotein deficiency
alpha-methylcrotonyl-coenzyme A
  carboxylase
Alphamul
alpha-N-acetylgalactosaminidase
  deficiency
Alphanate
alpha-reductase deficiency
alpha-tocopherol concentration
Alphatrex Topical
alphavirus
Alport syndrome
alprazolam
Alprem formula
alprostadil
ALPS
  autoimmune lymphoproliferative
    syndrome
ALRI
  acute lower respiratory infection
AL-Rr Oral
ALRTI
  acute lower respiratory tract infection
ALS
  advanced life support
Alsoy formula
Alström-Hallgren syndrome
Alström syndrome
ALT
  alanine aminotransferase
  alanine transaminase
ALTE
  acute life-threatening event
  apparent life-threatening event
altered
  a. gastric motility
  a. sensorium
  a. state of consciousness (ASC)
alternans
  convergens a.
  electrical a.
  pulsus a.
Alternaria
alternate-cover test

NOTES

alternating
- a. breath test (ABT)
- a. hemiplegia
- a. hemiplegia of childhood

alternative communication device

aluminum
- a. acetate
- a. acetate solution
- a. chloride
- a. hydroxide
- a. intoxication
- a. toxicity

Alupent

alveolar
- a. capillary dysplasia
- a. consolidation
- a. cyst
- a. echinococcosis
- a. fibrinous exudate
- a. hydatidosis
- a. hypoxia
- a. lavage
- a. lymphangioma
- a. myofibroblast differentiation
- a. notch
- a. osteitis
- a. oxygen tension
- a. proteinosis
- a. recruitment
- a. ridge
- a. RMS
- a. saccule formation
- a. sarcoid
- a. soft part sarcoma
- a. stage
- a. stage of lung development
- a. ventilation

alveolar-arterial (A-a)
- a.-a. difference in partial pressure of oxygen (AADPPO)
- a.-a. oxygen gradient
- a.-a. pressure gradient

alveoli (*pl. of* alveolus)

alveolitis
- cryptogenic fibrosing a.
- extrinsic alveolar a.

alveolization
- abrogated neonatal a.

alveolus, pl. alveoli
- functional a.
- pulmonary a.

alymphocytosis

alymphoplasia
- thymic a.

Alzheimer II cell

a-2M
- a-2 macroglobulin
- a-2M coagulation inhibitor

amalonaticus
- *Citrobacter a.*

AMAN
- acute motor-axonal neuropathy

Amanita
- A. mushroom
- A. *phalloides*

a-mannosidosis type I, II

amantadine

amastia

amaurosis
- a. fugax
- Leber congenital retinal a.

amaurotic familial idiocy

AmBd
- amphotericin B deoxycholate

Ambi 10

ambient
- a. light
- a. sound
- a. temperature

ambiguity
- sexual a.

ambiguous
- a. external genitalia
- a. reference

ambiguus
- situs a.

AmBisome

amblyogenic stimulus

Amblyomma americanum

amblyopia
- ametropic a.
- anisometropic a.
- deprivation a.
- disuse a.
- image-degradation a.
- isoametropic a.
- occlusion a.
- strabismic a.
- transient a.

amblyopic eye

ambosexual area

ambulate

ambulatory
- a. blood pressure (ABP)
- a. blood pressure monitoring (ABPM)
- a. polysomnography

Ambu respirator

amcinonide

Amcort Injection

AMD
- acid maltase deficiency

AME
- apparent mineralocorticoid excess
- congenital AME

amebiasis
  cerebral a.
  hepatic a.
amebic
  a. colitis
  a. dysentery
  a. hepatic abscess
  a. liver abscess
  a. meningoencephalitis
amegakaryocyte
amegakaryocytic thrombocytopenia
amelia
  upper limb a.
ameliorate
amelioration
ameloblastoma
amelogenesis imperfecta
amendment
  Clinical Laboratory
    Improvements A.'s (CLIA)
  Education of the Handicapped A.'s
    of 1986
Amen Oral
amenorrhea
  primary a.
  secondary a.
amenorrhea-galactorrhea syndrome
amensic shellfish poisoning
Americaine
American
  A. Academy of Child and
    Adolescent Psychiatry (AACAP)
  A. Academy of Pediatrics (AAP)
  A. Association on Mental
    Deficiency (AAMD)
  A. Association on Mental
    Deficiency Adaptive Behavior
    Scale for Children and Adults
  A. Association on Mental
    Retardation (AAMR)
  A. Association of Poison Control
    Centers (AAPCC)
  A. Association for the Surgery of
    Trauma (AAST)
  A. Board of Psychiatry and
    Neurology (ABPN)
  A. Burkitt lymphoma
  A. College of Graduate Medical
    Education (ACGME)
  A. Diabetes Association (ADA)
  A. Diabetes Association diet

  A. Heart Association Step One
    Diet
  A. Institute of Ultrasound in
    Medicine (AIUM)
  A. Psychiatric Association (APA)
  A. Sign Language (ASL)
  A. Sleep Disorders Association
    (ASDA)
  A. trypanosomiasis
  A.'s with Disabilities Act (ADA)
americanum
  Amblyomma a.
americanus
  Ancylostoma a.
  Necator a.
A-methaPred Injection
amethocaine gel
Ametop gel
ametropic amblyopia
AMI
  acute myocardial infarction
  non-Q-wave AMI
Amicar
amicrobic pyuria
amifostine
amikacin sulfate
Amikin
amiloride
amine
  a. odor
  sympathomimetic a.
amino
  a. acid
  a. acid chromatography
  a. acid metabolism
  a. acid screening
  a. acid transport defect
aminoacetic analog
aminoacidemia
aminoacidopathy
aminoaciduria
  dibasic a.
  generalized a.
  hyperdibasic a.
  renal a.
aminoaciduriasis
aminocaproic acid
aminoglycoside
  antimicrobial a.
  a. nephrotoxicity
aminogram
  plasma a.

NOTES

aminoguanidine
Amino-Opti-E
aminophospholipid
Aminophyllin
aminophylline
5-aminosalicylic
    5-a. acid
aminotransferase
    alanine a. (ALT)
    aspartate a. (AST)
    branched-chain a.
    serum a.
amiodarone
amisulpride
Amitone
amitriptyline
AML
    acute myeloid leukemia
AMLA
    antimyolemmal antibody
AMM
    agnogenic myeloid metaplasia
Ammon horn sclerosis
ammonia
    plasma a.
    serum a.
ammonium
    a. chloride
    a. lactate
AMN
    acquired melanocytic nevus
amnesia
    hysterical a.
    posttraumatic a.
    retrograde a.
amniocentesis
amniogenesis
amnioinfusion therapy
amnion nodosum
amnioreduction
amniotic
    a. band disruption sequence
    a. banding
    a. band syndrome
    a. constriction band
    a. debris
    a. fluid (AF)
    a. fluid alpha fetoprotein (AFAFP)
    a. fluid index (AFI)
    a. infection syndrome
amobarbital
A-mode echocardiography
amotivational syndrome
amoxicillin
amoxicillin-clavulanate
amoxicillin-clavulanic acid
Amoxil

AMP
    amprenavir
amphetamine
    a. aspartate
    a. sulfate
Amphojel
amphotericin
    aerosolized a. B
    a. B
    a. B deoxycholate (AmBd)
    a. B lipid complete
    a. B lipid complex
    a. B liposome
ampicillin
    a. rash
    a. resistant
    a. and sulbactam
ampicillin-resistant *Escherichia coli*
ampicillin/sulbactam
Amplatz catheter
Amplatzer
    A. device
    A. septal occluder
amplification
    nucleic acid a. (NAA)
    nucleic acid sequence-based a. (NASBA)
    transcription-mediated a. (TMA)
amplitude
amplitude-integrated
    a.-i. EEG
    a.-i. electroencephalogram (aEEG)
amprenavir (AMP, VX-478)
ampulla of Vater
amputation
    congenital a.
    Syme a.
amrinone lactate
AMS
    ablepharon macrostomia syndrome
amsacrine (MAMSA, m-AMSA)
AMSAN
    acute motor-sensory axonal neuropathy
Amsel criteria
Amsterdam Depression List (ADL)
amygdala, pl. amygdalae
amygdalohippocampectomy
amyl
    A. Nitrate Vaporole
    a. nitrite
    A. Nitrite Aspirols
amylase
    human pancreatic a. (HPA)
    salivary a.
amyloidosis
    secondary a.
amylopectinosis
    branching enzyme deficiency a.

A

amyopathic
   a. JDM
   a. juvenile dermatomyositis
amyoplasia
   bimelic a.
   segmental a.
amyotonia congenita
amyotrophic
   a. lateral sclerosis
   a. lateral sclerosis-Parkinson-
      dementia complex
amyotrophy
AN
   anorexia nervosa
ANA
   antinuclear antibody
   positive antinuclear antibody
   ANA-negative lupus
   ANA seropositive
anabolic androgenic steroid
anabolism
Anacin
anaclitic
   a. depression
   a. depression of infancy
anaerobic
   a. cellulitis
   a. streptococcus
Anafranil
anagen effluvium
Ana-Kit
anal
   a. atresia
   a. canal
   a. dimple
   a. fissure
   a. index (AI)
   a. margin
   a. penetration
   a. pruritus
   a. sphincter
   a. sphincter paralysis
   a. thrombosis
   a. tone
   a. verge
   a. wink
analbuminemic
analeptic
analgesia
   epidural a.
   patient-controlled a. (PCA)
   procedural sedation and a. (PSA)

analgesic
analog, analogue
   aminoacetic a.
   nucleoside a.
   vasopressin a.
analysis, pl. analyses
   acylcarnitine a.
   applied behavior a. (ABA)
   aqueous a.
   bioelectrical impedance a. (BIA)
   bioimpedance a.
   blood gas a.
   capillary electrophoresis/frontal a.
      (CE/FA)
   chorionic villus haplotype a.
   chromosome a.
   cytogenetic a.
   deoxyribonucleic acid a.
   DNA a.
   fat a.
   FISH a.
   flow cytometric a.
   flow cytometry a.
   fragile X a.
   genetic linkage a.
   hair cotinine a.
   heart rate power spectral a.
      (HRSA)
   induced sputum a. (ISA)
   latent class a. (LCA)
   linear regression a.
   Newman-Keuls a.
   oligonucleotide probe a.
   photometric a.
   pleural fluid a.
   power spectral a. (PSA)
   restriction fragment length
      polymorphism a.
   RFLP a.
   Scatchard a.
   spectral power a.
   toxicologic a.
   transgenerational a.
   Trauma Score and Injury Severity
      Score A. (TRISS)
   white blood cell lysosomal
      enzyme a.
analyzer
   Bayer DCA2000 a.
   BiliCheck bilirubin a.
   Cobas fast centrifugal a.
   cooximeter a.

NOTES

25

analyzer *(continued)*
    CO-stat end tidal breath a.
    Elecsys 1010 a.
    Leadcare handheld blood lead a.
    NE-8000 a.
    STA a.
anamnestic immune response
anaphylactic
    a. purpura
    a. reaction
    a. shock
anaphylactoid
    a. purpura
    a. shock
anaphylatoxin
anaphylaxis
    biphasic a.
    gastrointestinal a.
anaplasia
anaplastic
    a. large cell lymphoma
    a. oligodendroglioma
    a. pathology
    a. pilocytic astrocytoma
Anaprox
anarthria
anasarca
Anaspaz
anastomosis, pl. **anastomoses**
    Damus-Kaye-Stansel a.
    descending aorta a.
    end-to-side a.
    esophageal a.
    extended end-to-end a.
    extracardiac conduit
      cavopulmonary a.
    Glenn a.
    ileal pouch-anal a. (IPAA)
    ileoanal a. (IAA)
    ileoileal a.
    intrarenal a.
    jejunojejunal a.
    lateral atrial tunnel
      cavopulmonary a.
    primary a.
    Roux-en-Y a.
    side-to-end a.
    staple a.
    total cavopulmonary a.
    Waterston aortopulmonary a.
anatomic
    a. asplenia
    a. profile (AP)
Anbesol Maximum Strength
ANCA
    antineutrophil cytoplasmic antibody
      cytoplasmic ANCA
      perinuclear ANCA

Ancef
anchoring
    a. fibril
    a. villus
Ancobon
Ancylostoma
    A. americanus
    A. braziliense
    A. caninum
    A. ceylanicum
    A. duodenale
ancylostomiasis
Andersen deficiency
Anderson
    A. disease
    A. syndrome
andersoni
    Dermacentor a.
Androderm Transdermal System
androgen
    attenuated a.
    a. binding
    a. insensitivity syndrome
    a. resistance
    a. resistance syndrome
androgenic steroid
android pattern
Andro-L.A. Injection
Andropository Injection
androstenediol
androstenedione
Anectine Chloride
anemia
    aplastic a.
    aregenerative a.
    autoimmune hemolytic a. (AIHA)
    Blackfan-Diamond a.
    B_6-responsive a.
    cardiac hemolytic a.
    chronic nonspherocytic hemolytic a.
    congenital aplastic a.
    congenital dyserythropoietic a.
      (CDA)
    congenital Heinz body a.
    congenital hypoplastic a.
    congenital nonspherocytic
      hemolytic a.
    congenital pernicious a.
    congenital sideroblastic a.
    Cooley a.
    Coombs-negative autoimmune
      hemolytic a.
    Coombs-positive isoimmune
      hemolytic a.
    copper deficiency a.
    a. of CRF
    Czerny a.
    Diamond-Blackfan a. (DBA)

erythroblastic a.
familial erythroblastic a.
Fanconi a. (FA)
Fanconi aplastic a.
fetal a.
globe cell a.
hemolytic a.
homozygous sickle cell a.
hypochromic a.
hypoplastic a.
iatrogenic a.
idiopathic acquired sideroblastic a.
  (IASA)
iron-deficiency a. (IDA)
juvenile pernicious a.
macrocytic a.
Mediterranean a.
megaloblastic a.
microangiopathic hemolytic a.
microcytic a.
mild a.
a. neonatorum
nonspherocytic a.
normochromic a.
normocytic a.
pernicious a.
physiologic a.
posthepatic aplastic a.
a. of prematurity
pyridoxine-refractory sideroblastic a.
refractory dyserythropoietic a.
schistocytic hemolytic a.
severe megaloblastic a.
sickle cell a.
sideroblastic a.
a. syndrome
thiamine-response sideroblastic a.
X-linked pyridoxine-responsive
  sideroblastic a.
anemic
anemicus
nevus a.
anencephalic
anencephaly
Anergan Injection
anergy
Anestacon Topical Solution
anesthesia
a. bag
general a.
hypotensive a.
local a.

neuraxial a.
saddle a.
anesthesiologist
anesthetic
eutectic mixture of local a.
  (EMLA)
Orajel Brace-Aid Oral A.
a. skin lesion
anetoderma of prematurity
aneuploidy
segmental a.
aneurysm
arterial a.
berry a.
cerebral artery a.
circle of Willis a.
cirsoid a.
CNS a.
congenital cerebral a.
coronary a.
coronary artery a. (CAA)
dissecting aortic a.
fusiform a.
giant coronary artery a.
intracerebral a.
intracranial arterial a.
left ventricular apical a.
mycotic a.
ruptured sinus of Valsalva a.
vein of Galen a.
a. of vein of Galen
ventricular a.
aneurysmal bone cyst
Anexsia
ANF
atrial natriuretic factor
Angelman syndrome
angel's kiss
anger stage
angiectatic skin rash
angiitic luminal compromise
angiitis
granulomatous a.
hypersensitivity a.
leukoclastic a.
leukocytoclastic a.
lupus a.
angina
Ludwig a.
nocturnal a.
Vincent a.

NOTES

angiocardiogram
Elema a.
Angiocath catheter
angiodysplasia
angioedema
acquired a. (type I, II)
episodic a.
hereditary a. (type I)
recurrent a.
angiofibroma
juvenile nasopharyngeal a.
angiofollicular lymph node hyperplasia
angiogenesis
angiogram
superior mesenteric a.
angiography
catheter a.
cerebral a.
digital subtraction a.
fluorescein fundus a.
magnetic resonance a. (MRA)
radioisotope a.
selective a.
angiokeratoma
a. circumscriptum
a. corporis diffusum
Mibelli a.
a. of Mibelli
angioma
capillary a.
cavernous venous a.
cutaneous a.
facial a.
port-wine stained a.
retinal a.
spider a.
subependymal cryptic a.
venous a.
angiomatosis
bacillary a. (BA)
encephalofacial a.
encephalotrigeminal a.
leptomeningeal a.
meningeal a.
angiomatous involuting nevus
angiomyolipoma
angioneurotic edema
angioosteohypertrophy syndrome
angiopathy
vulvar congenital dysplastic a.
angioplasty
percutaneous transluminal a.
pulmonary artery a.
angiostrongyliasis
Angiostrongylus cantonensis
angiotensin-converting
a.-c. enzyme (ACE)
a.-c. enzyme inhibitor

angiotensin II
angiotensinogen
angle
adductor a.
anterior chamber a.
calcaneotibial a.
center edge a.
A. classification
A. classification of occlusion
corneoscleral a.
costovertebral a. (CVA)
decreased talocalcaneal a.
femoral-tibial a.
foot-progression a. (FPA)
hip-knee-ankle a.
a. of His
knee a.
left costovertebral a.
metaphyseal-diaphyseal a.
neck-shaft a. (NSA)
popliteal a.
Q a.
talar to first metatarsal a.
talocalcaneal a. (TCA)
thigh-foot a. (TFA)
thigh-leg a. (TLA)
transmalleolar axis a. (TMA)
angular
a. cheilitis
a. cheilosis
a. movement
a. stomatitis
angulation
congenital anterolateral tibial a.
congenital posteromedial tibial a.
flow a.
metaphysis a.
volar a.
anhedonia
anhidrosis
ipsilateral a.
neuropathic a.
anhidrotic
a. ectodermal dysplasia
a. sweating
anhydramnion
anhydrous
betaine a.
ANI
autoimmune neutropenia of infancy
ani (*pl. of* anus)
anicteric
a. hepatitis
a. leptospirosis
aniline dye
animal
a. antisera
a. bite

a. dander
a. scabies
animal-assisted therapy (AAT)
anion
competing a.
a. gap
aniridia
nonfamilial a.
sporadic a.
aniridia-Wilms tumor
anismus
anisocoria
ipsilateral a.
simple central a.
anisocytosis
anisomelia
anisometropia
anisometropic amblyopia
anisotropic
ankle
dancer's a.
a. equinus
jogger's a.
a. stability
a. stirrup splint
ankle-foot orthosis (AFO)
ankyloglossia
ankylosing
a. spondylitis
a. spondyloarthropathy
ankylosis
artificial a.
interbody a.
ankyrin
anlage
fibrous a.
ventral pancreatic a.
ANLL
acute nonlymphoblastic leukemia
ANN
alloimmune neonatal neutropenia
Ann Arbor Staging System
annual
a. goal
a. review
annular
a. band
a. erythema antigen
a. lesion
a. pancreas
a. stenosis
a. testis

annulare
granuloma a.
perforating granuloma a.
subcutaneous granuloma a.
annulati
pili a.
pseudopili a.
annuloaortic ectasia
annuloplasty
De Vega tricuspid a.
annulus
ano
fissure in a.
anodontia
Anodynos-DHC
anogenital wart
anomalad
Poland a.
anomalous
a. coronary artery
a. pulmonary vein
a. pulmonary venous drainage
a. pulmonary venous return
a. right pulmonary vein
dextroposition
anomaly
acyanotic cardiac a.
Alder a.
Alexander a.
Arnold-Chiari a.
Axenfeld a.
branchial cleft a.
cloacal plate a.
coloboma, heart disease, atresia
choanae, retarded growth, genital
anomalies, ear a.'s (CHARGE)
congenital a.
conotruncal facial a.
craniofacial a.
development and/or central nervous
system a.'s, genital hypoplasia,
ear a.'s
DiGeorge a.
duplication a.
ear a.
Ebstein a.
extracardiac a.
Greig cephalopolysyndactyly a.
gyral a.
intraspinous vascular a.
May-Hegglin a.
Michel a.

NOTES

anomaly *(continued)*
> Mondini a.
> morning glory disk a.
> pancreaticobiliary a.
> partial DiGeorge a.
> Peters a.
> Poland a.
> Rieger a.
> Scheibe a.
> skeletal a.
> sling a.
> Sprengel a.
> Taussig-Bing a.
> thymic hypoplasia a.
> umbilical a.
> valvuloplasty and angioplasty of congenital a.'s (VACA)
> vertebral defects, anal atresia, tracheoesophageal fistula with esophageal atresia, radial and renal a.'s (VATER)

anomeric
anonychia
anophthalmos
anoplasty
anorchia
anorchism
anorectal
> a. agenesis
> a. manometry
> a. plug
> a. stenosis

anorectoplasty
> anterior sagittal a.
> laparoscopically assisted a.
> Pena midsagittal a.
> posterior sagittal a.

anorectum
anorexia
> a. athletica
> infantile a.
> a. nervosa (AN)

anosmia
anotia
anovulation
> chronic a.

anoxia
> cerebral a.
> tissue a.

anoxic seizure
ANP
> atrial natriuretic peptide

ANRBC
> absolute nucleated red blood cell

ANS
> antenatal corticosteroid treatment
> autonomic nervous system

Ansaid Oral

ANSD
> autonomic nervous system dysfunction

anserinus
> pes a.

ANSWER System Questionnaire
Antabuse
antacid
antagonism
antagonist
> bradykinin a.
> calcium channel a.
> coactivated a.'s
> folate a.
> histamine H_2 receptor a.
> leukotriene receptor a. (LTRA)
> proton pump a.
> serotonin receptor a.

antagonistic muscle
antalgic
> a. gait
> a. limp

antecedent
> plasma thromboplastin a.

ante cibum (before meals) (a.c.)
antecubital
> a. space
> a. vein

antegrade
> a. continence enema (ACE)
> a. continence enema procedure

antenatal
> a. corticosteroid treatment (ANS)
> a. disease process
> a. steroid

antepartum
anterior
> a. chamber
> a. chamber angle
> a. chamber cleavage syndrome
> a. chamber dysgenesis syndrome
> a. cricoid split (ACS)
> a. cricoid split procedure
> a. cruciate ligament (ACL)
> a. drawer test
> a. fontanelle
> a. horn cell degeneration
> a. horn cell disease
> a. lenticonus
> a. microphthalmia
> a. nasal packing
> a. nasal septum
> a. neural tube closure
> a. rectoperineal fistula
> a. resection rectopexy
> a. sagittal anorectoplasty
> a. spinal fusion
> a. spinal instrumentation
> a. superior iliac spine

A

a. synechia
a. talofibular ligament (ATFL)
a. thoracic wall
a. tibial bowing
a. tibialis transfer
a. translation
a. translation of knee
anteriorly displaced anus
anterolateral tibial bowing
anteroposterior (AP)
a. laxity
a. view
antetorsion
femoral a.
anteversion
acetabular a. (AA)
bilateral increased femoral a.
femoral a. (FA)
increased femoral a.
anteverted naris
anthelminthic drug
anthracycline
anthrax
cutaneous a.
anthropi
Ochrobactrum a.
anthropometric measure
anthropometry
anthropomorphic measurement
anti-ACh antibody
antiadrenal antibody
anti-A isohemagglutinin
antiangiogenic therapy
antianxiety
a. agent
a. drug
antiarrhythmic
antiasthmatic
antibacterial drug
antibasement membrane antibody
antibiotic
broad-spectrum a.
a. drug
a. infusion therapy
preventive a.
prophylactic a.
a. prophylaxis
a. treatment
antibiotic-associated diarrhea (AAD)
AntibiOtic Otic
antibiotic-resistant gram-negative
organism (ARGNO)

anti-B isohemagglutinin
antibody
ADB a.
AH a.
anti-ACh a.
antiadrenal a.
antibasement membrane a.
anticardiolipin a.
anticentromere a.
anticholera toxin a.
anti-CMV a.
anti-cytomegalovirus a.
anti-D a.
anti-DNase B a.
antidrug IgE a.
anti-EBNA a.
antiendomysium a. (AEA)
anti-Epstei-Barr nuclear antigen a.
anti-GBM a.
antigliadin a. (AGA)
antihistone a.
anti-*Histoplasma* a.
antihyaluronidase a.
antiidiotype a.
antiinsulin a.
antimitochondrial a.
antimyolemmal a. (AMLA)
antineutrophil a.
antineutrophil cytoplasmic a.
(ANCA, c-ANCA)
antinuclear a. (ANA)
antiovarian a.
antiphospholipid a.
antiplatelet a.
antireticulin a.
antiribosomal P a.
anti-*Saccharomyces cerevisiae* a.
anti-smooth-muscle a.
anti-SS-A a.
anti-SS-B a.
antithyroid a.
anti-TNF a.
antitoxocaral a.
ASO a.
celiac a.
cold a.
complement-fixing serum a.
conjugated antichlamydial
monoclonal a.
Coombs a.
a. deficiency
direct fluorescent a. (DFA)

NOTES

31

antibody *(continued)*
    endomysium a. (EMA)
    fluorescent treponemal a.
    glutamic acid decarboxylase a.
    hantavirus immunoglobulin M a.
    hemagglutination inhibition a. (HIA)
    a. to hepatitis A virus (anti-HAV)
    hepatitis B core a. (HBcAb)
    a. to hepatitis B core antigen
      (anti-HBc, anti-HBcAg)
    hepatitis B early a. (HBeAb)
    hepatitis B surface a. (HBsAb)
    a. to hepatitis B surface antigen
      (anti-HBs, anti-HBsAg)
    heterophil a.
    HI a.
    humoral a.
    IgA antiendomysium a.
    IgA antireticulin a.
    IgE a.
    IgM a.
    immunofluorescent a. (IFA)
    immunoglobulin a.
    indirect fluorescent a. (IFA)
    a. induction therapy
    intrathecal anti-HIV a.
    islet cell a. (ICA)
    Jo-1 a.
    maternal antithyroid a.
    maternal-fetal transmission of a.
    maternal IgG a.
    monoclonal a. (MAb)
    monoclonal antiendotoxin a.
    monoclonal anti-IgE a.
    mycoplasmal a.
    parietal cell a.
    perinuclear antineutrophil
      cytoplasmic a. (p-ANCA)
    polyclonal antiendotoxin anticore a.
    positive antinuclear a. (ANA)
    a. production assay
    a. replacement therapy
    S 100 a.
    serum antienterocyte a.
    sperm surface a.
    streptococcal a.
    titer of anti-ragweed IgE a.
    transglutaminase a.
    a. transplacental transfer
    vibriocidal a.
    virus-neutralizing a. (VNA)
    VZV-specific IgM a.
    warm a.
**antibody-dependent cell-mediated
cytotoxicity (ADCC)**
antibody-secreting cell (ASC)
anticardiolipin antibody
anticentromere antibody

anticholera toxin antibody
anticholinergic drug
anticholinesterase medication
anticipation
anticipatory
    a. anxiety
    a. grief
anti-CMV antibody
anticoagulant
    circulating a.
    lupus a.
anticonvulsant
    a. drug
    a. hypersensitivity syndrome
    a. intoxication
    a. treatment
anti-cytomegalovirus antibody
anti-D
    a.-D antibody
    a.-D globulin treatment
    a.-D therapy
anti-deoxyribonucleic acid (anti-DNA)
antidepressant
    a. drug
    heterocyclic a.
    a. poisoning
    tricyclic a. (TCA)
antidiuresis
antidiuretic hormone (ADH)
anti-DNA
    anti-deoxyribonucleic acid
anti-DNase
    a.-D. B (ADB)
    a.-D. B antibody
    a.-D. B titer
antidote
antidromic conduction
antidrug IgE antibody
antidysrhythmic agent
anti-EBNA antibody
antiemetic medication
antiendomysial
    IgA a.
antiendomysium antibody (AEA)
antiepileptic drug (AED)
**anti-Epstein-Barr nuclear antigen
antibody**
antifungal
    Absorbine A.
    Absorbine Jr. A.
    a. azoles
    Breezee Mist A.
    a. drug
Anti-Gas
    Maalox A.-G.
anti-GBM antibody
antigen
    A a.

annular erythema a.
antibody to hepatitis B core a.
  (anti-HBc, anti-HBcAg)
antibody to hepatitis B surface a.
  (anti-HBs, anti-HBsAg)
antigen-specific a.
Australia a.
B a.
C a.
carcinoembryonic a.
cryptococcal a.
a. detection test
Duffy a.
E a.
Epstein-Barr nuclear a.
fetal histocompatibility a.
hantavirus a.
hepatitis B a.
hepatitis B surface a. (HBsAg)
histocompatibility leukocyte a.
  (HLA)
histone a.
HLA-B27 a.
human leukocyte a. (HLA)
Kell a.
La/SSB a.
lipoglycan a.
O a.
Pm-Scl a.
polysaccharide group-specific a.
RBC P a.
recombinant K29 a.
red cell a.
respiratory syncytial virus a.
ribonucleoprotein a.
Ro/SSA a.
RSV a.
sclerodermatomyositis a.
Sm a.
Thomsen-Friedenreich a.
T-independent a.
Toxoplasma a.
viral capsid a. (VCA)
viral p24 a.
von Willebrand factor a.
antigen-antibody complex
antigenemia
antigenic
  a. mimicry
  a. stimulus
antigen-presenting cell (APC)
antigen-specific antigen

antigenuria
antigliadin
  a. antibody (AGA)
  IgA a.
antiglobulin test
antiglomerular basement membrane
  antibody disease
antigravity
  a. activity
  a. position
anti-HAV
  antibody to hepatitis A virus
  IgG anti-HAV
anti-HBc, anti-HBcAg
  antibody to hepatitis B core antigen
anti-HBs, anti-HBsAg
  antibody to hepatitis B surface antigen
  anti-HBs concentration
antihelical fold
antihemophilic factor (AHF)
antihepatitis A virus immunoglobulin G
Antihist-1
antihistamine
  a. drug
  histamine-1 a.
antihistone antibody
anti-*Histoplasma* antibody
antihyaluronidase (AH)
  a. antibody
  a. titer
antihypertensive
antiidiotype antibody
antiimmunoglobulin reagent
antiinflammatory
  a. effect
  a. intervention
  a. therapy
  a. treatment
antiinsulin antibody
anti-Jo1
antileukemic therapy
antilewisite
  British a. (BAL)
antilipolysis
Antilirium Injection
antilymphocyte
  a. globulin
  a. sera
antimalarial
antimanic treatment
antimetabolite

NOTES

antimicrobial
- a. agent
- a. aminoglycoside
- a. prophylaxis
- a. susceptibility testing
- a. therapy
- a. treatment

Antiminth
antimitochondrial antibody
antimongoloid eye slant
antimycobacterial
antimycoplasma titer
antimyolemmal antibody (AMLA)
antineutrophil
- a. antibody
- a. cytoplasmic antibody (ANCA, c-ANCA)
- a. cytoplasmic antibody titer

antinociception
antinuclear antibody (ANA)
anti-O-specific polysaccharide
antiovarian antibody
antioxidant
- a. enzyme
- a. therapy

antiperistaltic intestinal interposition
antiphospholipid
- a. antibody
- a. antibody syndrome
- a. syndrome (APS)

antiplasmin (AP)
- a-2 antiplasmin (a-2AP)
- a. deficiency

antiplatelet
- a. agent
- a. antibody

antipsychotic drug
antipyretic therapy
antipyrine and benzocaine
antirabies serum
antirespiratory syncytial virus (anti-RSV)
antireticulin antibody
antiretroviral
- a. medication
- a. resistance
- a. therapy

antiribosomal P antibody
anti-RSV
- antirespiratory syncytial virus

anti-*Saccharomyces cerevisiae* antibody
anti-Scl-70
- antitopoisomerase-1
- anti-Scl-70 autoantibody

antisense
- a. nucleotide
- a. oligodeoxynucleotide

antisera
- animal a.

antiserum
- tetanus a.

antisiphon device
anti-smooth-muscle antibody
antisocial
- a. behavior
- a. personality disorder (ASPD)

Antispas Injection
antispastic drug
anti-SS-A antibody
anti-SS-B antibody
anti-ssDNA
antistaphylococcal
- a. agent
- a. IgE
- a. penicillin

antistreptolysin
- a. O (ASO)
- a. O assay
- a. O response
- a. titer

antithrombin
- a. II
- a. III (AT-III)
- a. III coagulation inhibitor
- a. III deficiency
- protein S a.

antithymocyte gamma globulin (ATGAM, ATG)
antithyreoperoxidase
antithyroid antibody
anti-TNF antibody
antitopoisomerase-1 (anti-Scl-70)
antitoxin
- botulinum a. (type A, B, E)
- diphtheria a.
- equine a.
- scarlatina a.
- tetanus a. (TAT)

antitoxocaral antibody
anti-*Toxoplasma*
- serum immunoglobulin G a.-*T.*

antitragus
antitrypsin
- a-2 a. (a-2AT)

antituberculosis chemotherapy
antituberculous therapy
Anti-Tuss Expectorant
antitussive medication
antivenin (crotalidae) polyvalent
antivenom
Antivert
antiviral therapy
Antizol
Antley-Bixler syndrome
Antopol disease

antral
    a. choanal polyp
    a. gastritis
    a. lavage
    a. stenosis
    a. washout
Antrizine
antrum
    aditus admission a.
    nasal a.
ANUG
    acute necrotizing ulcerative gingivitis
Anumed
anuria
anuric
anus, pl. **ani**
    adequate caliber of a.
    anteriorly displaced a.
    ectopic a.
    high imperforate a.
    imperforate a.
    low imperforate a.
    pruritus ani
    spastic levator ani
    supralevator imperforate a.
    translevator imperforate a.
Anusol
    A. HC-1 Topical
    A. HC-2.5% Topical
Anusol-HC Suppository
anvil
Anxanil Oral
anxiety
    anticipatory a.
    childhood a.
    a. depression
    a. disorder
    A. Disorder Interview for Children
    a. management
    a. rating for children (ARC)
    a. sensitivity index (ASI)
    separation a.
    stranger a.
anxiety-withdrawal scale
anxiogenic
anxiolytic
    a. agent
    a. drug
    a. medication
anxious look
Anzemet

AOD
    alcohol and other drugs
AOM
    acute otitis media
AOP
    apnea of prematurity
AOPP
    advanced oxidation protein product
aorta, pl. **aortae**
    coarctation of a.
    a. dilation
    overriding a.
    traumatic rupture of thoracic a.
     (TRA)
aortic
    a. arch
    a. arch coarctation (CoA)
    a. arch rupture
    a. blood pressure
    a. bruit
    a. bud
    a. coarctation
    a. cusp prolapse
    a. dissection
    a. ejection click
    a. insufficiency
    a. knob
    left atrial to a. (LA:Ao)
    a. oxygen content
    a. regurgitation
    a. root
    a. runoff
    a. stenosis (AS)
    a. valve
    a. valve stenosis
    a. valvotomy
aorticopulmonary
    a. septation
    a. window defect
aortic-to-pulmonary shunt
aortitis
aortogram
    thoracic a.
aortopexy
aortoplasty
    prosthetic patch a.
    subclavian flap a. (SFA)
aortopulmonary
    a. collateral coil embolization
    a. shunt
    a. transposition
    a. window

NOTES

AP
>anatomic profile
>anteroposterior
>antiplasmin
>appendiceal perforation
>>AP diameter

APA
>American Psychiatric Association

Apacet

APACHE
>Acute Physiology and Chronic Health
>Evaluation

apathy

APC
>antigen-presenting cell
>atrial premature contraction

APE
>Ara-C, Platinol, etoposide

Apert-Crouzon
>A.-C. disease
>A.-C. syndrome

Apert syndrome

aperture
>supraglottic a.

apex, pl. **apices**
>a. of intussusception
>prolapsing a.

APGAR
>adaptability, partnership, growth,
>affection, resolve
>>family APGAR

Apgar score

APGN
>acute postinfectious glomerulonephritis

aphakia
>pediatric a.

aphasia
>acquired epileptic a.
>Broca a.
>expressive a.
>global a.
>infantile acquired a.
>migraine with a.
>receptive a.
>thymic a.
>Wernicke a.

apheresis
>LDL a.

aphonia

aphrodisiac

aphrophilus
>*Haemophilus a.*

aphtha, pl. **aphthae**
>Bednar a.

aphthosis
>perianal a.

aphthous
>a. oral ulcer

>a. stomatitis
>a. ulceration

A1PI
>alpha-1 proteinase inhibitor

APIB
>Assessment of Preterm Infants Behavior

apical
>a. ectodermal ridge
>a. four-chamber view
>a. heave
>a. impulse
>a. pleural stripping
>a. presystolic murmur
>a. pulse
>a. vertebra

apices (*pl. of* apex)

apista
>*Pandoraea a.*

A.P.L.

aplasia
>Alexander a.
>a. axialis extracorticalis congenita
>B19-induced red cell a.
>bone marrow a.
>complete cerebellar a.
>complete radial a.
>congenital cutis a.
>congenital RBC a.
>congenital skin a.
>congenital vaginal a.
>cutis a.
>a. cutis congenita
>gonadal a.
>idiosyncratic marrow a.
>Leydig cell a.
>Michel a.
>Mondini a.
>optic nerve a.
>parvovirus B19 red cell a.
>pulmonary acinar a.
>pure red cell a.
>radial ray a.
>Scheibe a.
>selective a.
>thyroid a.

aplastic
>a. anemia
>a. crisis
>a. leukemia
>a. pancytopenia

Apley compression test

APLS
>advanced pediatric life support
>>APLS model

apnea
>a. and bradycardia
>central sleep a.
>expiratory a.

idiopathic a.
a. of infancy
initial a.
late a.
mixed sleep a.
a. monitor
neonatal a.
a. neonatorum
obstructive a.
obstructive sleep a. (OSA)
pathologic a.
pathological a.
postoperative a.
posttussive a.
a. of prematurity (AOP)
secondary a.
sleep a.
unrecognized a.

apnea-bradycardia
apnea-hypopnea combination
apnea/hypoventilation
obstructive sleep a./h. (OSA/H)
apneic
a. event
a. seizure
apneustic center
apobetalipoprotein
apoB gene
apocrine
a. chromhidrosis
a. duct
a. gland of Moll
apoenzyme deficiency
apoferritin
apolipoprotein
serum a.
aponeurosis
epicranial a.
gastrocnemius a.
apophyseal space
apophysis, pl. apophyses
apophysitis
calcaneal a.
iliac crest a.
olecranon a.
traction a.
apoptosis
postasphyxial a.
apoptotic
a. body
a. cell death
apositional ossification

apotransferrin infusion
apparatus
figure-of-eight a.
Golgi a.
vestibular a.
apparent
a. exophthalmos
a. life-threatening event (ALTE)
a. mineralocorticoid excess (AME)
a. paresis
appearance
apple-peel a.
bag of worms a.
bat wing a.
bird's beak a.
bread-and-butter a.
cobblestone a.
copper-wire a.
corkscrew a.
drooping lily a.
Erlenmeyer flask a.
hair-on-end a.
hatchet face a.
honeycombed a.
Hurler-like facial a.
lamellated a.
onion-skin a.
puppetlike a.
salt-and-pepper a.
silver-wire a.
slapped-cheek a.
soap-bubble a.
sporotrichoid a.
stacked-coin a.
sunburst a.
toxic a.
water bottle a.
wing-beating a.
worried facial a.
appendage
testicular a.
a. torsion
appendectomy
inversion-ligation a.
appendiceal
a. fecalith
a. intussusception
a. inversion
a. lumen
a. perforation (AP)
a. stump

NOTES

appendicitis
    acute a. (AA)
    gangrenous a.
    pelvic a.
    perforated a.
    ruptured a.
appendicolith
    calcified a.
appendicostomy
appendix
    ligation of a.
    obstruction of a.
    a. testis
    torsion of a.
    vascularized a.
    vermiform a.
apperception
appetite
    decreased a.
apple pattern
apple-peel
    a.-p. appearance
    a.-p. atresia
appliance
    dental speech a.
    lingual a.
    orthodontic a.
    orthopedic a.
applicator
    benzoin a.
applied behavior analysis (ABA)
applier
    vascular clip a.
apprehension
    a. sign
    a. test
approach
    Greenspan a.
    Kahn a.
    quasi-experimental research a.
    staircase a.
appropriate
    a. blood pressure cuff size
    a. for gestational age (AGA)
    a. learning experience
APPT
    Adolescent and Pediatric Pain Tool
apraxia
    buccolingual a.
    congenital ocular motor a.
    gait a.
    oculomotor a.
apraxic
Apresoline
    A. Injection
    A. Oral
Aprodine
aprosencephaly

aprotinin
APS
    antiphospholipid syndrome
APSGN
    acute poststreptococcal
    glomerulonephritis
Aptamil formula
Apt-Downey test
aptitude-2
    Detroit Test of Learning A.-2
APTT
    activated partial thromboplastin time
    APTT coagulation test
aP vaccine
AQ
    Beconase AQ
    Nasacort AQ
    Vancenase AQ
aqua
    A. Glycolic
    A. Tar
Aquachloral Supprettes
AquaMEPHYTON
Aquaphor
Aquaphyllin
Aquasol
    A. A
    A. E
    A. E Oral
Aquatar gel
aqueduct
    cochlear a.
    a. of Sylvius
aqueductal
    a. forking
    a. gliosis
    a. stenosis
aqueous
    a. analysis
    A. AVP
    a. beclomethasone
    a. crystalline penicillin
    a. crystalline penicillin G
    a. humor
AR
    autosomal recessive
arabinoside
    cytosine a.
arabinosylcytosine (Ara-C, ARA-C, araC)
    cyclophosphamide, Oncovin,
    methotrexate, a. (COMA)
Ara-C, ARA-C, araC
    arabinosylcytosine
    Ara-C, Platinol, etoposide (APE)
arachidic acid
arachidonic acid
arachnid envenomation

arachnidism
 necrotic a.
arachnodactyly
 congenital contractural a. (CCA)
arachnoid
 a. granulation
 a. villus
arachnoiditis
 chronic adhesive a.
 posterior fossa a.
 spinal a.
 tuberculous spinal a.
Aralen Phosphate
Aran-Duchenne
 A.-D. disease
 A.-D. muscular dystrophy
araneus
 nevus a.
ARAS
 ascending reticular activating system
arborization
 dendritic a.
arboviral encephalitis
arbovirus
ARC
 anxiety rating for children
 Association for Retarded Citizens
arc
 xenon a.
Arcanobacterium haemolyticum
arch
 aortic a.
 brachial a.
 branchial a.
 double aortic a. (DAA)
 hypoplastic zygomatic a.
 a. insole pad
 interrupted aortic a. (type A, B)
 medial longitudinal a.
 right aortic a. (RAA)
 vertebral laminar a.
 zygomatic a.
architecture
 cortical a.
 crypt-villus a.
 dysplastic cortical a.
 lobular a.
 mixed cystic/solid a.
 sleep a.
arciform lesion

arcus
 a. corneae
 a. juvenilis
ARD
 acute respiratory disease
ARDS
 acute respiratory distress syndrome
area
 ambosexual a.
 body surface a. (BSA)
 Broca a.
 developmental a.
 flexural a.
 frontal pole a.
 infraclavicular a.
 inguinal a.
 intertriginous a.
 Kiesselbach a.
 Little a.
 social/emotional developmental a.
 subpulmonic a.
 total body surface a. (TBSA)
 triginous a.
 Wernicke a.
areal bone mineral density
areata
 alopecia a.
Aredia
areflexia
areflexic paraparesis
aregenerative anemia
Arenavirus
areolar enlargement
ARF
 acute renal failure
 acute rheumatic fever
  nonoliguric ARF
  oliguric ARF
  postrenal ARF
  prerenal ARF
Arfonad Injection
Argentine hemorrhagic fever
arginase deficiency
arginine
 a. hydrochloride
 plasma a.
 a. vasopressin (AVP)
 a. vasopressin regulation
arginine-insulin
 a.-i. stimulation test
 a.-i. tolerance test
argininosuccinate lyase

NOTES

39

argininosuccinic
- a. acid
- a. acid synthetase deficiency
- a. aciduria

ARGNO
- antibiotic-resistant gram-negative organism

argon diode

Argyll Robertson pupil

arhinencephaly

ARI
- acute respiratory infection

ariboflavinosis

Aristocort
- A. A Topical
- A. Forte Injection
- A. Intralesional Injection
- A. Oral

Aristospan
- A. Intra-articular Injection
- A. Intralesional Injection

arithmetic method

arm
- a. board
- a. circumference
- a. dysfunction
- parallel study a.
- a. span

Arm-a-Med
- A.-a-M. Isoproterenol
- A.-a-M. Metaproterenol

ARMS
- acoustic respiratory motion sensor

ARND
- alcohol-related neurodevelopmental disorder

Arnold-Chiari
- A.-C. anomaly
- A.-C. malformation
- A.-C. syndrome

aromatherapy

arousal
- confusional a.
- a. disorder
- a. level

ARPKD
- autosomal recessive polycystic kidney disease

ARPTH
- autosomal recessive renal proximal tubulopathy and hypercalciuria

array
- density spectral a. (DSA)

arrest
- cardiac a.
- circulatory a.
- deep hypothermia and total circulatory a. (DHCA)

growth a.
physeal a.
pubertal a.
respiratory a.
sinus a.

arrest/akinetic fit

arrested hydrocephalus

Arrestin Injection

arrhenoblastoma

arrhinencephaly

arrhythmia
- clinically significant a. (CSA)
- digitalis-induced a.
- late a.
- malignant a.
- nonspecific a. (NSA)
- primary cardiac a.
- respiratory sinus a.
- sinus a.
- Xylocaine HCl I.V. Injection for Cardiac A.'s

arrhythmic twitching

arrhythmogenesis

arrhythmogenic right ventricular dysplasia (ARVD)

Arrow catheter

ARSA
- aberrant right subclavian artery

arsenic
- a. nickel silicon
- a. poisoning

arsenical
- organic a.

ART
- assisted reproductive technology
- automated reagin test

Artane

Artemisinin

arterial
- a. to alveolar oxygen tension ratio (AaPO$_2$)
- a. aneurysm
- a. banding
- a. blood gas (ABG)
- a. blood pressure (ABP)
- a. catheter
- a. ectasia
- a. embolization
- a. fibrosing sclerosis
- a. lactate
- a. line
- a. line flush solution
- a. obstruction
- a. oxygen tension
- a. pressure
- a. retransposition
- a. rupture
- a. spasm

a. stick
a. switch operation
a. switch procedure
a. thrombosis
arterial-alveolar gradient
arterial-ascitic fluid pH gradient
arterialized blood
arteriogram
pulmonary a.
arteriography
selective pulmonary a.
arteriohepatic dysplasia
arteriolar occlusion
arteriole
pulmonary a.
arteriolitis
necrotizing a.
arteriomesenteric duodenal compression
syndrome
arteriopathy
arterioplasty
arterioportal fistula
arteriosclerosis
infantile a.
arteriosus
ductus a.
patent ductus a. (PDA)
right ductus a. (RDA)
truncus a.
arteriovenous
a. canal defect
a. fistula
a. fistula malformation (AVFM)
a. malformation (AVM)
arteritis
giant cell a.
inflammatory a.
necrotizing a.
Takayasu a. (TA)
a. umbilicalis
artery
aberrant coronary a.
aberrant right subclavian a.
(ARSA)
aberrant subclavian a.
absence of branch pulmonary a.
acinar a.
a. of Adamkiewicz
anomalous coronary a.
brachial a.
caliber-persistent a.
carotid a.

celiac a.
complete transposition of great a.'s
d-transposition of great a.'s (d-
TGA)
femoral a.
gastroepiploic a. (GEA)
iliofemoral a.
innominate a.
left main coronary a.
l-transposition of great a.'s
major aortopulmonary collateral a.
(MAPCA)
middle cerebral a. (MCA)
proximal pulmonary a.
pulmonary a. (PA)
radial a.
right common carotid a. (RCCA)
right femoral a. (RFA)
sinoatrial node a.
spiral endometrial a.
subclavian a.
thalamostriatic a.
transposition of great a.'s (TGA)
umbilical a.
Arthobacter globiformis
arthralgia
psychogenic a.
arthritis, pl. **arthritides**
candidal a.
degenerative a.
gonococcal a.
gouty a.
hematogenous septic a.
idiopathic chronic a.
juvenile a. (JA)
juvenile chronic a.
juvenile idiopathic a. (JIA)
juvenile idiopathic polyarticular a.
juvenile psoriatic a.
juvenile rheumatoid a. (type I, II)
(JRA)
Lyme a.
migratory peripheral a.
monarticular a.
mumps a.
neonatal septic a.
oligoarticular a.
pauciarticular juvenile chronic a.
pauciarticular juvenile rheumatoid a.
pauciarticular-onset a.
peripheral a.
polyarticular juvenile chronic a.

NOTES

arthritis *(continued)*
    polyarticular juvenile rheumatoid a.
    postenteritis a.
    postinfectious a.
    Pseudomonas septic a.
    psoriasis-associated a.
    psoriatic a.
    purulent a.
    reactive a.
    a. of rheumatic fever
    rheumatoid a. (RA)
    septic a.
    spondylitis, enthesitis, a. (SEA)
    suppurative a.
    systemic juvenile chronic a.
    systemic-onset juvenile
      rheumatoid a.
    viral a.
    Yersinia a.
arthritis-dermatitis syndrome
arthrocentesis
arthrochalasis multiplex congenita
  Ehlers-Danlos syndrome
arthrodesis
    Dennyson-Fulford extraarticular
      subtalar a.
    triple a.
arthrogram
    air a.
arthrography
arthrogryposis
    distal a. (type I, II)
    a. multiplex
    a. multiplex congenita
    skeletal a.
arthrogrypotic clubfoot
arthroophthalmopathy
    hereditary a.
arthropathy
    hemophilic a.
    human parvovirus a.
    sensory a.
    seronegativity, enthesopathy, a.
      (SEA)
arthropod-borne virus
arthropod-induced blister
arthrosis
Arthus reaction
articular
articulate
articulation
    calcaneonavicular a.
    compensatory a.
    cricoarytenoid a.
    a. disorder
Articulose-50 Injection
artifact
    point-spread a.

artificial
    a. ankylosis
    a. fever
    a. insemination by donor (AID)
    a. insemination donor (AID)
    a. insemination with donor
    a. lung-expanding compound
      (ALEC)
    a. respiration
    a. temperature
    a. vaginal epithelium
ARVD
    arrhythmogenic right ventricular
      dysplasia
aryepiglottic fold
arylsulfatase
    a. A (ASA)
arylsulfatase-activator deficiency
arytenoid
AS
    active sleep
    aortic stenosis
    Asperger syndrome
A.S.
    Crysticillin A.S.
a.s., AS
    auris sinistra (left ear)
ASA
    arylsulfatase A
    MSD Enteric Coated ASA
5-ASA
A.S.A.
Asacol Oral
ASC
    altered state of consciousness
    antibody-secreting cell
    asthma symptom checklist
A-scan
ascariasis
    pulmonary a.
ascaris
    A. lumbricoides
ascending
    a. cholangiopathy
    a. cholangitis
    a. radiculomyelitis
    a. reticular activating system
      (ARAS)
Aschoff
    A. body
    A. nodule
ascites
    biliary a.
    chylous a.
    congenital neonatal a.
    culture-negative neutrocytic a.
    eosinophilic a.
    exudative a.

fetal a.
massive a.
refractory a.
tense a.

ascitic fluid
ascorbate
ascorbic
a. acid
a. acid deficiency

Ascorbicap
Ascriptin
ASD
acute stress disorder
atrial septal defect
autism spectrum disorder
canal type ASD
ostium primum ASD
secundum ASD

ASDA
American Sleep Disorders Association

aseptic
a. fever
a. meningitis
a. meningitis syndrome
a. meningoencephalitis
a. necrosis
a. necrosis of bone
a. temperature

asexual
Asherman syndrome
Ashkenazi Jew
ash-leaf
a.-l. macule
a.-l. spot

Ashman phenomenon
Ashworth
A. score
A. score of spasticity

ASI
anxiety sensitivity index

Askin tumor
Ask-Upmark kidney
ASL
American Sign Language

ASLD
adenylosuccinate lyase deficiency

Asmalix
ASO
antistreptolysin O
ASO antibody
ASO titer

asparaginase

asparagine
aspartate
a. aminotransferase (AST)
amphetamine a.
a. transaminase (AST)

aspartic acid
aspartoacylase hydrolytic activity
aspartylglycosaminuria
A-Spas S/L
ASPD
antisocial personality disorder

Asperger
A. disorder (AD)
A. syndrome (AS)

aspergilloma
aspergillosis
allergic bronchopulmonary a.
(ABPA)
bronchopulmonary a.
cerebral a.
fatal cutaneous a.
ocular a.

Aspergillus
A. *flavus*
A. *fumigatus*
A. *nidulans*
A. *niger*
A. *terreus*

Aspergum
asphyxia
acute total a.
asphyxia, bacterial meningitis,
congenital perinatal infection
(cytomegalovirus, rubella, herpes,
toxoplasmosis, syphillis), defects
of head or neck, elevated
bilirubin exceeding indications for
exchange, family history of
childhood hearing impairment,
gram birth weight ≤500 g
birth a.
fetal a.
intrapartum a.
intrauterine a.
neonatal a.
a. neonatorum
perinatal a.
prenatal a.
prolonged partial a.

asphyxial
a. birth injury

NOTES

asphyxial *(continued)*
- a. brain injury
- a. event

asphyxiating
- a. thoracic dysplasia syndrome
- a. thoracic dystrophy
- a. thoracodystrophy syndrome

asphyxiation

aspiny interneuron

aspirate
- blood-flecked gastric a.
- bone marrow a. (BMA)
- bubo a.
- nasogastric a.
- nasopharyngeal a. (NPA)
- tracheal a.
- tracheobronchial a.

aspiration
- bone marrow a.
- caustic a.
- chronic a.
- epididymal sperm a.
- foreign body a.
- maxillary sinus a.
- meconium a.
- metaphyseal a.
- microsurgical epididymal sperm a. (MESA)
- percutaneous cyst a.
- percutaneous epididymal sperm a. (PESA)
- a. pneumonia
- pulmonary a.
- sperm a.
- subperiosteal a.
- suprapubic bladder a.
- a. syndrome
- transtracheal a.

aspirator
- mucus a.

aspirin
- Bayer A.
- oxycodone and a.
- a. triad

Aspirols
- Amyl Nitrite A.

asplenia
- anatomic a.
- congenital a.
- functional a.
- a. syndrome

asplenic

ASQ
- Ages and Stages Questionnaire

ASS
- Asthma Severity Score

assaultive
- verbally a.

assay
- AccuStat Strep A a.
- agglutination a.
- antibody production a.
- antistreptolysin O a.
- Bethesda a.
- CH_{50} a.
- Chiron branched DNA a.
- Clinitest a.
- C1q a.
- DNA hybridization a.
- dot immunobinding a. (DIA)
- electrophoretic mobility shift a. (EMSA)
- ELISPOT a.
- enzyme a.
- enzyme immunosorbent a. (EIA)
- enzyme-linked immunofiltration a. (ELIFA)
- enzyme-linked immunosorbent a. (ELISA)
- factor Xa inhibition a.
- genotypic a.
- hemagglutinin enzyme-linked immunosorbent a. (H(c)ELISA)
- Heptest Xa a.
- HIV-1 RNA PCR a.
- 5-hydroxyindoleacetic a.
- immunoblot a.
- immunofluorescent a. (IFA)
- immunofunctional a.
- immunosorbent agglutination a. (ISAGA)
- indirect immunofluorescence a.
- latex agglutination a.
- LCR a.
- ligase-chain reaction a.
- luciferase a.
- Lyme enzyme-linked immunosorbent a.
- measles virus enzyme-linked immunosorbent a. (MV(c)ELISA)
- NucliSens a.
- quantitative Bethesda a.
- quantitative serum drug a.
- radioantigen-binding a. (RABA)
- radioimmunoprecipitation a. (RIPA)
- Raji cell a.
- recombinant immunosorbent a. (RIBA)
- respiratory burst a.
- Roche Amplicor Monitor a.
- salivary cortisol a.
- serum hexosaminidase a.
- solid-phase enzyme-linked immunospot a.
- sperm penetration a. (SPA)
- Thomsen-Friedenreich antigen a.

TMA a.
transcription-mediated
  amplification a.
ultrasensitive a.
virologic a.
in vitro antibody production a.
assembly
brush border a.
infant nasal cannula a. (INCA)
assertive
assessment
ABCDE a.
abuse, sexuality, safety a.
behavioral a.
child and adolescent burden a.
  (CABA)
Child and Adolescent
  Psychiatric A. (CAPA)
Child and Adolescent Services A.
  (CASA)
clinical risk a. (CRA)
Dubowitz Neurological A.
Erhardt developmental prehension a.
gestational age a.
health-related quality-of-life a.
HRQOL a.
A. in Infancy Ordinal Scales of
  Psychological Development
neurodevelopmental a.
neuromuscular maturity a.
phallometric a.
preschool-age psychiatric a. (PAPA)
A. of Preterm Infants Behavior
  (APIB)
projective a.
quadrant a.
qualitative developmental a.
substance abuse, sexuality, safety a.
young adult psychiatric a. (YAPA)
assignment
gender a.
assimilation
atlas a.
assisted
a. reproductive technology (ART)
a. ventilation (AV)
assistive technology (AT)
association
American Diabetes A. (ADA)
American Psychiatric A. (APA)
American Sleep Disorders A.
  (ASDA)

CHARGE a.
a. reaction
A. for Retarded Citizens (ARC)
A. of Women's Health, Obstetrics,
  and Neonatal Nursing
  (AWHONN)
ASSQ
autism spectrum screening questionnaire
AST
aspartate aminotransferase
aspartate transaminase
astasia-abasia
astatic seizure
asteatotic eczema
Astech Peak Flow Meter
Astelin Nasal Spray
astemizole
asterixis
asteroides
  Nocardia a.
asthenia
asthenozoospermia
asthma
allergen-induced a.
atopic a.
bronchial a.
cardiac a.
chronic a.
a. exacerbation
exercise-induced a. (EIA)
infantile a.
intrinsic a.
labile a.
a. morbidity
nocturnal a.
perennial a.
seasonal a.
A. Severity Score (ASS)
a. symptom checklist (ASC)
a. with vasculitis
AsthmaHaler Mist
AsthmaNefrin
asthmatic
a. bronchitis
a. response
asthmaticus
status a.
astigmatism
astragalus
Astramorph PF Injection
astrocyte footplate
astrocytic gliosis

NOTES

astrocytoma
> anaplastic pilocytic a.
> chiasmatic pilocytic a.
> diffuse a.
> fibrillary a.
> a. (grade I–IV)
> juvenile pilocytic a.
> low-grade diffuse a.
> low-grade fibrillary a.
> malignant pilocytic a.
> pilocytic fibrillary a.

astrogliosis
Astrovirus
asymbolia to pain
asymmetric
> a. crying facies
> a. hyperopia
> a. IUGR
> a. nystagmus
> a. palatal paresis
> a. small foramen magnum
> a. tonic neck reflex (ATNR)

asymmetrical
asymmetros
> duplicitas a.

asymmetry
> left/right a.
> truncal a.

asymptomatic
asynchronously
asynchrony
> marked a.

asynergia
> cerebellar a.

asystole
AT
> assistive technology
> ataxia-telangiectasia

Atarax Oral
AT1, AT2 receptor
ataxia
> acute cerebellar a.
> acute childhood a.
> acute recurrent a.
> adult-onset spinocerebellar a.
> cerebellar a.
> chronic progressive a.
> episodic a. (1, 2)
> Friedreich a.
> gait a.
> hereditary paroxysmal a.
> infantile-onset spinocerebellar a.
> Machado-Joseph a.
> myoclonic a.
> spastic a.
> spinocerebellar a. (type 1) (SCA)
> transient cerebellar a.
> truncal a.

> a. with isolated vitamin E
> deficiency

ataxia-telangiectasia (AT)
ataxic cerebral palsy
atelectasis
> congenital a.
> massive a.
> obstructive a.
> primary a.
> resorption a.
> subsegmental a.

atelectrauma
atelencephaly
atelosteogenesis
atenolol
ATFL
> anterior talofibular ligament

ATGAM, ATG
> antithymocyte gamma globulin

Atgam
athelia
atherectomy
> directional coronary a. (DCA)

atherogenesis
atherogenic
atherosclerosis
> accelerated a.

athetoid
> a. cerebral palsy
> a. movement

athetosis
> congenital a.

athetotic
> a. movement disorder
> a. posturing

athlete's foot
athletica
> anorexia a.

athyrotic
> a. hypothyroidism
> a. neonate

AT-III
> antithrombin III
> AT-III coagulation inhibitor

Ativan
Atlanta Scottish Rite Hospital orthosis
atlantoaxial (AA)
> a. dislocation
> a. instability
> a. subluxation

atlantodens interval (ADI)
atlantooccipital dislocation
atlas
> a. assimilation
> Gruelich and Pyle a.

ATLL
> adult T-cell leukemia/lymphoma

Got a Good Word for STEDMAN'S?

Help us keep STEDMAN'S products fresh and up-to-date with new words and new ideas! How can we make your STEDMAN'S product the best medical word reference possible for you?

Do we need to add or revise any items? Is there a better way to organize the content?

Be specific! Fill in the lines below with your thoughts and recommendations and FAX the page to **ATTENTION STEDMANS, 410-528-4153.**

You are our most important contributor, and we want to know what's on your mind. Thanks!

Please tell us a little bit about yourself:

Name/Title: _____

Company: _____

Address: _____

City/State/Zip: _____

Day Telephone No.: (_____) _____

E-mail Address: _____

TERMS YOU BELIEVE ARE INCORRECT:

Appears as: Suggested revision:

_____   _____

_____   _____

_____   _____

NEW TERMS/WORDS YOU WOULD LIKE US TO ADD:

_____

_____

Other comments:

_____

_____

_____

May we quote you?   ☐ Yes   ☐ No

All done? Great, just FAX this page to the attention of STEDMAN'S at 410-528-4153 or MAIL the page to us at:

Lippincott Williams & Wilkins
ATTN: STEDMAN'S EDITORIAL
351 West Camden Street
Baltimore, MD 21201-2436

OR enter your information
ONLINE at **www.stedmans.com**

Thanks again!

PEDS 730570

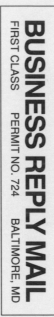

ATLS
    advanced trauma life support
ATN
    acute tubular necrosis
ATNR
    asymmetric tonic neck reflex
ATOD
    alcohol, tobacco, and other drugs
Atolone Oral
atomic absorption spectrometer
Atomlab 200 dose calibrator
atonic
    a. cerebral palsy
    a. seizure
atonic-astatic diplegia
atony
    bowel a.
    diaphragmatic a.
    gastric a.
atopic
    a. asthma
    a. dermatitis
    a. diaper rash
    a. eczema
    a. erythroderma
atopy
atovaquone
Atozine
ATP
    adenosine triphosphate
    deoxy ATP
atra
    Stachybotrys a.
atracurium
atransferrinemia
    congenital a.
atresia
    anal a.
    apple-peel a.
    aural a.
    bilateral a.
    biliary a. (BA)
    bronchial a.
    a. choanae
    choanal a.
    congenital aural a.
    congenital duodenal a.
    de la Cruz classification of
      congenital aural a.
    distal esophageal a.
    duodenal a.
    esophageal a. (EA)

    extrahepatic biliary a.
    functional pulmonary a.
    gastrointestinal a.
    ileal a.
    intestinal a.
    intrahepatic biliary a.
    jejunal a.
    jejunoileal a.
    laryngeal a.
    a. of larynx
    oocyte a.
    primary repair of esophageal a.
    pulmonary artery a.
    pure esophageal a.
    pyloric a.
    Schuknecht classification of
      congenital aural a. (type A–D)
    small bowel a.
    tracheal a.
    tracheoesophageal a.
    tricuspid a.
    urethral a.
    vaginal a.
atretic
    a. extrahepatic bile duct resection
    a. gallbladder
    a. ureter
    a. vagina
atria (*pl. of* atrium)
atrial
    a. contraction
    a. fibrillation
    a. flutter
    a. hypertrophy
    a. inversion procedure
    a. natriuretic factor (ANF)
    a. natriuretic peptide (ANP)
    a. premature contraction (APC)
    a. premature depolarization
    a. septal defect (ASD)
    a. septectomy
    a. septoplasty procedure
    a. septostomy
    a. septostomy procedure
    a. septum excision
    a. shunt
    a. switch operation
    a. switch procedure
    a. tachyarrhythmia
    a. tachycardia
atriotomy
atrioventricular (AV)

NOTES

atrioventricular *(continued)*
    a. canal
    a. canal defect
    a. dissociation
    a. nodal reentrant tachycardia
      (AVNRT)
    a. node
    a. node function
    a. reciprocating tachycardia (AVRT)
    a. valve
at-risk
    Carolina Curriculum for
      Handicapped Infants and
      Infants A.-r.
    a.-r. infant
atrium, pl. **atria**
    common a.
    left a.
    ventricles to a.
Atropair Ophthalmic
atrophia bulborum hereditaria
atrophic
    a. patch
    a. vaginal mucosa
atrophicae
    striae a.
atrophicans
    acrodermatitis chronica a.
atrophicus
    lichen sclerosus et a.
atrophy
    Behr optic a.
    brain a.
    central a.
    congenital microvillus a.
    cortical a.
    corticosteroid-induced a.
    cutaneous a.
    Dejerine-Sottas a.
    dentatorubral a.
    disuse muscular a.
    familial muscular a.
    Fazio-Londe a.
    focal a.
    frontotemporal cortical a.
    gastric a.
    generalized gray matter a.
    generalized white matter a.
    gyral a.
    gyrate a.
    hereditary dentatorubral-
      pallidoluysian a.
    hereditary optic neuron a.
    hereditary spinal muscular a.
    infantile spinal muscular a.
    intestinal villous a.
    juvenile spinal muscular a.
    Leber hereditary a.

    leg a.
    Leydig cell a.
    limb a.
    macular a.
    microvillus a. (MVA)
    muscle a.
    muscular a.
    neurogenic a.
    olivopontocerebellar a. (OPCA)
    optic nerve a.
    Parrot a.
    partial villus a.
    perifascicular a.
    peroneal muscular a.
    primary macular a.
    secondary macular a.
    spinal muscle a.
    spinal muscular a. (SMA)
    Sudeck a.
    syndrome of cerebral a.
    testicular a.
    total villous a.
    tubular a.
    villous a.
atropine
    a. cromolyn
    diphenoxylate and a.
    a. sulfate
Atropine-Care Ophthalmic
Atropisol Ophthalmic
Atrovent
    A. Aerosol Inhalation
    A. Inhalation Solution
    A. Nasal Spray
A/T/S Topical
attaching process
attachment
    abnormal aortic valve a.
    dismissing a.
    a. disorder
    disturbance of a.
    gubernacular a.
    maternal-infant a.
    nonautonomous a.
    a. parenting
    prosthetic a.
    secure a.
    testicular a.
attack
    absence a.
    cataplectic a.
    drop a.
    grand mal a.
    lightning a.
    migrainous a.
    narcoleptic a.
    panic a.
    paroxysmal hypercyanotic a.

petit mal a.
shuddering a.
sleep a.
Stokes-Adams a.
attapulgite
attempted suicide
attending skill
attention
a. deficit
a. deficit disorder (ADD)
A. Deficit Disorders Evaluation
Scale
a. deficit hyperactivity disorder
(ADHD)
joint a.
a. span
Test of Variables of A. (TOVA)
attentional difficulty
attention-distractibility problem
attenuated
a. androgen
live a.
a. pyloric canal
attenuation
attrition
acute-phase a.
a. rate scale
attunement
affect a.
ATV
all-terrain vehicle
atypia
nuclear a.
atypica
Veillonella a.
atypical
a. absence seizure
a. depression
a. hemolytic uremia syndrome
a. interest
a. Kawasaki disease
a. measles
a. melanocytic nevus
a. mycobacteria
a. petit mal seizure
a. teratoid/rhabdoid tumor
a. teratoid tumor
a. teratoma
a.u., AU
aures unitas (both ears)
auris uterque (each ear)
audible stridor

audiogram
audiological testing
audiologist
audiology
audiometer
Pilot a.
audiometric
a. evaluation
a. examination
a. testing
audiometry
behavioral a.
behavioral observation a. (BOA)
brainstem evoked response a.
(BSERA)
evoked response a. (ERA)
impedance a.
visual reinforcement a. (VRA)
visual response a. (VRA)
AudioScope
Welch Allyn A.
AUDIT
Alcohol Use Disorders Inventory Test
auditory
a. agnosia
a. brainstem response (ABR,
ABSR)
a. canal
a. discrimination
a. dysfunction
a. evoked potential (AEP)
a. evoked response (AER)
a. impairment
integrated visual and a. (IVA)
a. integration thinking (AIT)
a. integration training (AIT)
a. learner
a. meatus
a. nerve
a. ossicles
a. response to bell
a. response cradle
a. training
audouinii
Microsporum a.
Auerbach plexus
Aufricht nasal retractor
augmentation
bladder a.
colocecal bladder a.
intestinal bladder a.
a. ureterocystoplasty

NOTES

augmentative
- a. and alternative communication (AAC)
- a. communication device

augmented
- a. voltage unipolar left arm lead (aVL)
- a. voltage unipolar left foot lead (aVF)
- a. voltage unipolar right arm lead (aVR)

Augmentin
- A. ES

aura
- epileptic a.
- migraine with a.
- migraine without a.
- somatosensory a.
- viscerosensory a.
- visual a.

aural
- a. atresia
- a. microtia
- a. polyp
- a. temperature

Auralgan
auramine
auramine-rhodamine stain
auranofin
aures unitas (both ears) (a.u., AU)
aureus
- borderline-resistant *Staphylococcus a.* (BRSA)
- methicillin-resistant *Staphylococcus a.* (MRSA)
- *Staphylococcus a.*
- *Streptococcus a.*
- vancomycin intermediate resistant *Staphylococcus a.*

auricle
- accessory a.

auricular
- a. abscess
- a. hematoma
- a. seroma

auris
- a. dextra (right ear) (a.d., AD)
- a. sinistra (left ear) (a.s., AS)
- a. uterque (each ear) (a.u., AU)

Auro Ear Drops
Aurolate
aurothioglucose
Auroto
auscultation
Auspitz sign
Austin Flint murmur
Australia antigen

australis
- *Rickettsia a.*

autism
- a. diagnostic interview (ADI)
- A. Diagnostic Interview-Revised (ADI-R)
- A. Diagnostic Observation Schedule (ADOS)
- early infantile a.
- high-functioning a. (HFA)
- infantile a.
- a. spectrum disorder (ASD)
- a. spectrum screening questionnaire (ASSQ)

autistic
- a. behavior
- a. spectrum disorder
- a. syndrome

autistic-like behavior
autoamputate
autoamputation
- a. of ovary

autoantibody
- anti-Scl-70 a.

autoaugmentation
- laparoscopic laser-assisted a.

autobiographical memory
autoclave
autocrine-acting growth factor
autocrine/paracrine-acting growth factor
autoeczematization
autofluorescent
autograft
- free tracheal a.

autohemolysis
autoimmune
- a. disease
- a. enteropathy (AIE)
- a. glomerulonephritis
- a. hemolytic anemia (AIHA)
- a. hepatitis
- a. interstitial nephritis
- a. lymphoproliferative syndrome (ALPS)
- a. myasthenia gravis
- a. neutropenia (AIN)
- a. neutropenia of infancy (ANI)
- a. polyendocrine syndrome
- a. thyroiditis

autoinfarction
Auto-Injector
- LidoPen I.M. Injection A.-I.

autoinjector
autoinoculation
autologous
- a. BMT
- a. bone marrow transplantation

a. cord blood
a. stem cell transplantation
automated
a. auditory brainstem response (AABR, A-ABR)
a. auditory brainstem response hearing screening
a. hematocrit
a. radiometric technique
a. reagin test (ART)
automatic
a. atrial tachycardia
a. movement reaction
a. reflex
automatism
motor a.
autonomic
a. crisis
a. dysregulation
a. nerve tumor
a. nervous system (ANS)
a. nervous system dysfunction (ANSD)
a. neuropathy
a. seizure
a. walking reflex
autonomy
auto-PEEP
auto-positive end-expiratory pressure
autoprothrombin I
autoradiograph
autoradiography
autoreaction
Autoread centrifuge hematology system
autoregulation
autosomal
a. congenital tubular dysgenesis
a. dominant (AD)
a. dominant disorder
a. dominant inheritance
a. dominant medullary cystic kidney disease (ADMCKD)
a. dominant polycystic disease
a. dominant polycystic kidney disease (ADPKD)
a. gene
a. heredity
a. recessive (AR)
a. recessive disorder
a. recessive mutation
a. recessive ocular Ehlers-Danlos syndrome

a. recessive polycystic kidney disease (ARPKD)
a. recessive renal proximal tubulopathy and hypercalciuria (ARPTH)
autosome
autosplenectomized
autosplenectomy
Auto Syringe
auxiliary orthotopic liver transplantation
auxometry
auxotyping
AV
assisted ventilation
atrioventricular
AV nodal reentry tachycardia
AV node dysfunction
avascularity
periungual a.
avascular necrosis (AVN)
Aveeno Cleansing Bar
Aventyl Hydrochloride
average
a. for gestational age (AGA)
pure-tone a. (PTA)
aversive
aVF
augmented voltage unipolar left foot lead
AVFM
arteriovenous fistula malformation
Avita
avium
Mycobacterium a.
avium-intracellulare
Mycobacterium a.-i. (MAI)
aVL
augmented voltage unipolar left arm lead
Avlosulfon
AVM
arteriovenous malformation
AVN
avascular necrosis
AVNRT
atrioventricular nodal reentrant tachycardia
avoidance
phobic a.
school a.
avoidant disorder
Avonex

NOTES

AVP
    arginine vasopressin
        Aqueous AVP
AVPU
    alertness, response to voice, response to
      pain, unresponsive
aVR
    augmented voltage unipolar right arm
      lead
AVRT
    atrioventricular reciprocating tachycardia
avulse
avulsion
        dental a.
        a. fracture
awake and active state
awareness
        inadequate body a.
AWHONN
    Association of Women's Health,
      Obstetrics, and Neonatal Nursing
Axenfeld anomaly
axes (*pl. of* axis)
axetil
        cefuroxime a. (CAE)
axial
        a. acetabular index (AAI)
        a. hypertonia
        a. load
        a. traction
Axid AR Acid Reducer
axilla
axillary
        a. freckling
        a. hair
        a. temperature
        a. vein
axis, pl. **axes**
        celiac a.
        a. deviation
        hypothalamic-pituitary a. (HPA)
        hypothalamic-pituitary-adrenal a.
          (HPA)

        hypothalamic-pituitary-ovarian a.
        long a.
        neural a.
        P-wave a.
        QRS a.
        short a.
        thigh-foot a.
        transmalleolar a.
        T-wave a.
axonal
        a. degeneration
        a. injury
        a. retraction ball
        a. type
axonotmesis
axon reflex
Aygestin
Ayr
        A. Nasal
        A. saline drops
        A. saline nasal mist
Azactam
5-azacytidine
azar
        kala a.
azatadine
azathioprine
azelastine
azidothymidine (AZT)
azithromycin
Azmacort Oral Inhaler
azole
        antifungal a.'s
        a. therapy
Azo-Standard
azotemia
        prerenal a.
azotemic osteodystrophy
AZT
    azidothymidine
aztreonam
Azulfidine EN-tabs
azygous

B

B antigen
B cell
B chromosome
B lymphocyte
B symptoms

B-100

familial defective apolipoprotein B-100

B19

Coxsackie B19
HPV B19
human parvovirus B19
B19-induced red cell aplasia
parvovirus B19

B₆

B_6 deficiency
vitamin B_6

B₁₂

vitamin B_{12}

BA

bacillary angiomatosis
biliary atresia

babbling
Babee Teething
Babesia

B. divergens
B. microti
B. WA1 type

babesiosis
Babinski

B. reflex
B. response
B. sign

Babinski-Fröhlich syndrome
baby

B. Air mesh netting
b. bottle syndrome
bronze b.
B. CareLink system
Clinical Risk Index for B.'s (CRIB)
collodion b.
B. Doe Regulations
drug b.
febrile b.
gray b.
jittery b.
B. Sense monitor
sling b.
b. teeth
well-hydrated b.

BABYbird respirator
BabyFace

Babylog

B. 8000 oscillator
B. 8000 respirator

baby's day diary
Babytherm IC
Bacid
Baciguent Topical
Baci-IM Injection
bacillary

b. angiomatosis (BA)
b. dysentery
enteric gram-negative b. (EGNB)
b. meningitis
b. peliosis
b. peliosis hepatis

bacille

b. Calmette-Guérin (BCG)
b. Calmette-Guérin vaccination
b. Calmette-Guérin vaccine

bacilli (*pl. of* bacillus)
bacilliformis

Bartonella b.

Bacillus

B. cereus
B. megaterium
B. subtilis

bacillus, pl. **bacilli**

acid-fast b.
b. Calmette-Guérin
gram-negative b.

bacitracin

neomycin, polymyxin B, b.
b. and polymyxin B

back

flat b.

back-knee deformity
backpack

AirPacks b.
AirTEC model b.

backscatter

dipyridamole stress integrated b.

back-selected T cell
backward chaining
backwardness

general reading b. (GRB)

backwash ileitis
baclofen
Bactec blood-culturing system
bacteremia

afebrile b.
catheter-associated b.
clostridial b.
coagulase-negative b.
CoNS b.

bacteremia *(continued)*
    occult b.
    streptococcal b.
**bacteremia-associated pneumococcal
  pneumonia (BAPP)**
bacteremic shock
bacteria, sing. **bacterium**
    coliform b.
    intracerebral seeding of b.
    pyogenic b.
    Salmonella b.
    Shigella b.
    Streptococcus b.
bacterial
    b. cervical adenitis
    b. conjunctivitis
    b. endocarditis
    b. enteritis
    b. inhibition assay method of
      Guthrie
    b. keratitis
    b. labyrinthitis
    b. laryngotracheobronchitis
    b. meningitis
    b. meningoencephalitis
    b. overgrowth syndrome
    b. parotitis
    b. pericarditis
    b. peritonitis
    b. plaque
    b. pneumonia
    b. rhinosinusitis
    b. sepsis
    b. sinusitis
    b. soilage
    b. tracheitis
    b. vaginosis
bactericidal, bacteriocidal
    b. drug
**bactericidal/permeability-increasing
  protein (BPI)**
bacteriologic
bacteriostatic drug
bacterium (*sing. of* bacteria)
bacteriuria
    rapid filter testing for b.
bacteroide
Bacteroides fragilis
bacteroidosis
Bacticort Otic
Bactine
Bactocill
BactoShield
Bactrim DS
Bactroban cream
BAEP
    brainstem auditory evoked potential

BAER
    brainstem auditory evoked response
      BAER test
bag
    anesthesia b.
    B. balm
    Douglas b.
    manual ventilation b. (MVB)
    b. and mask
    Rusch b.
    b., valve, mask (BVM)
    b. of worms
    b. of worms appearance
    zinc-free plastic b.
bag-and-mask resuscitation
bagged urinalysis
bagging
bag-valve-mask
    b.-v.-m. device
    b.-v.-m. ventilation
Baker cyst
BAL
    British antilewisite
    bronchoalveolar lavage
      BAL fluid
      BAL in Oil
Balamuthia
    B. mandrillaris
    B. meningoencephalitis
balance
    macronutrient b.
    negative b.
    b. reaction
balancing
    soft tissue b.
balanitis
    circinate b.
balanoposthitis
Balantidium coli
baldness
    frontal b.
ball
    axonal retraction b.
    fungal b.
    fungus b.
    renal fungus b.
    Stycar graded b.'s
    TheraGym exercise b.
Ballantyne-Runge syndrome
Ballard
    B. Assessment Score (BAS)
    B. score
Baller-Gerold syndrome
ballismus
balloon
    b. atrial septostomy (BAS)
    gastric b.
    pediatric b.

B

b. pulmonary valvuloplasty
Rigiflex b.
b. septostomy
b. septostomy catheter
b. tamponade
transurethral self-detachable b.
b. valvotomy
ballooning
balloon-tipped catheter
ballottement
abdominal b.
ball-valve effect
balm
Bag b.
lemon b.
Balmex cream
Balo disease
balsa vaginal form
BALT
bronchus-associated lymphoid tissue
Balthazar Scales of Adaptive Behavior
Baltic myoclonus
bamboo
b. hair
b. spine
bambooing of digit
BAMO
behavioral, anxiety, mood, and other
types of disorders
BAMO scale
banana
b.'s, rice, applesauce, tea, toast
(BRATT)
b.'s, rice cereal, applesauce, tea,
toast diet
b.'s, rice cereal, applesauce, toast
(BRAT)
b.'s, rice cereal, applesauce, toast
diet
b. sign
Bancap HC
band
adhesive b.
amniotic constriction b.
annular b.
b. cell
congenital intestinal b.
congenital peritoneal b.
dense b.
b. form neutrophil
b. heterotopia
iliotibial b.

b. keratopathy
Ladd b.
lucent b.
pelvic b.
vitreous b.
Z b.
bandage
Tubigrip b.
Velpeau b.
Webril b.
bandaging
elastic b.
bandemia
banding
amniotic b.
arterial b.
proximal pulmonary artery b.
pulmonary arterial b.
pulmonary artery b.
banging
head b.
Bankart lesion
banked milk
banking
cord blood b.
Bannayan syndrome
Bannwarth syndrome
Banophen Oral
Banti syndrome
BAPP
bacteremia-associated pneumococcal
pneumonia
bar
Aveeno Cleansing B.
bilateral b.'s
calcaneonavicular b.
Denis Browne b.
Fostex B.
PanOxyl B.
pectus b.
stabilizing b.
syndet cleaning b.
talocalcaneal b.
unilateral b.
barbae
sycosis b.
Barbidonna
Barbita
barbiturate intoxication
Barc shampoo
Bardet-Biedl syndrome
Bard PDA Umbrella

NOTES

bare lymphocyte syndrome
bargaining stage
Baridium
barium
> b. contrast
> b. enema
> b. esophagogram
> b. esophagography
> b. esophagram
> b. swallow

barking cough
barky cough
barley
> b. allergy
> b. malt

Barlow
> B. disease
> B. maneuver
> B. and Ortolani test
> B. sign
> B. syndrome
> B. technique

Barnes Akathisia Scale (BAS)
Barophen
baroreceptor
baroreflex
barotitis
> acute b.

barotrauma
barovolutrauma
barrel
> b. chest
> b. chest deformity

barrel-shaped upper central incisor
Barré sign
barrier
> blood-brain b. (BBB)
> b. contraceptive
> b. method

Bartholin
> B. gland
> B. gland abscess
> B. gland cyst

Barth syndrome
Bartonella
> B. bacilliformis
> B. henselae
> B. henselae infection
> B. quintana

Bart syndrome
Bartter syndrome
BAS
> Ballard Assessment Score
> balloon atrial septostomy
> Barnes Akathisia Scale

basal
> b. arterial occlusion
> b. body temperature (BBT)

> b. cell carcinoma
> b. cell epithelioma
> b. cell nevus syndrome
> b. cistern
> b. ganglia calcification
> b. ganglia disorder
> b. ganglia necrosis
> b. ganglion
> b. lamina
> b. membrane (BM)
> b. metabolic rate (BMR)
> b. perivillous fibrin
> b. pleural abrasion
> b. skull fracture

basalis
> decidua b.

Basaljel
BASC
> Behavioral Assessment Scale for Children
> BASC monitor

base
> broad nasal b.
> hydrocortisone b.
> methylprednisolone b.
> thickened b.

baseball finger
baseline
> b. visual acuity
> zero-voltage b.

basement membrane
basic
> b. fibroblast growth factor (bFGF)
> b. life support (BLS)
> b. skill

basicranium
basilar
> b. artery migraine
> b. consolidation
> b. impression
> b. invagination
> b. meningitis
> b. pleural abrasion

basis
> b. pontis
> B. soap

basket cell
basolateral membrane transport system
basophil
> b. cell

basophilic
> b. leukemia
> b. stippling

Bassen-Kornzweig
> B.-K. disease
> B.-K. syndrome

bassinet

bath
- hexachlorophene b.
- pHisoHex b.
- b. seat
- sitz b.

Battelle Developmental Inventory (BDI)

Batten-Bielschowsky
- B.-B. type
- B.-B. type of late infantile and juvenile amaurotic idiocy

Batten disease

Batten-Mayou disease

battery
- MacArthur Story Stem B. (MSSB)
- Vulpe Assessment B.
- Woodcock-Johnson Psychoeducational B.

battle
- b. neurosis
- B. sign

bat wing appearance

Baxa oral dispenser

Bayer
- B. Aspirin
- B. DCA2000 analyzer

Bayley
- B. cognitive outcome
- B. Developmental Scale
- B. mental developmental index
- B. Mental Scale
- B. Motor Score
- B. and Pinneau height-predicting method
- B. Psychomotor Developmental Index
- B. Scales of Infant Development (BSID)
- B. Scales of Infant Development-II (BSID-II)
- B. Scales of Infant Development-Motor, 2nd edition

Baylisascaris procyonis

bayonet forceps

Bazett formula

Bazex syndrome

Bazin
- erythema induration of B. (EIB)

BBB
- blood-brain barrier
- BBB syndrome

BBT
- basal body temperature

BC Cold Powder Non-Drowsy Formula

B-cell
- B-c. dysfunction
- B-c. lineage
- B-c. lymphoma

BCFA
- branched-chain fatty acid

BCG
- bacille Calmette-Guérin
- BCG vaccine

BCI
- blunt cardiac injury

bcl-2 protein

BCNU
- bis-chloroethylnitrosourea

bcr
- breakpoint cluster region

B-D
- Breslow-Day

BDD
- body dysmorphic disorder

B_6-dependent convulsion

BDI
- Battelle Developmental Inventory
- Beck Depression Inventory

bDNA
- branched deoxyribonucleic acid

BDNF
- brain-derived neurotrophic factor

BD test

bead
- Prader b.

beak
- medial metaphyseal b.

beaked nose

Beall valve

BEAM
- brain electrical activity mapping

bean
- cassava b.
- fava b.
- b. gum

bear
- InterMed B.
- b. tracks
- b. walk

beard ringworm

beat
- dropped b.
- left ventricular paced b.

NOTES

B

beat-to-beat
    b.-t.-b. continuous blood pressure monitoring
    b.-t.-b. variability
Beau line
beaveri
    Brugia b.
Bebelac
    B. FL formula
    B. #1 formula
Beck
    B. Depression Inventory (BDI)
    B. triad
Becker
    B. disease
    B. dystrophy
    B. melanosis
    B. muscular dystrophy (BMD)
    B. nevus
Beckwith syndrome
Beckwith-Wiedemann syndrome (BWS)
beclomethasone
    aqueous b.
    b. dipropionate
    b. propionate
Beclovent Oral Inhaler
Beconase
    B. AQ
    B. AQ Nasal Inhaler
bed
    hypoplastic pulmonary vascular b.
    Ohio b.
    Ultra Dream Ride car b.
    vascular b.
Bednar aphtha
bedwetting
Beepen-VK
bee sting challenge
BEF
    Byrne and Euler formula
behavior
    adaptive b.
    aggressive b.
    antisocial b.
    Assessment of Preterm Infants B. (APIB)
    B. Assessment System for Children monitor
    autistic b.
    autistic-like b.
    Balthazar Scales of Adaptive B.
    catatonic b.
    cognitive b.
    b. contract
    disorganized b.
    dysregulated b.
    externalizing b.
    b. family therapy

    fire-setting b.
    functional b.
    hypersexual b.
    b. modification
    obsessive-compulsive b. (OCB)
    b. pattern
    B. Rating Scale (BRS)
    risk b.
    risk-taking b.
    self-comforting b.
    self-injurious b. (SIB)
    self-mutilating b.
    stereotypic b.
    withdrawn b.
behavioral
    b., anxiety, mood, and other types of disorders (BAMO)
    b. assessment
    B. Assessment Scale for Children (BASC)
    b. audiometry
    b. disturbance
    B. and Emotional Rating Scale (BERS)
    b. family systems therapy (BFST)
    b. inhibition
    b. observation audiometry (BOA)
    b. state
    b. stress
    b. therapy
Behçet
    B. disease
    B. syndrome
Behr
    B. disease
    B. optic atrophy
beigelii
    Trichosporon b.
bejel
belching
Belix Oral
bell
    auditory response to b.
    B. palsy
    b. stethoscope
bell-clapper deformity
belli
    Isospora b.
belly
    b. crawl
    prune b.
belt mark
Bena-D Injection
Benadryl
    B. Injection
    B. Oral
    B. Topical
Ben-Allergin-50 Injection

Ben-Aqua
Bence Jones protein
bend
    deep-knee b.
    b. deformity
    b. fracture
Bender Visual Motor Gestalt Test
beneficence
Benemid
benign
    b. childhood epilepsy
    b. congenital hypotonia
    b. external hydrocephalus
    b. familial neonatal convulsion
      (BFNC)
    b. familial neonatal seizure
    b. familial recurrent cholestasis
    b. fructosuria
    b. hepatic adenoma
    b. hyperphenylalaninemia
    b. idiopathic neonatal convulsion
    b. infantile familial convulsion
      (BIFC)
    b. infantile hypotonia
    b. intracranial hypertension
    b. jaundice
    b. juvenile melanoma
    b. lymphoid hyperplasia
    b. maturation delay
    b. migratory glossitis
    b. myoclonic epilepsy
    b. myoclonus of infancy
    b. nasopharyngeal fibroma
    b. neonatal convulsion
    b. neutropenia
    b. nonprogressive familial chorea
    b. papillomatosis
    b. paroxysmal torticollis
    b. paroxysmal torticollis of infancy
    b. paroxysmal vertigo (BPV)
    b. partial epilepsy
    b. partial epilepsy with
      centrotemporal spike (BPEC)
    b. pineal cyst
    b. recurrent hematuria
    b. rolandic epilepsy (BRE)
    b. teratoma
    b. transient gynecomastia
    b. vascular neoplasm
    b. venous hum
Benisone
Bennett PR-2 ventilator

Benoxyl
bent finger
Benton Visual Retention Test
Bentyl
    B. Hydrochloride Injection
    B. Hydrochloride Oral
Benylin
    B. Cough Syrup
    B. DM
    B. Expectorant
    B. Pediatric
Benzac
    B. AC Gel
    B. AC Wash
    B. W Gel
    B. W Wash
5-Benzagel
Benzamycin
benzathine
    b. penicillin
    penicillin G b.
    b. penicillin G (BPG)
benzene
benzimidazole
benzoate
    benzyl b.
    sodium phenylacetate and
      sodium b.
benzocaine
    antipyrine and b.
    b. lozenge
Benzocol
Benzodent
benzodiazepine
benzoin applicator
benzoyl peroxide
benztropine mesylate
benzyl
    b. alcohol
    b. benzoate
benzylpenicilloyl-polylysine
bepridil
beractant
Berardinelli-Seip syndrome
Berens 3-character test
Berger disease
bergeriae
    Gemella b.
Bergmeister papilla
beriberi
    infantile b.

NOTES

Berlin
  B. edema
  B. score
Bernard-Soulier syndrome
Berne criteria
berry aneurysm
BERS
  Behavioral and Emotional Rating Scale
Berubigen
best
  B. disease
  b. practice
beta
  b. blocker
  b. cell adenoma
  b. cell adenomatosis
  b. lactamase
  b. lactamase stable drug
  b. thalassemia
  transforming growth factor b.
  (TGF-B)
beta-adrenergic
  b.-a. agonist
  b.-a. blockade
  b.-a. drug
  b.-a. receptor
beta-2 agonist
beta-aminoisobutyric aciduria
beta-chemokine receptor
Betachron E-R
Betadine First Aid Antibiotics +
  Moisturizer
17-beta-estradiol
beta-galactosidase
Betagan Liquifilm Ophthalmic
beta-hCG
  beta-human chorionic gonadotropin
beta-hemolytic streptococcal coinfection
11-beta-HSD2 deficiency
beta-human chorionic gonadotropin
  (beta-hCG)
11-beta-hydroxysteroid dehydrogenase
  type 2 deficiency
betaine
  b. anhydrous
  b. hydrochloride
Betalene Topical
Betalin S
betamethasone dipropionate
betamimetic agent
Betapen-VK
Betasept
Betaseron
beta-spectrin
betasympathomimetic
beta-thalassemia
  Hb E b-t.
  sickle b-t.
Betatrex Topical

Beta-Val Topical
bethanechol
Bethesda
  B. assay
  B. classification system
  B. unit
Betke stain
Betz cell
bexarotene
bezoar
Bezold abscess
Bezold-Jarisch reflex
bFGF
  basic fibroblast growth factor
BFNC
  benign familial neonatal convulsion
BFST
  behavioral family systems therapy
BFU-E
  burst-forming units-erythroid
BH$_4$
  tetrahydrobiopterin cofactor
  BH$_4$ loading test
BHS
  Bogalusa Heart Study
BIA
  bioelectrical impedance analysis
bias
biatriatum
  cor triloculare b.
Biaxin
bibasilar
bicarbonate (HCO$_3$)
  b. concentration
  b. infusion
  plasma b. (PHCO$_3$)
  sodium b. (NaHCO$_3$)
  b. wasting
bicarbonaturia
biceps
  b. femoris muscle
  b. reflex
Bicillin
  B. C-R
  B. L-A
bicipital tuberosity
Bicitra
BiCNU
biconcave vertebra
bicornuate uterus
bicuculline-induced seizure
bicuspid
  b. aortic valve
  first b.
  second b.
bicycle ergometer
bicycling movement
b.i.d.
  bis in die (twice a day)

B

bidirectional
  b. Glenn procedure
  b. Glenn shunt
  b. shunting
Bielschowsky-Jansky disease
Bielschowsky syndrome
Biemond syndrome
bieneusi
  Enterocytozoon b.
Bieri scale
bifascicular block
BIFC
  benign infantile familial convulsion
bifid
  b. cervix
  b. clitoris
  b. earlobe
  b. P wave
  b. scrotum
  b. spinal cord
  b. uterus
  b. uvula
bifida
  spina b.
Bifidobacterium
  B. adeloscentis
  B. bifidum
  B. breve
  B. catenulatum
  B. infantis
  B. longum
bifidum
  Bifidobacterium b.
  cranium b.
bifidus
  Lactobacillus b.
bifurcate
bifurcation
bigeminy
Biglieri syndrome
biguanide
  polyhexamethyl b. (PHMB)
bilabial
  b. closure
  b. speech sound
bilateral
  b. acoustic neuromas
  b. atresia
  b. atresia of external auditory
    meatus
  b. bars
  b. cephalhematomas

  b. choreoathetosis
  b. congenital ptosis
  b. conjunctivitis
  b. corticobulbar disruption
  b. cryptorchidism
  b. ductus
  b. flank masses
  b. gonadal failure
  b. hearing impairment
  b. increased femoral anteversion
  b. lung hypoplasia
  b. myringotomy tubes
  b. optic neuritis
  b. otitis media with effusion
    (BOME)
  b. PC-IOL implantation
  b. periventricular nodular
    heterotopia
  b. pyramidal tract signs
  b. retinoblastomas
  b. schizencephalic cleft
  b. slowing
  b. spasticity
  b. subcostal incisions
  b. ureteral diversion
bile
  b. acid
  b. acid flux
  b. acid malabsorption
  b. acid sequestration
  b. acid synthesis
  b. chenodeoxycholic acid level
  b. duct
  b. duct catheter
  b. duct paucity
  b. duct resection
  b. duct stenosis
  b. ductule
  inspissated b.
  b. peritonitis
  b. pigment
  b. salt
  b. salt-stimulated lipase (BSSL)
  b. stasis
  supersaturation of b.
bile-stained emesis
bilevel positive airway pressure (BiPAP)
biliary
  b. abscess
  b. ascites
  b. atresia (BA)
  b. cirrhosis

NOTES

biliary *(continued)*
    b. colic
    b. hypoplasia
    b. lithiasis
    b. microhamartoma
    b. microlithiasis
    b. perforation
Bilibed
Biliblanket Phototherapy System
BiliBottoms
BiliCheck bilirubin analyzer
bililights
Bili mask
bilineal category
bilingual
bilious
    b. emesis
    b. vomiting
    b. vomitus
bilirubin
    conjugated b.
    cord blood b.
    direct b.
    direct-reacting b.
    elevated conjugated b.
    b. encephalopathy
    hour-specific total serum b.
    b. infarct
    b. lights
    serum b.
    total b.
    total serum b. (TSB)
    transcutaneous b. (TcB)
    unconjugated b.
bilirubin-albumin binding
bilirubin-induced
    b.-i. neurologic dysfunction (BIND)
    b.-i. neurologic dysfunction score
bilirubinometer
    BiliTest transcutaneous b.
BiliTest transcutaneous bilirubinometer
biloba
    ginkgo b.
biloculare
    cor b.
biloma
Biltricide
bimelic amyoplasia
bimodal pattern
binasal prongs
BIND
    bilirubin-induced neurologic dysfunction
    BIND score
binding
    androgen b.
    bilirubin-albumin b.
    C1q b.

    protein b.
    b. protein
    b. protein-2 insulinlike growth factor
    b. protein-3 insulinlike growth factor
binge
    b. eating
    b. eating syndrome
binocular
    b. function
    b. vision
binomial
bioactivity
biobehavioral shift
Biocef
biochemical
biochemistry
bioelectrical
    b. impedance
    b. impedance analysis (BIA)
biofeedback
biofilm
bioimpedance analysis
Biojector
biologically plastic femora
biological risk
biologic satiation curve
biology
biomedical factor
BioMerieux Vitek system
biomicroscopy
    slit-lamp b.
Biomox
biophysical profile (BPP)
biopsy
    bone marrow b.
    chorionic villus b.
    ciliary b.
    core needle b.
    endomyocardial b.
    fine-needle aspiration b. (FNAB)
    frozen b.
    jejunal b.
    mucosal b.
    muscle b.
    open b.
    open lung b. (OLB)
    percutaneous renal b.
    pleural b.
    quadriceps femoris muscle b.
    small bowel b.
    sural nerve b.
    synovial b.
biopsychosocial syndrome
biopterin
Bioself fertility indicator

Biostar
    B. Flu OIA
    B. Flu optical immunoassay
biosynthesis
    inborn error of bile acid b.
Bio-Tab
biotin
    b. factor
    B. Forte
    B. Forte Extra Strength
biotinidase deficiency
Bio-Tn
biotyping
BiPAP
    bilevel positive airway pressure
    BiPAP machine
biparietal
    b. bulge
    b. diameter (BPD)
bipartite patella
bipedal
    b. lymphangiography
    b. posture
biphasic
    b. anaphylactic reaction
    b. anaphylaxis
    b. fever
    b. P wave
    b. response
    b. temperature pattern
biplane cineangiocardiography
bipolar
    b. depression
    b. disorder (type 1, 2) (BPD)
bipolarity
    prepubertal-onset b.
Bipp paste
Birbeck
    B. granule
    B. granule-positive cell
birch tree pollen
bird
    b. beak appearance
    B. respirator
bird-headed dwarf syndrome
birdlike facies
18-item Birleson Depression Inventory
birth
    b. asphyxia
    breech b.
    b. canal
    b. defect

    b. length
    multiple b.
    b. trauma
    b. trauma theory
    b. weight
    b. weight for gestational age (BWGA)
    b. weight Z score
    year of b. (YOB)
birthmark
BIS
    budesonide inhalation suspension
Bisac-Evac
bisacodyl
    b. suppository
    b. tablet
Bisacodyl Uniserts
bis-chloroethylnitrosourea (BCNU)
Bisco-Lax
bis in die (twice a day) (b.i.d.)
bisexual
    gay, lesbian, b. (GLB)
bisferiens
    pulsus b.
Bishop-Koop
    B.-K. ileostomy
    B.-K. procedure
bishydroxycoumarin
Bismatrol
bismuth
    b. subsalicylate
    b. toxicity
bisphosphonate
bis(piareloyloxymethyl) (bis-POM)
bis-POM
    bis(piareloyloxymethyl)
bite
    animal b.
    b. cell
    chigger b.
    closed b.
    open b.
    b. reflex
    stork b.
bitemporal
    b. aplasia cutis congenita
    b. hemianopia
bithionol
biting
    tongue b.
bitolterol
Bitot spot

NOTES

bivalved cast
bivariate
biventricular hypertrophy
Björnstad syndrome
BK
    papovavirus BK
BL
  Burkitt lymphoma
  BL pattern
black
    b. dot
    b. dot ringworm
    B. Draught
    b. hairy tongue
    b. measles
    b. pigmentation
    b. spot
    b. widow spider
Blackfan-Diamond
    B.-D. anemia
    B.-D. syndrome
blackhead
blackout
    weight-lifter b.
blackwater fever
bladder
    b. augmentation
    b. catheterization
    Christmas tree b.
    defunctionalized b.
    b. diverticulum
    b. exstrophy
    iatrogenic b.
    b. instrumentation
    kidneys, ureters, b. (KUB)
    low pressure b.
    neurogenic b.
    neuropathic b.
    nonneurogenic neurogenic b.
    occult neurogenic b.
    b. pressure
    psychologic nonneuropathic b.
    radiolucent circular shadow in b.
    b. sphincter paralysis
    b. stretching
    b. tap
    uninhibited b.
    urinary b.
    in utero drainage of fetal b.
    walnut-shaped b.
blade
    laryngoscope b.
    Miller b. (#0, #1)
Blalock-Hanlon
    B.-H. atrial septostomy procedure
    B.-H. operation
Blalock-Taussig
    B.-T. operation

B.-T. shunt
    B.-T. shunt procedure
blanch
Blanche
    B. sign
    B. sign of Steele
blanching
    cutaneous b.
    episodic b.
    b. macule
    b. pallor
    b. wheal and flare lesion
Bland-Garland-White syndrome
blanket
    cooling b.
    forced-air b.
    plastic b.
    space b.
    b. swinging
Blaschko line
blast
    b. crisis
    leukemic b.
blastema
    renal b.
Blastocystis hominis
blastoma
    pleuropulmonary b. (PPB)
Blastomyces dermatitidis
blastomycosis
    Brazilian b.
    Lutz-Splendore-Almeida b.
    South American b.
blastomycosis-like pyoderma
bleb
    pulmonary b.
    venous b.
bleed
    brain b.
    fetomaternal b.
    intraparenchymal b.
    intraventricular b.
    joint b.
bleed-back valve
bleeding
    abnormal vaginal b.
    b. diathesis
    dysfunctional uterine b. (DUB)
    GI b.
    gum b.
    mucosal b.
    severe gastrointestinal b. (SGIB)
    subependymal b.
    withdrawal b.
BlemErase Lotion
blennorrhagicum
    keratoderma b.
Blenoxane

B

bleomycin
Bleph-10
blepharitis
    seborrheic b.
    simple squamous b.
    staphylococcal b.
    ulcerative b.
blepharoconjunctivitis
blepharophimosis
blepharophimosis-ptosis syndrome
blepharoptosis
blepharospasm
blepharostenosis
BLES
    bovine lavage extract surfactant
blind
    legally b.
    b. loop syndrome
    b. trachea
    b. vagina
blinded challenge
blind-ending vagina
blindness
    congenital stationary night b.
    cortical b.
    night b.
    transient cortical b.
blinking
    paroxysmal b.
    rapid b.
blink reflex
blister
    arthropod-induced b.
    b. cell
    fever b.
    intraepidermal b.
    recurrent b.
    rosettelike b.
    subepidermal b.
    sucking b.
    suprabasal b.
    tense b.
blistering
    b. distal dactylitis
    b. sunburn
Blistik
Blizzard syndrome
BLL
    blood lead level
        capillary BLL
bloat
    gas b.

bloated abdomen
Blocadren Oral
Bloch-Sulzberger syndrome
block
    bifascicular b.
    congenital complete AV b.
    congenital complete heart b.
        (CCHB)
    Corsi b.
    b. design test
    dorsal penile nerve b. (DPNB)
    enzymatic b.
    field b.
    first-degree atrioventricular b.
    heart b.
    iatrogenic complete heart b.
    left bundle branch b.
    Mobitz I, II b.
    nerve b.
    radial nerve b.
    regional nerve b.
    right bundle branch b. (RBBB)
    second-degree heart b.
    sinoatrial b.
    spinal subarachnoid b.
    Super B.
    supraorbital nerve b.
    third-degree AV b.
    ulnar nerve b.
    b. vertebra
    Wenckebach heart b.
blockade
    beta-adrenergic b.
    neuromuscular b.
    serotonergic reuptake b.
    serotonin receptor b.
    splenic Fc b.
blockage
    shunt b.
blocked premature atrial complex
blocker
    beta b.
    calcium channel b.
    H_2 b.
    serotonin reuptake b.
Block-Sulzberger incontinentia pigmenti
blood
    b. agar
    b. ammonia level
    arterialized b.
    autologous cord b.
    cord b.

NOTES

blood *(continued)*
    b. count
    b. culture
    b. extravasation
    fetal cord b.
    b. gas
    b. gas analysis
    b. gas determination
    b. glycine
    b. group
    b. group incompatibility
    b. group isoimmunization
    b. lactate
    b. lead
    b. lead level (BLL)
    b. loss
    occult b.
    oxygenated b.
    peripheral b.
    b. PHE
    b. pressure (BP)
    b. pressure cuff size
    b. pressure gradient
    b. pressure measurement
    b. pressure monitor
    b. relationship
    b. relative
    b. sample
    b. sampling
    b. smear
    b. spot
    b. sugar
    swallowed maternal b.
    b. type
    b. type A, AB, B, O
    unoxygenated b.
    b. urea nitrogen (BUN)
    b. vessel
    b. vessel elasticity
    b. volume
blood-borne pathogen
blood-brain barrier (BBB)
blood-flecked gastric aspirate
bloodstream infection (BSI)
bloody
    b. CSF
    b. diarrhea
Bloom syndrome
blot
    enzyme-linked immunotransfer b.
      (EITB)
    Northern b.
    Western b.
Blount
    B. disease
    B. syndrome

blow-by
    b.-b. oxygen
    b.-b. through tubing
blowing decrescendo diastolic murmur
blowout
    b. fracture
    b. injury
    orbital b.
BLS
    basic life support
Bluboro
blue
    b. baby syndrome
    brilliant cresyl b.
    b. diaper syndrome
    b. dot sign
    b. histiocyte syndrome
    methylene b.
    b. papule
    Prussian b.
    b. rubber bleb nevus
    b. rubber bleb nevus syndrome
      (BRBNS)
    b. sclera
    b. scleral hue
    b. spell
blueberry
    b. muffin nodule
    b. muffin rash
    b. muffin skin lesion
    b. muffin syndrome
blue-cell sarcoma
blue-green algae
blues
bluish-black macule
bluish discoloration of flank
blunt
    b. cardiac injury (BCI)
    b. chest trauma
blurred vision
blurring of left psoas margin
blush
    ciliary b.
    erythematous b.
    terminal b.
    tumor b.
BM
    basal membrane
BMA
    bone marrow aspirate
BMC
    bone mineral content
BMD
    Becker muscular dystrophy
    bone mineral density
BMI
    body mass index

B

BMM
  bone mineral mass
BMR
  basal metabolic rate
BMT
  bone marrow transplant
  bone marrow transplantation
    allogenic BMT
    autologous BMT
BN
  bulimia nervosa
BNAS
  Brazelton Neonatal Assessment Scale
BNBAS
  Brazelton Neonatal Behavioral
    Assessment Scale
BOA
  behavioral observation audiometry
board
    arm b.
    communication b.
    prone b.
    recumbent infant b.
    scooter b.
    vestibular b.
Bobath
    B. response
    B. therapy
bobbing
    head b.
    ocular b.
bobble-head doll syndrome
Bochdalek
    congenital diaphragmatic hernia
      of B.
    B. hernia
Bockhart impetigo
body
    b. alignment
    apoptotic b.
    Aschoff b.
    b. composition
    concentric amyloid b.
    b. conscious
    Cowdry type A inclusion b.
    Creola b.
    cytoid b.
    b. dysmorphic disorder (BDD)
    extracranial foreign b.
    foreign b.
    b. habitus
    Heinz b.

    b. homeostasis
    Howell-Jolly b.
    hyaline b.
    b. image
    inclusion b.
    intracranial foreign b.
    intranuclear inclusion b.
    b. jacket
    ketone b.
    Lafora b.
    lamellar b. (LB)
    lamellar inclusion b.
    b. language
    lateral geniculate b.
    b. lead burden
    loose b.
    b. louse
    lyssa b.
    b. mass index (BMI)
    b. measurement
    Negri b.
    osmiophilic b.
    b. phenotype
    pineal b.
    b. ringworm
    b. rocking
    b. shell
    b. size
    striate b.
    b. surface area (BSA)
    b. temperature
    vertebral b.
    vitreous b.
    Weibel Palade b.
    zebra b.
bodybuilding
Bogalusa Heart Study (BHS)
boggy synovial effusion
Bohn nodule
Boix-Ochoa
    B.-O. procedure
    B.-O. score (BOS)
Bolivian hemorrhagic fever
bolster
bolt
    subarachnoid b.
bolus
    b. dose
    fecal b.
    fluid b.
    isotonic b.
    b. tube feeding

NOTES

Bombay erythrocyte phenotype
BOME
   bilateral otitis media with effusion
Bonamil with Iron formula
bonding
   maternal-infant b.
bone
   b. age determination
   b. ALP
   aseptic necrosis of b.
   b. avascular necrosis
   capitate b.
   cortical b.
   craniobasal b.
   cuneiform b.
   b. densitometry
   b. density measurement
   b. dysplasia
   ethmoid b.
   fiber b.
   flat frontal b.
   fragmentation of necrotic b.
   b. graft
   b. hemangioma
   high frontal b.
   hyoid b.
   lacrimal b.
   lamellar b.
   long b.
   b. marrow
   b. marrow aplasia
   b. marrow aspirate (BMA)
   b. marrow aspiration
   b. marrow biopsy
   b. marrow cytogenetics
   b. marrow dysfunction
   b. marrow puncture
   b. marrow relapse
   b. marrow stem cell
   b. marrow suppression
   b. marrow toxicity
   b. marrow transplant (BMT)
   b. marrow transplantation (BMT)
   b. matrix
   maxillary b.
   b. mineral content (BMC)
   b. mineral density (BMD)
   b. mineral mass (BMM)
   b. mineral measurement
   b. mineral metabolism
   b. mineral uptake
   nasal b.
   navicular b.
   omovertebral b.
   b. pain
   parietal b.
   b. quantitative ultrasound velocity
   b. remodeling
   b. resorption
   round iliac b.
   b. scan
   b. sclerosis
   short metacarpal b.
   small maxillary b.
   sphenoid b.
   b. strength measurement
   tubular b.
   turbinate b.
   wormian b.
   woven b.
   zygomatic b.
bone-age determination method
bone-specific alkaline phosphatase
Bonferroni
   B. correction
   B. correlation
Bonferroni-Dunn correction
Bonine
Bonnet-Dechaume-Blanc syndrome
Bonnevie-Ullrich syndrome
bony
   b. dysplasia
   b. erosion
   b. projection
   b. spur
book
   communication b.
Boom syndrome
BOOP
   bronchiolitis obliterans organizing
      pneumonia
booster
Boost nutritional supplement
boot-shaped heart
borborygmus, pl. **borborygmi**
border
   serpiginous b.
borderline
   Child Version of the Retrospective
      Diagnostic Interview for B.'s
   b. diabetes
   b. intelligence
   b. lepromatous leprosy
   b. lepromatous pattern
   b. personality disorder
   b. tuberculoid (BT)
   b. tuberculoid leprosy
   b. tuberculoid pattern
borderline-resistant *Staphylococcus*
   aureus **(BRSA)**
Bordetella
   B. bronchiseptica
   B. parapertussis
   B. pertussis
Bordet-Gengoi medium
boredom

Borna disease virus
Bornholm disease
boron
Boropak
Borrelia
    B. afzelii
    B. burgdorferi
    B. burgdorferi sensu lato
    B. burgdorferi sensu stricto
    B. garinii
    B. recurrentis
BOS
    Boix-Ochoa score
Bosma Henkin Christiansen syndrome
bossing
    frontal b.
    occipital b.
Boston
    B. exanthem
    B. Naming Test
    B. orthosis
Boston-type craniosynostosis
Botox
Botryoid
botryoides
    sarcoma b.
Botryomycosis
bottle
    disposable b.
    Mead Johnson b.
    Nursette prefilled disposable b.
    prefilled disposable b.
    b. propping
    b. tooth decay
botulinum
    b. antitoxin (type A, B, E)
    Clostridium b.
    b. immune globulin
    b. toxin
    b. toxin A (BTA)
botulinus
    b. intoxication
    b. neurotoxin
botulism
    Clostridium b.
    infantile b. (IB)
    b. toxin
    wound b.
bougie dilator
bougienage
boulardii
    Saccharomyces b.

bouncing
bounding pulse
Bount disease
Bourneville disease
Bourns infant ventilator
boutonneuse fever
boutonniere finger
bovine
    b. lavage extract surfactant (BLES)
    pegademase b.
    b. pericardium patch
    b. spongiform encephalopathy
    b. tuberculosis
bovis
    Mycobacterium b.
    Streptococcus b.
bow
    posteromedial b.
bowel
    b. adaptation
    aganglionic b.
    b. atony
    b. clean-out
    echogenic b.
    impacted b.
    b. infarction
    invaginated b.
    b. lengthening procedure
    b. loop resection
    malrotation of b.
    neurogenic b.
    b. obstruction
    proximal b.
    b. segment resection
    short small b. (SSB)
    b. sound
    b. stasis
Bowen Hutterite syndrome
bowenoid papulosis
bowing
    anterior tibial b.
    anterolateral tibial b.
    congenital posteromedial b.
    b. deformity
    b. fracture
    lateral tibial b.
    posteromedial tibial b.
    b. reflex
    tibial b.
    traumatic b.
bowleg
    physiological b.

B

NOTES

Bowman
    B. capsule
    B. layer
    B. space
bowstringing of tendon
box
    head b.
boxer's fracture
boydii
    Pseudallescheria b.
BP
    blood pressure
BPD
    biparietal diameter
    bipolar disorder (type 1, 2)
    bronchopulmonary dysplasia
BPEC
    benign partial epilepsy with
      centrotemporal spike
BPF
    bronchopulmonary fistula
BPG
    benzathine penicillin G
BPI
    bactericidal/permeability-increasing
      protein
BPP
    biophysical profile
BPS
    bronchopulmonary sequestration
BPV
    benign paroxysmal vertigo
bra
    lead b.
braakii
    Citrobacter b.
brace
    cast boot b.
    Charleston b.
    Counter Rotation System b. (CRS)
    Cruiser hip abduction b.
    Friedman Splint b.
    b. management
    Milwaukee b.
    Rhino Triangle b.
    Risser b.
    b. treatment
brachial
    b. arch
    b. artery
    b. plexopathy
    b. plexus
    b. plexus palsy
brachiocephalic vessel
brachioradialis reflex
brachioskeletal-genital syndrome
Brachmann-de Lange syndrome
brachycephalic configuration

brachycephaly
brachydactyly
brachymetacarpalism
brachytherapy
bradyarrhythmia
bradycardia
    apnea and b.
    feeding b.
    prolonged b.
    sinus b.
    vagotonic b.
bradycardia-tachycardia syndrome
bradykinin antagonist
brain
    b. atrophy
    b. bleed
    coning of b.
    b. damage
    b. death
    b. dysfunction
    b. edema
    b. electrical activity mapping
      (BEAM)
    b. function
    b. herniation
    b. imaging technique
    b. injury
    b. lesion
    b. mapping
    b. sparing
    b. swelling
    b. tumor
    b. wart
    water on b.
    b. wave
brain-derived neurotrophic factor
  (BDNF)
brainstem
    b. auditory evoked potential
      (BAEP)
    b. auditory evoked response
      (BAER, BSAER)
    b. auditory evoked response test
    b. auditory tract
    b. compression
    b. encephalitis
    b. evoked response (BSER)
    b. evoked response audiometry
      (BSERA)
    b. function
    b. glioma
    b. herniation
    b. lesion
branched
    b. chain ketoacid
    b. deoxyribonucleic acid (bDNA)
    b. DNA

branched-chain
  b.-c. amino acid
  b.-c. amino acidemia
  b.-c. aminotransferase
  b.-c. fatty acid (BCFA)
  b.-c. ketoaciduria
  b.-c. ketonuria
brancher deficiency
branchial
  b. arch
  b. arch syndrome
  b. cleft
  b. cleft anomaly
  b. cleft cyst
  b. cleft fistula
  b. cleft sinus
  b. cyst
  b. pouch
branching
  airway b.
  b. enzyme deficiency
  b. enzyme deficiency
    amylopectinosis
  b. morphogenesis
  b. pattern
branchiootorenal syndrome
Brandt syndrome
Branhamella catarrhalis
brash
  weaning b.
brasiliensis
  Nocardia b.
  Paracoccidioides b.
brassy cough
BRAT
  bananas, rice cereal, applesauce, toast
  BRAT diet
BRATT
  bananas, rice, applesauce, tea, toast
  BRATT diet
Bratton-Marshall test
Braun tympanic thermometer
brawny
  b. dermatitis
  b. edema
  b. scaling
Brazelton
  B. Neonatal Assessment Scale
    (BNAS)
  B. Neonatal Behavioral Assessment
    Scale (BNBAS)
Brazilian blastomycosis

braziliense
  Ancylostoma b.
braziliensis
  Leishmania b.
BRBNS
  blue rubber bleb nevus syndrome
BRE
  benign rolandic epilepsy
bread-and-butter appearance
breakpoint cluster region (bcr)
breakthrough varicella
breast
  b. abscess
  b. bud
  b. enlargement
  b. milk
  pigeon b.
  supernumerary b.
breastfed
breastfeed
breastfeeding
  failed b.
  b. jaundice
breast-milk jaundice
breaststroker's knee
breath
  fetid b.
  b. holding
  b. H$_2$ test
  b. hydrogen excretion test
  b. hydrogen study
  malodorous b.
  b. sound
  strep b.
  b. testing
  B. Tracker
  uriniferous b.
breathe
  B. Easy foam pad
  B. Free
breath-holding spell
breath-hold MR cholangiography
breathing
  abdominal b.
  intermittent positive-pressure b.
    (IPPB)
  mouth b.
  mouth-to-mask b.
  paradoxical b.
  b. pattern
  patterned b.
  periodic b.

B

NOTES

breathing *(continued)*
    rescue b.
    seesaw b.
    sleep-disordered b.
    spontaneous periodic b.
    stridulous b.
    tidal b.
    tubular b.
    upper airway sleep-disordered b.
    work of b.
breathing-related sleep disorder
breech
    b. birth
    b. deformation sequence
    b. delivery
    midfoot b.
    b. position
    b. presentation
Breezee
    B. Mist Aerosol
    B. Mist Antifungal
Brenner tumor
Breonesin
brequinar
Breslow-Day (B-D)
    B.-D. test
B₆-responsive anemia
Brethaire
Brethine
Brett
    B. epileptogenic encephalopathy
    B. syndrome
bretylium
Bretylol
breve
    Bifidobacterium b.
Brevibloc
brevis
    Demodex b.
Brevital Sodium
Bricanyl
bridge
    flat nasal b.
    low nasal b.
    nasal b.
    physeal b.
    B. Reading Program
bridging
    b. physis
    b. vein
brief
    b. reactive psychosis
    b., small, abundant motor-unit
      action potential (BSAP)
    b. tonic seizure
Brigance Diagnostic Inventory of Early Development
Briggs T-adapter

bright thalamus syndrome
Brill disease
brilliant cresyl blue
Brill-Zinsser disease
British antilewisite (BAL)
brittle
    b. diabetes
    b. hair
    b. nail
brittle-bone disease
broad
    b. débridement
    b. flat nose
    b. forehead
    b. nasal base
    b. nasal root
    b. physis
    b. P wave
    b. thumb
    b. toe
broad-band scale
broad-based gait
broad-spectrum
    b.-s. antibiotic
    b.-s. white light
Broca
    B. aphasia
    B. area
Brodie abscess
Bromaline Elixir
Bromanate Elixir
Bromarest
Bromatapp Relief 4 Hour Tablet
Brombay
Bromfed
bromhidrosis
    eccrine b.
    plantar eccrine b.
bromide
    diphenyl tetrazolium b.
    ipratropium b.
    pancuronium b.
    pyridostigmine b.
    vecuronium b.
bromium
bromocriptine
Bromphen Elixir
brompheniramine and phenylpropanolamine
bronchi (*pl. of* bronchus)
bronchial
    b. asthma
    b. atresia
    b. breath sound
    b. mucous cast
    b. provocation
    b. provocation challenge
    b. provocation testing

b. tree
b. tube
b. wall thickening
bronchiectasis
congenital b.
bronchiolar thickening
bronchiole
ruptured b.
terminal b.
bronchiolectasia
bronchiolitis
acute b.
b. obliterans
b. obliterans organizing pneumonia
(BOOP)
obliterative fibroproliferative b.
respiratory syncytial virus b.
(RSVB)
RSV b.
viral necrotizing b.
bronchiseptica
Bordetella b.
bronchitis
acute b.
asthmatic b.
chronic obstructive b.
follicular b.
obliterative b.
plastic b.
wheezy b.
bronchoalveolar
b. fluid
b. lavage (BAL)
bronchobiliary fistula
bronchoconstriction
bronchodilation
bronchodilator
b. drug
inhaled b.
oral b.
short-acting beta-2 agonist b.
bronchoesophageal fistula
bronchogenic cyst
bronchogram
bronchomalacia
bronchomotor tone
bronchophony
bronchopleural fistula
bronchopneumonia
bronchopulmonary
b. aspergillosis
b. dysplasia (BPD)

b. fistula (BPF)
b. lavage
b. malformation
b. sequestration (BPS)
bronchorrhea
bronchoscope
Storz infant b.
bronchoscopy
fiberoptic b.
flexible fiberoptic b.
open-tube b.
virtual b.
bronchospasm
exercise-induced b. (EIB)
bronchospastic cough
bronchovesicular breath sound
bronchus, pl. **bronchi**
main b.
bronchus-associated lymphoid tissue
(BALT)
Bronitin Mist
Bronkaid Mist
Bronkodyl
Bronkosol Inhalation Solution
Brontex
bronze
b. baby
b. baby syndrome
b. diabetes
Broselow
B. chart
B. tape
Brotane
broth
b. culture
Lim b.
Todd-Hewitt b.
Broviac catheter
brow
olympian b.
b. presentation
brown
B. and Harris interview
B. nodule
b. recluse spider
b. skin lesion
B. superior oblique tendon sheath
syndrome
Browne
testis within superficial inguinal
pouch of Denis B.
Brown-Hopp tissue Gram stain

NOTES

73

Brown-Séquard syndrome
BRS
  Behavior Rating Scale
BRSA
  borderline-resistant *Staphylococcus aureus*
brucei
  Trypanosoma b.
Brucella
  B. abortus
  B. agar plate
  B. canis
  B. melitensis
  B. suis
brucellosis
Brudzinski sign
Bruel and Kjaer sonometer
Brugada syndrome
Brugia
  B. beaveri
  B. lepori
Bruininks-Oseretsky
  B.-O. test
  B.-O. Test of Motor Proficiency
bruisabilty
  easy b.
bruit
  abdominal b.
  aortic b.
  carotid b.
  cranial b.
Brun
  layer of B.
Brunner gland
brush border assembly
Brushfield spot
Bruton
  B. agammaglobulinemia
  B. disease
Bruton/B-cell tyrosine kinase gene
bruxism
  sleep b.
Bryant traction
BSA
  body surface area
BSAER
  brainstem auditory evoked response
BSAP
  brief, small, abundant motor-unit action potential
BSER
  brainstem evoked response
BSERA
  brainstem evoked response audiometry
BSI
  bloodstream infection
BSID
  Bayley Scales of Infant Development

BSID-II
  Bayley Scales of Infant Development-II
BSSL
  bile salt-stimulated lipase
BT
  borderline tuberculoid
  BT pattern
BTA
  botulinum toxin A
B-T shunt
bubble
  extraluminal gas b.
bubble-boy disease
bubbler humidifier
bubbly
  b. crackle
  b. lungs
  b. lung syndrome
bubo, pl. **buboes**
  b. aspirate
bucca, pl. **buccae**
buccal
  b. cellulitis
  b. feeding technique
  b. mucosa
  b. mucosa graft
  Nitrogard B.
buccolingual apraxia
buccomandibular dystonia
bucket-handle pattern of fracture
buckle fracture
buckshot calcification
bud
  aortic b.
  breast b.
  epithelial b.
  pulmonary b.
  taste b.
  tooth b.
Budd-Chiari syndrome
buddy taping
budesonide
  b. inhalation suspension (BIS)
  b. Turbuhaler
buffalo hump
buffer
buffered lidocaine
Bufferin
buffy-coat
  b.-c. examination
  b.-c. layer
buffy coat
bulb
  femoral b.
  b. syringe
bulbar
  b. conjunctiva
  b. conjunctival injection

b. hereditary motor neuropathy (type I, II)
b. palsy
b. paralysis
b. polioencephalitis
b. poliomyelitis
bulbo ponto mesencephalic region
bulbospinal poliomyelitis
bulbous nasal tip
bulboventricular foramen
bulbus cordis
bulgaricus
    Lactobacillus b.
bulge
biparietal b.
parietal b.
precordial b.
bulging
b. flank
b. fontanelle
bulimia nervosa (BN)
bulimorexia
bulk
b. flow
Modane B.
muscle b.
bulla, pl. **bullae**
sausage-shaped b.
scaling b.
transparent b.
bullosa
acantholysis b.
albopapuloid Pasini form of dominant dystrophic epidermolysis b.
Cockayne-Touraine variant of dominant dystrophic epidermolysis b.
concha b.
dermolysis b.
dominant dystrophic epidermolysis b.
dystrophic epidermolysis b.
epidermolysis b. (EB)
generalized atrophic benign epidermolysis b.
junctional epidermolysis b.
recessive dystrophic epidermolysis b. (RDEB)
varicella b.

bullous
b. congenital ichthyosiform erythroderma
b. dermatosis
b. drug eruption
b. erythema multiforme
b. impetigo
b. mastocytosis
b. myringitis
b. pemphigoid
b. reaction
b. varicella
bumetanide
Bumex
Buminate
Bumpa Bed crib bumper pad
BUN
blood urea nitrogen
bundle
His b.
b. of His
papillomacular b.
b. of Probst
bungarotoxin
bunion
adolescent b.
dorsal b.
bunionette deformity
bunny hopping
Bunostomum phlebotomum
Bunyaviridae
Bunyavirus
Buphenyl
buphthalmos
bupivacaine
buprenorphine
bupropion hydrochloride
burden
body lcad b.
b. of care interview for children
tumor b.
Burg algorithm
burgdorferi
    Borrelia b.
buried penis
Burkholderia
    B. cepacia
    B. gladioli
    B. mallei
    B. multivorans
    B. norimbergensis
    B. pickettii

NOTES

B

Burkholderia (*continued*)
  B. *pseudomallei*
  B. *vietnamiensis*
Burkitt
  B. lymphoma (BL)
  B. sarcoma
  B. tumor cell
burn
  circumferential b.
  deep partial-thickness b.
  b. encephalopathy
  first-degree b.
  flame b.
  full-thickness b.
  immersion b.
  partial-thickness b.
  second-degree b.
  splash b.
  third-degree b.
burned
  TBSA b.
  total body surface area b.
burner
burnetii
  Coxiella b.
burnlike dermatitis
burnout
  mother b.
Burow solution
burp
  wet b.
burping
burrow
  pus b.
burr-shaped erythrocyte
bursa, pl. **bursae**
  gastrocnemius-semimembranosus b.
  greater trochanteric b.
  iliopectineal b.
bursitis
  pes anserina b.
  prepatellar b.
  septic b.
  suppurative b.
burst
  suppression b.
burst-forming units-erythroid (BFU-E)
bursting fracture
burst-suppression pattern
Burton gum lead line

Burt Word Reading Test
Buschke
  scleredema of B.
Buschke-Ollendorf syndrome
BuSpar
buspirone hydrochloride
bus transport
busulfan
butoconazole 2% cream
butterfly
  b. distribution
  b. drain
  b. flap
  b. rash
  b. scalp vein needle
  b. vertebra
button
  gastrostomy b.
  B. gastrostomy device
Button-One Step gastrostomy device
buttonpexy fixation
butt paste
buttress
  facial b.
  b. response
butyrate
  hydrocortisone b.
  b. therapy
butyrophenone
BVM
  bag, valve, mask
BWGA
  birth weight for gestational age
BWS
  Beckwith-Wiedemann syndrome
by
  b. mouth feeding
  b. mouth (per os) (p.o.)
  b. way of rectum (p.r.)
Byclomine Injection
Bydramine Cough Syrup
Byler
  B. disease
  B. syndrome
bypass
  cardiopulmonary b.
  jejunoileal b.
  ventricular b.
Byrne and Euler formula (BEF)
bystander effect

C1
- C1 to C2 dislocation
- C1 esterase inhibitor
- C1 esterase inhibitor deficiency

C$_4$
- leukotriene C$_4$ (LTC$_4$)

CA
- cardiac-apnea
- child abuse
- chorioamnionitis
- community-acquired
  - CA monitor

Ca
- calcium

CAA
- coronary artery aneurysm

CAAT
- computer-assisted axial tomography

CABA
- child and adolescent burden assessment

cabergoline

CaBF
- carotid blood flow

cable
- twister c.

cachexia

cadaveric donor

cadence

CAE
- cefuroxime axetil

CAF
- coronary artery fistula

CAFAS
- Child and Adolescent Functional Assessment Scale

Cafatine
- Ergotamine Tartrate and Caffeine C.

Cafatine-PB

Cafcit

café-au-lait (CAL)
- c.-a.-l. spot

Cafergot

Cafetrate

caffeine
- c. citrate
- c. terbutaline
- c. therapy

caffeinism

Caffey
- C. disease
- C. syndrome

Caffey-Silverman syndrome

CAFMHS
- Child, Adolescent, and Family Mental Health Service

cage
- manual splinting of thoracic c.

CAH
- congenital adrenal hyperplasia

Caisson disease

Caitlin mark

CAIV
- cold-attenuated intranasal influenza vaccine

CAIV-T
- cold-adapted influenza virus vaccine, trivalent

Cajal-Retzius neuron

CAL
- café-au-lait
- coronary artery lesion

cal
- calorie

Caladryl for Kids

calamine lotion

Calan SR

calcaneal
- c. apophysitis
- c. compartment
- c. fracture
- c. prominence
- c. tendon
- c. view

calcanel (*pl. of* calcaneus)

calcaneocuboid ligament

calcaneofibular ligament (CFL)

calcaneonavicular (CN)
- c. articulation
- c. bar
- c. coalition
- c. fusion

calcaneotibial angle

calcaneovalgus
- c. flatfoot
- c. foot
- c. foot deformity
- talipes c.

calcaneus, pl. **calcanei**

Cal Carb-HD

Calci-Chew

Calciday-667

calcidiol

Calciferol

calcification
- adrenal c.
- basal ganglia c.
- buckshot c.

C

calcification *(continued)*
cervical disk space c.
hepatic capsular c.
intervertebral disk c. (IDC)
intracranial c.
perivascular c.
provisional c.
subcutaneous c.
zone of preparatory c. (ZPC)
calcified
c. appendicolith
c. bacterial plaque
c. exostosis
c. fecalith
c. matrix
calcifying
c. epithelioma
c. vasopathy
Calcijex
Calcimar
Calci-Mix
calcineurin inhibitor
calcinosis
c. cutis, Raynaud phenomenon, sclerodactyly, telangiectasia (CRST)
c., Raynaud phenomenon, esophageal dysmotility, sclerodactyly, telangiectasia (CREST)
calcipotriene
calcitonin
calcitriol
calcium (Ca)
c. alginate
c. alginate swab
c. carbonate
c. channel antagonist
c. channel blocker
c. chloride
cisplatin, 5-fluorouracil, leucovorin c. (CFL)
c. crystal
death by c.
c. deficiency
C. Disodium Versenate
c. glubionate
c. gluconate
c. leukovorin
c. phosphate
c. rich
c. salt
calcivirus
calcofluor white stain
calculus, pl. **calculi**
indinavir calculi
renal c.

CaldeCort
C. Anti-Itch Topical Spray
C. Topical
Caldesene Topical
Caldwell view
calfactant
calf lung surfactant extract (CLSE)
Calgiswab
caliber
caliber-persistent artery
calibrated
calibration
calibrator
Atomlab 200 dose c.
calicivirus
human c. (HuCV)
California
C. encephalitis
C. Verbal Learning Test-Children's Version
caliper
callosal
c. agenesis
c. inhibition
callosum
agenesis of corpus c.
corpus c.
calmers
Robitussin Cough C.
Sucrets Cough C.
Calmette-Guérin
bacille C.-G. (BCG)
bacillus C.-G.
Calmol 4
Calm-X Oral
calomel
caloric
c. challenge
c. intake
calorie (cal)
20-calorie formula
24-calorie formula
calorimeter
DeltaTrac II indirect c.
calorimetry
indirect c.
infrared thermographic c. (ITC)
resting c.
Cal-Plus
Caltrate 600
Caltrate, Jr.
calvarial osteomyelitis
calvarium
Calvé-Legg-Perthes syndrome
Calvé-Perthes disease
Calymmatobacterium granulomatis
calyx
renal c.

CAM
    cell adhesion molecule
    complementary and alternative medicine
    cystic adenomatoid malformation
      CAM tent
Cameco syringe holder
camera
    video c.
Camino monitor
cAMP
    cyclic adenosine monophosphate
      cAMP test
Campbell Soup kid facies
campesterol
camptobrachydactyly
camptodactylia
camptodactyly
camptomelic
    c. dysplasia
    c. syndrome
Campylobacter
    C. coli
    C. concisus
    C. cryaerophilia
    C. curvus
    C. enteritis
    C. fetus
    C. fetus intestinalis
    C. fetus jejuni
    C. gastroenteritis
    C. gracilis
    C. hyointestinalis
    C. infection
    C. jejuni subspecies *doylei*
    C. lari
    C. mucosalis
    C. pylori
    C. sputorum
    C. upsaliensis
camsylate
    trimethaphan c.
Camurati-Englemann syndrome
Canadian
    C. Acute Respiratory Illness and
      Flu Scale (CARIFS)
    C. Crohn Relapse Prevention Trial
canal
    anal c.
    atrioventricular c.
    attenuated pyloric c.
    auditory c.
    birth c.

    ear c.
    external auditory c.
    Hunter c.
    Kohn c.
    Lambert c.
    medullary c.
    c. of Nuck
    Schlemm c.
    semicircular c.
    c. type ASD
canalicular
    c. stage
    c. stage of lung development
    c. testis
canaliculus, pl. canaliculi
    pili trianguli et canaliculi
Canavan disease
c-ANCA
    antineutrophil cytoplasmic antibody
cancer
    c. family syndrome
    hereditary nonpolyposis colorectal c.
    c. predisposition syndrome
    thyroid c.
Candida
    C. albicans
    C. diaper dermatitis
    C. guilliermondi
    C. krusei
    C. meningitis
    C. parapsilosis
    C. paratropicalis
    C. pseudotropicalis
    C. skin test
    C. stellatoides
    C. tropicalis
candidal
    c. arthritis
    c. diaper dermatitis
    c. diaper rash
    c. glossitis
    c. onychomycosis
    c. paronychia
candidate gene
candidemia
    transient c.
candidiasis
    acute atrophic c.
    acute pseudomembranous c.
    chronic mucocutaneous c.
    congenital c.
    cutaneous c.

NOTES

candidiasis *(continued)*
    disseminated c.
    esophageal c.
    hepatosplenic c.
    intertriginous c.
    invasive c.
    mucocutaneous c.
    neonatal c.
    oral c.
    oropharyngeal c. (OPC)
    renal c.
    systemic c.
    vulvovaginal c.
candidosis
    congenital cutaneous c.
    interdigital c.
    intertriginous c.
    oral c.
    perianal c.
    vaginal c.
candiduria
candle dripping
candlestick sign
canicola
    Leptospira c.
canimorsus
    Capnocytophaga c.
canine
    c. distemper
    c. scabies
    c. tooth
caninum
    Ancylostoma c.
canis
    Brucella c.
    Microsporum c.
    Pasteurella c.
    Toxocara c.
canker sore
cannabis
Cannabis sativa
cannonball lesion
cannula
    high-flow nasal c.
    nasal c.
cannulated screw
cannulation
    jugular venous c.
canthorum
    dystopia c.
canthus, pl. **canthi**
    heterochromia of inner c.
    inner c.
    lateral displacement of inner c.
    outer c.
C antigen
cantonensis
    Angiostrongylus c.

Cantrell
    pentalogy of C.
    C. syndrome
Cantwell-Ransley repair
cap
    cervical c.
    Compoz Gel C.'s
    cradle c.
    Drixoral Cough Liquid C.'s
    Dumas vault c.
    Prentif cavity-rim c.
    ProtectaCap c.
    Vimule c.
CAPA
    Child and Adolescent Psychiatric
    Assessment
capacity
    closing c. (CC)
    diffusing c.
    forced vital c. (FVC)
    functional residual c. (FRC)
    inspiratory c. (IC)
    iron-binding c.
    reduced bladder c.
    renal reserve filtration c. (RRFC)
    serum bilirubin-binding c.
    total lung c. (TLC)
    vital c. (VC)
CAPD
    central auditory processing disorder
    continuous ambulatory peritoneal dialysis
capillariasis
    hepatic c.
capillary, pl. **capillaries**
    c. angioma
    c. BLL
    dilated c.
    distended c.
    c. dropout
    c. electrophoresis
    c. electrophoresis/frontal analysis (CE/FA)
    c. end loop
    c. filling time
    c. hemangioma
    c. isoelectric focusing technique
    c. leak
    c. leak syndrome (CLS)
    nail-fold c.
    c. pattern
    c. refill
    c. refill time
    tortuous c.
capita (*pl. of* caput)
capital femoral epiphysis
capitate bone

capitellar
    c. epiphysis
    c. osteochondritis
capitellum
    osteochondritis of c.
capitis
    Pediculus humanus var c.
    tinea c.
caplet
    Miles Nervine C.'s
    Sinumist-SR C.'s
    TripTone C.'s
Capnocytophaga canimorsus
capnograph
    Microstream c.
capnography
    low-flow sidestream c.
capnometry
Capoten
capreomycin
Capronor
capsaicin
Capsin
capsulatum
    Histoplasma c.
capsule
    Bowman c.
    Crosby c.
    Crosby-Kugler pediatric c.
    Dexedrine Spansule c.
    Dialose Plus C.
    Dimetapp 4-Hour Liqui-Gel C.
    Glisson c.
    joint c.
    Norvir c.
    Watson c.
capsulotomy
    posterior knee c.
captopril
caput, pl. **capita**
    c. medusae
    c. succedaneum
Capzasin-P
Carafate
caramel test
carateum
    Treponema c.
carbamazepine (CBZ)
carbamide peroxide
carbamoyl
    c. phosphate synthetase (CPS)
    c. phosphate synthetase deficiency

carbapenem
carbenicillin
Carb-HD
    Cal C.-HD
carbimazole
carbinoxamine and pseudoephedrine
Carbiset Tablet
Carbiset-TR Tablet
Carbodec
    C. Syrup
    C. TR Tablet
carbohydrate
    c. homeostasis transporter
    c. malabsorption
    c. overloading
carbohydrate-deficient glycoprotein syndrome (type I) (CDGS)
carbohydrate-free
    Ross c.-f. (RCF)
carbon
    c. dioxide (CO_2)
    c. dioxide laser
    c. dioxide retention
    c. monoxide (CO)
    c. monoxide poisoning
    c. monoxide toxicity
    c. tetrachloride
carbon-14 test
carbonaceous sputum
carbonate
    calcium c.
    lithium c.
carbonic anhydrase inhibitor
carbon-13 urea breath test
carbonyl
carboplatin
carboxamide
    imidazole c. (DTIC)
carboxykinase
    phosphoenolpyruvate c. (PEPCK)
carboxylase
    acetyl-CoA c.
    alpha-methylcrotonyl-coenzyme A c.
    c. deficiency
    deficiency of pyruvate c.
carboxylation
carboxypeptidase E
carboxyterminal
    c. propeptide
    c. propeptide of type 1 procollagen (PICP)
carbuncle

C

NOTES

81

carcinoembryonic antigen
carcinogen
carcinogenesis
    pediatric thyroid c.
    radiation c.
carcinogenic
carcinoid syndrome
carcinoma
    acinic cell c.
    adrenal cortical c.
    basal cell c.
    childhood thyroid c.
    choroid plexus c. (CPC)
    embryonal c.
    fibrolamellar hepatocellular c.
    hepatocellular c. (HCC)
    keratinizing nasopharyngeal c.
    medullary thyroid c.
    mucoepidermoid c.
    nasopharyngeal c.
    primary hepatocellular c. (PHC)
    renal medullary c.
    thyroid c.
carcinomatosis
    meningeal c.
card
    Allen Kindergarten Picture C.'s
    neonatal Guthrie c.
    Peabody Developmental Motor
      Activity C.'s
    Sheridan-Gardiner c.'s
    Sonksen-Silver visual acuity c.
Cardec-S Syrup
cardiac
    c., abnormal facies, thymic
      hypoplasia, cleft palate,
      hypocalcemia syndrome
    c. abnormality
    c. abnormality, abnormal facies,
      thymic hypoplasia, cleft palate,
      hypocalcemia (CATCH 22)
    c. abnormality, T-cell deficit,
      clefting, hypocalcemia (CATCH)
    c. abnormality, T-cell deficit,
      clefting, hypocalcemia phenotype
    c. arrest
    c. asthma
    c. catheter
    c. catheterization
    c. cyanosis
    c. ejection fraction
    c. event monitor
    c. failure
    c. glycoside
    c. hemangioma
    c. hemolytic anemia
    c. lesion
    c. looping

    c. malformation
    c. malposition
    c. massage
    c. murmur
    c. output
    c. rhabdomyoma
    c. rhythm disorder
    c. rupture
    c. septal defect
    c. septation
    c. silhouette
    c. size
    c. standstill
    c. stun
    c. syncope
    c. tamponade
    c. troponin T
    c. twinning
    c. width
cardiac-apnea (CA)
    c.-a. monitor
cardiac-limb syndrome
cardinal vein
Cardiobacterium
cardiofacial syndrome
cardiofaciocutaneous syndrome
cardiogenesis
cardiogenic
    c. shock
    c. shot
cardiogram
    impedance c.
cardiologist
cardiology
cardiomegaly
cardiomyocyte
cardiomyopathy
    chronic chagasic c.
    diabetic c.
    dilated c.
    histiocytoid c.
    hypertrophic c.
    ipecac c.
    maternally inherited myopathy
      and c. (MIMyCA)
    restrictive c. (RCM)
    Sengers c.
    subaortic hypertrophic c.
    X-linked c.
cardioplegic solution
cardiopneumograph
cardioprotective
cardiopulmonary
    c. bypass
    c. dysfunction
    c. resuscitation (CPR)
Cardioquin
cardiorespiratory monitor

CardioSEAL device
cardioskeletal
    c. myopathy
    c. neutropenia
cardiospasm
cardiothoracic ratio
cardiothymic shadow
cardiotocography (CTG)
cardiotoxicity
cardiovascular
    c. collapse
    c. depression
    c. effect
    c. malformation (CVM)
    c. pertubation
    c. sequela
    c. shock
    c. system
cardiovascular/central nervous system syndrome
cardioversion
    synchronized DC c.
carditis
    acute rheumatic c.
    indolent c.
    rheumatic c.
Cardizem
    C. CD
    C. Injectable
    C. SR
    C. Tablet
care
    foster c.
    hospice c.
    kangaroo c.
    newborn intensive c. (NBIC)
    pediatric neurocritical c.
    respite c.
    substitute c.
    well-child c. (WCC)
caregiver
    primary c.
caretaker
    primary c.
Carey Temperament Scale
caries
    dental c.
    early childhood c. (ECC)
CARIFS
    Canadian Acute Respiratory Illness and Flu Scale
carina, pl. carinae

carinatum
    pectus c.
carinii
    Pneumocystis c.
C-arm
carmustine
Carnation
    C. Follow-Up
    C. Follow-Up soy formula
    C. Good Start formula
carnitine
    c. acylcarnitine translocase deficiency
    c. palmitoyltransferase (CPT)
    c. palmitoyltransferase I (CPT I)
    c. palmitoyltransferase II (CPT II)
    c. palmitoyltransferase II deficiency
    c. palmitoyltransferase I, II deficiency
Carnitor
carnivore
Carnoy fixative
carob
    c. gum
    c. seed flour
Caroli disease
Carolina
    C. Curriculum for Handicapped Infants and Infants At-Risk
    C. Curriculum for Infants and Toddlers with Special Needs
carotid
    c. artery
    c. artery-cavernous sinus fistula
    c. blood flow (CaBF)
    c. bruit
    left common c.
    right common c.
    c. sinus pressure
carotid-cavernous fistula
carpal navicular
carpectomy
    proximal row c.
Carpenter syndrome
carpopedal spasm
carpus, pl. carpi
carrier
    silent c.
CARS
    Childhood Autism Rating Scale
car sickness
Carter's Little Pills

NOTES

83

Cartesian system
cartilage
    costal c.
    c. hair hypoplasia (CHH)
    c. interposition
    c. oligomeric matrix protein
    (COMP)
    c. piercing
cartilaginous coalition
Carvajal formula
CAS
    central anticholinergic syndrome
    child assessment schedule
CASA
    Child and Adolescent Services
    Assessment
Casal necklace
casanthranol
    docusate and c.
cascade
    coagulation c.
    cytokine c.
    toxic c.
cascara sagrada
caseating necrosis
caseation
Casec
    C. formula
    C. powder
casein
    c. hydrolysate
    c. hydrolysate formula
    powdered c.
case manager
caseosa
    vernix c.
caseous node
caseum
CASH
    cortical androgen-stimulating hormone
cassava bean
casseliflavus
    Enterococcus c.
CAST
    childhood accidental spiral tibial
    Children of Alcoholics Screening Test
cast
    abduction c.
    bivalved c.
    c. boot brace
    bronchial mucous c.
    cellular c.
    clubfoot c.
    cylinder c.
    dense c.
    hip spica c.
    hypereosinophilic mucoid c.
    long leg c.

    Petrie c.
    red blood cell c.
    Risser localizer c.
    short leg walking c.
    spica c.
    C. syndrome
    thumb spica c.
castellani
    Acanthamoeba c.
casting
    inhibitive c.
    serial c.
Castleman disease
castor oil
castrated
castration
CAT
    Clinical Adaptive Test
    computed axial tomography
    CAT scanning
catabolism
    tissue c.
    unregulated c.
Cataflam Oral
catalase negative
catalytic
catamenial pneumothorax
cataplectic attack
cataplexy
Catapres Oral
Catapres-TTS Transdermal
cataract
    congenital bilateral c.
    developmental c.
    c. formation
    juvenile c.
    lenticular c.
    sunflower c.
    zonular c.
catarrhal
catarrhalis
    Branhamella c.
    Moraxella c.
catatonic
    c. behavior
    c. syndrome
CATCH
    cardiac abnormality, T-cell deficit,
    clefting, hypocalcemia
    CATCH phenotype
    CATCH 22 syndrome
CATCH 22
    cardiac abnormality, abnormal facies,
    thymic hypoplasia, cleft palate,
    hypocalcemia
    conotruncal cardiac defect, abnormal
    face, thymic hypoplasia, cleft palate

CAT/CLAMS
  Clinical Adaptive Test/Clinical Linguistic
    and Auditory Milestone Scale
cat dander
catecholamine
catechol oxidase
categorical placement
category
  bilineal c.
  unilineal c.
catenulatum
  Bifidobacterium c.
cathartic
  c. colon
  magnesium-containing c.
catheter
  Amplatz c.
  Angiocath c.
  c. angiography
  Arrow c.
  arterial c.
  balloon septostomy c.
  balloon-tipped c.
  bile duct c.
  Broviac c.
  cardiac c.
  central venous c. (CVC)
  Cook c.
  Corcath c.
  de Pezzer c.
  double-lumen c.
  elastomer c.
  c. embolization
  FΛE c.
  flexible Teflon c.
  Fogarty arterial embolectomy c.
  Fogarty atrioseptostomy c.
  Foley c.
  Hermed c.
  Hickman c.
  indwelling c.
  indwelling arterial c. (IAC)
  indwelling venous c. (IVC)
  Infuse-A-Port c.
  Judkins c.
  jugular bulb c.
  Kendall double-lumen c.
  Landmark c.
  large-bore c.
  Leonard c.
  MediPort c.
  Millar c.

  over-the-needle c.
  percutaneous central venous c.
    (PCVC)
  percutaneous femoral venous c.
  percutaneously inserted central
    line c. (PICC)
  peripheral arterial c.
  peripheral intravenous c.
  peripherally inserted c. (PIC)
  peripherally inserted central c.
    (PICC)
  Per-Q-Cath c.
  Pezzer c.
  pigtail c.
  PIV c.
  polyethylene c.
  Port-A-Cath c.
  c. pullback
  pulmonary thermodilution c.
  Raaf c.
  radial artery c.
  Raimondi c.
  Replogle suction c.
  c. reservoir
  scalp vein c.
  c. septostomy
  shearing of c.
  Silastic c.
  silicone c.
  Sones c.
  Swan-Ganz c.
  tracheal c.
  transtracheal c.
  umbilical artery c. (UAC)
  umbilical vein c.
  umbilical venous c. (UVC)
  umbilical vessel c.
  urinary c.
  venous c.
  ventricular c.
  water-perfused manometry c.
  Word c.
  Yankauer c.
catheter-associated bacteremia
catheter-in-a-catheter technique
catheterization
  bladder c.
  cardiac c.
  clean intermittent c. (CIC)
  jugular bulb c.
  radial artery c.
  scalp vein c.

NOTES

C

catheterization *(continued)*
    umbilical artery c.
    umbilical vein c.
    urinary c.
catheter-over-needle technique
catheter-over-wire technique
cathode ray oscilloscope (CRO)
cati
    Toxocara c.
cat's
    c. cry
    c. eye pupil
    c. eye reflex
    c. eye syndrome
    c. urine syndrome
cat-scratch
    c.-s. disease (CSD)
    c.-s. fever
    c.-s. fever disease
Cattell
    C. Infant Intelligence Scale
    C. Infant Intelligence Test
Catterall classification (grade 1–4)
cauda, pl. **caudae**
    c. equina
    c. equina syndrome
caudal
    c. agenesis
    c. chordamesoderm
    c. direction
    c. dysplasia
    c. dysplasia syndrome
    c. regression syndrome
caudate
    c. hypometabolism
    c. nucleus
caudocranial
causalgia
causation
causative
cause
    acute cerebellar ataxia of
        unknown c.
cause-and-effect activity
caustic
    c. aspiration
    c. ingestion
    c. injury
cauterization
    nasal c.
cautery
    endoscopic c.
    L-shaped c.
cava, pl. **cavae**
    inferior vena c. (IVC)
    superior vena c. (SVC)
    vena c.

CAVD
    congenital absence of vas deferens
C(aVDO$_2$)
    cerebral arteriovenous difference for
        oxygen
cave
    Meckel c.
Caverject
cavernosa
    corpus c.
cavernosal
    c. artery thrombosis
    c. fibrosis
    c. infarction
cavernous
    c. hemangioma
    c. sinus
    c. sinusitis
    c. sinus syndrome
    c. sinus thrombosis
    c. venous angioma
CAVH
    continuous arteriovenous hemofiltration
caviae
    Nocardia c.
cavitary
    c. lung disease
    c. tuberculosis
cavitation
cavity
    abdominal c.
    abscess c.
    chorionic c.
    coelomic c.
    oral c.
    peritoneal c.
    syringomyelic c.
    thoracic c.
    ventricles to peritoneal c. (VP)
CAVM
    cerebral arteriovenous malformation
cavovarus
    c. deformity
    c. foot
cavum
    c. septi pellucidum
    c. vergae
cavus
    c. foot
    pathological c.
    pes c.
    physiological c.
cayetanensis
    Cyclospora c.
Caylor cardiofacial syndrome
CBC
    complete blood count

CBCL
Child Behavior Checklist
C-beta-thal
CBF
cerebral blood flow
CBFV
cerebral blood flow velocity
Cbl
cobalamin
CBR
cord blood registry
CBRF
child behavior rating form
CBS
child behavioral study
CBT
cognitive behavioral therapy
cord blood transplantation
CBV
cerebral blood volume
CBZ
carbamazepine
CC
closing capacity
Adalat CC
hemoglobin CC
CCA
congenital contractural arachnodactyly
CCAI
Clinical Colitis Activity Index
CCAM
congenital cystic adenomatoid
malformation
CCAM (type 1–3)
C2, C3, C4, C5, C6, C7, C8, C9 deficiency
CCG
Children's Cancer Group
CCH
chronic cryptogenic hepatitis
CCHB
congenital complete heart block
CCHD
cyanotic congenital heart disease
CCHS
congenital central hypoventilation
syndrome
CCK
cholecystokinin
CCLO
child-centered literary orientation

CCNU
cyclohexylchloroethylnitrosurea
CCPD
continuous cyclic peritoneal dialysis
C-Crystals
CCS
Crippled Children's Services
CCSC
Children's Coping Strategies Checklist
CCSG
Children's Cancer Study Group
CCVM
congenital cardiovascular malformation
CD
celiac disease
cluster of differentiation
conduct disorder
Cardizem CD
Ceclor CD
CD4
cluster of differentiation 4
CD4 cell count
CD4 T-cell
CD4:CD8 ratio
CD4+ cell
CD8 T-cell
CDA
congenital dyserythropoietic anemia
CDAC
Clostridium difficile-associated diarrhea
CDC
Centers for Disease Control
Communicable Disease Center
CDD
childhood disintegrative disorder
CDFI
color Doppler flow imaging
CDGS
carbohydrate-deficient glycoprotein
syndrome (type I)
CDH
congenital diaphragmatic hernia
congenital dislocation of hip
congenital hip dysplasia
CDH repair
CDHNF
Children's Digestive Health and Nutrition
Foundation
CDI
Children's Depression Inventory
Cotrel-Dubousset instrumentation

NOTES

cDICA, C-DICA
Computerized Diagnostic Interview for
Children and Adolescents
CD4-IgG
cluster of differentiation 4
immunoglobulin G
cDNA
complementary deoxyribonucleic acid
complementary DNA
CDP
continuous distending pressure
CDRS-R
Children's Depression Rating Scale-
Revised
CE
conductive education
ceasmic
Cebid
cebocephaly
cecal pouch
Ceclor CD
cecocolic intussusception
Cecon
cecostomy
cecum
exstrophic c.
Cedax
CeeNU
CE/FA
capillary electrophoresis/frontal analysis
cefaclor
cefadroxil monohydrate
Cefadyl
Cefanex
cefazolin sodium
cefdinir
cefepime
cefixime
Cefizox
Cefobid
cefoperazone sodium
Cefotan
cefotaxime sodium
cefotetan
cefoxitin
cefpodoxime proxetil
cefprozil
ceftazidime
ceftibuten
Ceftin Oral
ceftizoxime
ceftriaxone
c. sodium
cefuroxime
c. axetil (CAE)
c. sodium
Cefzil
ceiling

Celestone
C. Oral
C. Phosphate Injection
C. Soluspan
celiac
c. antibody
c. artery
c. axis
c. disease (CD)
c. sprue
c. syndrome
cell
absolute nucleated red blood c.
(ANRBC)
activated T c.
c. adhesion molecule (CAM)
Alzheimer II c.
antibody-secreting c. (ASC)
antigen-presenting c. (APC)
B c.
back-selected T c.
band c.
basket c.
basophil c.
Betz c.
Birbeck granule-positive c.
bite c.
blister c.
bone marrow stem c.
Burkitt tumor c.
CD4+ c.
choroid plexus c.
circulating fetal c.
clue c.
crenated red c.
crypt c.
CTL c.
cytotoxic memory T c.
daughter c.
dendritic c.
desquamated epithelial c.
donor T c.
embryonic renomedullary
interstitial c.
encephalitogenic c.
endothelial c.
enterochromaffin c.
eosinophil c.
epithelial c.
erythroid progenitor c.
eukaryotic c.
fetal red c.
c. and flare
foam c.
ganglion c.
Gaucher c.
germ c.
giant c.

Haller c.
haploid c.
helper T c.
HLA-identical haploidentical bone marrow stem c.
hyperplasia of beta c.
inclusion c. (I-cell)
c. interaction gene
killer c.
Kupffer c.
lack of natural killer c.
Langerhans c.
Langhans giant c.
leukemic c.
Leydig c.
lymphocyte c.
mast c.
mastoid air c.
memory c.
Merkel c.
mesenchymal c.
metamyelocyte c.
monocyte c.
monster c.
multinucleated giant c.
myeloblast c.
myelocyte c.
natural killer c. (NKC)
natural killer T c.
neural crest c.
neuroblastoma c.
Niemann-Pick c.
NK c.
nonencephalitogenic c.
normoblast c.
nuclear factor of activated T c. (NFAT)
nucleated red blood c.
Opalski c.
packed red blood c. (PRBC)
pancreatic islet c.
peripheral blood mononuclear c. (PBMC)
peripheral blood stem c. (PBSC)
plasma c.
pneumatic c.
c. precursor
promyelocyte c.
pronormoblast c.
Purkinje c.
pyknotic c.
Raji c.

red blood c. (RBC)
Reed-Sternberg c.
renal tubular epithelial c.
reticuloendothelial c.
Rh null c.
Schwann c.
segmented neutrophil c.
Sertoli c.
sickle c.
c. sorting
spherocytic red blood c.
spiculated red c.
spindle c.
stellate c.
stem c.
syncytiotrophoblastic tumor giant c.
syngeneic stem c.
T c.
T-cell-depleted haploidentical bone marrow stem c.
technetium-labeled red blood c.
T-helper c.
triphasic pattern blastemal c.
white blood c. (WBC)
CellCept
cell-mediated immunity (CMI)
cellular
c. blue nevus
c. cast
c. debris
c. desmoplastic stroma
c. edema
c. hypoxia
c. immunodeficiency
c. infiltrate
c. and molecular regulation of lung development
c. proteolysis
c. regulation
cellulitis
anaerobic c.
buccal c.
Haemophilus influenzae c.
orbital c.
periorbital c.
peritonsillar c.
pneumococcal facial c.
preseptal c.
retropharyngeal c.
streptococcal c.
cellulosae
Cysticercus c.

NOTES

Celontin
Cel-U-Jec Injection
cementum
  dental c.
Cenafed Plus
Cena-K
center
  American Association of Poison
    Control C.'s (AAPCC)
  apneustic c.
  Children's National Medical C.
  Communicable Disease C. (CDC)
  C.'s for Disease Control (CDC)
  C.'s for Disease Control and
    Prevention
  c. edge angle
  c. edge angle of Wiberg
  C. for Epidemiological Studies
    Depression Scale for Children
  germinal c.
  hotline c.
  malleolar ossification c.
  pneumotaxic c.
  Poison Control C. (PCC)
  regional perinatal intensive care c.
    (RPICC)
  school-based health c. (SBHC)
centigray (cGy)
centimeters of water (cm H₂O)
central
  c. alveolar hypoventilation
  c. anticholinergic syndrome (CAS)
  c. atrophy
  c. auditory processing disorder
    (CAPD)
  c. cord lesion
  c. cord syndrome
  c. core disease
  c. cyanosis
  c. diabetes insipidus
  c. fat distribution pattern
  c. hypothyroidism
  c. hypoventilation syndrome
  c. incisor
  c. nervous system (CNS)
  c. nervous system/cardiovascular
    syndrome
  c. nervous system disease
  c. nervous system leukemia
  c. nervous system lymphoma
  c. neuroblastoma
  c. neurofibromatosis
  c. neurogenic hyperventilation
  c. pontine myelinolysis
  c. porencephaly
  c. precocious puberty (CPP)
  c. primitive neuroectodermal tumor
    (cPNET)

  c. respiratory drive
  c. serotonergic hyperactivity
  c. serotonin abnormality
  c. shunt
  c. sleep apnea
  c. venous access device (CVAD)
  c. venous catheter (CVC)
  c. venous line (CVL)
  c. venous nutrition (CVN)
  c. venous pressure (CVP)
  c. venous pressure line
  c. visual field
centralization
centrencephalic
  c. epilepsy
  c. system
centrifugation
  Ficoll-Hypaque c.
centrifugum
  leukoderma acquisitum c.
centrilobular necrosis
centripetal spread
centrizonal
  c. hypoxia
  c. sinusoidal distention
centromere
centronuclear myopathy
centrotemporal spike
CEP
  congenital erythropoietic porphyria
cepacia
  Burkholderia c.
  Pseudomonas c.
cephalexin
cephalhematoma
  bilateral c.'s
cephalic
  c. tetanus
  c. vein
cephalization
  primordial c.
cephalocaudal
  c. sequence
  c. sequence of development
cephalocele
cephalodactyly
  Vogt c.
cephalometric radiograph
cephalopelvic disproportion (CPD)
cephalopolysyndactyly
cephalosporin
  first-generation c.
cephalosporin-resistant pneumococcus
cephalostat
cephalothin sodium
cephapirin
cephradine
Cephulac

C

Ceptaz
ceramidase activity
ceramide
    c. trihexose
    c. trihexoside alpha galactosidase
ceramidosis
cercaria, pl. **cercariae**
cercarial skin penetration
Cercopithecine herpesvirus 1
cerebella (*pl. of* cerebellum)
cerebellar
    c. asynergia
    c. ataxia
    c. cerebral palsy
    c. degeneration
    c. dysfunction
    c. dysplasia
    c. encephalitis
    c. folia
    c. hemangioblastoma
    c. hemorrhage
    c. hypertrophy
    c. hypoplasia
    c. mutism
    c. neoplasm
    c. nucleus
    c. tonsils
    c. vermis
    c. vermis hypoplasia, oligophrenia,
      congenital ataxia, coloboma,
      hepatic fibrosis (COACH)
cerebellar-vestibular system
cerebelli
    vermis c.
cerebellitis
    acute c.
    postinfectious c.
    viral c.
cerebellum, pl. **cerebella**
    dysplastic gangliocytoma of c.
    inverse c.
cerebral
    c. amebiasis
    c. angiography
    c. anoxia
    c. arteriovenous difference for
      oxygen (C(aVDO$_2$))
    c. arteriovenous malformation
      (CAVM)
    c. artery aneurysm
    c. artery occlusion
    c. aspergillosis

    c. blood flow (CBF)
    c. blood flow velocity (CBFV)
    c. blood volume (CBV)
    c. compression
    c. contusion
    c. cortex
    c. cortical necrosis
    c. dysfunction
    c. dysfunction syndrome
    c. edema
    c. embolism
    c. falx
    c. function monitor (CFM)
    c. gigantism
    c. glucose metabolism
    c. hemisphere
    c. herniation
    c. hypoperfusion
    c. hypothermia
    c. injury
    c. ischemia
    c. laceration
    c. lactic alkalosis
    c. malaria
    c. oximetry
    c. palsy (CP)
    c. paragonimiasis
    c. peduncle
    c. perfusion pressure (CPP)
    c. resuscitation
    c. salt wasting (CSW)
    c. salt-wasting syndrome
    c. schistosomiasis
    c. swelling
    c. syncope
    c. trypanosomiasis
    c. vasospasm
    c. ventriculomegaly
cerebri
    pseudotumor c.
cerebritis
    lupus c.
cerebrohepatorenal syndrome (CHRS)
cerebromacular degeneration
cerebroocular muscular dystrophy
cerebrooculofacial-skeletal (COFS)
    c.-s. syndrome
cerebroprotective mechanism
cerebroside lipidosis
cerebrospinal
    c. fluid (CSF)
    c. fluid leak

NOTES

cerebrospinal *(continued)*
    c. fluid pleocytosis
    c. fluid procalcitonin
    c. fluid rhinorrhea
cerebrotendinous xanthomatosis
cerebrovascular accident (CVA)
cerebrovasculosa
cerebrum
Cerebyx
Ceredase
cereus
    Bacillus c.
cerevisiae
    Saccharomyces c.
ceroid lipofuscinosis
Certiva vaccine
Cerubidine
ceruleus
    locus c.
    noradrenergic locus c.
ceruloplasmin
    c. deficiency
    c. level
cerumen
Cerumenex Otic
Cervagem
cervical
    c. adenitis
    c. adenopathy
    c. agenesis
    c. cap
    c. collar
    c. cord tumor
    c. culture
    c. disk space calcification
    c. ectopy
    c. esophagostomy
    c. esophagus
    c. herpes
    c. incompetence
    c. lymphadenitis
    c. lymphadenopathy
    c. mucus
    c. rib
    c. sinus
    c. spine immobilization
    c. spine subluxation
cervices (*pl. of* cervix)
cervicitis
    mucopurulent c.
cervicofacial actinomycosis
cervicomedullary
    c. brainstem glioma
    c. compression
    c. junction
cervix, pl. **cervices**
    bifid c.
    congenital atresia of uterine c.

    incompetent c.
    strawberry c.
cesarean
    c. delivery
    c. section
CESD
    cholesterol ester storage disease
cesium iodide (CsI)
cessation
Cetacort Topical
Cetamide
Cetane
Cetaphil
cetirizine hydrochloride
cetyl alcohol
Cevalin
Cevi-bid
Ce-Vi-Sol
ceylanicum
    Ancylostoma c.
CF
    clubfoot
    cystic fibrosis
        CF test
CFE infarction
CFL
    calcaneofibular ligament
    cisplatin, 5-fluorouracil, leucovorin
        calcium
CFM
    cerebral function monitor
CFR
    coronary flow reserve
CFS
    chronic fatigue syndrome
CFTR
    cystic fibrosis transmembrane
        conductance regulator
    cystic fibrosis transmembrane regulator
CFU
    colony-forming unit
CGAS
    Children's Global Assessment Scale
CGD
    chronic granulomatous disease
    continuous gastric drip
CGI
    Clinical Global Impressions
    clinical global index
        CGI scale
cGMP-specific
    cGMP-s. phosphodiesterase
    cGMP-s. phosphodiesterase 5
cGy
    centigray
CH
    congenital hypothyroidism

CH$_{50}$
    hemolytic complement
        CH$_{50}$ assay
CHADD
    children and adults with attention deficit
        disorder
Chadwick sign
chaffeensis
        Ehrlichia c.
Chagas disease
chagasic encephalitis
chagoma
chain
        globin c.
        light c.
        c. reaction
        sympathetic c.
chaining
        backward c.
        forward c.
chair
        adaptive c.
        child's c.
        corner c.
        Kid-EXO 2 child's c.
chalasia
chalazion
challenge
        bee sting c.
        blinded c.
        bronchial provocation c.
        caloric c.
        cow's milk c.
        double-blind, placebo-controlled
            food c. (DBPCFC)
        exercise bronchial c.
        gluten c.
        methacholine c.
chamber
        anterior c.
        holding c.
        infundibular c.
        respiratory c.
        vitreous c.
Chamberlain line
chameleon tongue
chamomile
Chanarin-Dorfman syndrome
Chance fracture
chancre
        trypanosomal c.
        tuberculous c.

chancroid ulcer
change
        harlequin color c.
        lumbosacral skin pigment c.
        papulosquamous skin c.
        personality c.
        postasphyxial c.
        pupillary c.
        rachitic c.
        retinal c.
        ST c.
        wave c.
channel
        common c.
        sinusoidal c.
channelopathy
        chloride c.
        sodium c.
2-channel pneumogram
CHAOS
        congenital high airway obstruction
            syndrome
chaotic
        c. atrial tachycardia
        c. eye movement
characteristic
        c. electroencephalogram pattern
        c. emotional response
        receiver operating c. (ROC)
Charcoaid
charcoal
        activated c.
        c. agar
        multidose activated c. (MDAC)
        c. polyp
charcoal-blood medium
Charcocaps
Charcot
        C. disease
        C. joint
        C. triad
Charcot-Leyden crystal
Charcot-Marie-Tooth
        C.-M.-T. disease
        C.-M.-T. disorder
        C.-M.-T. syndrome
Charcot-Marie-Tooth-Hoffmann
    syndrome
CHARGE
        coloboma, heart disease, atresia choanae,
            retarded growth, genital anomalies, ear
            anomalies

NOTES

CHARGE *(continued)*
  coloboma, heart disease, atresia choanae,
    retarded growth and retarded
    development, CNS anomalies, genital
    hypoplasia, ear anomalies and/or
    deafness
    CHARGE association
    CHARGE syndrome
Charleston brace
Charlevois-Saguenay syndrome
Char syndrome
chart
  Allen c.
  Broselow c.
  Down syndrome growth c.
  Genentech growth c.
  letter c.
  picture c.
  Ross growth c.
  Snellen acuity c.
  star c.
  Swedish national growth c.
  tumbling E c.
  Welch Allyn SureSight eye c.
chartarum
  Stachybotrys c.
chaser
  Scot-Tussin DM Dough C.'s
chasteberry
chat
  cri du c.
chatter
  cocktail c.
CHD
  congenital heart disease
  congestive heart disease
Cheadle disease
Chealamide
check
  developmental c.
  c. valve obstruction
checklist
  Achenbach Child Behavior C.
  asthma symptom c. (ASC)
  Child Behavior C. (CBCL)
  Children's Coping Strategies C.
    (CCSC)
  Developmental Behaviour C.
  Hopkins symptom c.
  life events c. (LEC)
  Pediatric Symptom C. (PSC)
  Swanson, Nolan, and Pelham c.
  Wing Autistic Disorder
    Interview C. (WADIC)
Chédiak-Higashi
  C.-H. deficiency
  C.-H. syndrome

cheek
  chipmunk c.'s
cheesy exudate
cheilitis
  angular c.
cheilosis
  angular c.
cheiroarthropathy
  diabetic c.
chelated gadolinium
chelation
  iron c.
  c. therapy
chelator
  iron c.
chelonae
  Mycobacterium c.
Chemet
chemical
  c. dependency
  c. pleurodesis
  c. pneumonia
  c. pneumonitis
  c. shift imaging (CSI)
chemically
  c. exposed
  c. exposed child
C-hemoglobinopathy
chemokine
chemoprophylactic
chemoprophylaxis
  selective intrapartum c. (SIC)
chemoreceptor
  c. sensitivity
  c. trigger zone (CTZ)
chemoreflex
  laryngeal c.
chemosis
chemotactic
  c. agent
  c. factor
chemotaxis
chemotherapeutic agent
chemotherapy
  antituberculosis c.
  CHOP c.
  cyclophosphamide,
    hydroxydaunorubicin, methotrexate,
    prednisone c.
  intraarterial c.
  marrow-ablative c.
  multidrug c.
  near-myeloablative c.
  c. protocol
  salvage c.
  VAMP c.
chemotherapy-related neutropenia

Cheracol
    C. D
cherry-red
    c.-r. macula
    c.-r. macular spot
    c.-r. spot myoclonus syndrome
cherubism
Chesapeake
    hemoglobin C.
Cheshire cat smile
chessboard pattern
chest
    barrel c.
    c. compression
    flail c.
    funnel c.
    keel c.
    c. mount
    c. pain
    c. percussion
    c. physical therapy (CPT)
    c. radiograph
    c. roentgenography
    shield-shaped c.
    c. syndrome
    c. trauma
    c. tube
    c. tube drainage
    c. wall motion
    c. wall rigidity
    c. width
    c. x-ray (CXR)
chewable
    E.E.S. C.
    Triaminic C.'s
chewing
    rotary c.
Cheyne-Stokes respiration
CHF
    congestive heart failure
CHH
    cartilage hair hypoplasia
CHI
    closed head injury
Chiari
    C. crisis
    C. deformity
    C. malformation (type I–IV)
    C. net
    C. procedure
Chiari-Arnold syndrome

chiasma
    optic c.
chiasmal glioma
chiasmatic
    c. cistern
    c. pilocytic astrocytoma
chiasmatic-hypothalamic glioma
CHIC
    Coping Health Inventory for Children
chicken ovalbumin upstream promoter (COUP)
chickenpox
    gestational c.
    c. vaccine
    c. virus
chickpea
chiclero ulcer
chigger bite
Chiggertox
chikungunya virus
Chilaiditi syndrome
chilblain
CHILD
    congenital hemidysplasia with ichthyosiform erythroderma and limb defects
child
    c. abuse (CA)
    c. abuse and neglect
    C. Abuse Prevention and Treatment Act
    c. and adolescent burden assessment (CABA)
    C., Adolescent, and Family Mental Health Service (CAFMHS)
    c. and adolescent forensic psychiatry
    C. and Adolescent Functional Assessment Scale (CAFAS)
    C. and Adolescent Psychiatric Assessment (CAPA)
    c. and adolescent psychiatrist
    C. and Adolescent Services Assessment (CASA)
    c. of alcoholic (COA)
    c. assessment schedule (CAS)
    c. behavioral study (CBS)
    C. Behavior Checklist (CBCL)
    c. behavior rating form (CBRF)
    c. chair
    chemically exposed c.
    Down syndrome c. (DSC)

NOTES

child *(continued)*
    C. Find
    C. Health and Illness Profile,
        Adolescent Edition (CHIP-AE)
    c. health questionnaire (CHQ)
    parent c.
    c. physical abuse
    c. protective agency
    C. Protective Services (CPS)
    c. restraint
    C. Sexual Behavior Inventory
        (CSBI)
    c. of substance abuser (COSA)
    C. Version of the Retrospective
        Diagnostic Interview for
        Borderlines
    very low birth weight c.
childbearing
childbed fever
child-centered literary orientation
   (CCLO)
child-directed instruction
childhood
    c. absence epilepsy
    c. accidental spiral tibial (CAST)
    alternating hemiplegia of c.
    c. anxiety
    C. Autism Rating Scale (CARS)
    C. Cancer Survivor Study
    chronic benign neutropenia of c.
    chronic bullous dermatosis of c.
    chronic bullous disease of c.
    chronic idiopathic arthritides of c.
        (CIAC)
    c. cicatricial pemphigoid
    c. disintegrative disorder (CDD)
    c. epileptic encephalopathy
    erythroblastic anemia of c.
    c. fibromyalgia
    c. idiopathic thrombocytopenic
        purpura
    localized vulvar pemphigoid of c.
        (LVPC)
    overanxious disorder of c.
    papular acrodermatitis of c. (PAC)
    progressive bulbar paralysis of c.
    c. progressive systemic sclerosis
    reactive attachment disorder of
        infancy or early c.
    recurring digital fibroma of c.
        (RDFC)
    c. schizophrenia
    c. severity of psychiatric illness
        (CSPI)
    small round blue cell tumor of c.
    c. thyroid carcinoma
    transient erythroblastopenia of c.
        (TEC)

    c. trauma questionnaire (CTQ)
    universal nose of c.
    unstable bladder of c.
childhood-onset schizophrenia (COS)
children
    c. and adults with attention deficit
        disorder (CHADD)
    Aid to Families with
        Dependent C. (AFDC)
    c. of alcoholics (COA)
    C. of Alcoholics Screening Test
        (CAST)
    Anxiety Disorder Interview for C.
    anxiety rating for c. (ARC)
    Behavioral Assessment Scale for C.
        (BASC)
    burden of care interview for c.
    Center for Epidemiological Studies
        Depression Scale for C.
    Coping Health Inventory for C.
        (CHIC)
    Developmental Programming for
        Infants and Young C.
    Diagnostic Interview Schedule
        for C. (DISC)
    Diagnostic Interview Schedule
        for C.-Revised (DISC-R)
    emergency medical services for c.
        (EMS-C)
    Functional Independence Measure
        for C. (WeeFIM)
    HIV Classification for C. (P0, P1,
        P2)
    Hospital for Sick C. (HSC)
    human immunodeficiency virus
        infected c.
    immune-competent c.
    Kaufman Assessment Battery
        for C. (KABC)
    Naldecon DX C.'s
    Neurological Examination for C.
        (NEC)
    Personality Inventory for C. (PIC)
    Schedule for Affective Disorders
        and Schizophrenia for School-
        Age C. (K-SADS)
    Silverman and Nelles Anxiety
        Disorders Interview Schedule
        for C.
    Stanford-Binet Intelligence Scale
        for C.
    State-Trait Anxiety Inventory
        for C.
    St. Joseph Aspirin-Free Cold
        Tablets for C.
    Trauma Symptom Checklist for C.
        (TSCC)
    traumatic aortic injuries in c.

treatment and education of autistic and related communications handicapped c. (TEACCH)

Tylenol Cold, C.'s

Wechsler Intelligence Scale for C. (WISC)

Wechsler Intelligence Scale for C. III (WISC-III)

Wechsler Intelligence Scale for C.-Revised (WISC-R)

C. with Special Health Care Needs (CWSN)

women, infants, c. (WIC)

Children's

C. Advil

C. Advil Suspension

C. Cancer Group (CCG)

C. Cancer Study Group (CCSG)

C. Coping Strategies Checklist (CCSC)

C. Depression Inventory (CDI)

C. Depression Rating Scale-Revised (CDRS-R)

C. Depression Scale

C. Digestive Health and Nutrition Foundation (CDHNF)

C. Global Assessment Scale (CGAS)

C. Health Insurance Program (CHIP)

C. Hold

C. Interview for Psychiatric Disorders (ChIPS)

C. Kaopectate

C. Manifest Anxiety Scale

C. Motrin

C. Motrin Suspension

C. National Medical Center

C. Silfedrine

children's service

CHIME

Collaborative Home Infant Monitoring Evaluation

CHIME study

chimeric protein

chimerism

chin

c. lift

underdeveloped c.

Chinese restaurant syndrome

CHIP

Children's Health Insurance Program

CHIP-AE

Child Health and Illness Profile, Adolescent Edition

chipmunk cheeks

ChIPS

Children's Interview for Psychiatric Disorders

Chiron branched DNA assay

chiropractic

chi square

chi-square test

Chlamydia

C. pecorum

C. pneumoniae

C. psittaci

C. sepsis

C. trachomatis (CT)

C. trachomatis pneumonia

chlamydia

chlamydial

c. conjunctivitis

c. pneumonia

c. urethritis

Chlo-Amine Oral

chloracne

chloral

c. hydrate

c. hydrate sedation

chlorambucil

chloramphenicol

Chloraseptic

Vicks Children's C.

Chlorate Oral

chlorcyclizine

chlordiazepoxide

chlorhexidine

c. gluconate

c. solution

chloride

Adrenalin C.

aluminum c.

ammonium c.

Anectine C.

calcium c.

c. channelopathy

ethyl c.

ferrous c.

Gebauer ethyl c.

isotonic sodium c.

magnesium c.

mercuric c.

obidoxime c.

NOTES

C

chloride *(continued)*
    polyvinyl c.
    potassium c. (KCl)
    sodium c.
    sweat c.
    tubocurarine c.
    vinyl c.
chloride-losing diarrhea
chloridometer
chloroma
Chloromycetin
Chloroptic Ophthalmic
chloroquine phosphate
chloroquine-resistant
    c.-r. malaria
    c.-r. *Plasmodium falciparum*
chloroquine-sensitive *Plasmodium falciparum*
chlorosis
chlorothiazide
Chlorphed
Chlorphed-LA Nasal Solution
chlorpheniramine
Chlor-Pro Injection
chlorpromazine
chlortetracycline
Chlor-Trimeton
    C.-T. Injection
    C.-T. Oral
chlorzoxazone
CHN
    congenital hypomyelinating neuropathy
choanae
    atresia c.
choanal
    c. atresia
    c. stenosis
chocolate agar
choice
    forced c.
choked disk
choke mark
Cholac
cholangiogram
    T-tube c.
cholangiography
    breath-hold MR c.
    magnetic resonance c. (MRC)
    non-breathhold MR c.
    percutaneous c.
cholangiopancreatography
    endoscopic retrograde c.
    magnetic resonance c. (MRCP)
cholangiopathy
    ascending c.
    infantile obstructive c.
    progressive obliterative c.

cholangitis
    ascending c.
    primary sclerosing c.
    recurrent c.
    sclerosing c.
    suppurative c.
cholecalciferol
    deficient hydroxylation of c.
cholecystitis
    acalculous c.
    acute acalculous c.
    hydropslike c.
cholecystokinin (CCK)
    fasting plasma c.
    postprandial plasma c.
choledochal
    c. cyst
    c. cyst-induced pancreatitis
choledochojejunostomy
    Roux-en-Y c.
choledocholithiasis
choledochus
    ductus c.
cholelithiasis
    cholesterol c.
cholera
    c. infantum
    c. vaccine
cholerae
    Vibrio c.
choleraesuis
    Salmonella c.
cholestasis
    benign familial recurrent c.
    familial intrahepatic c.
    hyperalimentation-associated c.
    intrahepatic c.
    neonatal c.
    progressive familial intrahepatic c. (PFIC)
    total parenteral nutrition-associated c.
cholestatic
    c. jaundice
    c. liver disease
    parenteral nutrition-associated c. (PNAC)
    c. syndrome
cholesteatoma
    congenital c.
cholesterol
    c. cholelithiasis
    c. ester
    c. ester storage disease (CESD)
    c. gallstone
    c. granuloma
    c. stone
    c. synthesis

cholestyramine resin
choline
    free c.
choline-magnesium trisalicylate
cholinergic
    c. crisis
    c. urticaria
cholinesterase
chondrification
chondroblastic osteosarcoma
chondroblastoma
chondrocyte
chondrodysplasia
    Jansen metaphyseal c.
    c. punctata
    rhizomelic c.
    Schmid-like metaphyseal c.
chondrodystrophia calcificans congenita
chondrodystrophic myotonia
chondrodystrophy
    myotonic c.
    primary c.
chondroectodermal dysplasia
chondroitin sulfate
chondrolysis
chondromalacia patella
chondromyxoid fibroma
chondroosteodystrophy
chondroplastic dwarfism
chondrosarcoma
Chooz
CHOP
    cyclophosphamide, hydroxydaunorubicin,
    methotrexate, prednisone
    CHOP chemotherapy
choramphenicol
chorda
    c. tympani
chordae
    c. tendineae
chordamesoderm
    caudal c.
chordee
    c. correction
    dorsal c.
    penile c.
chordoid sarcoma
chordoma
chorea
    benign nonprogressive familial c.
    Huntington c.
    c. magna

    c. minor
    Sydenham c.
chorea-acanthocytosis
choreic
    c. hand
    c. movement
choreiform movement
choreoathetoid
    c. cerebral palsy
    c. movement
choreoathetosis
    bilateral c.
    paroxysmal kinesigenic c.
choreoathetotic
    c. movement
    c. movement disorder
Chorex
chorioamnionitis (CA)
chorioamniotic infection
choriocarcinoma
choriomeningitis
    experimental lymphocytic c.
    lymphocytic c.
chorion
    smooth c.
    villous c.
chorionic
    c. cavity
    c. gonadotropin
    c. plate
    c. vessel thrombus
    c. villus biopsy
    c. villus haplotype analysis
    c. villus sampling (CVS)
chorioretinitis
    toxoplasmic c.
choroid
    c. plexus
    c. plexus carcinoma (CPC)
    c. plexus cell
    c. plexus cyst
    c. plexus papillocarcinoma
    c. plexus papilloma (CPP)
    c. plexus primordia
    c. plexus pulse effect
    c. tubercle
choroiditis
Choron
Chotzen syndrome
CHQ
    child health questionnaire

NOTES

C

Christmas
- C. disease
- C. factor
- C. tree bladder
- C. tree distribution
- C. tree distribution eruption
- C. tree pattern

Christ-Siemens-Touraine syndrome
chromaffinoma
Chroma-Pak
chromatography
- amino acid c.
- gas c.
- high-performance liquid c. (HPLC)
- high-power liquid c. (HPLC)
- high-pressure liquid c. (HPLC)
- thin-layer c. (TLC)

chromatolysis
chromhidrosis
- apocrine c.

chromium
chromophobe
chromophore
chromosomal
- c. abnormality
- c. defect
- c. deletion
- c. karyotype
- c. nondisjunction
- c. translocation

chromosome
- accessory c.
- acentric c.
- c. analysis
- B c.
- c. breakage test
- c. complement
- contiguous gene syndrome of c. 13
- c. 4 deletion
- c. 15 deletion
- fragile X c.
- heterotypical c.
- inactivated X c.
- long arm of c.
- c. microdeletion
- c. 17 mutation
- c. 1p deletion
- Philadelphia c.
- sex c.
- X c.
- Y c.

chronic
- c. active hepatitis
- c. adhesive arachnoiditis
- c. adrenal insufficiency
- c. anovulation
- c. aspiration

- c. aspiration syndrome
- c. asthma
- c. behavior problem
- c. benign neutropenia
- c. benign neutropenia of childhood
- c. biopsychosocial syndrome
- c. bullous dermatitis
- c. bullous dermatosis of childhood
- c. bullous disease of childhood
- c. chagasic cardiomyopathy
- c. compartment syndrome
- c. conjunctival infection
- c. cryptogenic hepatitis (CCH)
- c. cyanide toxicity
- c. eczematoid dermatitis
- c. fatigue syndrome (CFS)
- c. focal encephalitis
- c. Gaucher disease
- c. glomerulonephritis
- c. granulomatous amebic encephalitis
- c. granulomatous disease (CGD)
- c. headache
- c. hydrocephalus
- c. hyperreninemia
- c. hypertransfusion program
- c. hypervitaminosis A
- c. idiopathic arthritides of childhood (CIAC)
- c. idiopathic neutropenia
- c. idiopathic urticaria
- c. illness
- c. inflammatory demyelinating polyneuropathy (CIDP)
- c. inflammatory demyelinating polyradiculoneuropathy (CIDP)
- c. interstitial fibrosis
- c. intestinal pseudoobstruction
- c. intravascular hemolysis
- c. iridocyclitis
- c. ITP
- c. lung disease (CLD)
- c. lymphocytic leukemia (CLL)
- c. lymphocytic meningitis
- c. lymphocytic thyroiditis
- c. mastoiditis
- c. meningococcemia
- c. meningoradiculomyelitis
- c. mitral insufficiency
- c. motor tic disorder
- c. mucocutaneous candidiasis
- c. mumps encephalitis
- c. myelocytic leukemia
- c. myelogenous leukemia (CML)
- c. neuromuscular disease (CNMD)
- c. neuronopathic Gaucher disease
- c. non-A-E hepatitis
- c. nonspecific diarrhea

c. nonspecific diarrhea of infancy
c. nonspherocytic hemolytic anemia
c. obstructive bronchitis
c. osteomyelitis
c. otitis media (COM)
c. pancreatitis
c. papilledema
c. parvoviral infection
c. peripheral neuropathy
c. pneumonitis of infancy (CPI)
c. progressive ataxia
c. progressive encephalitis
c. progressive external
  ophthalmoplegia (CPEO)
c. pulmonary disease
c. pulmonary histoplasmosis
c. pulmonary insufficiency
c. pupillary syndrome
c. pyogenic lymphadenitis
c. recurrent multifocal osteomyelitis
  (CRMO)
c. rejection
c. relapsing polyradiculoneuropathy
c. renal failure (CRF)
c. renal insufficiency
c. respiratory acidosis
c. SCFE
c. schistosomiasis
c. sickle cell lung disease
c. sinusitis
c. spongiform encephalopathy
c. subglottic stenosis
c. suppurative otitis media (CSOM)
c. synovial inflammation
c. syphilitic meningitis
c. tic
c. tic disorder (CTD)
c. tonsillar herniation
c. unremitting
  polyradiculoneuropathy
c. vitamin A intoxication
chronica
  pityriasis lichenoides et c. (PLC)
chronicus
  lichen simplex c.
chronograph
chronological age
chronotherapy
  phase delay c.
chronotropic
  c. effect
  c. response

chronotropy
Chronulac
CHRS
  cerebrohepatorenal syndrome
Chryseobacterium
Chrysosporium
CHTN
  Cooperative Human Tissue Network
Chuen-Lin herbal tea
Churg-Strauss
  C.-S. syndrome
  C.-S. vasculitis
Chvostek sign
chyle
chyliform
chylomicron
  c. formation
  c. retention disease
chylomicronemia syndrome
chylopericardium
chylothorax
  congenital c.
chylous
  c. ascites
  c. liquid
  c. pleural effusion
chymopapain
CIAC
  chronic idiopathic arthritides of
  childhood
Cibacalcin
CIC
  clean intermittent catheterization
Cicatrene
cicatricial
  c. alopecia
  c. lesion
  c. retinal disease
cicatrix
CID
  combined immunodeficiency
  cytomegalic inclusion disease
cidofovir
CIDP
  chronic inflammatory demyelinating
  polyneuropathy
  chronic inflammatory demyelinating
  polyradiculoneuropathy
CIE
  counterimmunoelectrophoresis
Ciel
  Kay C.

NOTES

cigarette smoke
ciguatera
  c. fish poisoning
  c. intoxication
cilastatin
  imipenem and c.
cilia (*pl. of* cilium)
ciliaris
  tylosis c.
ciliary
  c. biopsy
  c. blush
  c. dyskinesia
  c. dysmotility
  c. flush
  c. function
  c. muscle
  c. nerve
  c. neurotrophic factor (CNTF)
  c. paralysis
  c. spasm
cilium, pl. **cilia**
  immotile c.
Ciloxan
  C. Ophthalmic
  C. ophthalmic solution
cimetidine
cineangiocardiography
  biplane c.
cineangiogram
  continuous c.
cineangiography
  radionuclide c.
cine magnetic resonance imaging (cine-
  MRI)
cine-MRI
  cine magnetic resonance imaging
cineradiography
cingulate gyrus
C1INH coagulation inhibitor
Cipro
  C. HC Otic
  C. Injection
  C. Oral
ciprofloxacin hydrochloride
circadian
  c. rhythm
  c. rhythm dyssomnia
circinate balanitis
circle
  c. of Willis
  c. of Willis aneurysm
circling disease
circuit
  failed Fontan c.
circular reaction
circulating
  c. anticoagulant

  c. fetal cell
  c. neutrophils
circulation
  airway, breathing, c. (ABC)
  collateral c.
  ductal-dependent systemic c.
  duct-dependent pulmonary c.
  duct-dependent systemic c.
  extracorporeal c.
  fetal-placental c.
  fetal pulmonary c.
  parallel c.
  persistence of fetal c.
  persistent fetal c. (PFC)
circulation-cavopulmonary connection
circulatory
  c. arrest
  c. collapse
  c. system
circumcision
  pharaonic c.
  c. status
  Sunna c.
circumduction
  c. gait
  c. movement
circumference
  arm c.
  head c. (HC)
  mean arm muscle c. (MAMC)
  midarm c. (MAC)
  midarm muscle c. (MAMC)
  occipitofrontal c. (OFC)
circumferential
  c. burn
  c. eversion
  c. eversion of urethral epithelium
circumflex
circumflexa
  ichthyosis linearis c.
circummarginate placenta
circumoral pallor
circumscribed neurodermatitis
circumscripta
  myositis ossificans c.
circumscriptum
  angiokeratoma c.
  lymphangioma c.
circumvallate placenta
cirrhonosus
cirrhosis
  biliary c.
  compensated c.
  cryptogenic c.
  decompensated c.
  endemic Tyrolean infantile c.
  end-stage c.
  hepatic c.

Indian childhood c. (ICC)
liver c.
macronodular c.
micronodular liver c.
postnecrotic c.
primary biliary c. (PBC)
progressive biliary c.
pseudolobular c.
cirsoid aneurysm
cisapride
cis-**atracurium**
cisplatin, 5-fluorouracil, leucovorin calcium (CFL)
cistern
basal c.
chiasmatic c.
cisternal puncture
cisterna magna
cisternography
radioisotope c.
citalopram
citizen
Association for Retarded C.'s (ARC)
Citracal
citrate
c. blood sample
caffeine c.
c. and citric acid
diphenhydramine c.
fentanyl c.
lithium c.
magnesium c.
oral transmucosal fentanyl c. (OTFC)
c. toxicity
citric acid cycle
Citrobacter
C. amalonaticus
C. braakii
C. diversus
C. farmeri
C. freundii
C. koseri
C. sedlakii
C. werkmanii
C. youngae
citrulline
plasma c.
citrullinemia
citrullinuria

C-IV
Pemoline C-IV
CJD
Creutzfeldt-Jakob disease
iatrogenic CJD
new variant CJD
CK
creatine kinase
CK-MB
myocardial muscle creatine kinase isoenzyme
CLA
conjugated linoleic acid
Cladosporium
cladribine
Claforan
clamp
DeBakey aortic c.
Gomco c.
Hoffmann c.
Mogen c.
pediatric bulldog c.
pediatric vascular c.
CLAMS
Clinical Linguistic and Auditory Milestone Scale
clamshell-type catheter occlusion device
Clara cell 16 protein
Clarion hearing implant
clarithromycin
Claritin
C. RediTab
C. syrup
Clarke column
Clarke-Hadfield syndrome
Clark mechanistic classification
clasp-knife
c.-k. phenomenon
c.-k. response
classic
c. celiac disease
c. medulloblastoma
c. migraine
c. migraine headache
c. plaque psoriasis
classical
c. lissencephaly
c. migraine
classification
Abramson c.
Angle c.
Catterall c. (grade 1–4)

NOTES

C

classification *(continued)*
    Clark mechanistic c.
    de la Cruz c.
    Delbet fracture c. (types I–IV)
    EULAR c.
    European League Against
      Rheumatism c.
    FAB classification
    French-American-British c.
    HIV c.
    ILAR peripheral arthritis c.
    International League Against
      Rheumatism peripheral arthritis c.
    King c.
    PAAS c.
    Pediatric Acute Admission
      Severity c.
    Reese-Ellsworth c.
    Risser c.
    Rye c.
    Salter-Harris c.
    Schuknecht c.
    Sillence c. of osteogenesis
      imperfecta (type I, IA, IB, II,
      III, IV, IVA, IVB)
    Zero to Three diagnostic c.
clastic lesion
clastogenic stress
Clatworthy mesocaval shunt
clavicle
clavicular
    c. fracture
    c. injury
    c. shaft
claviculectomy
    distal c.
clavulanate
    c. potassium
    ticarcillin c.
clawfoot
clawhand
    c. deformity
    c. deformity repair
    lobster c.
clawing
clawtoe
clay
    green c.
CLD
    chronic lung disease
    cytoplasmic lipid droplet
clean-catch technique
clean intermittent catheterization (CIC)
clean-out
    bowel c.-o.
Clear
clear
    C. Away Disc
    c. cell sarcoma
    C. Eyes
    c. mucoid sputum
    Scot-Tussin Senior C.
    C. Tussin 30
clearance
    creatinine c.
    mucociliary c.
    xenon c.
clear-cell adenocarcinoma
clearing
    throat c.
cleavage syndrome
cleft
    bilateral schizencephalic c.
    branchial c.
    complete c.
    c. hand
    incomplete c.
    intergluteal c.
    laryngeal c.
    laryngotracheoesophageal c.
    c. lip
    c. lip-nasal reconstruction
    c. lip and palate (CLP)
    nasal alar cartilage c.
    c. nasal deformity correction
    orofacial c.
    c. palate (CP)
    c. palate repair
    postalveolar c.
    c. premaxillary process
    submucous c.
    syndromic c.
cleidocranial
    c. dysplasia
    c. dysplasia syndrome
    c. dystosis
clemastine
clenched fist injury
Cleocin
CLIA
    Clinical Laboratory Improvements
    Amendments
click
    aortic ejection c.
    ejection c.
    hip c.
    midsystolic c.
    pulmonary ejection c.
    c. stimulus
Clifford syndrome
Climara Transdermal
clindamycin
Clindoxyl
clinical
    C. Adaptive Test (CAT)

C. Adaptive Test/Clinical Linguistic and Auditory Milestone Scale (CAT/CLAMS)
c. assessment in neuropsychology
c. cohort study
C. Colitis Activity Index (CCAI)
C. Evaluation of Language Fundamentals-Preschool
C. Evaluation of Language Fundamentals, 3rd edition
C. Global Impairment scale
C. Global Impressions (CGI)
C. Global Impressions scale
C. Global Improvement scale
c. global index (CGI)
c. grouping
C. Laboratory Improvements Amendments (CLIA)
C. Linguistic and Auditory Milestone Scale (CLAMS)
c. risk assessment (CRA)
C. Risk Index for Babies (CRIB)
c. type
clinically significant arrhythmia (CSA)
Clinitest assay
clinodactyly
Clinoril
clioquinol
clip
Fentendo c.
Filshie c.
Hulka c.
Clistin
clitoral
c. hypertrophy
c. length
clitoridectomy
clitoris
bifid c.
glans c.
c. tourniquet syndrome (CTS)
clivus, pl. **clivi**
inferior c.
CLL
chronic lymphocytic leukemia
CLO
congenital lobar overinflation
cloaca
cloacae
Enterobacter c.
cloacal
c. exstrophy

c. extrophy
c. membrane
c. plate anomaly
cloaking
periosteal c.
clobetasol propionate
Clocort Maximum Strength
clodronate
clofazimine
clomipramine hydrochloride
clonazepam
clone
clonic
c. movement
c. seizure
clonidine hydrochloride
cloning
functional c.
clonorchiasis
Clonorchis sinensis
clonus
sustained c.
clopamide
Clopra
clorazepate
closed
c. bite
c. comedo
c. endotracheal suctioning
c. endotracheal tube suctioning
c. head injury (CHI)
c. thoracotomy
closed-circuit video recording
closed-loop
c.-l. obstruction
c.-l. system passing electrode
closing
c. capacity (CC)
c. volume (CV)
clostridia (*pl. of* clostridium)
clostridial
c. bacteremia
c. myonecrosis
c. otitis media
c. toxin
Clostridium
C. *botulinum*
C. *botulinum* type A toxin
C. botulism
C. *difficile*
C. *difficile*-associated diarrhea (CDAC)

C

NOTES

105

Clostridium (continued)
>   C. freundii
>   C. perfringens
>   C. ramosum
>   C. septicum
>   C. spiroforme
>   C. tetani

clostridium, pl. **clostridia**
>   clostridia septicemia

closure
>   anterior neural tube c.
>   bilabial c.
>   delayed primary c.
>   ductus c.
>   early midsystolic c.
>   Gestalt c.
>   hysterical glottic c.
>   laryngeal c.
>   lip c.
>   neural tube c.
>   neurosurgical c.
>   palatal fistula c.
>   percutaneous patent ductus
>   arteriosus c.
>   physeal c.
>   posterior neural tube c.
>   premature c.
>   primary c.
>   secondary c.
>   tertiary c.
>   transcatheter c. (TCC)
>   ventricular septal defect patch c.

clot
>   friable c.

clotrimazole troche

clouding
>   corneal c.
>   infantile corneal c.
>   c. of lesion
>   mental c.
>   c. of sensorium

cloudy
>   c. cornea
>   c. mastoid
>   c. sputum

Clouston syndrome

cloverleaf
>   c. skull deformity
>   c. skull syndrome

cloxacillin

Cloxapen

clozapine

CLP
>   cleft lip and palate

CLS
>   capillary leak syndrome

CLSE
>   calf lung surfactant extract

CLTM
>   continuous long-term monitoring

club

clubbing
>   digital c.
>   c. of nails

clubfoot (CF)
>   adductus c.
>   arthrogrypotic c.
>   c. cast
>   congenital c.
>   c. deformity
>   c. dysplasia
>   equinus c.
>   idiopathic c.
>   medial rotation c.
>   neurogenic c.
>   positional c.
>   rigid c.
>   c. splint
>   Turco posteromedial release of c.
>   varus c.

clubhand
>   radial c.
>   ulnar c.

clue cell

clumsiness

clumsy child syndrome

clunk
>   hip c.

cluster
>   c. B disorder
>   c. of differentiation (CD)
>   c. of differentiation 4 (CD4)
>   c. of differentiation 4
>   immunoglobulin G (CD4-IgG)
>   c. headache

cluster-stratified sampling method

cluttering

Clutton joint

Clysodrast

CMA
>   cow's milk allergy

CMD
>   congenital muscular dystrophy
>   Fukuyama CMD

CMFTD
>   congenital muscle fiber-type
>   disproportion

cm H$_2$O
>   centimeters of water

CMI
>   cell-mediated immunity

CML
>   chronic myelogenous leukemia

CMV
>   cytomegalovirus

CMV enteritis
CMV retinitis
CMVIG
cytomegalovirus immune globulin
CMV-IGIV
cytomegalovirus immune globulin
intravenous
CMV-seronegative transplant patient
CN
calcaneonavicular
CNEP
continuous negative extrathoracic
pressure
CNF
congenital nephrotic syndrome, Finnish
CNLDO
congenital nasolacrimal duct obstruction
CNMD
chronic neuromuscular disease
CNPAS
congenital nasal pyriform aperture
stenosis
CNS
central nervous system
CNS aneurysm
CNS dysfunction
CNS hemorrhage
CNS infarction
CNS leukemia
CNS malignancy
primary angiitis of CNS (PACNS)
CNS tumor
CNTF
ciliary neurotrophic factor
CO
carbon monoxide
end-tidal CO
Co$_2$
carbon dioxide
end-tidal CO$_2$
pressure of CO$_2$ (PCO$_2$)
COA
child of alcoholic
children of alcoholics
CoA
aortic arch coarctation
coenzyme A
enzyme CoA

COACH
cerebellar vermis hypoplasia,
oligophrenia, congenital ataxia,
coloboma, hepatic fibrosis
COACH syndrome
coach's finger
Coactin
coactivated antagonists
coadministration
coagulase
coagulase-negative (CoNS)
c.-n. bacteremia
c.-n. *Staphylococcus*
coagulase-positive *Staphylococcus*
coagulation
c. cascade
disseminated intravascular c. (DIC)
c. study
coagulative myocytolysis
coagulopathy
consumption c.
consumptive c.
coagulum
necrotic c.
coalescent mastoiditis
coalition
calcaneonavicular c.
cartilaginous c.
congenital tarsal c.
fibrinous c.
osseous c.
tarsal c.
coal tar
coarctation
abdominal c.
c. of aorta
aortic c.
aortic arch c. (CoA)
complex c.
juxtaductal aortic c.
postductal c.
preductal c.
recurrent c.
residual c.
simple c.
coarse
c. facial features
c. tremor
coat
buffy c.
lipopolysaccharide c.

NOTES

C

Coat-a-Count neonatal 17
  hydroxyprogesterone kit
Coats disease
coaxial flow
cobalamin (Cbl)
    c. adenosyltransferase
    c. reductase deficiency
cobalt poisoning
Cobas fast centrifugal analyzer
Cobb
    C. measurement technique
    C. method
    C. syndrome
cobblestone
    c. appearance
    c. sessile polyp
cobblestoning of conjunctiva
co-bedding
Cobex
coca
    Erythroxylum c.
cocaine
    crack c.
    freebase c.
    c. hydrochloride powder
    liquified powder c.
    c. test
    tetracaine, adrenaline, c. (TAC)
    tetracaine, epinephrine, c.
coccidioidal
    c. granuloma
    c. placentitis
Coccidioides immitis
coccidioidin reaction
coccidioidomycosis
    disseminated c.
    c. meningitis
coccidiomycosis
coccobacillus
    HACEK c.
coccygeal fracture
coccyx
cochlea
cochlear
    c. aqueduct
    c. implant
Cochran-Mantel-Haenszel test
Cockayne syndrome (A, B)
Cockayne-Touraine variant of dominant
  dystrophic epidermolysis bullosa
cock-robin
    c.-r. position
    c.-r. sign
cocktail
    c. chatter
    lytic c.
    c. party patter

codeine
    Fioricet With C.
    guaifenesin and c.
    Guiatussin With C.
    Mallergan-VC With C.
    Phenergan VC With C.
    Pherazine With C.
    promethazine, phenylephrine, c.
    Tylenol With C.
    Tylenol With C. No. 2, 3, 4
codfish vertebra
coding
    phonological c.
Codman triangle
Codoxy
coefficient
    c. of fat absorption
    intraclass correlation c.
    K c.
    kappa c.
    Kendall c.
    Pearson correlation c.
    Spearman c.
coelom
coelomic cavity
coenzyme A (CoA)
coenzyme Q10
coercive feeding
coeur en sabot
cofactor
    c. deficiency
    heparin c. II (HCII)
    molybdenum c.
    tetrahydrobiopterin c. (BH$_4$)
coffee-ground
    c.-g. drainage
    c.-g. emesis
    c.-g. hematemesis
    c.-g. material
Coffin-Lowry syndrome
Coffin-Siris
    C.-S. defect
    C.-S. syndrome
COFS
    cerebrooculofacial-skeletal
    COFS syndrome
Cogan
    congenital ocular motor apraxia
      type C. (COMA)
    C. syndrome
Cogentin
Co-Gesic
cognition
    spatial c.
cognitive
    c. ability
    c. behavior
    c. behavioral therapy (CBT)

c. deficiency
c. delay
c. developmental milestone
c. disability
c. domain
c. therapy
c. toxicity
cognitive-behavioral psychotherapy
cognitive-diathesis model
cognitive-stress diathesis
cohabitation
Cohen
C. procedure
C. syndrome
C. transtrigonal technique
Cohens criteria
cohesion
lexical c.
referential c.
cohort
Dunedin birth c.
c. study
coil
Dacron fiber-coated c.
DuctOcclud c.
MRCP using HASTE with a
phased array c.
c. occlusion
coin
esophageal c.
c. lesion
coinfection
beta-hemolytic streptococcal c.
coining
coital contact
coitarche
Coke-colored urine
COL7A1 gene
COLA
Commission on Office Laboratory
Accreditation
Colace
cola-colored urine
Co-Lav
colchicine
cold
c. abscess
c. agglutinin
c. agglutinin disease
c. antibody
common c.
c. hemagglutinin disease

c. intolerance
c. nodule
c. panniculitis
c. stress
c. urticaria
c. water near drowning
cold-adapted influenza virus vaccine,
trivalent (CAIV-T)
cold-attenuated intranasal influenza
vaccine (CAIV)
cold-induced myotonia
Coldloc
colectomy
Cole-Hughes macrocephaly-mental
retardation syndrome
colfosceril palmitate
coli
ampicillin-resistant *Escherichia c.*
Balantidium c.
Campylobacter c.
enterohemorrhagic *Escherichia c.*
(EHEC)
enteropathogenic *Escherichia c.*
(EPEC)
enterotoxigenic *Escherichia c.*
(ETEC)
Escherichia c.
familial adenomatous polyposis c.
hemorrhagic *Escherichia c.*
pterygium c.
Shiga toxin-producing
Escherichia c. (STEC)
colic
biliary c.
infantile c.
Monday morning c.
non-Wessel c.
Wessel c.
colicky abdominal pain
coliform
c. bacteria
c. organism
colistin
colitis
acute fulminant c.
acute infectious c.
allergic c.
amebic c.
Crohn c.
eosinophilic allergic c.
fulminant ulcerative c.
granulomatous c.

C

NOTES

colitis *(continued)*
    hemorrhagic c.
    Hirschsprung c.
    infectious c.
    inflammatory c.
    mild ulcerative c.
    moderate ulcerative c.
    necrotizing c.
    protein-induced eosinophilic c.
      (PEC)
    pseudomembranous c.
    steroid-dependent c.
    tuberculous c.
    ulcerative c.
collaborative
    C. Home Infant Monitoring
      Evaluation (CHIME)
    C. Home Infant Monitoring
      Evaluation study
    C. Perinatal Study (CPS)
collagen
    C-terminal propeptide of type I c.
    c. I, III, IV, V, X
    c. vascular disease
    c. vascular disorder
collagenosis
    reactive perforating c. (RPC)
collapse
    acute circulatory c.
    cardiovascular c.
    circulatory c.
collapse-consolidation lesion
collar
    c. button ulcer
    cervical c.
    Philadelphia c.
    sebaceous c.
collarette of rash
collateral
    c. circulation
    c. ligament stability
    systemic venous c. (SSVC)
collateralization
    coronary c.
collection
    24-hour urine c.
    72-hour stool c.
    first-morning urine c.
    subphrenic gas c.
colliculus, pl. **colliculi**
    inferior c.
collimation
    pinhole c.
collimator
collinearity
Collins law
collodion baby
colloid cyst

coloboma
    congenital iris c.
    c., heart disease, atresia choanae,
      retarded growth, genital
      anomalies, ear anomalies
      (CHARGE)
    c., heart disease, atresia choanae,
      retarded growth and retarded
      development, CNS anomalies,
      genital hypoplasia, ear anomalies
      and/or deafness (CHARGE)
    ocular c.
colobomatous defect
colocecal bladder augmentation
colocolic intussusception
colon
    aganglionic c.
    cathartic c.
    giant c.
    nervous c.
    c. pouch
    spastic c.
colonic
    c. B-cell lymphoma
    c. conduit diversion
    c. dysmotility
    c. interposition
    c. plug
    c. polyp
    c. polyposis
    c. stasis
    c. stricture
colonization
    stool c.
colonopathy
    fibrosing c.
colonoscopy
    surveillance c.
colony count
colony-forming unit (CFU)
colony-stimulating factor
color
    c. analog scale
    c. Doppler flow imaging (CDFI)
    flight of c.
    C. Trails Test
    c. vision
Colorado tick fever
color-coded duplex Doppler
3-color immunofluorescence
ColorMate TLc BiliTest System
colostomy
    diverting c.
    double-barrel c.
    c. formation
    protective c.
    transverse loop c.
colostration

colostrum
Colovage
colposcopic examination
Columbia Impairment Scale
column
    Clarke c.
    spinal c.
    vertebral c.
Coly-Mycin
CoLyte
CoLyte-Flavored
COM
    chronic otitis media
COMA
    congenital ocular motor apraxia type
    Cogan
    cyclophosphamide, Oncovin,
    methotrexate, arabinosylcytosine
coma
    diabetic c.
    hepatic c.
    hyperammonemic hepatic c.
    hyperosmolar c.
    myxedema c.
    nonketotic hyperosmolar c.
    pentobarbital c.
comatose
combat crawl
combination
    apnea-hypopnea c.
    consonant-vowel c.
    C-V c.
    xanthan/guar c.
combined
    c. immunodeficiency (CID)
    c. nevus
Combitude
Comby sign
comedo, pl. comedos, comedones
    closed c.
    comedones extractor
    open c.
comedonicus
    nevus c.
Comfort Ophthalmic
comitant strabismus
commando crawl
comma-shaped organism
comminuted fracture
Commission on Office Laboratory
  Accreditation (COLA)

commissural
    c. lip pit
    c. separation
commissure
commissurotomy
committee
    National Vaccine Advisory C.
    (NVAC)
common
    c. atrium
    c. blue nevus
    c. channel
    c. cold
    c. hepatic duct
    c. migraine
    c. migraine headache
    c. sheath reimplant
    c. variable hypogammaglobulinemia
    c. variable immunodeficiency (CVI,
    CVID)
    c. wart
common-inlet single right ventricle
commotio
    c. cordis
    c. retinae
communal traumatic experiences
  inventory (CTEI)
communicable
    c. disease
    C. Disease Center (CDC)
    c. illness
communicating hydrocephalus
communication
    c. aid
    augmentative and alternative c.
    (AAC)
    c. board
    c. book
    c. disorder
    c. domain
    facilitated c. (F/C)
    fistulous vascular c.
    interatrial c. (IAC)
    nonverbal c.
    total c.
Communication-Handicapped
    Project Treatment and Education of
    Autistic and Related C.-H.
communicative development inventory
community-acquired (CA)
comorbid anxiety disorder

C

NOTES

comorbidity
    psychological c.
COMP
    cartilage oligomeric matrix protein
    cyclophosphamide, Oncovin,
      methotrexate, prednisone
      COMP drug regimen
Companion 318 Nasal CPAP System
comparison view
compartment
    adductor interosseous c.
    calcaneal c.
    extracellular fluid c.
    lateral c.
    medial c.
    superficial c.
    c. syndrome
compartmentalization
compassionate use
Compazine
compensated
    c. cirrhosis
    c. hydrocephalus
    c. shock
compensatory
    c. antiinflammatory syndrome
    c. articulation
    c. erythropoiesis
    c. gliosis
    c. movement
    c. scoliosis
competence
    cultural c.
competing anion
complaint
    psychosomatic c.
    somatic c.
Compleat
    C. Modified formula
    C. Pediatric formula
complement
    c. chemotactic factor
    chromosome c.
    c. C3 level
    c. deficiency
    c. deposition
    c. fixation
    c. fixation test
    hemolytic c. (CH_{50})
    c. receptor (CR1)
    serum c.
    total hemolytic c.
complementary
    c. and alternative medicine (CAM)
    c. deoxyribonucleic acid (cDNA)
    c. DNA (cDNA)
complement-fixing serum antibody

complete
    amphotericin B lipid c.
    c. blood count (CBC)
    c. cerebellar aplasia
    c. cleft
    c. cord transection
    c. DiGeorge syndrome
    c. fracture
    c. hernia
    c. radial aplasia
    c. rectal prolapse
    c. subtalar release (CSTR)
    c. suppression pattern
    c. transposition
    c. transposition of great arteries
    c. transposition of great vessels
    c. vulvar duplication
complex
    amphotericin B lipid c.
    amyotrophic lateral sclerosis-
      Parkinson-dementia c.
    antigen-antibody c.
    blocked premature atrial c.
    c. coarctation
    C. 15 cream
    disseminated *Mycobacterium*
      avium c. (DMAC)
    Eisenmenger c.
    c. enteral feeding
    epispadias-exstrophy c.
    c. febrile seizure
    gene c.
    generalized bilaterally synchronous
      sharp-wave and slow-wave c.'s
    Ghon c.
    c. heart defect
    human factor IX c.
    immune c. (IC)
    iron dextran c.
    lap belt c.
    lateral collateral ligament c.
    limb-body wall c. (LBWC)
    major histocompatibility c. (MHC)
    membrane attack c.
    c. motor tic
    Mycobacterium avium c. (MAC)
    Mycobacterium avium-
      intracellulare c. (MAC)
    Mycobacterium fortuitum c.
    c. myoclonic epilepsy
    ostiomeatal c.
    c. partial epilepsy
    c. partial seizure (CPS)
    c. partial status epilepticus
    QRS c.
    QS c.
    Rh c.
    sicca c.

c. syndactyly
triangular fibrocartilaginous c. (TFCC)
tuberous sclerosis c. (TSC)
c. unroofed coronary sinus (CUCS)
c. vocal tic
von Meyenburg c.

compliance
pulmonary c.
tympanic membrane c.

complicated
c. gastroesophageal reflux
c. meconium ileus
c. migraine
c. migraine headache

complication
end-organ c.
late c.

Comply formula
compomelic dwarfism
component
diastolic c.
systolic c.
terminal complement c.

composite allograft
composition
body c.

compound
artificial lung-expanding compound (ALEC)
c. nevus
pteridine ring c.
C. W

Compoz
C. Gel Caps
C. Nighttime Sleep Aid

compressed air-driven nebulizer
compression
brainstem c.
cerebral c.
cervicomedullary c.
chest c.
c. fracture
c. injury
intrauterine c.
joint c.
c. myelopathy
spinal cord c.
tracheobronchial c.
vertebral artery c.

compression-rarefaction strain

compressor
Pari Proneb Turbo c.

compromise
angiitic luminal c.
microcirculatory c.
neurovascular c.
severe respiratory c.

compulsion
compulsive
c. echolalia
c. self-mutilation

computed
c. axial tomography (CAT)
c. tomography (CT)
c. tomography scan

computer-assisted axial tomography (CAAT)
computerized
C. Diagnostic Interview for Children and Adolescents (cDICA, C-DICA)
c. tomographic scan
c. tomography scanning

Comtrex Cough Formula
Comvax vaccine
conal muscle
concave temporalis muscle
concavity
concealed
c. penis
c. rectal prolapse

conceive
PreCare C.

concentrate
protein C. c.

concentrated
c. oral sucrose
c. urine

concentration
alpha-tocopherol c.
anti-HBs c.
bicarbonate c.
cord blood leptin c.
cord leptin c.
cortisol c.
elevated sweat chloride c.
fetal leptin c.
fetal thrombopoietin c.
glucose c.
hemoglobin c.
hepatic iron c. (HIC)
hydrogen in c. (pH)

NOTES

C

concentration *(continued)*
intracellular hydrogen ion c. (pHi)
mean cell hemoglobin c. (MCHC)
mean corpuscular hemoglobin c.
(MCHC)
minimal bacterial c. (MBC)
minimal inhibitory c. (MIC)
minimum inhibitory c.
plasma amino acid c.
plasma bilirubin c. (PBC)
plasma histamine c.
plasma phosphate c.
plasma retinol c.
plasma theophylline c.
plasma vitamin A c.
platelet c.
pulmonary tissue c. (PTC)
serum albumin c.
serum amino acid c.
serum ferritin c.
serum inhibit B c.
serum lactate dehydrogenase c.
serum melatonin c.
serum protein c.
sweat chloride c.
concentric
c. amyloid body
c. sclerosis
concentrica
encephalitis periaxialis c.
concept
conceptus
Concerta
concha bullosa
concisus
Campylobacter c.
concomitans
strabismus c.
concomitant
concordance
concussion
labyrinthine c.
spinal c.
condition
nonangiitic vasculopathic c.
nonvertiginous c.
Questionnaire for Identifying
Children with Chronic C.'s
(QuICCC)
vertiginous c.
conditioned orientation reflex (COR)
conditioning regimen
condom
conductance
airway c.
conduct disorder (CD)
conduction
antidromic c.

c. defect
orthodromic c.
conductive
c. education (CE)
c. hearing impairment
c. hearing loss
c. tissue
conductivity
total body electrical c. (TOBEC)
conduit
fetal vascular c.
homograft c.
ileal c.
condyle
lateral c.
medial c.
condyloma, pl. **condylomata**
c. acuminatum
condylomata lata
vulvar c.
Condylox solution
confetti lesion
configuration
brachycephalic c.
hourglass c.
conflict
confluent
c. eyebrows
c. plaque
confusion
postictal c.
confusional
c. arousal
c. migraine
congenita
alopecia totalis c.
amyotonia c.
aplasia axialis extracorticalis c.
aplasia cutis c.
arthrogryposis multiplex c.
bitemporal aplasia cutis c.
chondrodystrophia calcificans c.
cutis marmorata telangiectatica c.
dyskeratosis c.
erythropoietic porphyria c.
myotonia c.
pachyonychia c.
paramyotonia c.
spondyloepiphyseal dysplasia c.
Thomsen myotonia c.
X-linked dyskeratosis c.
congenital
c. abducens facial paralysis
c. absence
c. absence of iron-binding protein
c. absence of lactase
c. absence of vas deferens
(CAVD)

c. adrenal hyperplasia (CAH)
c. adrenal lipoid hyperplasia
c. aganglionic megacolon
c. aleukia
c. alveolar dysplasia
c. alveolar proteinosis
c. amblyogenic stimulus
c. AME
c. amegakaryocytic thrombocytopenia
c. amputation
c. anemia of newborn
c. anemia syndrome
c. anomaly
c. anterolateral tibial angulation
c. aortic stenosis
c. aplastic anemia
c. asplenia
c. atelectasis
c. athetosis
c. atransferrinemia
c. atresia of bile duct
c. atresia of uterine cervix
c. aural atresia
c. bilateral cataract
c. bronchiectasis
c. bronchopulmonary malformation
c. bullous urticaria pigmentosa
c. candidiasis
c. cardiac disease
c. cardiovascular malformation (CCVM)
c. central hypoventilation
c. central hypoventilation syndrome (CCHS)
c. cerebral aneurysm
c. choledochal dilation
c. cholesteatoma
c. chylothorax
c. clubfoot
c. complete AV block
c. complete heart block (CCHB)
c. condylar deformity
c. contractural arachnodactyly (CCA)
c. corneal dystrophy
c. cutaneous candidosis
c. cutis aplasia
c. cystic adenomatoid malformation (CCAM)
c. cystic adenomatoid malfunction
c. cytomegalovirus

c. defect of phosphofructokinase
c. diaphragmatic hernia (CDH)
c. diaphragmatic hernia of Bochdalek
c. dislocation
c. dislocation of hip (CDH)
c. dislocation of patella
c. duodenal atresia
c. dyserythropoietic anemia (CDA)
c. ectodermic scalp defect
c. elephantiasis
c. enamel abnormality
c. erythropoietic porphyria (CEP)
c. esophageal stenosis
c. esotropia
c. eventration
c. extremity lymphedema
c. familial lymphedema with ocular findings
c. fibrosarcoma
c. fibular hemimelia
c. generalized lipodystrophy
c. generalized phlebectasia
c. glaucoma
c. glenoid dysplasia
c. goitrous hypothyroidism
c. growth hormone deficiency
c. Guillain-Barré syndrome
c. hearing loss
c. heart defect
c. heart defect syndrome
c. heart disease (CHD)
c. Heinz body anemia
c. hemidysplasia with ichthyosiform erythroderma and limb defects (CHILD)
c. hemiparesis
c. hemiplegia
c. hepatic fibrosis
c. hereditary retinoschisis
c. herpes
c. heterochromia
c. high airway obstruction syndrome (CHAOS)
c. hip disease
c. hip disorder
c. hip dysplasia (CDH)
c. hydronephrosis
c. hypertrophic pyloric stenosis
c. hypogammaglobulinemia
c. hypogonadotropic hypogonadism
c. hypomagnesemia

NOTES

C

115

congenital *(continued)*

c. hypomyelinating neuropathy (CHN)
c. hypopituitarism
c. hypoplasia
c. hypoplastic anemia
c. hypothyroidism (CH)
c. hypothyroidism syndrome
c. hypotonia
c. ichthyosiform
c. ichthyosiform erythroderma
c. ichthyosis
c. insensitivity
c. insensitivity to pain
c. intestinal aganglionosis
c. intestinal band
c. intrinsic factor deficiency
c. iris coloboma
c. jerky nystagmus
c. kyphosis
c. lacrimal duct obstruction
c. lactase deficiency
c. lactic acidosis
c. laryngeal stridor
c. laxity of ligament
c. LCMV syndrome
c. lesion
c. lethal hypophosphatasia
c. leukemia
c. lipase/colipase deficiency
c. lip pit
c. lobar emphysema
c. lobar overinflation (CLO)
c. longitudinal deficiency
c. longitudinal deficiency of fibula
c. longitudinal deficiency of tibia
c. long QT syndrome
c. lymphedema
c. macular degeneration
c. melanocytic nevus
c. mesoblastic nephroma
c. metatarsus adductus
c. metatarsus varus
c. microvillus atrophy
c. miosis
c. multiple myofibromatosis
c. muscle fiber-type disproportion (CMFTD)
c. muscular dystrophy (CMD)
c. muscular torticollis
c. myasthenia
c. myasthenia gravis
c. mydriasis
c. myopathy
c. myotonic dystrophy
c. nasal pyriform aperture stenosis (CNPAS)

c. nasolacrimal duct obstruction (CNLDO)
c. neonatal ascites
c. nephrotic syndrome
c. nephrotic syndrome, Finnish (CNF)
c. nerve deafness
c. neutropenia
c. nonhemolytic unconjugated hyperbilirubinemia
c. nonspherocytic hemolytic anemia
c. obstruction of nasolacrimal duct
c. ocular motor apraxia
c. ocular motor apraxia type Cogan (COMA)
c. oculofacial paralysis
c. osteopetrosis
c. palatopharyngeal incompetence (CPI)
c. paretic neurosyphilis
c. paroxysmal atrial tachycardia
c. pendular nystagmus
c. perilymphatic fistula
c. peritoneal band
c. pernicious anemia
c. photosensitive porphyria
c. pigmental nevus
c. pneumonia
c. portosystemic venous shunt
c. posteromedial bowing
c. posteromedial tibial angulation
c. pseudarthrosis
c. pseudoarthrosis
c. pseudoarthrosis of tibia
c. pulmonary lymphangiectasia
c. pulmonary lymphangiectasis
c. RBC aplasia
c. rocker-bottom foot
c. rubella
c. rubella infection
c. rubella syndrome (CRS)
c. scoliosis
c. sensory neuropathy
c. sideroblastic anemia
c. skin aplasia
c. sodium diarrhea
c. spherocytosis
c. stationary night blindness
c. stippled epiphysis
c. suprabulbar paresis
c. syphilis
c. syphilitic infection
c. tarsal coalition
c. TC II deficiency
c. tendo Achillis contracture
c. tertiary neurosyphilis
c. 6th nerve palsy
c. thyroid deficiency

c. thyroid deficiency with muscular
   hypertrophy
c. tibial hemimelia
c. toxoplasmosis
c. tracheal stenosis
c. transcobalamin II deficiency
c. trypsinogen deficiency
c. tuberculosis
c. unilateral lower lip paralysis
c. vaginal aplasia
c. varicella syndrome
c. vertical talus

congenitale
poikiloderma c.

congestion
passive venous c.
pulmonary vascular c.
vascular c.

congestive
c. gastropathy
c. heart disease (CHD)
c. heart failure (CHF)

conglobata
acne c.

Congo virus
conical teeth
conidial forest
conidium, pl. **conidia**
coning of brain
conization
conjoined twin
conjugate
meningococcal c. (MenCon)
c. pneumococcal vaccine
c. pupil
c. upward gaze
7-valent pneumococcal c. (7VPnC)

conjugated
c. antichlamydial monoclonal
   antibody
c. bilirubin
c. equine estrogen
c. hyperbilirubinemia
c. linoleic acid (CLA)

conjugation activity
conjunctiva, pl. **conjunctivae**
bulbar c.
cobblestoning of c.
palpebral c.
xerosis c.

conjunctival
c. hyperemia

c. infection
c. injection
c. nevus
c. scraping
c. suffusion
c. telangiectasis

conjunctivitis
acute epidemic c.
acute hemorrhagic c.
acute perinatal c.
acute purulent c.
allergic c.
bacterial c.
bilateral c.
chlamydial c.
exudative c.
follicular c.
gonococcal c.
inclusion body of chlamydial c.
membranous c.
neonatal c.
palpebral c.
pediatric gonococcal c.
pseudomembranous c.
purulent c.
shipyard c.
silver nitrate c.
vernal c.
viral c.

conjunctivitis-otitis syndrome
connatal form
connection
circulation-cavopulmonary c.
total anomalous pulmonary
   venous c. (TAPVC)

connective
c. tissue
c. tissue disease
c. tissue disorder
c. tissue nevus

connector
domino c.
T c.
tube c.
Y c.

Conners
C. Abbreviated Parent Questionnaire
C. Hyperactivity indices
C. Rating Scale (CRS)

connexin
Conn syndrome

NOTES

117

conorii
  Rickettsia c.
conotruncal
  c. abnormality
  c. anomaly face syndrome
    (CTAFS)
  c. cardiac defect, abnormal face,
    thymic hypoplasia, cleft palate
    (CATCH 22)
  c. cardiac malformation
  c. facial anomaly
  c. facial syndrome
  c. septum
conotruncus
Conradi
  C. disease
  C. syndrome
Conradi-Hünermann syndrome
CoNS
  coagulase-negative
  CoNS bacteremia
consanguineous
consanguinity
conscious
  body c.
  c. sedation
consciousness
  altered state of c. (ASC)
  level of c. (LOC)
  loss of c.
consensus
consolability
  face, legs, activity, cry, c.
    (FLACC)
consolidation
  alveolar c.
  basilar c.
  pneumonic c.
consonant
  glide c.
  nasal c.
consonant-vowel (C-V)
  c.-v. combination
constancy
  object c.
constant
  c. exotropia
  c. flow end-inspiratory airway
    occlusion
  Michaelis-Menten dissociation c.
  c. positive airway pressure (CPAP)
  c. strabismus
  c. tidal volume
constellates
  Streptococcus c.
Constilac

constipation
  functional c.
  idiopathic c.
constituent
constitutional
  c. dwarfism
  c. growth delay
  c. short stature
constriction
  ainhumlike c.
  c. band syndrome
  ring c.
  c. ring
constrictive pericarditis
construct
  solid rod segmental c.
construction
  Davydov vagina c.
  Frank vaginal c.
Constulose
consumption
  c. coagulopathy
  oxygen c. per minute (Vo$_2$)
consumptive
  c. coagulopathy
  c. thrombocytopenia
Contac Cough Formula Liquid
contact
  c. allergen
  coital c.
  c. dermatitis
  c. factor
  heater probe thermal c.
  kangaroo c.
  c. sensitization
  c. vulvovaginitis
contagion
  c. factor
  symptom c.
contagiosa
  impetigo c.
contagiosum
  molluscum c.
contagious
containment
  surgical c.
contamination
content
  aortic oxygen c.
  bone mineral c. (BMC)
  fatty acid c.
  mixed venous oxygen c.
  poverty of c.
  pulmonary arterial oxygen c.
  pulmonary venous oxygen c.
  quantitative analysis of fat c.
  total body iron c.

contiguous
    c. gene deletion syndrome
    c. gene syndrome of chromosome 13
    c. pigmentation
contingent reinforcement
continua
    epilepsia partialis c.
continuant
continuous
    c. ambulatory peritoneal dialysis (CAPD)
    c. arteriovenous hemofiltration (CAVH)
    c. blood gas monitoring
    c. cineangiogram
    c. cyclic peritoneal dialysis (CCPD)
    c. distending pressure (CDP)
    c. gastric drip (CGD)
    c. long-term monitoring (CLTM)
    c. milk infusion
    c. negative extrathoracic pressure (CNEP)
    C. Performance Task
    c. performance test (CPT)
    c. positive airway pressure (CPAP)
    c. shunt murmur
    c. tracheal gas insufflation
    c. tube feeding
    c. venovenous hemodialysis (CVVHD)
    c. venovenous hemofiltration (CVVH)
    c. wave Doppler
    c. wave Doppler interrogation
continuum
    infantile Refsum disease c.
contraception
    postcoital c.
contraceptive
    all-progestin c.
    barrier c.
    progestin-only c.
contract
    behavior c.
contractile
contractility
    LV c.
contraction
    atrial c.
    atrial premature c. (APC)

premature atrial c. (PAC)
    c. stress test (CST)
    ventricular premature c. (VPC)
    volume c.
contractural arachnodactyly syndrome
contracture
    congenital tendo Achillis c.
    flaccid c.
    flexion c.
    gastrocnemius c.
    general triceps c.
    heel-cord c.
    joint c. (JC)
    Volkmann ischemic c.
contraindication
contralateral
    c. hernia
    c. hypertrophy
    c. hypertrophy of testis
    c. reflux
contrast
    barium c.
    c. esophagogram
    c. venography
contrecoup injury
control
    Centers for Disease C. (CDC)
    head c.
    motor c.
    Pepto Diarrhea C.
    poor head c.
    trunk c.
    waitlist c.
controlled intubation
controller
    Pepcid AC Acid C.
controversial
contused tissue
contusion
    cerebral c.
    iliac crest c.
    myocardial c.
Contuss
conus
    c. medullaris syndrome
    subaortic c.
convalescent
    c. sera
    c. serum
convection-warmed incubator
convergence
    poor c.

C

NOTES

convergens alternans
convergent
    c. nystagmus
    c. squint
    c. strabismus
conversion
    c. disorder
    c. reaction
    skin test c.
convoluted tubule
convolution
convulsion
    afebrile c.
    B_6-dependent c.
    benign familial neonatal c. (BFNC)
    benign idiopathic neonatal c.
    benign infantile familial c. (BIFC)
    benign neonatal c.
    epileptic c.
    febrile c.
    focal c.
    gelastic c.
    generalized c.
    multifocal clonic c.
    myoclonic c.
    tonic-clonic c.
convulsive
    c. seizure
    c. status epilepticus
cooing
Cook catheter
Cookie Insert
Cooley anemia
cooling blanket
cool-mist
    c.-m. humidifier
    c.-m. vaporizer
cool shock
Coombs
    C. antibody
    C. positive
    C. test
Coombs-negative autoimmune hemolytic anemia
Coombs-positive isoimmune hemolytic anemia
cooperative
    C. Human Tissue Network (CHTN)
    C. Study of Sickle Cell Disease (CSSCD)
coordination
    eye-hand c.
    hand-eye c.
    poor c.
    visual-motor c.
coordinator
    service c.
cooximeter analyzer

Copaxone
Copeland Symptom Checklist for Attention Deficit Disorders
Cophene-B
coping
    C. Health Inventory for Children (CHIC)
    c. self-statement
copper
    c. deficiency
    c. deficiency anemia
    c. deposition
    hepatic c.
    c. homeostasis
    c. metabolism
    serum c.
    c. sulfate ingestion
    c. toxicosis
    urinary c.
copper-histidine
copper-induced rhabdomyolysis
copper-wire appearance
coprolalia
coproporphyria
    hereditary c. (HCP)
coproporphyrin
    c. excretion
    urinary c.
    urinary c. I
copropraxia
COR
    conditioned orientation reflex
cor
    c. biloculare
    c. pulmonale
    c. triatriatum
    c. triloculare biatriatum
coracoclavicular ligament
Corcath catheter
cord
    bifid spinal c.
    c. blood
    c. blood acidosis
    c. blood banking
    c. blood bilirubin
    c. blood hemoglobin
    c. blood leptin concentration
    c. blood registry (CBR)
    c. blood sample
    c. blood transplantation (CBT)
    false vocal c.
    heel c.
    hemisection of c.
    c. IgG level
    c. leptin concentration
    c. lipoma
    milking of umbilical c.
    noncoiled c.

c. plasma leptin
c. prolapse
prolapsed c.
spermatic c.
spinal c.
c. stem cell marrow transplantation
tethered spinal c.
tight heel c.
c. transection
umbilical c.
vocal c.
Cordarone
Cordguard II
cordis
bulbus c.
commotio c.
ectopia c.
thoracoabdominal ectopia c.
Cordis-Hakim shunt
cordocentesis
Cordran
core
c. needle biopsy
c. temperature
corectopia
Corgard
Corgonject
Coricidin-D Tablets
Coricidin Tablets
Cori disease
Cori-Forbes disease
corkscrew
c. appearance
c. conjunctival blood vessel
cornea, pl. **corneas**
arcus corneae
cloudy c.
c. verticillata
wetting defect of c.
xerosis c.
corneal
c. abrasion
c. clouding
c. dystrophy
c. edema
c. enlargement
c. haze
c. hypoesthesia
c. light reflex test
c. opacification
c. opacity
c. scarring

c. stippling
c. ulcer
c. ulceration
Cornelia de Lange syndrome
corneocyte
corneoscleral angle
corner
c. chair
c. fracture
corneum
stratum c.
cornification
cornified
Cornsweet
double staircase method of C.
coronal
c. suture
c. synostosis
corona radiata
coronary
c. aneurysm
c. arteriovenous fistula
c. artery aneurysm (CAA)
c. artery fistula (CAF)
c. artery lesion (CAL)
c. collateralization
c. flow reserve (CFR)
c. heart disease
c. sinus
c. sinusoid
coronary-cameral fistula
coronavirus
corpora (*pl. of* corpus)
corporal cavernosal patch
corporis
pediculosis c.
Pediculus humanus c.
tinea c.
corpus, pl. **corpora**
c. callosum
c. callosum agenesis
c. callosum hypoplasia, retardation, adducted thumbs, spastic paraplegia, hydrocephalus (CRASH)
c. callosum hypoplasia, retardation, adducted thumbs, spastic paraplegia, hydrocephalus syndrome
c. cavernosa
corpora quadrigemina

NOTES

121

corpus *(continued)*
   c. spongiosum
   c. subthalamicum
corpuscle
   Hassall c.
correctable lesion
corrected gestational age
correction
   Bonferroni c.
   Bonferroni-Dunn c.
   chordee c.
   cleft nasal deformity c.
   Dwyer c.
   endoscopic c.
   loss of c.
   spectacle c.
Correct-Revised
   Percentage of Consonants C.-R. (PCC-R)
correlate
correlation
   Bonferroni c.
   Fisher c.
   mean intercriterion c. (MIC)
   Pearson c.
   point biserial c.
   Spearman c.
Corrigan sign
corrodens
   Eikenella c.
corrupting
Corsi block
CortaGel Topical
Cortatrigen Otic
Cort-Dome
   C.-D. High Potency Suppository
   C.-D. Topical
Cortef
   C. Feminine Itch Topical
   C. Oral
Cortenema
cortex, pl. cortices
   adrenal c.
   cerebral c.
   frontoparietal sensorimotor c.
   irregular c.
   mastoid c.
   metaphyseal c.
   motor c.
   nociferous c.
   renal c.
   visual c.
cortical
   c. agenesis
   c. androgen-stimulating hormone (CASH)
   c. architecture
   c. atrophy

   c. blindness
   c. bone
   c. dysgenesis
   c. dysplasia
   c. hyperostosis
   c. necrosis
   c. nephron
   c. reflex myoclonus
   c. scintigraphy
   c. spreading depression
   c. thrombophlebitis
   c. thumbing
   c. tuber
   c. vision
   c. visual impairment (CVI)
corticalis
   agenesia c.
cortices (*pl. of* cortex)
corticography
corticomedullary
   c. differentiation
   c. junction
corticospinal tract dysfunction
corticosteroid
   inhaled c. (ICS)
   c. therapy
   c. treatment
corticosteroid-induced atrophy
corticosterone
corticostriatal
corticotropin
corticotropin-releasing hormone (CRH)
cortin
   double c.
cortisol
   c. concentration
   plasma c.
   salivary c.
   urinary free c.
cortisol-binding globulin
cortisol-cortisone shuttle
cortisone
Cortisporin
   C. Ophthalmic Suspension
   C. Otic
   C. Otic Suspension
   C. Topical Cream
Cortizone-5 Topical
Cortizone-10 Topical
Cortone Acetate
Cortrosyn stimulation test
corynebacteria
Corynebacterium
   C. diphtheriae
   C. haemolyticum
   C. minutissimum
coryza

COS
: childhood-onset schizophrenia

COSA
: child of substance abuser

co-sleeping

Cosmegen

cosmetic acne

cost
: response c.

costal
: c. cartilage
: c. cartilage interposition
: c. margin

CO-stat end tidal breath analyzer

costochondral junction

costochondritis

costovertebral
: c. angle (CVA)
: c. angle tenderness
: c. angle tenderness to percussion

cosyntropin

Cotazym

Cotazym-S

cotinine level

co-transporter-1
: sodium/glucose c.-t.-1 (SGLT1)

Cotrel-Dubousset instrumentation (CDI)

Cotrim
: C. DS

cotrimoxazole trimethoprim

cotton
: c.-ball exudate
: c. pledget
: c. swab method

cotton-tipped swab

cotton-wool spot (CWS)

cotyledons

cough
: barking c.
: barky c.
: brassy c.
: bronchospastic c.
: croupy c.
: Diphen C.
: habit c.
: harassing c.
: psychogenic c.
: c. receptor
: rhonchorous c.
: seallike c.
: Silphen C.
: staccato c.

staccato-like c.
: c. syncope
: c. tic
: whooping c.

Cough-Cold
: PediaCare C.-C.

Cough/Cold
: Vicks Children's Nyquil Nighttime C.

coughing
: paroxysmal c.
: voluntary c.

Cough-X lozenge

Coumadin

coumadinization

council
: Interagency Coordinating C. (ICC)

counselor
: genetic c.

count
: absolute band c. (ABC)
: absolute CD4 c.
: absolute lymphocyte c.
: absolute neutrophil c.
: blood c.
: CD4 cell c.
: colony c.
: complete blood c. (CBC)
: granulocyte c.
: Guthrie c.
: hemolysis, elevated liver enzymes, low platelet c. (HELLP)
: platelet c.
: reticulocyte c.
: white blood cell c.

counter
: over the c. (OTC)
: C. Rotation System brace (CRS)
: Sysmex NE8000 cell c.

counterimmunoelectrophoresis (CIE)

counterpulsation
: intraaortic balloon c.

counterrotation

COUP
: chicken ovalbumin upstream promoter

coup injury

couplet

coupling defect

course
: aberrant c.

covariate

Covera-HS

C

NOTES

123

covering
    epidermal c.
Covermark
cover test
covert loss
Cowden
    C. disease
    C. syndrome
Cowdry
    C. type A inclusion body
    C. types A, B
cowlick
cow's
    c. milk allergy (CMA)
    c. milk challenge
    c. milk protein
COX
    cyclooxygenase
COX-2
    cyclooxygenase-2
    COX-2 inhibitor
Cox
    C. proportional hazard
    C. proportional hazard model
coxa, pl. **coxae**
    c. magna
    c. plana
    c. valga
    c. vara
    c. vara deformity
coxarthrosis
Coxiella burnetii
Coxsackie
    C. A16 infection
    C. B19
    C. viral meningitis
Coxsackievirus
    C. A9, A16, A21
    C. B, B5
    C. infection
CP
    cerebral palsy
    cleft palate
C-palmitic acid
CPAP
    constant positive airway pressure
    continuous positive airway pressure
    CPAP machine
    nasal CPAP
CPC
    choroid plexus carcinoma
CPD
    cephalopelvic disproportion
CPE
    cytopathic effect
CPEO
    chronic progressive external
      ophthalmoplegia

c-peptic
C-peptide level
CPI
    chronic pneumonitis of infancy
    congenital palatopharyngeal
      incompetence
CPK
    creatinine phosphokinase
cPNET
    central primitive neuroectodermal tumor
CPP
    central precocious puberty
    cerebral perfusion pressure
    choroid plexus papilloma
CPR
    cardiopulmonary resuscitation
CPS
    carbamoyl phosphate synthetase
    Child Protective Services
    Collaborative Perinatal Study
    complex partial seizure
CPT
    carnitine palmitoyltransferase
    chest physical therapy
    continuous performance test
      CPT deficiency
      CPT I, II deficiency
CPT I
    carnitine palmitoyltransferase I
CPT II
    carnitine palmitoyltransferase II
cPVL
    cystic periventricular leukomalacia
C1q
    C1q assay
    C1q binding
    deficiency of C1q
CR
    Norpace CR
C-R
    Bicillin C-R
CR1
    complement receptor
CRA
    clinical risk assessment
crab louse
crack cocaine
cracked mucous membrane
cracked-pot
    c.-p. head
    c.-p. sign
    c.-p. sound
crackle
    bubbly c.
    fine inspiratory c.
cradle
    auditory response c.
    c. cap

cradleboard
cramp
    nocturnal leg c.
    writer's c.
cranberry
Crandall ectodermal dysplasia syndrome
crania (*pl. of* cranium)
cranial
    c. bruit
    c. echoencephalography
    c. encephalocele
    c. epidural abscess
    c. fasciitis
    c. hypothermia
    c. meningocele
    c. molding helmet
    c. nerve defect
    c. nerve (II–XII)
    c. nerve nucleus
    c. nerve palsy
    c. nerve testing
    c. neuritis
    c. orthosis
    c. space
    c. suture
    c. ultrasound
craniectomy
    endoscopic strip c.
craniobasal bone
CranioCap cranial orthosis
craniocarpotarsal syndrome
craniocaudal
craniocerebral trauma
craniocervical
    c. dystonia
    c. myelopathy
craniodiaphyseal dysplasia
craniofacial
    c. anomaly
    c. disproportion
    c. dissociation
    c. dysostosis
    c. tumor
craniofacies
craniolacunia
craniometaphyseal dysplasia
craniopharyngioma
cranioplasty
craniospinal rachischisis
craniostenosis
craniostosis

craniosynostosis
    Boston-type c.
    metopic c.
    primary c.
    sagittal c.
    secondary c.
    single-suture c.
    syndromic c.
craniosynostosis-marfanoid habitus
craniosynostotic syndrome
craniotabes
craniotomy
cranium, pl. **crania**
    c. bifidum
    c. bifidum cysticum
    c. bifidum occultum
crankshaft phenomenon
CRASH
    corpus callosum hypoplasia, retardation, adducted thumbs, spastic paraplegia, hydrocephalus
    CRASH syndrome
craving
    salt c.
crawl
    belly c.
    combat c.
    commando c.
crawling aid
CRCT
    creamatocrit
    volume percent of cream in milk
C1r deficiency
C-reactive protein (CRP)
cream
    Bactroban c.
    Balmex c.
    butoconazole 2% c.
    Complex 15 c.
    Cortisporin Topical C.
    Cutivate c.
    Decadron Phosphate C.
    Elimite C.
    EMLA c.
    emollient c.
    Eucerin c.
    Exact C.
    gentamicin c.
    LCD c.
    lidocaine-prilocaine c.
    liquor carbonis detergens c.
    Neosporin C.

NOTES

cream (continued)
    Nivea c.
    Nutraderm c.
    permethrin 5% c.
    Purpose c.
    RVPaque c.
    silver sulfadiazine c.
    SSD C.
    stearin-lanolin c.
    Sulfamylon c.
    vasodilator c.
    Zonalon Topical C.

creamatocrit (CRCT)

crease
    allergic c.
    earlobe c.
    flexural c.
    palmar c.
    simian c.
    single transverse palmar c.
    sole c.
    transversal nasal c.

crease/pit
    ear c.

creatine
    c. deficiency
    c. kinase (CK)
    c. kinase MB
    c. phosphokinase

creatinine
    c. aldolase
    c. clearance
    c. phosphokinase (CPK)

Credé
    C. maneuver
    C. prophylaxis

creep

creeping eruption

cremasteric
    c. reflex
    c. response

creme
    Eucerin Plus C.
    Fungoid C.
    Vite E C.

crenated red cell

Creola body

Creon 10, 20

Creo-Terpin

crepitation

crepitus

crescendo murmur

crescent formation

crescentic
    c. glomerulonephritis
    c. lesion

CREST
    calcinosis, Raynaud phenomenon, esophageal dysmotility, sclerodactyly, telangiectasia
    CREST syndrome

crest
    iliac c.
    posterior iliac c.
    superior iliac c.

cretinism
    endemic c.
    c. idiocy

cretinoid dysplasia

Creutzfeldt-Jakob
    C.-J. disease (CJD)
    C.-J. syndrome

CRF
    chronic renal failure
    anemia of CRF

CRH
    corticotropin-releasing hormone

CRIB
    Clinical Risk Index for Babies
    CRIB score

crib death

Crib-O-Gram

cribriform
    c. fracture
    c. hymen
    c. plate

cribrosa
    lamina c.

cricoarytenoid
    c. articulation
    c. joint

cricoid
    c. split
    c. split procedure

cricopharyngeal incoordination of infancy

cricothyroidectomy

cricothyroid membrane

cricothyroidotomy
    needle c.

cricothyrotomy
    needle c.
    surgical c.

cri du chat
    c. d. c. syndrome

CRIES
    crying, requires, increased, expression, sleepless
    CRIES Neonatal Postoperative Pain Scale

Crigler-Najjar
    C.-N. disease (type I, II)
    C.-N. syndrome (type I, II)

Crimean-Congo hemorrhagic fever

criminology
Crippled Children's Services (CCS)
crisis
- acute adrenal c.
- acute splenic sequestration c.
- addisonian c.
- adrenal c.
- aplastic c.
- autonomic c.
- blast c.
- Chiari c.
- cholinergic c.
- encephalopathic c.
- Fabry c.
- hemolytic c.
- hepatic c.
- hypertensive c.
- megaloblastic c.
- oculogyric c.
- scleroderma renal c.
- sequestration c.
- sickle cell c.
- sickling c.
- splenic sequestration c.
- thyroid c.
- thyrotoxic c.
- transient aplastic c. (TAC)
- vasoocclusive c.

crista supraventricularis
criteria
- Amsel c.
- Berne c.
- Cohens c.
- family history research diagnostic c. (FH-RDC)
- ICSD c.
- International Classification of Sleep Disorders c.
- Jones rheumatic fever diagnostic c.
- Joshi c.
- Lorber c.
- Norris-Carrol c.
- Oxford diagnostic c.
- Ranson c.
- revised Jones c.
- Rochester c.
- Shimada c.
- Sydenham chorea c.

criterion
- Katz-Wachtel c.
- c. overlap

criterion-referenced test
critical
- c. aortic stenosis
- c. illness neuromuscular disease
- c. pulmonic stenosis
- c. temperature

Criticare H formula
Crixivan
CRMO
- chronic recurrent multifocal osteomyelitis

CRO
- cathode ray oscilloscope

Crohn
- C. colitis
- C. disease

Crolom
cromoglycate
- disodium c.
- sodium c.

cromolyn
- atropine c.
- c. sodium
- c. sodium inhalation aerosol

Cronbach values
Cronkhite-Canada syndrome
crop
- c. of macules
- c. of papules
- rash c.

Crosby capsule
Crosby-Kugler pediatric capsule
crossbite
crossed
- c. adductor reflex
- c. fused ectopia

cross-eye
crosslink
- TSRH c.

Cross-McKusick-Breen syndrome
cross-modal fluency
cross-section
Cross syndrome
cross-table lateral film
crotamiton
crouch gait
croup
- diphtheritic c.
- membranous c.
- C. Score
- spasmodic c.

croupy cough

C

NOTES

Crouzon
    C. disease
    C. syndrome
crowded teeth
crowding
    dental c.
    fetal c.
    c. theory
Crowe sign
crown-heel length
CRP
    C-reactive protein
CRS
    congenital rubella syndrome
    Conners Rating Scale
    Counter Rotation System brace
CRST
    calcinosis cutis, Raynaud phenomenon,
      sclerodactyly, telangiectasia
    CRST syndrome
Cruex Topical
Cruiser hip abduction brace
cruising
crunch
    mediastinal c.
cruris
    tinea c.
crusta lacteal
crusted
    c. lesion
    c. scabies
crusting telangiectasia keratosis
crutches
    Lofstrand c.
crux
cruzi
    Trypanosoma c.
Cruz trypanosomiasis
cry
    cat's c.
    hoarse c.
    voiceless c.
    weak c.
cryaerophilia
    Campylobacter c.
crying
    c., requirement for oxygen
      supplementation, increases in heart
      rate and blood pressure
    c., requires, increased, expression,
      sleepless (CRIES)
cryofibrinogenemia
cryoglobulin
    polyclonal c.
cryoglobulinemia
cryoprecipitate
cryopreserved valved allograft
cryothalamectomy

cryotherapy
crypt
    c. abscess
    c. cell
    c. cell mitosis
    c. depth
    c. hyperplasia
    c. hypoplasia
    c. of Lieberkuhn
cryptic
    c. hemangioma
    c. tuber
cryptococcal
    c. antigen
    c. meningitis
cryptococcosis
    cutaneous c.
    extrapulmonary c.
    pulmonary c.
Cryptococcus
    C. neoformans var. *neoformans*
cryptogenic
    c. cirrhosis
    c. fibrosing alveolitis
    c. hepatitis
    c. infantile spasm
cryptophthalmia-syndactyly syndrome
cryptophthalmia syndrome
cryptophthalmos syndrome
cryptorchidism
    bilateral c.
    unilateral c.
cryptorchid testis
cryptosporidial endocholecystitis
cryptosporidiosis
Cryptosporidium parvum
crypt-villus architecture
crystal
    calcium c.
    Charcot-Leyden c.
    indinavir c.
crystallina
    Miliaria c.
crystalline lens
crystalloid
    miliaria c.
    c. solution
crystalluria
    renal tubular c.
Crystamine
Crysticillin A.S.
C&S
    culture and sensitivity
CSA
    clinically significant arrhythmia
CsA
    cyclosporin A
Csaba stain

CSBI
  Child Sexual Behavior Inventory
CSD
  cat-scratch disease
CSF
  cerebrospinal fluid
    bloody CSF
    CSF glycine
    CSF lymphocytic pleocytosis
    CSF otorrhea
    CSF pleocytosis
    CSF rhinorrhea
    CSF VDRL
    xanthochromic CSF
C-shaped curve
CSI
  chemical shift imaging
CsI
  cesium iodide
C-Solve-2
CSOM
  chronic suppurative otitis media
CSPI
  childhood severity of psychiatric illness
CSSCD
  Cooperative Study of Sickle Cell Disease
CST
  contraction stress test
CSTR
  complete subtalar release
CSW
  cerebral salt wasting
CT
  Chlamydia trachomatis
  computed tomography
    CT scan
    CT scanning
CTAFS
  conotruncal anomaly face syndrome
CTD
  chronic tic disorder
CTEI
  communal traumatic experiences inventory
C-terminal propeptide of type I collagen
CTG
  cardiotocography
CTL
  cytotoxic lymphocyte
  cytotoxic T lymphocyte

    CTL cell
    CTL response
CTNS gene
CTQ
  childhood trauma questionnaire
CTS
  clitoris tourniquet syndrome
CTX
  cyclophosphamide
CTZ
  chemoreceptor trigger zone
cubitus varus
cuboid
CUCS
  complex unroofed coronary sinus
cue
    C. Fertility Monitor
cued speech
cuff
    muscular c.
cuffed
    c. endotracheal tube
    c. ET tube
cuffing
    pericapillary inflammatory c.
cuirass respirator
culbertsoni
    Acanthamoeba c.
Culex
    C. nigripalpus
    C. pipiens
    C. quinquefasciatus
    C. tarsalis
Culiseta melanura
Cullen sign
cultivable virus
cultural competence
culture
    blood c.
    broth c.
    cervical c.
    epiglottic surface c.
    fibroblast c.
    GBS screening c.
    gonorrhea c.
    nasal swab c.
    purified chick embryo cell c. (PCEC)
    screening c.
    c. and sensitivity (C&S)
    shell vial c.
    sputum c.

NOTES

C

culture *(continued)*
    test-of-cure c.
    urine c.
cultured skin fibroblast
culture-negative neutrocytic ascites
culturing
    viral c.
cumulative
    c. parental dysfunction
    c. sum (CUSUM)
    c. sum test
cuneiform bone
cup
    cut-away c.
    cut-out c.
    c. feeding
    heel c.
    zinc-free plastic specimen c.
Cupid's
    C. bow curve
    C. bow upper lip
cupped metaphysis
cupping
    optic nerve c.
    c. of optic nerve head
Cuprimine
cupriuria
cuprophane hemodialyzer membrane
cuproprotein
curare
curative
C-urea
    C-u. breath test
    C-u. serology
[13]C-urea breath test
[14]C-urea breath test
curettage
curette
Curling ulcer
curly toe
Curosurf intratracheal suspension
currant jelly stool
Currarino triad
Curretab Oral
Curschmann spiral
curse
    Ondine c.
    c. of Ondine
curtsey sign
curvature
    abnormal penile c.
    dorsal penile c.
    excessive penile c.
    lateral c.
    penile c.
    c. of spine
curve
    biologic satiation c.

    C-shaped c.
    Cupid's bow c.
    flow-volume c.
    growth c.
    hemoglobin-oxygen dissociation c.
    Kaplan-Meier survival c.
    lumbar c.
    Risser c.
    saddleback temperature c.
    c. of Spee
    S-shaped c.
curved finger
Curvularia lunata
curvus
    Campylobacter c.
Cushing
    C. disease
    C. effect
    C. syndrome
    C. triad
    C. ulcer
cushingoid
    c. body habitus
    c. facies
    c. syndrome
cushion
    endocardial c.
cusp
cuspid
CUSUM
    cumulative sum
        CUSUM test
cutaneous
    c. albinism
    c. angioma
    c. anthrax
    c. atrophy
    c. blanching
    c. candidiasis
    c. cryptococcosis
    c. dimple
    c. diphtheria
    c. ectoderm
    c. fibrosis
    c. hemangioma
    c. hepatic porphyria
    c. larva migrans
    c. leishmaniasis
    c. lesion
    c. mastocytosis
    c. melanoma
    c. melanosis
    c. mucormycosis
    c. nevus
    c. nodule
    c. pyelostomy
    c. shunt
    c. sporotrichosis

c. tag
c. telangiectasis
c. tuberculosis
c. ureterostomy
c. urticaria
c. vasculitis
c. vesicostomy

cut-away cup

cutdown
greater saphenous vein c.

cut-down liver

cutis
c. aplasia
c. elastica
c. hyperelastica
c. laxa
c. marmorata
c. marmorata alba
c. marmorata telangiectatica
c. marmorata telangiectatica
congenita
tuberculosis verrucosa c.
c. verticis gyrata
xanthosis c.

Cutivate cream

cutoff sign

cut-out cup

cutting

Cuvier
duct of C.

CV
closing volume

C-V
consonant-vowel
C-V combination

CVA
cerebrovascular accident
costovertebral angle
CVA tenderness

CVAD
central venous access device

CVC
central venous catheter

CVI
common variable immunodeficiency
cortical visual impairment

CVID
common variable immunodeficiency

CVL
central venous line
tunneled CVL

CVM
cardiovascular malformation

CVN
central venous nutrition

CVP
central venous pressure

CVS
chorionic villus sampling

CVVH
continuous venovenous hemofiltration

CVVHD
continuous venovenous hemodialysis

CWS
cotton-wool spot

CWSN
Children with Special Health Care Needs

CXR
chest x-ray

cyanide toxicity

cyanocobalamin

Cyanoject

cyanosis
acral c.
cardiac c.
central c.
differential c.
nail bed c.
oral mucosa c.
peripheral c.
pulmonary c.
slate-gray c.

cyanotic
c. breathholding spell
c. congenital heart disease (CCHD)
c. congenital heart lesion
c. flush
c. heart disease
c. newborn

cyclase
adenylate c.

cycle
citric acid c.
ectopic P-P c.
itch-scratch c.
Krebs c.
c. length
periodic breathing c. (PBC)
respiratory c.
urea c.

cyclic
c. adenosine monophosphate
(cAMP)

NOTES

C

cyclic *(continued)*
    c. adenosine monophosphate test
    c. antidepressant poisoning
    c. guanosine monophosphate-specific phosphodiesterase 5 (PDE5)
    c. neutropenia
    c. vomiting
    c. vomiting syndrome
cycling
cyclizine
Cyclocort
cyclocryotherapy
cyclodestructive procedure
Cyclofem
Cyclogyl
cyclohexylchloroethylnitrosurea (CCNU)
cyclohydrolase
    guanosine triphosphate c.
cyclomethycaine
Cyclomydril
cyclooxygenase (COX)
cyclooxygenase-2 (COX-2)
    c. inhibitor
cyclopentolate hydrochloride
cyclophosphamide (CTX)
    c., doxorubicin (Adriamycin), Oncovin (vincristine), prednisone
    c., hydroxydaunorubicin, methotrexate, prednisone (CHOP)
    c., hydroxydaunorubicin, methotrexate, prednisone chemotherapy
    c., Oncovin, methotrexate, arabinosylcytosine (COMA)
    c., Oncovin, methotrexate, prednisone (COMP)
cyclopia
cycloplegic
Cyclo-Provera
cycloserine
Cyclospora cayetanensis
cyclosporiasis
cyclosporin A (CsA)
cyclosporine
cyclosporine-induced gingival overgrowth
cyclothymia
cyclothymic disorder
Cycrin Oral
Cyklokapron
Cylert
Cylex
Cylexin
cylinder
    c. cast
    muscle c.
Cynapin
Cyomin
CYP21 genotyping

cypionate
    hydrocortisone c.
cyproheptadine
cyst
    acne c.
    alveolar c.
    aneurysmal bone c.
    Baker c.
    Bartholin gland c.
    benign pineal c.
    branchial c.
    branchial cleft c.
    bronchogenic c.
    choledochal c.
    choroid plexus c.
    colloid c.
    Dandy-Walker c.
    dental lamina c.
    dentigerous c.
    dermoid c.
    duplication c.
    Echinococcus granulosus hydatid c.
    enterogenous c.
    epidermal inclusion c.
    epidermoid c.
    eruptive vellus hair c.
    extraaxial arachnoid c.
    gingival c.
    hydatid c.
    inclusion c.
    intraabdominal c.
    keratinized c.
    leptomeningeal c.
    mesonephric c.
    mucous retention c.
    multilocular thymic c. (MTC)
    neurenteric c.
    noncommunicating c.
    omental c.
    ovarian c.
    paraurethral c.
    parenchymal c.
    pilar c.
    pilonidal c.
    popliteal c.
    porencephalic c.
    posterior fossa arachnoid c.
    pseudoporencephalic c.
    renal cortex c.
    retrocerebellar arachnoidal c.
    second branchial cleft c.
    skin c.
    solitary bone c.
    sperm-containing c.
    subepidermal keratin c.
    suprasellar arachnoid c.
    thyroglossal duct c.

trichilemmal c.
unicameral bone c.
Cystadane
cystadenocarcinoma
Cystagon
cystathionine
   c. synthase
   c. synthase deficiency
cystathioninuria
cystatin C
cysteamine
cysteine hydrochloride
cystic
   c. adenomatoid malformation
     (CAM)
   c. adenomatoid malformation of
     lung
   c. brainstem glioma
   c. cerebellar neoplasm
   c. degeneration
   c. dilation
   c. dilation of intrahepatic bile duct
   c. encephalomalacia
   c. fibrosis (CF)
   c. fibrosis transmembrane
     conductance regulator (CFTR)
   c. fibrosis transmembrane
     conductance regulator protein
   c. fibrosis transmembrane regulator
     (CFTR)
   c. hydatid disease
   c. hygroma
   c. leukomalacia
   c. medial necrosis
   c. nephroma
   c. periventricular leukomalacia
     (cPVL)
   c. PVL
   c. renal disease
   c. teratoma
cystica
   osteitis fibrosis c.
   osteogenesis imperfecta c.
   spina bifida c.
cysticercosis
   parenchymatous cerebral c.
Cysticercus cellulosae
cysticum
   cranium bifidum c.
   epithelioma adenoides c.
   lymphangioma c.
cyst-induced pancreatitis

cystine
   c. deposition
   c. stone
cystinosis
   infantile neuropathic c.
   neuropathic c.
   ocular nonnephropathic c.
cystinuria
   transient neonatal c.
cystitis
   acute c.
   eosinophilic c.
   hemorrhagic c.
cystoduodenostomy
cystogastrostomy
cystogram
   sleep c.
cystography
   indirect c.
   voiding c.
cystojejunostomy
cystometrogram
cystometrography
cystometry
cystoperitoneal shunt
cystoscopy
Cystospaz
Cystospaz-M
cystostomy
   suprapubic c.
cystourethrogram
   voiding c. (VCUG)
cystourethrograph
   voiding c. (VCUG)
cystourethrography
   voiding c. (VCUG)
cystourethroscopy
cytarabine
cytoarchitectonic
cytoarchitectural development
cytoarchitecture
cytobrush
cytochalasin
cytochrome
   c. *b* system
   c. *c* oxidase
   91kD c. b peptide
   c. oxidase deficiency
   P450 c.
cytochrome *b*
cytochrome-*c*-oxidase deficiency
cytochrome-*c* oxidative enzyme

C

NOTES

CytoGam
cytogenetic analysis
cytogenetics
  bone marrow c.
cytoid body
cytokine
  c. cascade
  c. modulator
  proinflammatory c.
cytokinemia
  fetal c.
  maternal c.
cytokine-related dysmotility
cytology
cytolysis
cytomegalic inclusion disease (CID)
cytomegalovirus (CMV)
  congenital c.
  c. disease
  c. immune globulin (CMVIG)
  c. immune globulin intravenous
    (CMV-IGIV)
  c. infection
  prenatal c.
  transfusion-associated c.
cytomegaly syndrome
Cytomel Oral
cytometer
  Epics XL flow c.
cytometry
  flow c.
cytopathic effect (CPE)

cytopathy
  mitochondrial c.
cytoplasm
cytoplasmic
  c. ANCA
  c. lipid droplet (CLD)
  c. membrane
cytoreduction
Cytosar-U
cytosine
  c. arabinoside
  c. nucleotide
cytosol
Cytotec
cytotoxic
  c. edema
  c. lymphocyte (CTL)
  c. lymphocyte response
  c. memory T cell
  c. T lymphocyte (CTL)
cytotoxicity
  antibody-dependent cell-mediated c.
    (ADCC)
cytotoxin
  vero c.
cytotrophoblast
Cytovene
Cytoxan
Czerny anemia

D₂
$$D_2$$
prostaglandin D_2
D₄
leukotriene D_4 (LTD₄)
DA
dextroamphetamine
DAA
digital auditory aerobics
double aortic arch
dacarbazine
Adriamycin (doxorubicin),
bleomycin, vinblastine, d. (ABVD)
dacliximab
Dacodyl
Dacron fiber-coated coil
dacryoadenitis
dacryocystitis
acute d.
dacryocystorhinostomy
dacryocystostenosis
dacryostenosis
dactinomycin
dactylitis
blistering distal d.
sickle cell d.
tuberculous d.
DAI
diffuse axonal injury
Dalalone
D. D.P. Injection
D. L.A. Injection
dalfopristin
Dalmane
Dalrymple sign
damage
brain d.
minimal brain d.
neuronal d.
vestibular d.
virus-induced epithelial d.
white matter d. (WMD)
DAMP
deficits in attention, motor control,
perception
D-amphetamine
Damus-Kaye-Stansel
D.-K.-S. anastomosis
D.-K.-S. operation
D.-K.-S. procedure
danazol
dance
hilar d.
D. sign
St. Vitus d.
dancer's ankle

dancing
d. eye movement
d. eyes
d. eye syndrome
d. feet
dander
animal d.
cat d.
Dandy-Walker
D.-W. cyst
D.-W. deformity
D.-W. formation
D.-W. malformation
D.-W. syndrome
Dane particle
dangerousness
Dantrium
dantrolene sodium
DAP
diastolic arterial pressure
Dapa
Dapacin
dapsone
Daraprim
Darier
D. disease
D. sign
Darier-White disease
darkened reflex
darkfield
d. examination
d. microscopy
dark urine
Darrow-Gamble syndrome
darting tongue
Darvocet
Darvocet-N
D.-N. 100
Darvon
Darvon-N
DAT
direct antiglobulin test
data
hemodynamic d.
oximetric d.
sociodemographic d.
database
Vermont-Oxford Neonatal D.
datalink
Vaccine Safety D. (VSD)
date
small for d.'s
daughter cell
daunorubicin
Davidenkow syndrome

D

Davydov vagina construction
Dawson
> D. disease
> D. encephalitis

DAX1 gene
day
> bis in die (twice a d.) (b.i.d.)
> d. of life (DOL)
> quaque altera die (every other d.)
> (q.o.d.)
> quaque die (every d.) (q.d.)
> quater in die (four times a d.)
> (q.i.d.)
> ter in die (three times a d.)
> (t.i.d.)

daycare
daze
dB
> decibel

DBA
> Diamond-Blackfan anemia

d-Biotin
DBPCFC
> double-blind, placebo-controlled food
> challenge

DBS
> diffuse brain swelling

DCA
> directional coronary atherectomy

DCCT
> Diabetes Control and Complications Trial

DCD
> developmental coordination disorder

DCFS
> Department of Children and Family
> Services

DCL
> diffuse cutaneous leishmaniasis

DCS
> Department of Children's Services

DC 240 Softgel
DD
> developmental disability

DDAVP
> 1-desamino-8-D-arginine vasopressin
> desmopressin
> > DDAVP nasal spray

ddC
> zalcitabine

DDH
> developmental dysplasia of hip

ddI
> didanosine

D-dimer
DDST
> Denver Developmental Screening Test

DE
> diatomaceous earth
> > DE slurry

de
> de la Chapelle dysplasia
> de la Cruz classification
> de la Cruz classification of
> congenital aural atresia
> de Lange syndrome
> de Morsier-Gauthier syndrome
> de Morsier syndrome
> de novo
> de novo deletion
> de Pezzer catheter
> De Sanctis-Cacchione syndrome
> de Toni-Fanconi-Debré syndrome
> de Toni-Fanconi syndrome
> De Vega tricuspid annuloplasty

dead
> d. space
> d. space technique

deaf-blindness
deafness
> adventitious d.
> coloboma, heart disease, atresia
> choanae, retarded growth and
> retarded development, CNS
> anomalies, genital hypoplasia, ear
> anomalies and/or d. (CHARGE)
> congenital nerve d.
> diabetes insipidus, diabetes mellitus,
> optic atrophy, d. (DIDMOAD)
> eighth nerve d.
> goitrous hypothyroidism with d.
> growth and d.
> keratitis, ichthyosis, d. (KID)
> lentigines, electrocardiographic
> abnormalities, ocular hypertelorism,
> pulmonary stenosis, abnormalities
> of genitalia, retardation of
> growth, d. (LEOPARD)
> maturity onset d.
> neurosensory d.
> d., onychodystrophy, osteodystrophy,
> mild to severe mental retardation
> (DOOR)
> prelingual d.
> retardation of growth and d.
> sensorineural d.

Deal syndrome
deaminase
> adenosine d. (ADA)
> polyethylene glycol-modified
> adenosine d. (PEG-ADA)

death
> apoptotic cell d.
> brain d.
> d. by calcium

crib d.
fetal d.
postoperative sudden d.
sudden d.
sudden infant d.
sudden unexpected d. (SUD)
DEB
diepoxybutane
DeBakey aortic clamp
debrancher deficiency
debranching enzyme deficiency
Debré-Fibiger syndrome
Debré-Sémélaigne syndrome
débridement
broad d.
thoracoscopic pleural d.
debriefing
debris
amniotic d.
cellular d.
keratinous d.
keratotic d.
nuclear d.
Debrox Otic
debt
sleep d.
Decadron
D. Oral
D. Phosphate Cream
D. Phosphate Injection
D. Phosphate Nasal Turbinaire
D. Phosphate Ophthalmic
D. Respihaler
D. Turbinaire
Decadron-LA Injection
Decaject Injection
Decaject-LA Injection
decancellation
talar d.
decanoate
Haldol D.
decarboxy
decarboxylase
glutamic acid d. (GAD)
ornithine d.
decarboxylation
Decaspray Topical Aerosol
decay
bottle tooth d.
tooth d.
decay-accelerating factor

deceleration
early d.
d. injury
late d.
variable d.
decerebrate
d. posturing
d. rigidity
decerebration
decibel (dB)
decidua basalis
decidual floor
deciduitis
deciduous teeth
Declomycin
decoding stage
Decofed Syrup
decompensated cirrhosis
decompression
silo d.
decongestant
nasal d.
decontamination
gastrointestinal d.
decorticate posturing
decortication
pleural d.
decreased
d. anal tone
d. appetite
d. attending skill
d. breath sound
d. commissural separation
d. gastrointestinal motility
d. mucosal surface
d. propulsion
d. red cell survival
d. sphincter tone
d. talocalcaneal angle
d. urine output
decrescendo diastolic murmur
decubitus ulcer
decussation
dedicated Doppler probe
deep
d. hypothermia and total circulatory arrest (DHCA)
d. partial-thickness burn
d. set eyes
d. sleep
d. systemic hypothermia
d. tendon reflex (DTR)

NOTES

deep *(continued)*
    d. tendon reflex delayed relaxation phase
    d. venous thrombosis (DVT)
deep-knee bend
DEET
    diethyltoluamide
    n,n-diethyl-m-toluamide
defasciculation
defecation
defect
    acyanotic congenital d.
    amino acid transport d.
    aorticopulmonary window d.
    arteriovenous canal d.
    atrial septal d. (ASD)
    atrioventricular canal d.
    birth d.
    cardiac septal d.
    chromosomal d.
    Coffin-Siris d.
    colobomatous d.
    complex heart d.
    conduction d.
    congenital ectodermic scalp d.
    congenital heart d.
    congenital hemidysplasia with ichthyosiform erythroderma and limb d.'s (CHILD)
    congenital d. of phosphofructokinase
    coupling d.
    cranial nerve d.
    dehalogenase d.
    dental d.
    endocardial cushion d.
    enzyme d.
    erythrocyte acquired d.
    eustachian tube d.
    fibrocortical d.
    fibrous cortical d.
    Hartnup d.
    heart d.
    hydroxylase enzyme d.
    intercalary d.
    intracardiac d.
    intrauterine positional d.
    laterality d.
    lobulation d.
    metaphyseal fibrous d.
    midline facial d.
    mitochondrial respiratory chain d.
    nail d.
    neural tube d. (NTD)
    nonneural congenital d.
    opsonin d.
    ostium primum d.
    ostium secundum d.
    ostium venosus d.
    peroxidase d.
    Pi-type ZZ d.
    radial ray d.
    recessive disorder d.
    red blood cell membrane d.
    relative afferent d.
    septal d.
    sinus venosus d.
    skeletal d.
    skin d.
    spinal d.
    subclavian artery d.
    supracristal ventricular septal d.
    T-cell activation d.
    testis migration d.
    unbalanced AV canal d.
    unrestrictive ventricular septal d.
    urea cycle enzyme d.
    urinary concentrating d.
    ventricular septal d. (VSD)
    vertebral arch d.
    vertebral column d.
    visual field d.
defectiva
    Abiotrophia d.
defective
    d. eye abduction
    d. primary platelet aggregation
    d. purine metabolism
    d. tryptophan absorption
defensiveness
    oral tactile d.
    tactile d.
deferens
    congenital absence of vas d. (CAVD)
    vas d.
deferiprone
deferoxamine challenge test
defervescence
defiant
defibrillation
deficiency
    abdominal muscular d.
    acid ceramidase d.
    acid maltase d. (AMD)
    acquired antithrombin III d.
    acquired C1 INH d.
    acquired growth hormone d.
    acquired protein C, S d.
    adenosine deaminase d.
    adenylosuccinate d.
    adenylosuccinate lyase d. (ASLD)
    aldosterone d.
    alpha-antilysin d.
    alpha-1 antitrypsin d.
    alpha-glucosidase d.

alpha-lipoprotein d.
alpha-N-acetylgalactosaminidase d.
alpha-reductase d.
American Association on
  Mental D. (AAMD)
Andersen d.
antibody d.
antiplasmin d.
antithrombin III d.
apoenzyme d.
arginase d.
argininosuccinic acid synthetase d.
arylsulfatase-activator d.
ascorbic acid d.
ataxia with isolated vitamin E d.
B_6 d.
11-beta-HSD2 d.
11-beta-hydroxysteroid
  dehydrogenase type 2 d.
biotinidase d.
brancher d.
branching enzyme d.
calcium d.
carbamoyl phosphate synthetase d.
carboxylase d.
carnitine acylcarnitine translocase d.
carnitine palmitoyltransferase II d.
carnitine palmitoyltransferase I,
  II d.
d. of C4-binding protein
C2, C3, C4, C5, C6, C7, C8,
  C9 d.
ceruloplasmin d.
C1 esterase inhibitor d.
Chédiak-Higashi d.
cobalamin reductase d.
cofactor d.
cognitive d.
complement d.
congenital growth hormone d.
congenital intrinsic factor d.
congenital lactase d.
congenital lipase/colipase d.
congenital longitudinal d.
congenital TC II d.
congenital thyroid d.
congenital transcobalamin II d.
congenital trypsinogen d.
copper d.
CPT d.
CPT I, II d.
C1r d.

creatine d.
cystathionine synthase d.
cytochrome-c-oxidase d.
cytochrome oxidase d.
debrancher d.
debranching enzyme d.
dense body d.
dihydropteridine reductase d.
disaccharidase d.
enterokinase d.
enzyme d.
epinephrine d.
erythrocyte glutathione
  peroxidase d.
erythrocyte pyruvate kinase d.
essential fatty acid d.
factor I d.
factor II d.
factor V d.
factor VIII d.
factor X d.
factor XI d.
factor XIII d.
d. of factor B, D
factor D d.
factor H d.
familial APOA-I d.
familial lecithin:cholesterol
  acyltransferase d.
femoral d.
fibrinogen d.
folate folic acid d.
folic acid d.
formiminotransferase d.
fructose galactokinase d.
GABA transaminase d.
galactokinase d.
galactose-1-phosphate uridyl
  transferase d.
gamma-aminobutyric acidemia
  transaminase d.
genetic isolated CD59 d.
glucoamylase d.
glucocorticoid d.
glucose-6-phosphate dehydrogenase
  enzyme d.
glucuronyl transferase d.
glutamate formiminotransferase d.
glutathione synthetase d.
glycogen synthetase d.
gonadotropic d.
G6PD d.

D

NOTES

deficiency *(continued)*
    granule d.
    growth hormone d. (GHD)
    growth hormone receptor d.
      (GHRD)
    HCS d.
    heparin cofactor II d.
    hepatic lipase d.
    hexosaminidase-A d.
    high molecular weight kininogen d.
    holocarboxylase synthetase d.
    humoral antibody d.
    11-hydroxylase d.
    21-hydroxylase d.
    idiopathic growth hormone d.
    IgA d.
    IgG2 d.
    IgG4 d.
    IgM d.
    IL-7R d.
    immune d.
    immunoglobulin A d.
    immunoglobulin G subclass d.
    insulin d.
    iron d.
    isolated gonadotropin d.
    isolated growth hormone d.
      (IGHD)
    lactase d.
    lactate dehydrogenase d.
    lactose d.
    LCAD/VLCAD d.
    LCHAD d.
    leukocyte adherence d.
    leukocyte adhesion d. (LAD)
    lipoprotein lipase d.
    liver phosphorylase d.
    long-chain 3-hydroxyacyl-CoA
      dehydrogenase d.
    long-chain very long-chain acyl-
      CoA dehydrogenase d.
    longitudinal d.
    long- and medium-chain fatty acid
      coenzyme-A dehydrogenase d.
      (LCAD/MCAD)
    LPL d.
    luteal phase d.
    magnesium d.
    MCAD d.
    medium-chain acyl-CoA
      dehydrogenase d.
    mental d.
    merosin d.
    methionine synthase d.
    MHC class I antigen d.
    micronutrient d.
    mineralocortical d.
    molybdenum cofactor d. (MCD)

    MPO d.
    multiple acyl-coenzyme A
      dehydrogenase d. (MADD)
    multiple carboxylase d.
    multiple pituitary hormone d.
      (MPHD)
    multiple sulfatase d.
    muscle adenosine monophosphate
      deaminase d.
    muscle carnitine
      palmityltransferase d.
    muscle phosphofructokinase d.
    myeloperoxidase d.
    myophosphorylase d.
    N-acetylglutamate d.
    neuraminidase d.
    neutrophil actin d.
    neutrophil chemotactic d.
    neutrophil G6PD d.
    d. of C1q
    ornithine-ketoacid
      aminotransferase d.
    ornithine transcarbamylase d.
    5-oxoprolinase d.
    PAI d.
    pancreatic exocrine d.
    PEPCK d.
    peroxisomal d.
    PFK d.
    phosphoenolpyruvate
      carboxykinase d.
    phosphofructokinase d.
    phosphorylase kinase d.
    placental progesterone d.
    plasminogen activator inhibitor d.
    PNP d.
    postinfectious secondary lactase d.
    prekallikrein d.
    primary carnitine d.
    primary immune d. (PID)
    primary neuraminidase d.
    prolidase d.
    properdin d.
    propionyl CoA carboxylase d.
    protein C, S d.
    proximal focal femoral d.
    pseudocholinesterase d.
    purine nucleoside phosphorylase d.
    pyridoxine d.
    d. of pyruvate carboxylase
    pyruvate dehydrogenase complex d.
    pyruvate kinase d.
    RAG1 d.
    RAG2 d.
    riboflavin d.
    SCAD d.
    SCOT d.
    secondary carnitine d.

selective IgA d.
serotonin d.
sphingolipid activator protein d.
steroid sulfatase d.
STS d.
succinyl CoA:3-ketoacid CoA
  transferase d.
sucrase-isomaltase d.
sulfite oxidase d.
surfactant protein d.
systemic carnitine d.
systemic fatty acid d.
TBG d.
terminal complement component d.
tetany of vitamin D d.
tetrahydrobiopterin d.
thiamine d.
thiopurine methyltransferase d.
thyroid d.
thyroid-binding globulin d.
thyroxine-binding globulin d.
tocopherol d.
TPI d.
TPMT d.
transcobalamin II d.
transglutaminase d.
trifunctional protein d. (TFP)
triose phosphate isomerase d.
upper limb d.
urocanase d.
vitamin A d. (VAD)
vitamin B_{12} d.
vitamin C d.
vitamin D d.
vitamin E d.
vitamin K d.
d. of xylulose dehydrogenase
zinc d.
deficiency-1
leukocyte adhesion d.-1 (LAD-1)
deficiency-2
leukocyte adhesion d.-2 (LAD-2)
deficient hydroxylation of cholecalciferol
deficit
attention d.
d.'s in attention, motor control,
  perception (DAMP)
dichotic listening d.
focal neurologic d.
hemisensory d.
lexical-syntactic d.
naming speed d.

neurodevelopmental d.
posterior column sensory d.
pragmatic and semantic-
  pragmatic d.'s
spinothalamic sensory d.
d. therapy
Deficol
deflection
QRS-T d.
defoaming
deformans
dystonia musculorum d. (DMD)
deformation
shear-strain d.
deformational occipital plagiocephaly
deformity
adduction d.
back-knee d.
barrel chest d.
bell-clapper d.
bend d.
bowing d.
bunionette d.
calcaneovalgus foot d.
cavovarus d.
Chiari d.
clawhand d.
cloverleaf skull d.
clubfoot d.
congenital condylar d.
coxa vara d.
Dandy-Walker d.
equinovarus pes d.
equinus d.
fixed flexion d.
genu varum d.
gooseneck d.
gunstock d.
habit tic d.
hindfoot valgus d.
hyperextension d.
inversion d.
Jaccoud d.
jaw d.
kleeblattschädel d.
lobster claw d.
lordotic d.
Madelung d.
mitten-hand d.
neurogenic equinus d.
pes cavus d.
ping-pong ball d.

D

NOTES

deformity *(continued)*
    protuberant step d.
    pseudo-Hurler d.
    rachitic bone d.
    recurvatum d.
    rigid supination d.
    rocker-bottom foot d.
    round back d.
    sabre shin d.
    saddle-nose d.
    shepherd crook d.
    silver fork d.
    spinning top d.
    Sprengel d.
    static d.
    supratip nasal tip d.
    talipes equinovarus d.
    thumb in palm d.
    torsional d.
    Volkmann d.
    windswept d.
    wry neck d.
defunctionalized bladder
degeneration
    anterior horn cell d.
    axonal d.
    cerebellar d.
    cerebromacular d.
    congenital macular d.
    cystic d.
    dying-back axonal d.
    hepatolenticular d.
    hypobetalipoproteinemia,
      acanthocytosis, retinitis
      pigmentosa, and pallidal d.
      (HARP)
    infantile neuronal d.
    joint d.
    myocardial fiber d.
    nuclear d.
    oligodendroglial d.
    olivopontocerebellar d.
    pallidal d.
    pulpal d.
    retinal pigmentary d.
    spinocerebellar d.
    spongy d.
    subacute combined d.
    tapetoretinal d.
    wallerian d.
    white matter d.
degenerative
    d. arthritis
    d. osteoarthritis
Degest 2 Ophthalmic
degloving injury
deglutition

degradation
    ganglioside d.
    glycoprotein d.
degranulation
45-degree skin traction
dehalogenase defect
dehydrated
dehydration
    d. fever
    hypernatremic d.
    hyperosmolar d.
    hypertonic d.
    hyponatremic d.
    hypotonic d.
    isonatremic d.
    isotonic d.
    mild d.
    moderate d.
    d., poisoning, trauma (DPT)
    severe d.
7-dehydrocholesterol
dehydroepiandrosterone (DHEA)
    d. sulfate (DHEAS)
dehydrogenase
    acetyl-CoA d.
    deficiency of xylulose d.
    electron transfer flavoprotein d.
      (ETF-DH)
    glucose-6-phosphate d. (G6PD)
    hydroxysteroid d. type 2 (HSD2)
    isovaleryl-CoA d.
    lactate d. (LDH)
    long-chain acyl-CoA d. (LCAD)
    long-chain 3-hydroxyacyl-CoA d.
      (LCHAD)
    long-chain hydroxyacyl-coenzyme
      A d. (LCHAD)
    long- and very-long-chain acyl-
      CoA d. (LCAD/VLCAD)
    medium-chain acyl-CoA d.
      (MCAD)
    pyruvate d.
    short-chain acyl coenzyme A d.
      (SCAD)
    short-chain hydroxyacyl-coenzyme
      A d. (SCHAD)
    succinate d.
    very long chain acyl-CoA d.
      (VLCAD)
dehydrogenation
    pyruvate d.
5-dehydrotachysterol
dehydroxylase
    phenylalanine d.
déjà vu
Dejerine disease
Dejerine-Klumpke syndrome

Dejerine-Sottas
    D.-S. atrophy
    D.-S. disease
    D.-S. syndrome
Dekasol Injection
Dekasol-L.A. Inject
Del
    D. Aqua-5 Gel
    D. Aqua-10 Gel
Delatest Injection
Delatestryl Injection
delavirdine (DLV)
Delaxin
delay
    adaptive d.
    benign maturation d.
    cognitive d.
    constitutional growth d.
    developmental d.
    global developmental d.
    growth d.
    language d.
    neurodevelopmental d.
    physiologic d.
    pubertal d.
    radial-femoral d.
    speech d.
delayed
    d. bone age
    d. deep tendon reflex
    d. gastric emptying
    d. motor development
    d. myelopathy
    d. neuropsychological sequela (DNS)
    d. orthostatic intolerance
    d. primary closure
    d. puberty
    d. relaxation phase
    d. repair
    d. sexual maturation
    d. sleep phase syndrome (DSPS)
    d. tooth eruption
    d. transfusion reaction
    d. union
delayed-phase computed tomography
delayed-type hypersensitivity (DTH)
Delbet fracture classification (types I–IV)
Delcort Topical
Delestrogen

deletion
    chromosomal d.
    chromosome 4 d.
    chromosome 15 d.
    chromosome 1p d.
    de novo d.
    elastin gene d.
    interstitial d.
    4p d. syndrome
    22q11.2 d. syndrome
    d. syndrome
    Xp d.
delinquency
delinquent
delirium
Deliver formula
delivery
    breech d.
    cesarean d.
    normal spontaneous vaginal d. (NSVD)
    normal vaginal d.
    precipitate d.
    precipitous d.
    preterm d.
    route of d.
Delorme procedure
Delsym
delta
    d. phalanx
    D. shunt
    d. sleep
    D. Valve
    d. wave
Delta-Cortef Oral
Deltasone
DeltaTrac II indirect calorimeter
Delta-Tritex Topical
deltoid
    d. insertion
    d. muscle
    d. paralysis
delusion
    grandiose d.
Del-Vi-A
Demadex
    D. Injection
    D. Oral
demander
    entitled d.
Demazin
demeclocycline

NOTES

dementia
  Heller d.
Demerol
demineralization
demise
  fetal d.
Demodex
  D. brevis
  D. follicurum
demographic
demyelinating encephalopathy
demyelination
  inflammatory d.
  symmetric d.
demyelinative
denature
dendritic
  d. arborization
  d. cell
  d. keratitis
denervation
dengue
  d. fever
  d. hemorrhagic fever
  d. shock syndrome
  d. virus
denial stage
Denis
  D. Browne bar
  D. Browne clubfoot splint
  D. Browne night splint
Dennie
  D. line
  D. lines of lower eyelids
Dennie-Morgan fold
Dennyson-Fulford extraarticular subtalar arthrodesis
Denorex
dens
  hypoplastic d.
densa
  sublamina d.
dense
  d. band
  d. body deficiency
  d. cast
  d. striation
densitometry
  bone d.
  dynamic spiral CT lung d.
density
  areal bone mineral d.
  bone mineral d. (BMD)
  increased bone d.
  lamellar body number d.
  soft-tissue d.
  d. spectral array (DSA)

  volumetric bone mineral d.
    (vBMD)
dental
  d. avulsion
  d. caries
  d. cementum
  d. crowding
  d. defect
  d. enamel hypoplasia
  d. extrusion
  d. extrusion/lateral luxation
  d. intrusion
  d. lamina cyst
  d. speech appliance
  d. trauma
dental-alveolar abscess
dentate
  d. line
  d. nucleus
dentatorubral atrophy
dentatorubrothalamocortical system
dentigerous cyst
dentin
dentinogenesis imperfecta
dentition
  permanent d.
  primary d.
dentoalveolar unit
Denver
  D. Developmental Screening Test
    (DDST)
  D. Developmental Screening Test
    II
  D. Home Screening Questionnaire
  D. II screening
Denys-Drash syndrome
deossification
deoxyadenosine
deoxyadenosylcobalamin
deoxy ATP
deoxycholate
  amphotericin B d. (AmBd)
deoxyhemoglobin
deoxynucleotide triphosphate
deoxyribonuclease (DNAse, DNase)
deoxyribonucleic
  d. acid (DNA)
  d. acid analysis
15-deoxyspergualin
Depacon
Depakene
Depakote sprinkle
depAndro Injection
department
  D. of Children and Family
    Services (DCFS)
  D. of Children's Services (DCS)
  pediatric emergency d. (PED)

D. of Public Social Services
(DPSS)
Depen
dependence
vitamin D d.
dependency
chemical d.
pyridoxine d.
dependent pooling
depersonalization
depGynogen
depigmentation
depigmented nevus
depigmentosus
nevus d.
depilation
depleted
lymphocyte d.
depletion
germ-cell d.
intravascular volume d.
T-cell d.
depMedalone Injection
Depo-Estradiol
Depogen
Depoject Injection
depolarization
atrial premature d.
ventricular premature d.
Depo-Medrol Injection
depomedroxyprogesterone acetate
(DMPA)
depo-MPA
Deponit Patch
Depopred Injection
Depo-Provera Injection
deposit
electron-dense subepithelial d.
granular osmiophilic d.
deposition
complement d.
copper d.
cystine d.
fat d.
fibrin d.
hemosiderin d.
IgΛ mesangial d.
immunoglobulin d.
neonatal elastin d.
depot
Lupron D.
Sandostatin LAR D.

Depotest Injection
Depo-Testosterone Injection
depressed
d. fontanelle
d. scar
d. sensorium
d. skull fracture
depression
anaclitic d.
anxiety d.
atypical d.
bipolar d.
cardiovascular d.
cortical spreading d.
double d.
melancholic d.
ping-pong ball d.
posteromedial articular d.
postictal d.
postnatal d. (PND)
prepubertal d.
psychotic d.
d. rating scale
respiratory d.
D. Self-Rating Scale
d. stage
treatment-refractory d.
unipolar d.
depressive
d. disorder
d. symptom
depressor
d. anguli oris
d. anguli oris muscle
tongue d.
torque d.
deprivation
d. amblyopia
idiocy by d.
oxygen d.
social d.
depth
crypt d.
d. perception
d. relationship
derangement
internal d.
derealization
derecruitment
derepressed gene
derivative
purified protein d. (PPD)

D

NOTES

145

Dermablend
Dermabond
dermabrasion
Dermacentor
    D. *andersoni*
    D. *variabilis*
Dermacort Topical
dermal
    d. erythropoiesis
    d. melanocytosis
    d. nevus
    d. sinus
    d. sinus tract
    d. vasculitis
    d. vitiligo
Dermarest Dricort Topical
Derma-Smoothe/FS Topical
dermatan
    d. sulfate
    d. sulfate accumulation
dermatitic
dermatitidis
    Blastomyces d.
dermatitis
    allergic contact d.
    atopic d.
    brawny d.
    burnlike d.
    Candida diaper d.
    candidal diaper d.
    chronic bullous d.
    chronic eczematoid d.
    contact d.
    diaper d.
    eczematoid d.
    d. enteropathica
    d. exfoliativa infantum
    exfoliative d.
    follicular d.
    friction d.
    d. gangrenosa infantum
    d. herpetiformis (DH)
    d. herpetiformis-associated gluten-
      sensitive enteropathy
    infectious eczematoid d.
    infective d.
    irritant contact d.
    irritant diaper d.
    Jacquet erosive diaper d.
    juvenile plantar d.
    mask of atopic d.
    monilial diaper d.
    neonatal bullous d.
    nickel d.
    nummular d.
    occlusion d.
    perianal d.

    photosensitive d.
    psoriatic d.
    rhus d.
    scalp seborrheic d.
    scaly d.
    seborrheic d.
    shoe contact d.
    tide mark d.
    d. venenata
    weeping d.
dermatofibroma
dermatofibrosis lenticularis disseminata
dermatoglyphic abnormality
dermatoglyphics
dermatology
    neonatal d.
    pediatric d.
dermatomal distribution
dermatomegaly
dermatomyositis (DM)
    amyopathic juvenile d.
    juvenile d. (JDM, JDMS)
dermatomyositis/polymyositis
dermatophyte
    d. infection
    d. lesion
    d. test media (DTM)
dermatophytid reaction
dermatophytosis
dermatosis, pl. **dermatoses**
    acute febrile neurophilic d.
    bullous d.
    ichthyosiform d.
    idiopathic d.
    juvenile plantar d.
    d. of kwashiorkor
    linear IgA d.
    plantar d.
dermis
    thinned d.
dermoepidermal junction
dermographism
    white d.
dermoid
    d. cyst
    epibulbar d.
Dermolate Topical
dermolipoma
dermolysis bullosa
Dermoplast
Dermtex HC with Aloe Topical
derotation
    d. femoral osteotomy
    d. osteotomy
DES
    diethylstilbestrol
25-desacetyl rifapentine

desalination
1-desamino-8-D-arginine vasopressin
   (DDAVP)
desaturate
desaturation
   red d.
Descemet membrane
descending
   d. aorta anastomosis
   left anterior d. (LAD)
descent
   aberrant course of testicular d.
   spontaneous d.
   testicular d.
Desenex
desensitization
   imaginal d.
desert rheumatism
Desferal Mesylate
desferrioxamine therapy
desflurane
desiccate
designation
   eligibility d.
designed
   Dortmund Nutritional and
      Anthropometrical Longitudinally D.
      (DONALD)
designer
   Pharsight Trial D.
desipramine
Desmarres retractor
desmethylimipramine
desmoplasia
   intratumoral d.
desmoplastic
   d. medulloblastoma
   d. small round cell tumor
      (DSRCT)
desmopressin (DDAVP)
   d. acetate
   d. acetate nasal spray
   intranasal d.
desmosome
Desogen
desonide
DesOwen Topical
desoximetasone
desoxycholate amphotericin B
Desoxyn
Despec
desquamated epithelial cell

desquamation
   follicular d.
   perineal d.
   periungual d.
desquamative
   d. interstitial pneumonia
   d. interstitial pneumonitis (DIP)
desquamativum
   erythroderma d.
Desquam-E Gel
Desquam-X
   D.-X Gel
   D.-X Wash
destruction
   hypothalamic-hypophyseal d.
   physeal d.
Desyrel
detachment
   exudative retinal d.
   retinal d.
   rhegmatogenous d.
   serous retinal d.
   tractional retinal d.
detector
   Pedi-cap d.
   piezoelectric PVDF d.
detergens
   liquor carbonis d. (LCD)
determinant
   sialyl Lewis X d.
determination
   blood gas d.
   bone age d.
   selective renal vein renin d.
   sweat chloride d.
detoxification
Detroit Test of Learning Aptitude-2
detrusor hyperreflexia
detrusorrhaphy
detrusor-sphincter dyssynergia
detumescence
devascularization
development
   adaptive d.
   alveolar stage of lung d.
   d. and/or central nervous system
      anomalies, genital hypoplasia, ear
      anomalies
   Assessment in Infancy Ordinal
      Scales of Psychological D.
   Bayley Scales of Infant D. (BSID)

D

NOTES

147

development *(continued)*
    Brigance Diagnostic Inventory of Early D.
    canalicular stage of lung d.
    cellular and molecular regulation of lung d.
    cephalocaudal sequence of d.
    cytoarchitectural d.
    delayed motor d.
    dissociated motor d.
    embryonic d.
    expressive language d.
    fine motor d.
    Griffiths Scale of Mental D.
    gross motor d.
    infant d.
    language d.
    lung growth and d.
    mental d.
    National Institute of Child Health and Human D. (NICHD)
    normal fetal d.
    Ordinal Scales of Intellectual D.
    phonological d.
    pseudoglandular stage of lung d.
    psychosocial d.
    pulmonary vascular d.
    receptive language d.
    saccular stage of lung d.
    social d.
    d. specialist
    speech d.
developmental
    d. age
    d. area
    d. assessment score
    D. Behaviour Checklist
    d. cataract
    d. check
    d. coordination disorder (DCD)
    d. delay
    d. disability (DD)
    d. disorder
    d. dysfluency
    d. dyslexia
    d. dysphasia
    d. dysplasia of hip (DDH)
    d. flatfoot
    d. genu varum
    d. hip disease
    d. hip dysplasia
    d. language disorder (DLD)
    d. milestone
    d. motor quotient (DMQ)
    D. Profile-II (DP-II)
    D. Programming for Infants and Young Children
    d. quotient (DQ)
    D. Test of Visual-Motor Integration
Development-II
    Bayley Scales of Infant D.-II (BSID-II)
deviant volitional movement
deviated septum
deviation
    axis d.
    eye d.
    jaw d.
    left axis d.
    right axis d.
    septal d.
    standard d.
Devic disease
device
    AeroChamber spacer d.
    alternative communication d.
    Amplatzer d.
    antisiphon d.
    augmentative communication d.
    bag-valve-mask d.
    Button gastrostomy d.
    Button-One Step gastrostomy d.
    CardioSEAL d.
    central venous access d. (CVAD)
    clamshell-type catheter occlusion d.
    double-umbrella d.
    dynamic orthotic cranioplasty d.
    ExacTech glucose measuring d.
    Finapres d.
    flutter d.
    Gianturco-Grifka vascular occlusion d.
    handheld flutter d.
    HemoCue AB hemoglobin measurement d.
    Ilizarov d.
    intrauterine d. (IUD)
    knee height measuring d.
    LactAid d.
    McMaster Family Assessment D.
    STARFlex d.
    umbrella d.
    ventricular assist d.
deworm
DEXA
    dual-energy x-ray absorptiometry
    DEXA scan
Dexacidin Ophthalmic
Dexacort
    D. Phosphate Respihaler Oral Inhaler
    D. Phosphate Turbinaire Intranasal Aerosol
Dex-A-Diet

dexamethasone
  methotrexate, bleomycin, doxorubicin, cyclophosphamide, Oncovin, d. (m-BACOD)
  d., neomycin and polymyxin B
  pulse d.
  d. suppression test
  d. suppression testing (DST)
  vincristine and d.
Dexameth Oral
Dexasone L.A. Injection
Dexasporin Ophthalmic
Dexatrim
Dexedrine Spansule capsule
dexfenfluramine
Dexone
  D. LA Injection
  D. Tablet
dexrazoxane
dexter
  oculus d. (right eye) (o.d., OD)
dextran
dextrans
  limit d.
dextrinosis
  limit d.
dextroamphetamine (DA)
  d. saccharate
  d. sulfate
dextrocardia
  mirror-image d.
dextro formula
dextromethorphan
  guaifenesin and d.
dextroposition
  anomalous right pulmonary vein d.
dextrose
Dextrostix reagent strip
Dey-Dose
  D.-D. Isoproterenol
  D.-D. Metaproterenol
Dey-Drop Ophthalmic Solution
Dey-Lute Isoetharine
DF
  diabetic fetopathy
DFA
  direct fluorescent antibody
  DFA staining
DFMO
  difluoromethyl ornithine
DH
  dermatitis herpetiformis

DHA
  docosahexaenoic acid
DHC
  Duradyne DHC
DHCA
  deep hypothermia and total circulatory arrest
DHEA
  dehydroepiandrosterone
DHEAS
  dehydroepiandrosterone sulfate
DHS Tar
DHT
  dihydrotestosterone
DI
  diabetes insipidus
DIA
  dot immunobinding assay
diabetes
  borderline d.
  brittle d.
  bronze d.
  D. Control and Complications Trial (DCCT)
  gestational d.
  d. insipidus (DI)
  d. insipidus, diabetes mellitus, optic atrophy, deafness (DIDMOAD)
  d. insipidus, diabetes mellitus, optic atrophy, deafness syndrome
  insulin-dependent d.
  juvenile-onset d.
  ketosis-prone d.
  ketosis-resistant d.
  latent d.
  lipoatrophic d.
  maternal d.
  maturity-onset d.
  d. mellitus (type 1, 2) (DM)
  non-insulin-dependent d.
  sugar d.
  transient neonatal d. (TND)
diabetic
  d. acidosis
  d. cardiomyopathy
  d. cheiroarthropathy
  d. coma
  d. embryopathy
  d. fetopathy (DF)
  d. ketoacidosis (DKA)
  d. retinopathy

D

NOTES

diabetic *(continued)*
   D. Tussin DM
   D. Tussin EX
diabeticorum
   necrobiosis lipoidica d. (NLD)
diacetate
   diflorasone d.
diacylglycerol
diadochokinesis
diagnosis
   established medical d.
   preimplantation genetic d. (PGD)
   prenatal d.
diagnostic
   D. Interview for Genetic Study
      (DIGS)
   D. Interview Schedule for Children
      (DISC)
   D. Interview Schedule for
      Children-Revised (DISC-R)
   d. overshadowing
   d. peritoneal lavage (DPL)
   d. procedure
   D. and Statistical Manual of
      Mental Disorders - 4th Edition
      (DSM-IV)
diakinesis
Dialose Plus Capsule
dialysate protein loss
dialysis
   continuous ambulatory peritoneal d.
      (CAPD)
   continuous cyclic peritoneal d.
      (CCPD)
   peritoneal d. (PD)
diameter
   AP d.
   biparietal d. (BPD)
   increased anteroposterior chest d.
   narrow bifrontal d.
   occipitofrontal d.
Diamine T.D. Oral
diamniotic
Diamond-Blackfan
   D.-B. anemia (DBA)
   D.-B. syndrome
diamond-shaped murmur
Diamox Sequels
diapedetic leukocyte
diaper
   d. dermatitis
   d. rash
   zinc-free plastic-lined d.
diaphanous
   Drosophila melanogaster gene d.
diaphoresis
diaphoretic

diaphragm
   duodenal d.
   eventration of d.
   d. palsy
   d. paralysis
   plication of d.
diaphragmatic
   d. atony
   d. eventration
   d. hernia
   d. hiatus
   d. injury
   d. plication
diaphyseal
   d. aclasis
   d. dysplasia
   d. fibular osteotomy
   d. fracture
   d. osteomyelitis
diaphysis
Diar-aid
diarrhea
   antibiotic-associated d. (AAD)
   bloody d.
   chloride-losing d.
   chronic nonspecific d.
   Clostridium difficile-associated d.
      (CDAC)
   congenital sodium d.
   explosive watery d.
   infantile d.
   nosocomial d.
   osmotic d.
   pediatric viral d.
   protracted d.
   secretory d.
   toddler's d.
   traveler's d. (TD)
   watery d.
**diarrhea-associated hemolytic uremic
   syndrome**
diarrheal shellfish poisoning
diarrheic
diarthrodial
   d. joint
   d. muscle
diary
   baby's day d.
   headache d.
DiaScreen reagent strip
Diasorb
diastasis
   d. recti
   d. recti abdominis
   symphysis pubis d.
diastatic fracture
Diastat Rectal Delivery System
diastematomyelia

diastole
diastolic
  d. arterial pressure (DAP)
  d. blood pressure
  d. component
  d. gradient
  d. murmur
  d. overload
  d. overload pattern
  d. thrill
diastomyelia
diastrophic
  d. dwarf
  d. dwarfism
  d. dysplasia
diathermy loop excision
diathesis
  bleeding d.
  cognitive-stress d.
  hemorrhagic d.
diatomaceous
  d. earth (DE)
  d. earth slurry
diatrizoate
  meglumine d.
Diazemuls Injection
diazepam
Diazepam Intensol
diazo reaction
diazoxide
dibasic
  d. amino acid
  d. aminoaciduria
Dibbell cleft lip-nasal reconstruction
Dibent Injection
Dibenzyline
dibucaine
DIC
  disseminated intravascular coagulation
Dicarbosil
dichotic
  d. listening
  d. listening deficit
dichotomy
Dick test
diclofenac
dicloxacillin
dicumarol
dicyclomine hydrochloride
didactic material
didanosine (ddI)

DIDMOAD
  diabetes insipidus, diabetes mellitus,
    optic atrophy, deafness
  DIDMOAD syndrome
Didronel
Dieckmann intraosseous needle
diencephalic
  d. syndrome (DS)
  d. syndrome of infancy
  d. system n
diencephalon
Dientamoeba fragilis
diepoxybutane (DEB)
diet
  ADA d.
  ad libitum d.
  American Diabetes Association d.
  American Heart Association Step
    One D.
  bananas, rice cereal, applesauce,
    tea, toast d.
  bananas, rice cereal, applesauce,
    toast d.
  BRAT d.
  BRATT d.
  elemental d.
  elimination d.
  fluid d.
  galactose-free d.
  glutamine-supplemented d.
  gluten-free d. (GFD)
  glycemic index d.
  high-calorie d.
  high-phosphate d.
  K d.
  K+2 d.
  ketogenic d.
  Lorenzo oil d.
  low-branched-chain amino acid d.
  low-phenylalanine d.
  polymeric d.
  protein-sparing modified fast d.
  PSMF d.
  pureed d.
  semifluid d.
  traffic-light d.
dietary
  d. protein enterocolitis
  d. supplement
Dieterle stain
diethylcarbamazine

D

NOTES

151

diethylenetetramine pentaacetic acid radionuclide scan
diethylenetriamine pentaacetic acid (DTPA)
diethylstilbestrol (DES)
diethyltoluamide (DEET)
diet-induced hypochloremic metabolic alkalosis
dietitian
Dieulafoy
    D. gastric lesion
    D. lesion
DIF
  direct immunofluorescence
  DIF test
difference
  gender d.
differential
    d. agglutination test
    d. cyanosis
    d. detection hypothesis
    manual d.
    d. treatment hypothesis
differentiation
    alveolar myofibroblast d.
    cluster of d. (CD)
    cluster of d. 4 (CD4)
    corticomedullary d.
    ganglionic d.
    hematopoietic d.
    lymphopoietic d.
    schwannian d.
    terminal lung d.
Differin gel
difficile
    Clostridium d.
difficulty
    attentional d.
    feeding d.
    d. sleeping
    swallowing d.
diffuse
    d. astrocytoma
    d. axonal injury (DAI)
    d. brain swelling (DBS)
    d. cortical thrombophlebitis
    d. cutaneous leishmaniasis (DCL)
    d. cutaneous mastocytosis
    d. cystic polycystic kidney disease
    d. esophageal spasm
    d. fasciitis
    d. glomerular sclerosis
    d. hyperpigmentation
    d. intestinal polyp
    d. mesangial sclerosis (DMS)
    d. mixed lymphocytic plasmacytic disease

    d. morbilliform rash
    d. neonatal hemangiomatosis
    d. nonmalignant lymphadenopathy
    d. periaxial encephalitis
    d. proliferative glomerulonephritis
    d. proliferative lupus nephritis
    d. small cell cleaved lymphoma
    d. tensor brain MRI
diffusing
    d. capacity
    d. capacity of lung for carbon monoxide (DL_{co})
diffusion
diffusion-weighted
    d.-w. imaging (DWI)
    d.-w. magnetic resonance imaging
diffusum
    angiokeratoma corporis d.
diflorasone diacetate
Diflucan
difluoromethyl ornithine (DFMO)
DiGeorge
    D. anomaly
    D. syndrome
digestion
Digibind
DigiScope
digit
    ainhumlike constriction of d.
    bambooing of d.
    hypoplastic d.
    rudimentary-type d.
    sausage d.
    D. Span Subtest
    supernumerary d.
    d. syndactyly
    trigger d.
digital
    d. auditory aerobics (DAA)
    d. clubbing
    d. fibroma
    d. pitting
    d. pulp
    d. radiography
    d. subtraction angiography
    d. tuft
    d. ulceration
digitalis effect
digitalis-induced arrhythmia
digitorenocerebral syndrome
digitoxin
Digitrapper portable pH recorder
digoxin
    d. immune fab
    d. monotherapy
DIGS
  Diagnostic Interview for Genetic Study

dihydrochloride
    quinine d.
    triethylene tetramine d.
dihydropteridine
    d. reductase
    d. reductase deficiency
dihydrotachysterol
dihydrotestosterone (DHT)
1,25-dihydroxycholecalciferol
9-13-dihydroxypropoxymethyl guanine
Dihyrex Injection
diiodothyronine
diisopropyl iminodiacetic acid (DISIDA)
Dilacor XR
Dilantin
dilatation (*var. of* dilation)
dilated
    d. bowel loop resection
    d. capillary
    d. cardiomyopathy
    d. cisterna magna
    d. intestinal loop
    d. posterior urethra
    d. renal pelvis
    d. vein
dilating reflux
dilation, dilatation
    aorta d.
    congenital choledochal d.
    cystic d.
    esophageal d.
    fusiform d.
    gastric d.
    pneumatic d.
    posthemorrhagic ventricular d.
      (PHVD)
    saccular d.
    urinary tract d.
dilator
    bougie d.
    iris d.
Dilaudid
    D. Cough Syrup
    D. Injection
    D. Oral
    D. Suppository
Dilaudid-HP Injection
dilemma
    taxonomic and assessment d.
Dilocaine Injection
Dilomine Injection

diltiazem
dilute
    d. Surfaxin
    d. urine
diluted formula
Dimaphen Elixir
dimeglumine
    gadopentetate d.
dimenhydrinate
dimension
    hyperactive/impulsive d.
    inattention d.
    left ventricular end-diastolic d.
    left ventricular end-systolic d.
dimer
    metalloprotein d.
dimercaprol
dimercaptosuccinic acid
Dimetabs Oral
Dimetane Extentabs
Dimetapp
    D. DM
    D. Elixir
    D. 4-Hour Liqui-Gel
    D. 4-Hour Liqui-Gel Capsule
    D. Tablets
dimethyl
    d. phthalate
    d. sulfoxide (DMSO)
diminazene
diminished fremitus
dimorphism
dimorphous leprosy
dimple
    anal d.
    cutaneous d.
    lumbosacral d.
    pilonidal d.
    pretibial skin d.
    sacral d.
Dinate Injection
dinitrate
    isosorbide d. (ISDN)
dinitrochlorobenzene
dinitrophenylhydrazine
dinucleotide
    flavin adenine d. (FAD)
Diocto
Diocto-C
Diocto-K Plus
Dioctolose Plus

D

NOTES

153

diode
   argon d.
   light-emitting d.
dioesophageal junction
Dioeze
Dioralyte
DIOS
   distal intestinal obstruction
Dioval
diovular twin
dioxide
   carbon d. (CO_2)
   end-tidal carbon d. (E_TCO_2)
   pressure of carbon d. (PCO_2)
   sulfur d.
DIP
   desquamative interstitial pneumonitis
dipalmitoyl phosphatidylcholine
Dipentum
diphasic
Diphenacen-50 Injection
Diphen Cough
diphencyprone
Diphenhist
diphenhydramine citrate
diphenoxylate and atropine
Diphenylan Sodium
diphenylhydantoin
diphenyl tetrazolium bromide
diphosphate
   galactose uridine d.
   uridine d. (UDP)
diphtheria
   d. antitoxin
   cutaneous d.
   laryngeal d.
   nasal d.
   pharyngeal d.
   tetanus and d. (Td)
   d., tetanus, acellular pertussis vaccine
   d., tetanus, pertussis
   d., tetanus, pertussis vaccine
   tetanus toxoid and d.
   d., tetanus toxoid, acellular pertussis
   d., tetanus toxoid, acellular pertussis vaccine
   d., tetanus toxoid, pertussis (DTP)
   d., tetanus (toxoids), accelerated pertussis vaccine
   d., tetanus toxoids, whole-cell pertussis vaccine
   d. toxin (DT)
diphtheriae
   Corynebacterium d.
diphtheria-pertussis-tetanus (DPT)

diphtheria-tetanus
   d.-t. toxoids-acellular pertussis (DTaP)
   d.-t. toxoid with pertussis (DTwP)
diphtheria-tetanus-pertussis immunization
diphtheritic
   d. croup
   d. membrane
   d. toxic myocarditis
diphtheroid
diphthong
diphyllobothriasis
Diphyllobothrium latum
DIPI
   direct intraperitoneal insemination
dipivefrin
dipivoxil
   adefovir d.
diplegia
   atonic-astatic d.
   facial d.
   faciolingual-masticatory d.
   infantile d.
   spastic d.
diplococcus, pl. diplococci
   gram-positive d.
Diplococcus pneumoniae
diploid
diplomyelia
Diplopagus
diplopia
   monocular d.
dipole
Diprivan Injection
Diprolene AF Topical
dipropionate
   beclomethasone d.
   betamethasone d.
Diprosone Topical
dipstick
   leukocyte esterase d.
   d. test
   urine d.
dipyridamole
   d. myocardial scintigraphy
   d. stress integrated backscatter
dipyrone
diquotidian fever
direct
   d. antiglobulin test (DAT)
   d. bilirubin
   d. Coombs test
   d. egg injection
   d. fluorescent antibody (DFA)
   d. fluorescent antibody stain
   d. fluorescent antibody staining
   d. hyperbilirubinemia
   d. immunofluorescence (DIF)

d. immunofluorescent staining
d. immunohistochemical staining
d. intraperitoneal insemination (DIPI)
d. laryngoscopy
d. ophthalmoscope
d. orbital floor fracture
d. stimulation
d. stimulation of pancreas
d. suicide risk (DSR)
d. wet mount

Directigen Flu A
direction
caudal d.
rostral d.
directional coronary atherectomy (DCA)
directly observed therapy (DOT)
direct-reacting bilirubin
Dirofilaria
D. immitis
D. tenuis
disability
cognitive d.
developmental d. (DD)
intellectual d.
learning d. (LD)
motor d.
National Joint Committee on Learning D.'s (NJCLD)
nonverbal learning d. (NVLD)
reading d.
selective reading d.
social-emotional learning d.
specific reading d.
disabled
orthopedically d.
disaccharidase deficiency
disaccharide intolerance
Disanthrol
disarray
myofiber d.
panlobar d.
disassociation
DISC
Diagnostic Interview Schedule for Children
Disc
Clear Away D.
disc (*var. of* disk)
discharge
epileptiform d.
foul-smelling d.

frothy d.
generalized epileptogenic d.
hypersynchronous d.
hypersynchrony of neural d.'s
interictal d.
neural d.
partial epileptogenic d.
polyspike d.
purulent nasal d.
sharp-wave d.
vaginal d.
disciform keratitis
discitis (*var. of* diskitis)
discoid
d. eczema
d. lateral meniscus
d. lesion
d. lupus
d. lupus erythematosus
d. meniscus
d. rash
discoloration
heliotropic d.
prominent skin d.
skin d.
discomfort
suprapubic d.
discontinuity
ossicular d.
discontinuous lesion
DISC-R
Diagnostic Interview Schedule for Children-Revised
discrepancy
leg length d. (LLD)
discrepant
discrete subaortic stenosis (DSS)
discrete-trial
d.-t. learning
d.-t. teaching
discrimination
auditory d.
right-left d.
tactile d.
two-point d.
DISCUS
Dyskinesia Identification System: Condensed User Scale
discus
Advair D.
Serevent D.

NOTES

disease
ABO hemolytic d.
acid lipase deficiency d.
acid peptic d.
acquired heart d.
acute biliary d.
acute fulminant d.
acute graft-versus-host d. (AGVHD, aGVHD)
acute neuronopathic Gaucher d.
acute pelvic inflammatory d.
acute respiratory d. (ARD)
acyanotic congenital heart d.
Addison d.
adult-onset polycystic kidney d.
adult polycystic d.
adult Refsum d.
Aicardi-Goutiéres d.
Albers-Schönberg d.
Alexander d.
allergic bowel d.
Alpers d.
alpha-1 antitrypsin d.
Anderson d.
anterior horn cell d.
antiglomerular basement membrane antibody d.
Antopol d.
Apert-Crouzon d.
Aran-Duchenne d.
atypical Kawasaki d.
autoimmune d.
autosomal dominant medullary cystic kidney d. (ADMCKD)
autosomal dominant polycystic d.
autosomal dominant polycystic kidney d. (ADPKD)
autosomal recessive polycystic kidney d. (ARPKD)
Balo d.
Barlow d.
Bassen-Kornzweig d.
Batten d.
Batten-Mayou d.
Becker d.
Behçet d.
Behr d.
Berger d.
Best d.
Bielschowsky-Jansky d.
Blount d.
Bornholm d.
Bount d.
Bourneville d.
Brill d.
Brill-Zinsser d.
brittle-bone d.
Bruton d.

bubble-boy d.
Byler d.
Caffey d.
Caisson d.
Calvé-Perthes d.
Canavan d.
Caroli d.
Castleman d.
cat-scratch d. (CSD)
cat-scratch fever d.
cavitary lung d.
celiac d. (CD)
central core d.
central nervous system d.
Chagas d.
Charcot d.
Charcot-Marie-Tooth d.
Cheadle d.
cholestatic liver d.
cholesterol ester storage d. (CESD)
Christmas d.
chronic Gaucher d.
chronic granulomatous d. (CGD)
chronic lung d. (CLD)
chronic neuromuscular d. (CNMD)
chronic neuronopathic Gaucher d.
chronic pulmonary d.
chronic sickle cell lung d.
chylomicron retention d.
cicatricial retinal d.
circling d.
classic celiac d.
Coats d.
cold agglutinin d.
cold hemagglutinin d.
collagen vascular d.
communicable d.
congenital cardiac d.
congenital heart d. (CHD)
congenital hip d.
congestive heart d. (CHD)
connective tissue d.
Conradi d.
Cooperative Study of Sickle Cell D. (CSSCD)
Cori d.
Cori-Forbes d.
coronary heart d.
Cowden d.
Creutzfeldt-Jakob d. (CJD)
Crigler-Najjar d. (type I, II)
critical illness neuromuscular d.
Crohn d.
Crouzon d.
Cushing d.
cyanotic congenital heart d. (CCHD)
cyanotic heart d.

cystic hydatid d.
cystic renal d.
cytomegalic inclusion d. (CID)
cytomegalovirus d.
Darier d.
Darier-White d.
Dawson d.
Dejerine d.
Dejerine-Sottas d.
developmental hip d.
Devic d.
diffuse cystic polycystic kidney d.
diffuse mixed lymphocytic
  plasmacytic d.
disseminated adenovirus d.
Dorfman-Chanarin d.
duct-dependent heart d.
Dukes d.
Duncan d.
Duroziez d.
early-onset d.
end-stage liver d.
end-stage renal d. (ESRD)
Erdheim d.
Eulenburg d.
exanthematous d.
exertional reactive airway d.
extraabdominal organ system d.
Fabry d.
Fahr d.
familial Creutzfeldt-Jakob d.
Farber d.
Fazio-Londe d.
Feer d.
fibrocystic d.
fifth d.
Filatov-Dukes d.
first d.
Folling d.
Fordyce d.
Fox-Fordyce d.
Freiberg d.
Fukuyama d.
fulminant d.
gallbladder d.
Gambian d.
gastroesophageal reflux d. (GERD)
Gaucher d. (type 1–3)
gay bowel d.
genetotrophic d.
gestational trophoblastic d.
Gianotti d.

Gilbert d.
Gitelman d.
glandular d.
Glanzmann d.
glomerular renal d.
glomerulocystic d.
glycogen storage d. (type Ia, Ib,
  II–VII) (GSD)
Goldstein d.
graft-versus-host d. (GVHD)
granulomatous d.
Graves d.
group B streptococcus d.
Günther d.
Hallervorden-Spatz d.
hand-foot-and-mouth d. (HFMD)
Hand-Schüller-Christian d.
Hartnup d.
heart d.
helminthic d.
hemoglobin sickle cell d.
hemolytic d.
hemorrhagic d.
hepatic glycogen storage d.
hepatobiliary d.
hepatocellular d.
hereditary d.
heredodegenerative d.
Hers d.
Hirschsprung d.
Hodgkin d.
hookworm d.
horn cell d.
Huntington d. (HD)
hyaline membrane d. (HMD)
hydatid d.
hydrocephaloid d.
hypophosphatemic bone d.
iatrogenic Creutzfeldt-Jakob d.
I-cell d.
idiopathic peptic ulcer d.
immune complex d.
immunoproliferative small
  intestinal d.
inclusion cell d.
infantile Alexander d.
infantile celiac d.
infantile Gaucher d.
infantile motor neuron d.
infantile polycystic d.
infantile Refsum d.
inflammatory bowel d. (IBD)

NOTES

D

157

disease *(continued)*

International Classification of D.'s (ICD)
interstitial lung d. (ILD)
intranuclear hyaline inclusion d.
ischemic heart d. (IHD)
isoimmune hemolytic d.
Jansky-Bielschowsky d.
juvenile Alexander d.
juvenile hereditary motor neuron d.
juvenile neuronopathic Gaucher d.
juvenile-onset inflammatory bowel d.
juvenile-onset multisystem inflammatory d. (JOMID)
juvenile Paget d.
juvenile Parkinson d.
Kashin-Beck d.
Kawasaki d.
Keshan d.
Kienböck d.
Kikuchi d.
Kimmelstiel-Wilson d.
kinky-hair d. (KHD)
Kirner d.
kissing d.
Köhler bone d.
Kostmann d.
Krabbe d.
Kufs d.
Kugelberg-Welander d.
kuru d.
KW d.
kwashiorkor d.
Kyasanur Forest d.
Lafora body d.
late hemorrhagic d.
latent celiac d.
Leber d.
Legg-Calvé-Perthes d. (LCPD)
Legg-Perthes d.
Legionnaires d.
Leigh d.
Leiner d.
Letterer-Siwe d.
Lhermitte-Duclos d.
Libman-Sacks d.
linear IgA d.
lipid storage d.
Little d.
lower airway d.
Luft d.
Lyell d.
Lyme d.
lymphocyte-depleted Hodgkin d.
lymphocyte-predominant Hodgkin d.
lymphohematogenous d.
lymphoproliferative d.
lymphoproliferative/myeloproliferative d.
lysosomal storage d.
Machado-Joseph d.
maple syrup urine d. (MSUD)
marble bone d.
Marburg d.
Marion d.
mast cell d.
McArdle d.
medullary cystic d.
Melnick-Needles d.
Menetrier d.
Ménière d.
Menkes kinky-hair d.
Merzbacher-Pelizaeus d.
metabolic bone d.
metastatic Crohn d. (MCD)
microvillus inclusion d. (MID)
Miege d.
Mikulicz d.
milk precipitin d.
Milroy d.
Minamata d.
minimal change d.
mitochondrial d.
mixed cellularity Hodgkin d.
mixed connective tissue d. (MCTD)
Moeller-Barlow d.
Morquio d.
motor neuron d.
moyamoya d.
Mucha-Habermann d.
multicentric Castleman d.
multicystic kidney d.
Münchausen d.
muscle-eye-brain d.
nemaline rod d.
neonatal chest d.
neonatal cyanotic congenital heart d.
neonatal gonococcal d.
neonatal iron-storage d. (NISD)
neurogenic hip d.
neurologic demyelinating d.
neutral lipid storage d.
new variant Creutzfeldt-Jakob d. (nvCJD)
Niemann-Pick d. (NPD)
Niemann-Pick C d.
Niemann-Pick d. type A (NPA)
Niemann-Pick d. type B (NPB)
Niemann-Pick d. type C (NPC)
Niemann-Pick d. type D (NPD)
Niemann-Pick d. (type I, II)
nodular sclerosing Hodgkin d.
noncirrhotic ascitic d.

noncyanotic congenital heart d.
Norrbottnian Gaucher d.
Norrie d.
Oasthouse urine d.
obliterative coronary artery d.
obstructive respiratory d.
occlusive vascular d.
oligoarticular d.
Ollier d.
Oppenheim d.
optic nerve d.
oral Crohn d.
organic brain d.
organic heart d.
Osgood-Schlatter d. (OSD)
Osler-Weber-Rendu d.
Owren d.
oxidative phosphorylation d.
Paas d.
Paget d.
Panner d.
parenchymal lung d.
parenteral nutrition-associated
  cholestatic liver d.
Parkinson d.
Pediatric Spectrum of D. (PSD)
Pelizaeus-Merzbacher d. (PMD)
pelvic inflammatory d. (PID)
peptic ulcer d. (PUD)
periodontal d.
peripheral arterial d.
peroxisomal d.
Perthes d.
pink d.
Pityrosporum d.
platelet-type von Willebrand d.
PNAC liver d.
polycystic kidney d. (PKD)
polycystic ovarian d. (PCOD)
polycystic ovary d. (POD)
polyglandular autoimmune d. (type
  I, II)
Pompe glycogen storage d. (type I,
  II)
postrheumatic valve d.
posttransplant lymphoproliferative d.
  (PTLD)
Pott d.
Potter d.
prion d.
pseudo-von Willebrand d.
puff-of-smoke d.

pulmonary parenchymal d.
pulmonary venoocclusive d.
pulseless d.
Pyle d.
pyramidal tract d.
radiation-induced heart d. (RIHD)
Ramstedt d.
Raynaud d.
reactive airway d.
Recklinghausen d.
refractory Crohn d.
Refsum d.
renal cystic d.
Rendu-Osler-Weber d.
restrictive lung d.
restrictive respiratory d.
rheumatic valvular heart d.
Rh isoimmune hemolytic d.
Rh d. of newborn
rickettsial d.
Riga-Fede d.
rippling muscle d.
Ritter d.
Rosai-Dorfman d.
Rotor d.
Roussy-Lévy d.
Salla d.
Sandhoff d.
Santavuori d.
Saunders d.
Scheuermann d.
Schilder d.
Schindler d.
Schwartz-Jampel d.
secondary moyamoya d.
Seitelberger d.
Sever d.
severe combined
  immunodeficiency d. (SCID)
sexually transmitted d. (STD)
sickle cell d. (SCD)
sickle cell-hemoglobin C d.
sickle cell-hemoglobin D d.
sickle cell-thalassemia d.
silent celiac d.
silo filler's d.
sixth d.
Sly d.
sphingolipid storage d.
Spielmeyer-Vogt d.
sporadic Creutzfeldt-Jakob d.
Stargardt d.

D

NOTES

disease *(continued)*
 startle d.
 Steinert d.
 Sticker d.
 Still d.
 storage d.
 stress-related peptic ulcer d.
 Sturge-Weber d.
 subacute neuronopathic Gaucher d.
 Swift d.
 Takayasu d.
 Tangier d.
 Tarui d.
 Tay-Sachs d.
 T-cell-mediated d.
 Terson d.
 Thiemann d.
 thin basement membrane d.
  (TBMD)
 Thompson d.
 Thomsen d.
 thrombohemolytic d.
 Tourette d.
 transplant coronary artery d.
 triglyceride storage d. (type I)
 ulceroglandular d.
 Ullrich d.
 Underwood d.
 Unverricht d.
 Unverricht-Lundborg d.
 upper motor neuron d.
 Urbach-Wiethe d.
 urea cycle d.
 uveomeningitic d.
 vascular d.
 venoocclusive d. (VOD)
 Vogt-Spielmeyer d.
 Volkmann d.
 von Gierke glycogen storage d.
 von Hippel-Lindau d.
 von Recklinghausen d.
 von Willebrand d.
 Waldenström d.
 Werdnig-Hoffmann d.
 Wernicke d.
 wet lung d.
 Whipple d.
 Wilkie d.
 Wilkins d.
 Wilson d.
 Winckel d.
 Wolman d.
 woolly hair d.
 X-linked chronic granulomatous d.
 X-linked lymphoproliferative d.

 Zellweger d.
 Zinsser d.
disease-modifying antirheumatic drug (DMARD)
disequilibrium
 transmission d.
disfigurement
DISIDA
 diisopropyl iminodiacetic acid
disinfection
 vaginal d.
disinhibited
disinhibition
disintegrate
disintegration
disk, disc
 choked d.
 dragged d.
 EMLA anesthetic d.
 glandular d.
 herniated d.
 d. herniation
 intervertebral d. (IVD)
 neovascularization of d. (NVD)
 optic d.
 tilted d.
 trilaminar embryonic d.
Diskhaler metered-dose inhaler
diskitis, discitis
 intervertebral d.
Diskus inhaler
dislocated
 d. hip
 d. mandible
 d. patella
 d. testis
dislocating patella
dislocation
 atlantoaxial d.
 atlantooccipital d.
 C1 to C2 d.
 congenital d.
 elbow d.
 facet d.
 femoral head d.
 Galeazzi fracture d.
 habitual shoulder d.
 lens d.
 mandibular d.
 metacarpophalangeal d.
 Monteggia fracture d.
 multiple d.'s
 peroneal d.
 radial head d.
 subluxation d.
 teratologic d.
 testicular d.
dismissing attachment

dismutase
 recombinant human superoxide d.
  (rhSOD)
dismutase-1
 superoxide d.-1
disodium
 d. cromoglycate
 edetate calcium d.
 etidronate d.
 ticarcillin d.
disomy
 uniparental d. (UPD)
Disonate
disopyramide
disorder
 acid-base d.
 acquired platelet d.
 acute stress d. (ASD)
 adjustment d.
 aggressive conduct d.
 alcohol-related
  neurodevelopmental d. (ARND)
 antisocial personality d. (ASPD)
 anxiety d.
 arousal d.
 articulation d.
 Asperger d. (AD)
 athetotic movement d.
 attachment d.
 attention deficit d. (ADD)
 attention deficit hyperactivity d.
  (ADHD)
 autism spectrum d. (ASD)
 autistic spectrum d.
 autosomal dominant d.
 autosomal recessive d.
 avoidant d.
 basal ganglia d.
 behavioral, anxiety, mood, and
  other types of d.'s (BAMO)
 bipolar d. (type 1, 2) (BPD)
 body dysmorphic d. (BDD)
 borderline personality d.
 breathing-related sleep d.
 cardiac rhythm d.
 central auditory processing d.
  (CAPD)
 Charcot-Marie-Tooth d.
 childhood disintegrative d. (CDD)
 children and adults with attention
  deficit d. (CHADD)

 Children's Interview for
  Psychiatric D.'s (ChIPS)
 choreoathetotic movement d.
 chronic motor tic d.
 chronic tic d. (CTD)
 cluster B d.
 collagen vascular d.
 communication d.
 comorbid anxiety d.
 conduct d. (CD)
 congenital hip d.
 connective tissue d.
 conversion d.
 Copeland Symptom Checklist for
  Attention Deficit D.'s
 cyclothymic d.
 depressive d.
 developmental d.
 developmental coordination d.
  (DCD)
 developmental language d. (DLD)
 Diagnostic and Statistical Manual
  of Mental D.'s - 4th Edition
  (DSM-IV)
 disruptive behavior d.
 dissociative d.
 dysthymic d.
 dystonic dyskinetic d.
 eating d.
 embryogenic induction d.
 emotional d.
 endocrine d.
 factitious d.
 familial d.
 fatty acid oxidation d.
 full-syndrome eating d.
 gastrointestinal d.
 gender identity d. (GID)
 generalized anxiety d. (GAD)
 genetic d.
 glomerular d.
 GSH pathway d.
 Hartnup d.
 hepatic parenchymal d.
 heredodegenerative d.
 histiocytic d.
 human leukocyte antigen
  associated d.
 hyperkinetic d.
 impulse spectrum d.
 inherited bleeding d.

D

NOTES

disorder *(continued)*
International Classification of
Sleep D.'s (ICSD)
intersex d.
intestinal d.
language d.
laterality d.
learning d.
lipid storage d.
lymphoproliferative d.
lysosomal storage d.
major depressive d. (MDD)
manic-depressive d.
metabolic d.
Methods for Epidemiology of
Child and Adolescent Mental D.'s
(MECA)
mixed receptive-expressive
language d. (MRELD)
monogenic d.
mood d.
motility d.
multifactorial d.
multiple complex developmental d.
(MCDD)
National Organization for
Rare D.'s (NORD)
neural tube d.
neurocutaneous d.
neurological d.
neuromuscular d.
neuronal migration d.
neuropsychiatric d.
nonspecific esophageal motility d.
(NEMD)
nonverbal perceptual-organization-
output d.
obsessive-compulsive d. (OCD)
obsessive-compulsive personality d.
(OCPD)
oppositional d.
oppositional defiant d. (ODD)
overanxious d. (OAD)
oxidation d.
pain d.
panic d.
paranoid personality d.
parkinsonian movement d.
partial-syndrome eating d.
periodic movement d.
peripheral auditory d.
peroxisomal d.
peroxisome import d.
personality d. (PD)
pervasive developmental d. (PDD)
petit mal-like seizure d.
phonological d.

phytanic acid oxidation d.
posttransplant lymphoproliferative d.
(PTLD)
posttraumatic stress d. (PTSD)
Practice Parameters for the
Assessment and Treatment of
Anxiety D.'s
premenstrual dysphoric d.
primary bullous d.
recurrent affective d.
REM sleep behavior d.
Rett d.
rhythmic movement d.
rumination d.
schizoaffective d.
schizoid personality d.
schizophreniform d.
Screen for Child Anxiety-Related
Emotional D.'s (SCARED)
seasonal affective d. (SAD)
seizure d.
semantic-pragmatic d.
separation anxiety d. (SAD)
sex-linked d.
sickling d.
sleep terror d.
sleep-wake transition d.
sleepwalking d.
social anxiety d.
somatization d.
somatoform d.
speech d.
stereotypical movement d.
storage d.
substance-induced psychotic d.
substance use d. (SUD)
test of variables of attention
deficit d.
thought d.
tic d.
Tourette d. (TD)
transient myeloproliferative d.
transient tic d.
unifactorial d.
urea cycle d.
vesicobullous d.
voice d.
Werdnig-Hoffmann d.
within-the-infant depressive d.
X-linked dominant d.
X-linked recessive d.
year 7 conduct d.
disordered renal acidification
disorganized
d. behavior
d. brainstem nuclei
Disotate

dispar
>   *Entamoeba d.*
>   *Veillonella d.*

Di-Spaz
>   D.-S. Injection
>   D.-S. Oral

dispenser
>   Baxa oral d.
>   Exacta-Med oral d.

dispersion
>   Taylor d.

displaced pinna

displacement
>   inner canthus d.
>   rotatory d.

disposable
>   d. bottle
>   d. 23-gauge butterfly needle
>   d. wipe

Dispos-a-Med Isoproterenol

disproportion
>   cephalopelvic d. (CPD)
>   congenital muscle fiber-type d.
>   (CMFTD)
>   craniofacial d.
>   fiber-type d.
>   limb d.

disproportionate dwarfism

disruption
>   bilateral corticobulbar d.
>   inferior vena cava d.
>   ossicular d.
>   synchondrosis d.
>   tubular d.

disruptive
>   d. behavior disorder
>   D. Behavior Disorder Scale

dissecans
>   osteochondritis d. (OCD)

dissecting aortic aneurysm

dissection
>   aortic d.
>   inverted-Y detrusor d.
>   partial zonal d. (PZD)

disseminata
>   dermatofibrosis lenticularis d.

disseminated
>   d. adenovirus disease
>   d. candidiasis
>   d. coccidioidomycosis
>   d. gonorrhea
>   d. granuloma

>   d. granulomatous vasculitis
>   d. hemangiomatosis
>   d. histoplasmosis
>   d. intravascular coagulation (DIC)
>   d. lupus erythematosus
>   d. *Mycobacterium avium complex*
>   (DMAC)
>   d. sclerosis
>   d. tuberculosis
>   d. varicella

dissemination

disseminatus
>   lupus erythematosus d.

dissimilar twin

dissociate

dissociated
>   d. motor development
>   d. movement

dissociation
>   albuminocytologic d.
>   atrioventricular d.
>   craniofacial d.
>   electroclinical d.
>   electromechanical d. (EMD)
>   immune complex d. (ICD)

dissociative
>   d. disorder
>   d. phenomenon
>   d. symptom

dissolution

distal
>   d. arthrogryposis (type I, II)
>   d. claviclectomy
>   d. collecting duct
>   d. dilated bowel segment resection
>   d. esophageal atresia
>   d. esophageal pH monitoring
>   d. femoral skeletal traction
>   d. humeral physeal fracture
>   d. ileum
>   d. intestinal obstruction (DIOS)
>   d. intestinal obstruction syndrome
>   d. jejunum
>   d. onycholysis
>   d. RTA
>   d. splenorenal shunt
>   d. symmetric sensorimotor
>   neuropathy
>   d. trichorrhexis nodosa
>   d. triradius
>   d. tuft
>   d. vagina

D

NOTES

distance
> Euclidean d.
> d. vision

distemper
> canine d.

distended
> d. abdomen
> d. capillary

distending pressure

distensae
> striae cutis d.

distention, distension
> abdominal d.
> centrizonal sinusoidal d.
> gaseous d.
> jugulovenous d. (JVD)
> lacrimal sac d.

distractibility

distractible
> hyperactive d.

distraction

distress
> respiratory d.

distribution
> butterfly d.
> Christmas tree d.
> dermatomal d.
> gaussian d.
> malar d.
> d. pattern
> trigeminal nerve d.
> watershed d.

distributive
> d. justice
> d. shock

disturbance
> d. of attachment
> behavioral d.
> feeding d.
> growth d.
> immunologic d.
> serious emotional d. (SED)
> sleep d.
> thought d.

disturbed
> emotionally d.

disuse
> d. amblyopia
> d. muscular atrophy
> d. syndrome

dithiothreitol

Ditropan XL

diuresis
> glycosuric d.
> osmotic d.
> solute d.

diuretic
> loop d.

> mercurial d.
> potassium-sparing d.
> d. renography

Diurigen

Diuril

diurnal enuresis

diurnus
> pavor d.

divalproex sodium

divergens
> *Babesia* d.

divergent
> d. rectus muscle
> d. strabismus

diversion
> bilateral ureteral d.
> colonic conduit d.
> ileal loop d.
> ileocecal conduit d.
> Koch pouch d.
> loop d.
> Mainz pouch d.
> partial external biliary d. (PEBD)

diversus
> *Citrobacter* d.

diverticulum, pl. **diverticula**
> bladder d.
> Meckel d.
> porencephalic d.

diverting
> d. colostomy
> d. colostomy with pull-through
> procedure
> d. enterostomy

diving reflex

division
> meiotic d.
> d. of pancreatic ring
> urethral plate d.

divisum
> pancreas d.

divorce

Dizac Injectable Emulsion

Dizmiss

dizygotic twin

dizziness
> orthostatic d.

DKA
> diabetic ketoacidosis

DL$_{co}$
> diffusing capacity of lung for carbon
> monoxide

DLD
> developmental language disorder

d-loop

DLV
> delavirdine

DM
dermatomyositis
diabetes mellitus (type 1, 2)
Benylin DM
Diabetic Tussin DM
Dimetapp DM
Fenesin DM
Genatuss DM
Guaifenex DM
Guiatuss DM
Halotussin DM
Hold DM
Koffex DM
Mytussin DM
Silphen DM
Siltussin DM
Tolu-Sed DM
Uni-tussin DM
DMAC
disseminated *Mycobacterium avium complex*
DMARD
disease-modifying antirheumatic drug
DMD
Duchenne muscular dystrophy
dystonia musculorum deformans
DMD/BMD
Duchenne muscular dystrophy/Becker muscular dystrophy
DMD/BMD gene
D-Med Injection
DMP-266
efavirenz
DMPA
depomedroxyprogesterone acetate
DMQ
developmental motor quotient
fine motor total DMQ
gross motor total DMQ
DMS
diffuse mesangial sclerosis
DMSO
dimethyl sulfoxide
DNA
deoxyribonucleic acid
DNA analysis
branched DNA
complementary DNA (cDNA)
DNA hybridization
DNA hybridization assay
kinetoplast DNA
DNA library

DNA ligase
mitochondrial DNA (mtDNA)
DNA nucleotidylexotransferase
DNA nucleotidyltransferase
DNA polymerase
DNA probe
synthetic DNA
Watson-Crick double-helix DNA
DNA-based testing
DNA-directed
DNA-d. polymerase
DNA-d. RNA polymerase
DNAse, DNase
deoxyribonuclease
DNAse B factor
human recombinant DNase
DNS
delayed neuropsychological sequela
Dobrava virus
dobutamine hydrochloride
Dobutrex
Dochez serum test
docosahexaenoic acid (DHA)
docosapentaenoic acid
doctor
medical d. (MD)
d. of medicine
docusate
d. and casanthranol
sodium d.
dog
neck of Scotty d.
Scotty d.
d. tick
Doktors Nasal Solution
DOL
day of life
Dolacct
dolasetron
Dolene
dolichocephalic
dolichocephaly
dolichostenomelia
doll's
d. eye maneuver
d. eye phenomenon
d. eye reflex
d. eye response
d. head maneuver
Dolophine
Dolorac

NOTES

domain
>adaptive d.
>cognitive d.
>communication d.
>fine motor d.
>gross motor d.
>hyperactivity/impulsivity d.
>inattention d.
>language d.
>perceptual d.
>Revised Gesell Language D.
>self-help d.
>social/emotional d.

Domeboro solution
domestic violence
dominance
>eye d.

dominant
>autosomal d. (AD)
>d. dystrophic epidermolysis bullosa
>d. gene
>d. hand
>d. inheritance
>X-linked d. (XLD)

dominantly
>d. hyperactive
>d. hyperactive impulsive type

Dominic-R questionnaire
domino connector
domperidone
Donahue syndrome
DONALD
>Dortmund Nutritional and Anthropometrical Longitudinally Designed
>DONALD study

Donath-Landsteiner cold hemolysin
Done nomogram
dong quai
Donnagel
Donnamar
Donnan equilibrium
Donnapine
Donna-Sed
Donnatal
Donnazyme
donor
>artificial insemination d. (AID)
>artificial insemination by d. (AID)
>artificial insemination with d.
>cadaveric d.
>intrafamilial genoidentical d.
>d. T cell
>d. venous graft

Donphen

DOOR
>deafness, onychodystrophy, osteodystrophy, mild to severe mental retardation
>DOOR syndrome

dopamine hydrochloride
dopaminergic system
Dopar
dopa-responsive dystonia (DRD)
Doppler
>color-coded duplex D.
>continuous wave D.
>D. echocardiography
>D. flow study
>D. myocardial performance index
>D. probe
>pulsed wave D.
>D. scanning
>transcranial D. (TCD)
>D. ultrasonography
>D. ultrasound
>D. velocimetry

Dopram
d'orange
>peau d.

Dorcol
Dorfman-Chanarin disease
dormant basket cell hypothesis
Dormarex 2 Oral
Dormin Oral
dornase alfa
dorsal
>d. bunion
>d. chordee
>d. extension splint
>d. hood
>d. kyphosis
>d. myeloschisis
>d. penile curvature
>d. penile nerve block (DPNB)
>d. rhizotomy

dorsalis
>d. pedis
>d. pedis pulse
>tabes d.

dorsiflexion
dorsogluteal
dorsum
Dortmund
>D. Nutritional and Anthropometrical Longitudinally Designed (DONALD)
>D. Nutritional and Anthropometrical Longitudinally Designed study

DORV
>double-outlet right ventricle

Doryx

dose
>bolus d.
>minimal effective d. (MED)
>priming d.
>rescue d.

dosing
>extended internal d.

DOS Softgel

DOT
>directly observed therapy

dot
>black d.
>d. ELISA test
>glistening d.
>d. immunobinding assay (DIA)
>Mittendorf d.

double
>d. aortic arch (DAA)
>d. collecting system
>d. cortex syndrome
>d. cortin
>d. depression
>d. diaper treatment
>d. elevator palsy
>d. epiphyses
>d. hemiplegia
>d. staircase method of Cornsweet
>d. strength (XX)

double-bank phototherapy

double-barrel colostomy

double-blind
>d.-b., placebo-controlled food challenge (DBPCFC)
>d.-b. study

double-bubble
>d.-b. gas shadow
>d.-b. sign
>d.-b. ventriculoperitoneal shunt

double-catheter technique

double-contrast CT scan

doublecortin

double-freeze technique

double-inlet
>d.-i. left ventricle
>d.-i. right ventricle

double-insulated incubator

double-lumen
>d.-l. airway
>d.-l. catheter
>d.-l. venovenous ECMO

double-lung transplantation

double-onlay preputial flap

double-orifice mitral valve

double-outlet
>d.-o. right ventricle (DORV)
>d.-o. ventricle

double-sandwich ELISA

double-switch procedure

double-tract sign

double-umbrella device

double-walled incubator

doughnut-shaped mass

doughy
>d. mass
>d. skin

Douglas bag

doula

Dowling-Meara epidermolysis bullosa simplex

Down
>D. stigmata
>D. syndrome
>D. syndrome child (DSC)
>D. syndrome growth chart

downbeat nystagmus

Downes score

downgaze
>tonic d.

downregulate

downslant

downslanting
>d. eyes
>d. palpebral fissure

downturned mouth

downward gaze

doxacurium

doxapram hydrochloride

doxepin

doxorubicin

Doxy-200

Doxy-Caps

Doxychel

doxycycline hyclate

Doxy-Tabs

doylei
>*Campylobacter jejuni* subspecies *d.*

D-penicillamine

DPI
>dry powder inhaler
>dynamic pulmonary imaging

DP-II
>Developmental Profile-II

DPL
>diagnostic peritoneal lavage

D

NOTES

DPNB
    dorsal penile nerve block
DPSS
    Department of Public Social Services
DPT
    dehydration, poisoning, trauma
    diphtheria-pertussis-tetanus
        DPT vaccine
DQ
    developmental quotient
dracunculiasis
Dracunculus medinensis
Dräger thermal gel mattress
dragged disk
dragging of retina
drain
    butterfly d.
    Penrose d.
    peritoneal d.
drainage
    anomalous pulmonary venous d.
    chest tube d.
    coffee-ground d.
    felon d.
    incision and d. (I&D)
    d., irrigation, fibrinolytic therapy
      (DRIFT)
    mastoid d.
    nasogastric d.
    open flap d.
    open pericardial d.
    percutaneous catheter d.
    postural d. (PD)
    primary peritoneal d. (PPD)
    d. procedure
    syringopleural d.
    syringosubarachnoid d.
    thoracic duct d.
    in utero d.
draining otitis media
Dramamine II
Dramilin Injection
Dramoject Injection
Drapanas mesocaval shunt
Drash syndrome
draught
    Black D.
Draw-a-Person Test
drawing
    human figure d. (HFD)
    line d.
DRD
    dopa-responsive dystonia
dressing
    occlusive d.
Dri-Dot
    Monosticon D.-D.

DRIFT
    drainage, irrigation, fibrinolytic therapy
drilling
    zonal d.
drip
    continuous gastric d. (CGD)
    intravenous d. (IVD)
    postnasal d.
    sterile water gastric d. (SWGD)
dripping
    candle d.
Drisdol
Dristan
    D. Long Lasting Nasal Solution
    D. Saline Spray
drive
    central respiratory d.
    respiratory d.
    d. for thinness
    ventilatory d.
driving
    Mothers Against Drunk D.
    (MADD)
Drixoral
    D. Cough Liquid Caps
    D. Non-Drowsy
dronabinol
drooling
drooping
    d. lily appearance
    d. lily appearance of lower
      collecting system
drop
    Afrin Children's Nose D.'s
    Allerest Eye D.'s
    Allergen Ear D.'s
    d. attack
    Auro Ear D.'s
    Ayr saline d.'s
    E-R-O Ear D.'s
    foot d.
    head d.
    methylcellulose d.'s
    Murine Ear D.'s
    Naldecon DX Pediatric D.'s
    Naldecon EX Pediatric D.'s
    parasympathomimetic d.
    Phazyme infant d.'s
    Robitussin-DM infant d.'s
    Rondec D.'s
    saline nose d.
    d. seizure
    silver nitrate d.'s
    sympatholytic d.
    Triaminic Infant D.'s
    Vitamin C D.'s
droperidol and fentanyl
dropfoot

droplet
    cytoplasmic lipid d. (CLD)
    d. infection
dropout
    capillary d.
    d. of capillary end loop
    echo d.
dropped beat
Drosophila
    D. melanogaster gene diaphanous
    D. mutation
Drotic Otic
drowning
    cold water near d.
    dry d.
    freshwater near d.
    near d.
    saltwater near d.
    very cold water near d.
    warm water near d.
    wet d.
drowsiness
Droxia Hydrea
DRSP
    drug-resistant *Streptococcus pneumoniae*
drug
    acetylcysteine d.
    alcohol and other d.'s (AOD)
    alcohol, tobacco, and other d.'s
      (ATOD)
    anthelminthic d.
    antianxiety d.
    antibacterial d.
    antibiotic d.
    anticholinergic d.
    anticonvulsant d.
    antidepressant d.
    antiepileptic d. (AED)
    antifungal d.
    antihistamine d.
    antipsychotic d.
    antispastic d.
    anxiolytic d.
    d. baby
    bactericidal d.
    bacteriostatic d.
    beta-adrenergic d.
    beta lactamase stable d.
    bronchodilator d.
    disease-modifying antirheumatic d.
      (DMARD)
    d. fever

    gateway d.
    narcotic d.
    neuroleptic d.
    nonsteroidal antiinflammatory d.
      (NSAID)
    orphan d.
    ototoxic d.
    parasympatholytic d.
    prenatally exposed to d.'s (PED)
    d. prophylaxis
    psychedelic d.
    psychotropic d. (PTD)
    d. resistant
    stimulant d.
    tocolytic d.
    tranquilizer d.
drug-induced
    d.-i. acne
    d.-i. dystonia
    d.-i. gynecomastia
    d.-i. neonatal goiter
    d.-i. pancreatitis
    d.-i. rash
drug-resistant *Streptococcus pneumoniae*
  (DRSP)
drunk
drusen
dry
    d. crab yaws
    d. drowning
    d. eye
    d. eye syndrome
    d. mucous membrane
    d. pericarditis
    d. pleurisy
    d. powder inhaler (DPI)
    d. skin
    d. socket
    d. weight
Dryox
    D. Gel
    D. Wash
Drysol
DS
    diencephalic syndrome
      Bactrim DS
      Cotrim DS
      K-Lyte DS
      Septra DS
      Sulfatrim DS
      Tolectin DS
      Uroplus DS

D

NOTES

DSA
density spectral array
DSC
Down syndrome child
Parafon Forte DSC
DSMC Plus
DSM-IV
Diagnostic and Statistical Manual of
Mental Disorders - 4th Edition
DSPS
delayed sleep phase syndrome
DSR
direct suicide risk
DSRCT
desmoplastic small round cell tumor
DSS
discrete subaortic stenosis
D-S-S
D-S-S Plus
DST
dexamethasone suppression testing
DT
diphtheria toxin
d4T
stavudine
DTaP
diphtheria-tetanus toxoids-acellular
pertussis
DTaP vaccine
d-TGA
d-transposition of great arteries
DTH
delayed-type hypersensitivity
DTIC
imidazole carboxamide
DTIC-Dome
DTM
dermatophyte test media
DTP
diphtheria, tetanus toxoid, pertussis
DTP vaccine
DTPA
diethylenetriamine pentaacetic acid
DTPA scan
DTR
deep tendon reflex
d-transposition of great arteries (d-TGA)
D-tube feeding
DTwP
diphtheria-tetanus toxoid with pertussis
dual-energy
d.-e. x-ray
d.-e. x-ray absorptiometry (DEXA)
d.-e. x-ray absorptiometry scan
Duane retraction syndrome
DUB
dysfunctional uterine bleeding

Dubin-Johnson syndrome
dublin
Salmonella d.
Dubowitz
D. examination
neonatal maturity classification
of D.
D. Neurological Assessment
D. Scale for Infant Maturity
D. score
D. syndrome
Dubowitz/Ballard Exam for Gestational Age
Duchenne
D. muscular dystrophy (DMD)
D. muscular dystrophy/Becker
muscular dystrophy (DMD/BMD)
Duckett transverse preputial island flap
duckfeet
ducreyi
Haemophilus d.
duct
apocrine d.
bile d.
common hepatic d.
congenital atresia of bile d.
congenital obstruction of
nasolacrimal d.
d. of Cuvier
cystic dilation of intrahepatic
bile d.
distal collecting d.
eccrine sweat d.
follicular d.
Gartner d.
intrahepatic bile d.
lacrimal d.
lactiferous d.
müllerian d.
nasolacrimal d.
omphalomesenteric d.
pilosebaceous d.
sebaceous d.
stenotic nasolacrimal d.
Stensen d.
sweat d.
thyroglossal d.
vanishing bile d.
vitelline d.
wolffian d.
ductal
d. plate malformation
d. shunt
d. shunting
ductal-dependent systemic circulation
duct-dependent
d.-d. heart disease
d.-d. pulmonary blood flow

d.-d. pulmonary circulation
d.-d. systemic circulation
DuctOcclud coil
ductule
bile d.
ductus
d. arteriosus
bilateral d.
d. choledochus
d. closure
d. venosus
d. Wirsungianus
Duffy antigen
Duhamel procedure
Dukes disease
Dulbecco media
Dulcolax
Dull-C
dullness
flank d.
d. to percussion
shifting d.
span of liver d.
Dumas vault cap
dumbbell tumor
Dumex Infant Formula
dumping syndrome
Duncan
D. disease
D. syndrome
D. test
Dunedin
D. birth cohort
D. longitudinal study
DuoCet
duodenal
d. atresia
d. diaphragm
d. fluid
d. ileus
d. obstruction
d. resection
d. revacuolization
d. stenosis
d. ulcer
duodenale
Ancylostoma d.
duodenitis
duodenum
Z-shaped d.
Duofilm
Duo-Trach Injection

Duphalac
duplex
d. kidney
d. ultrasound
duplicated
d. elastic lamina
d. ureter
d. vagina
duplicate uterus
duplication
d. anomaly
complete vulvar d.
d. cyst
foregut d.
d. of gallbladder
gastric d.
d. of ileum
intestinal d.
penile d.
ureteral d.
urethral d.
duplication-deficiency syndrome
duplicitas asymmetros
dura
d. mater
d. mater allograft
Duraclon Injection
Duradyne DHC
Dura-Estrin
Duragesic Transdermal
Dura-Gest
dural
d. ectasia
d. sinus thrombosis
d. venous thrombosis
Duralone Injection
Duramist Plus
Duramorph Injection
Dura-Tabs
Quinaglute D.-T.
Duratears
Duratest Injection
Durathate Injection
duration
D. Nasal Solution
QRS d.
Duratuss-G
Duricef
Duroziez disease
Durrax Oral
dusky

NOTES

dust
    d. mite
    nuclear d.
Dutch Baby Food formula
Duvoid
DVSS
    dysfunctional voiding scoring system
DVT
    deep venous thrombosis
    silent DVT
dwarf
    diastrophic d.
dwarfism
    achondroplastic d.
    chondroplastic d.
    compomelic d.
    constitutional d.
    diastrophic d.
    disproportionate d.
    Kniest d.
    Langer mesomelic d.
    Laron-type d.
    lethal neonatal d.
    metatropic d.
    pituitary d.
    psychosocial d.
    rhizomelic d.
    short-limb d.
    thanatophoric d.
DWI
    diffusion-weighted imaging
Dwyer
    D. correction
    D. correction of scoliosis
DX
    Naldecon Senior DX
d-xylose
dyadic
    D. Adjustment Scale
Dycill
Dyclone
dyclonine
dye
    aniline d.
    d. decolorization test
    d. disappearance test
    formazan d.
    triple d.
Dyggve-Melchior-Clausen syndrome
dying-back axonal degeneration
Dyke-Davidoff syndrome
Dymenate Injection
Dynacin
Dyna-Hex
dynamic
    d. exercise testing
    family d.'s
    flow velocity d.

    d. mutation
    d. orthotic cranioplasty device
    d. pes varus
    d. pulmonary imaging (DPI)
    d. spiral CT lung densitometry
    d. splint
    toxic d.'s
Dynapen
dynein
    left/right d.
Dyrenium
dysacousia
dysacusis
dysarthria
dysarthritic speech
dysautonomia
    familial d.
dysbetalipoproteinemia
dyscalculia
dyschezia
dyschondroplasia
dyschondrosteosis
dyscontrol
    episodic d.
dyscoria
dyscrasia
    sonography blood d.
dysdiadochokinesis
dysenteriae
    Shigella d. (type 1)
dysentery
    amebic d.
    bacillary d.
    Shigella d.
dyserythropoiesis
dysfibrinogenemia
dysfibronectinemic Ehlers-Danlos syndrome
dysfluency
    abnormal d.
    developmental d.
dysfluent speech
dysfolliculogenesis
dysfunction
    arm d.
    auditory d.
    autonomic nervous system d. (ANSD)
    AV node d.
    B-cell d.
    bilirubin-induced neurologic d. (BIND)
    bone marrow d.
    brain d.
    cardiopulmonary d.
    cerebellar d.
    cerebral d.
    CNS d.

corticospinal tract d.
cumulative parental d.
endocrine pancreatic d.
erectile d. (ED)
eustachian tube d.
exocrine pancreatic d.
family d.
gait d.
global neurologic d.
gonadal d.
hypothalamic d.
hypothalamic-pituitary d.
left ventricular d. (LVD)
LV d.
metabolic disorder with hepatic d.
metabolic disorder with
 neurologic d.
microcirculatory d.
minimal brain d. (MBD)
minimal cerebral d.
minor cerebral d.
motor perception d.
neuromotor d.
neutrophil actin d.
oculomotor d.
oral-motor d.
palatorespiratory d.
pancreatic d.
papillary muscle d.
psychosexual d.
renal d.
serotonergic d.
sinus node d. (SND)
social-occupational d.
spinal cord d.
sudomotor d.
T-cell d.
temporomandibular joint d.
testicular d.
thyroid gland d.
transient pharyngeal muscle d.
vocal cord d. (VCD)
voiding d.

dysfunctional
d. family
d. uterine bleeding (DUB)
d. voiding
d. voiding scoring system (DVSS)

dysgammaglobulinemia

dysgenesia
reticular d.

dysgenesis
autosomal congenital tubular d.
cortical d.
familial pure gonadal d.
gonadal d.
mixed gonadal d. (MGD)
ovarian d.
partial gonadal d.
penile d.
renal d.
reticular d.
seminiferous tubule d.
d. syndrome
tubular d.

dysgenetic
d. gonad
d. ovotestis
d. testis

dysgerminoma
ovarian d.

dysgeusia

dyshepatia
lipogenic d.

dyshidrosis

dyshidrotic eczema

dyshormonogenesis

dyskeratoma
warty d.

dyskeratosis congenita

dyskinesia
ciliary d.
exertion-induced d.
D. Identification System: Condensed
 User Scale (DISCUS)
kinesigenic paroxysmal d.
orofacial d.
primary ciliary d. (PCD)
sleep-induced d.
tardive d.
withdrawal d.

dyskinetic cerebral palsy

dyslexia
developmental d.

dyslexic

dyslipidemia

dysmaturative myopathy

dysmature
d. infant

dysmegakaryocytopoiesis

dysmenorrhea
primary d.

D

NOTES

dysmetria
　　ocular motor d.
dysmorphic
　　d. erythrocyte
　　d. face
　　d. syndrome
dysmorphism
　　facial d.
dysmorphologist
dysmorphology
dysmotile cilia syndrome
dysmotility
　　ciliary d.
　　colonic d.
　　cytokine-related d.
　　gastric d.
　　gastrointestinal d.
　　small bowel d.
　　d. syndrome
dysmotility-sclerodactyly-telangiectasia
dysmyelinatus
　　status d.
dysmyelopoiesis
dysnomia
dysosmia
dysostosis
　　acrofacial d.
　　acrofacial d. (Nager type)
　　craniofacial d.
　　mandibulofacial d.
　　metaphyseal d.
　　d. multiplex
　　Nager acrofacial d.
　　orodigitofacial d.
dyspareunia
dyspepsia
dysphagia
　　motility-related d.
　　nonneurogenic d.
dysphasia
　　developmental d.
dysphonia
　　spasmodic d.
　　spastic d.
dysphoria
dysphoric
　　d. mood
　　d. reaction
dyspigmentation
dysplasia
　　acetabular d.
　　acromesomelic d.
　　agyria-pachygyria cortical d.
　　alveolar capillary d.
　　anhidrotic ectodermal d.
　　arrhythmogenic right ventricular d.
　　　(ARVD)
　　arteriohepatic d.

bone d.
bony d.
bronchopulmonary d. (BPD)
camptomelic d.
caudal d.
cerebellar d.
chondroectodermal d.
cleidocranial d.
clubfoot d.
congenital alveolar d.
congenital glenoid d.
congenital hip d. (CDH)
cortical d.
craniodiaphyseal d.
craniometaphyseal d.
cretinoid d.
de la Chapelle d.
developmental hip d.
diaphyseal d.
diastrophic d.
dyssegmental d.
ectodermal d.
epiphyseal d.
d. epiphysealis hemimelia
d. epiphysealis punctata
fibromuscular d.
fibrous d.
focal cortical d.
focal facial ectodermal d.
frontometaphyseal d.
glenoid d.
gonadal d.
hereditary bone d.
hereditary ectodermal d.
hidrotic ectodermal d.
hip d.
hypohidrotic ectodermal d.
immunoosseous d.
intestinal neuronal d.
Kniest d.
Kozlowski spondylometaphyseal d.
Langer mesomelic d.
lymphatic d.
mandibular-acral d.
medullary d.
mesomelic d.
metaphyseal d.
metatropic d.
mild acetabular d.
multicystic renal d.
multiple epiphyseal d.
myxoid d.
nerve d.
neurogenic hip d.
neuronal d.
oculoauriculovertebral d.
oculodentodigital d.
optic nerve d.

osteofibrous d.
polyostotic fibrous d.
porencephaly cortical d.
pulmonary d.
punctate epiphyseal d.
radial d.
renal medullary d.
retinal d.
right ventricular d.
Robinow mesomelic d.
Schimke immunoosseous d.
Schmid metaphyseal d.
septooptic d.
septooptic-pituitary d.
Silverman-Handmaker
  dyssegmental d.
skeletal d.
sphenoid d.
spondyloepiphyseal d. (SED)
spondylometaphyseal d.
Stickler d.
Streeter d.
d. syndrome
thanatophoric d.
trichorhinophalangeal d.
urinary tract d.
valves, unilateral reflux, d.
  (VURD)
ventricular d.
vertebral (defects), (imperforate)
  anus, tracheoesophageal (fistula),
  radial and renal (d.) (VATER)

dysplasia-clefting
ectrodactyly-ectodermal d.-c. (EEC)

dysplastic
d. cortical architecture
d. gangliocytoma
d. gangliocytoma of cerebellum
d. kidney
d. nevus
d. nevus syndrome

dyspnea
paroxysmal nocturnal d. (PND)

dyspraxia
dysproteinemia
dysprothrombinemia
dysraphia
tectocerebellar d.

dysraphism
occult d.
occult spinal d.
spinal d.

dysregulated
d. behavior
d. insulin secretion

dysregulation
autonomic d.
hypothalamic-pituitary-adrenal
  axis d.
temperature d.

dysrhythmia
ventricular d.

dyssegmental dysplasia
dyssomnia
circadian rhythm d.
extrinsic d.
infant d.
intrinsic d.

dyssynergia
detrusor-sphincter d.

dystasia
hereditary areflexic d.

dysthymia
dysthymic disorder
dystocia
shoulder d.

dystonia
buccomandibular d.
craniocervical d.
dopa-responsive d. (DRD)
drug-induced d.
early-onset d.
focal d.
generalized d.
idiopathic torsion d.
d. musculorum deformans (DMD)
myoclonic d.
oromandibular d.
paroxysmal d.
primary d.
secondary d.
segmental d.
symptomatic d.
tardive d.
torsion d.
transient d.

dystonia-parkinsonism
rapid-onset d.-p.

dystonic
d. cerebral palsy
d. dyskinetic disorder
d. hyperextension
d. posturing

dystopia canthorum

D

NOTES

dystosis
  cleidocranial d.
  metaphyseal d.
dystrophic
  d. epidermolysis bullosa
  d. nail
  d. tooth
dystrophinopathy
dystrophy
  Aran-Duchenne muscular d.
  asphyxiating thoracic d.
  Becker d.
  Becker muscular d. (BMD)
  cerebroocular muscular d.
  congenital corneal d.
  congenital muscular d. (CMD)
  congenital myotonic d.
  corneal d.
  Duchenne muscular d. (DMD)
  Duchenne muscular d./Becker
    muscular d. (DMD/BMD)
  early corneal d.
  Emery-Dreifuss muscular d.
  endothelial d.
  Erb juvenile muscular d.
  facioscapulohumeral muscular d.
    (FSHD)
  FSH muscular d.
  Fukuyama congenital muscular d.
  giant neuroaxonal d.
  humeroperoneal muscular d.

  infantile neuroaxonal d.
  Jeune thoracic d.
  juvenile muscular d.
  juvenile myotonic d.
  Landouzy d.
  Landouzy-Dejerine muscular d.
  Leyden-Möbius muscular d.
  limb-girdle d.
  muscular d.
  myotonic muscular d.
  nail d.
  neuroaxonal d.
  neurovascular d.
  ocular muscular d.
  oculocerebral d.
  oculocerebrorenal d.
  oculopharyngeal muscular d.
  peroneal muscular d.
  pseudohypertrophic muscular d.
  reflex sympathetic d. (RSD)
  scapulohumeral muscular d.
  scapuloperoneal d.
  secondary nail d.
  severe childhood autosomal
    recessive muscular d. (SCARMD)
  spinal muscular d.
  thoracic d.
  twenty-nail d.
dysuria
dysuria-pyuria syndrome

E
    E antigen
    E sign
    E test
44E
    Vicks Pediatric Formula 44E
E$_1$
    prostaglandin E$_1$
E$_4$
    leukotriene E$_4$ (LTE$_4$)
E$_{dyn}$
    respiratory system elastance
E$_{st}$
    static elastance
EA
    esophageal atresia
EAA
    excitotoxic amino acid
each (q.q.)
EAE
    experimental allergic encephalomyelitis
Eagle-Barrett syndrome
EAR
    early asthmatic response
car
    e. anomaly
    aures unitas (both e.'s) (a.u., AU)
    auris dextra (right e.) (a.d., AD)
    auris sinistra (left e.) (a.s., AS)
    auris uterque (each e.) (a.u., AU)
    e. canal
    e. crease/pit
    external e.
    glue e.
    inner e.
    laser office ventilation of e.'s
       (LOVE)
    left e.
    lop e.
    low-set e.'s
    malformed e.
    middle e.
    Otocalm E.
    outer e.
    prominent e.
    e. speculum
    swimmer's e.
    tugging at e.'s
    e. ventilation tube
EarCheck
eardrum
    perforated e.
    e. perforation
Earle media

earlobe
    bifid e.
    e. crease
early
    e. asthmatic response (EAR)
    e. childhood caries (ECC)
    E. Childhood Special Education
       Program
    e. congenital syphilis
    e. corneal dystrophy
    e. deceleration
    e. educator
    e. infantile autism
    e. infantile epileptic encephalopathy
    e. intervention
    e. interventionist
    e. intervention program (EIP)
    e. language milestone (ELM)
    E. Language Milestone scale
    e. mature
    e. midsystolic closure
    e. morning irritability
    E. and Periodic Screening,
       Diagnosis, and Treatment program
    e. satiety
early-onset
    e.-o. disease
    e.-o. dystonia
    e.-o. schizophrenia (EOS)
    e.-o. sepsis
earth
    diatomaceous e. (DE)
EAS
    Emotionality Activity Sociability Scale
Easprin
eastern equine encephalitis (EEE)
easy
    e. bruisabilty
    e. fatigability
eater
    picky e.
eating
    E. Attitudes Test
    binge e.
    e. disorder
    e. disorders examination (EDE)
    E. Disorders Inventory
    E. Disorders Inventory Score for
       Interoceptive Awareness Affect
Eaton-Lambert myasthenic syndrome
EB
    epidermolysis bullosa
EBCT
    electron-beam computed tomography

E

EBLL
elevation of blood lead level
Ebola hemorrhagic fever
Ebstein
E. anomaly
E. malformation
EBV
Epstein-Barr virus
EBV-related B-cell lymphoma
ECC
early childhood caries
eccentric
e. exercise
e. gaze
e. orifice
eccentrochondroplasia
ecchymosis
periorbital e.
postauricular e.
ecchymotic Ehlers-Danlos syndrome
eccrine
e. bromhidrosis
e. sweat duct
ECF
executive cognitive functioning
extracellular fluid
ECG, EKG
electrocardiogram
electrocardiography
echinococcosis
alveolar e.
Echinococcus
E. *granulosus*
E. *granulosus* hydatid cyst
E. *multilocularis*
echinocyte
ECHO
enteric cytopathogenic human orphan
ECHO 11 virus
echo
echocardiogram
echo Doppler gradient
echo dropout
echocardiogram (echo)
echocardiograph
echocardiography
A-mode e.
2D, 3D e.
Doppler e.
fetal e.
M-mode e.
real-time e.
transesophageal e. (TEE)
transpericardial e.
transthoracic e.
EchoCheck
echodensity

echoencephalography
cranial e.
echo-free zone
echogenic
e. bowel
e. focus
echogenicity
echo-guided balloon atrial septostomy
echolalia
compulsive e.
echolucency
periventricular e. (PVEL)
echolucent
echoplanar functional magnetic resonance imaging
echopraxia
Echo-Screen
echoviral meningitis
echovirus
E. 1, 6, 14, 16
e. 9 meningitis
E. type 9
Echovist
eclampsia
eclamptic idiocy
eclipse
Total E.
ECLS
extracorporeal life support
ECLT
euglobulin clot lysis time
ECM
erythema chronicum migrans
ECM rash
ECMO
extracorporeal membrane oxygenation
double-lumen venovenous ECMO
venovenous ECMO
E_TCO_2
end-tidal carbon dioxide
ECochG
electrocochleography
ECoG
electrocochleography
E-Complex-600
econazole
Econopred Plus Ophthalmic
Ecotrin
ECP
eosinophilic cationic protein
ecstasy
ECT
electroconvulsive therapy
ectasia
annuloaortic e.
arterial e.
dural e.
ectasis

ecthyma
- e. gangrenosa
- e. gangrenosum

ectoderm
- cutaneous e.

ectodermal
- e. dysplasia
- e. dysplasia of face
- e. dysplasia syndrome
- e. ridge

ectoparasite
ectopia
- e. cordis
- crossed fused e.
- e. lentis
- e. lentis et pupillae
- ureteral e.

ectopic
- e. anus
- e. atrial tachycardia
- e. gastric mucosa
- e. pancreatic rest
- e. pinealoma
- e. P-P cycle
- e. pregnancy
- e. testis
- e. thyroid
- e. ureter
- e. ureterocele

ectopy
- cervical e.

ectrodactyly
ectrodactyly-ectodermal
- c.-c. dysplasia-clefting (EEC)
- e.-e. dysplasia-clefting syndrome

ECV
- extracellular volume

eczema
- asteatotic e.
- atopic e.
- discoid e.
- dyshidrotic e.
- e. herpeticum
- infantile e.
- e. marginatum
- e. neonatorum
- nipple e.
- nummular e.
- plaque of nummular e.
- seborrheic e.
- e. vaccinatum

eczematization

eczematoid
- e. dermatitis
- e. lesion
- e. skin rash

eczematous
- e. halo nevus
- e. skin lesion

ED
- erectile dysfunction

EDAS
- encephaloduroarteriosynangios

EDE
- eating disorders examination

Edecrin
- E. Oral
- E. Sodium Injection

edema
- angioneurotic e.
- Berlin e.
- brain e.
- brawny e.
- cellular e.
- cerebral e.
- corneal e.
- cytotoxic e.
- focal cerebral e.
- hereditary e.
- high-altitude pulmonary e. (HAPE)
- idiopathic scrotal e.
- indurative e.
- intercellular e.
- interstitial e.
- ischemic e.
- laryngeal e.
- malignant brain e.
- e. neonatorum
- neurogenic pulmonary e.
- noncardiac pulmonary e.
- optic nerve e.
- periorbital e.
- peritonsillar e.
- pitting e.
- placental e.
- postasphyxial cerebral e.
- postthoracotomy pulmonary e.
- presternal e.
- pulmonary e.
- retinal e.
- scrotal e.
- segmental e.
- subglottic e.
- suborbital e.

E

NOTES

edema *(continued)*
    tonsillar e.
    vasogenic e.
    villous e.
edematous papilla
edetate calcium disodium
Edex
EDIN
    EDIN behavioral score
Edinburgh Postnatal Depression Scale (EPDS)
Edinger-Westphal nucleus
edition
    Bayley Scales of Infant Development-Motor, 2nd e.
    Child Health and Illness Profile, Adolescent E. (CHIP-AE)
    Clinical Evaluation of Language Fundamentals, 3rd e.
    Receptive-Expressive Emergent Language Scale, Second E. (REEL-2)
    Stanford-Binet Fourth E. (SBFE)
    Stanford-Binet Intelligence Scale, Fourth E.
    Stanford-Binet Memory Scale, 4th E.
    Wechsler Adult Intelligence Scale, 3rd e.
    Wechsler Intelligence Scale for Children, 3rd e.
Edmonston-Zagreb measles vaccine
edrophonium
EDS
    Ehlers-Danlos syndrome
ED-SPAZ
EDTA
    ethylenediaminetetraacetic acid
    EDTA-anticoagulated Vacutainer
educable
education
    E. for All Handicapped Children Act
    American College of Graduate Medical E. (ACGME)
    conductive e. (CE)
    E. of the Handicapped Amendments of 1986
    special e.
educator
    early e.
    infant e.
EDV
    end-diastolic velocity
    end-diastolic volume
    umbilical arterial EDV
Edwards-Gale syndrome
Edwards syndrome

EEC
    ectrodactyly-ectodermal dysplasia-clefting
    EEC syndrome
EEE
    eastern equine encephalitis
EEG
    electroencephalogram
    electroencephalography
    amplitude-integrated EEG
    interictal EEG
    EEG power value
EEG/polygraphic/video monitoring
EELV
    end-expiratory lung volume
EENT
    eyes, ears, nose, throat
EES
    erythromycin ethylsuccinate
    expandable esophageal stent
E.E.S.
    E.E.S. 200
    E.E.S. 400
    E.E.S. Chewable
    E.E.S. Granules
EFA
    essential fatty acid
efavirenz (DMP-266, EFV)
EFE
    endocardial fibroelastosis
    primary EFE
effect
    Accutane e.
    adiabatic e.
    antiinflammatory e.
    ball-valve e.
    bystander e.
    cardiovascular e.
    choroid plexus pulse e.
    chronotropic e.
    Cushing e.
    cytopathic e. (CPE)
    digitalis e.
    Eisenmenger e.
    fetal alcohol e. (FAE)
    first-pass e.
    halo e.
    iatrogenic e.
    inotropic e.
    mass e.
    mitogenic e.
    muscarinic e.
    side e.
    siphon e.
    waterhammer e.
    white coat e.
efferent limb
Effer-Syllium

Effexor
efficacious
efficacy
efficiency
    sleep e.
effluvium
    anagen e.
    telogen e.
effortless regurgitation
effusion
    bilateral otitis media with e.
        (BOME)
    boggy synovial e.
    chylous pleural e.
    hemorrhagic pleural e.
    lingular e.
    middle ear e. (MEE)
    otitis media with e. (OME)
    otitis media without e.
    parapneumonic pleural e.
    pericardial e.
    pleural e.
    subdural e.
    transudative pleural e.
    tuberculous pleural e.
Efidac/24
Efudex Topical
EFV
    efavirenz
EGD
    esophagogastroduodenoscopy
EGF
    epidermal growth factor
EGFR
    epidermal growth factor receptor
egg
    e. on a string
    e. phospholipid
eggbeater running pattern
EGNB
    enteric gram-negative bacillary
egodystonic
ego-oriented individual therapy (EOIT)
egophony
egosyntonic
egress
    neutrophil e.
EHEC
    enterohemorrhagic *Escherichia coli*
Ehlers-Danlos syndrome (EDS)
Ehrlichia
    E. chaffeensis

    E. phagocytophilia
    E. sennetsu
ehrlichiosis
    granulocytic e.
    human granulocytic e. (HGE)
    human monocytic e. (HME)
    sennetsu e.
EIA
    enzyme immunoassay
    enzyme immunosorbent assay
    exercise-induced asthma
EIB
    erythema induration of Bazin
    exercise-induced bronchospasm
eicosanoid
eicosapentaenoic acid
eight-ball hyphema
eight-drugs-in-one-day treatment series
eighth nerve deafness
Eikenella corrodens
EIM
    extraintestinal manifestation
EI/MV
    endotracheal intubation and mechanical
        ventilation
Einstein
    E. Neonatal Neurobehavioral
        Assessment Scale (ENNAS)
    E. screening test
EIP
    early intervention program
eIPV
    enhanced inactivated polio vaccine
Eisenmenger
    E. complex
    E. effect
    E. physiology
    E. syndrome
EITB
    enzyme-linked immunotransfer blot
ejection
    e. click
    e. reflex
EKC
    epidemic keratoconjunctivitis
EKG (*var. of* ECG)
ektacytometer
elastance
    respiratory system e. (E_{dyn})
    static e. (E_{st})
elastic
    e. bandaging

NOTES

elastic *(continued)*
    e. lamina
    e. tissue hyperplasia
elastica
    cutis e.
elasticity
    blood vessel e.
elasticum
    pseudoxanthoma e.
elastin (ELN)
    e. gene deletion
elastolysis
    generalized e.
elastomer catheter
elastosis perforans serpiginosa
Elavil
elbow
    e. dislocation
    Little League e.
    nursemaid's e.
    pitcher's e.
    prone on e.'s (POE)
    pulled e.
    tennis e.
ELBW
    extremely low birth weight
    ELBW infant
Eldecort Topical
EleCare
    E. formula
    E. nutritional supplement
Elecsys 1010 analyzer
electrical
    e. alternans
    e. stimulation
electrocardiogram (ECG, EKG)
electrocardiography (ECG, EKG)
electroclinical dissociation
electrocochleography (ECochG, ECoG)
    round window e. (RWECochG)
electroconvulsive therapy (ECT)
electrocortical silence
electroculography
electrode
    closed-loop system passing e.
    scalp e.
electrodesiccation
electrodialyzed whey formula
electroencephalogram (EEG)
    amplitude-integrated e. (aEEG)
electroencephalographic sleep study
electroencephalography (EEG)
    quantitative e. (qEEG)
    video e.
electrogastrography
electrographic background abnormality
electrolyte loss
electromechanical dissociation (EMD)

electromembrane
    therapeutic e. (TEM)
electromyogram (EMG)
    surface e.
electromyography (EMG)
electron
    e. microscopy
    e. microscopy of stool
    e. transfer flavoprotein (ETF)
    e. transfer flavoprotein
      dehydrogenase (ETF-DH)
electron-beam computed tomography
  (EBCT)
electron-dense subepithelial deposit
electronic
    e. communication aid
    e. scale
electronystagmography (ENG)
electrooculogram
electrophoresis
    capillary e.
    fluorophore-assisted carbohydrate e.
      (FACE)
    hemoglobin e.
    high-performance capillary e.
      (HPCE)
    Laurell rocket immune e.
    polyacrylamide gel e.
    pulsed field gel e. (PFGE)
    RNA e.
electrophoretic mobility shift assay
  (EMSA)
electrophrenic stimulation
electroporation
electroretinogram (ERG)
electroretinography (ERG)
electroshock
    maximal e. (MES)
electrospray ionization mass
  spectrometry (ESIMS)
electrosurgery
elegans
    Abiotrophia e.
Elejalde syndrome
Elek test
Elema angiocardiogram
elemental diet
elephantiasis
    congenital e.
elephant man
elevate
    rest, ice, compress, e.
elevated
    e. bile acid
    e. conjugated bilirubin
    e. fetal hemoglobin
    e. intracranial pressure
    e. renin

e. sweat chloride concentration
e. transaminase
elevation
e. of blood lead level (EBLL)
periosteal e.
posterior pharyngeal wall e.
rest, ice, compression, e. (RICE)
ST-segment e.
ELF
epithelial lining fluid
pulmonary ELF
elfin facies syndrome
elfinlike facies
ELIFA
enzyme-linked immunofiltration assay
eligibility designation
eligible
elimination diet
Elimite Cream
ELISA
enzyme-linked immunosorbent assay
double-sandwich ELISA
ELISA test
ELISPOT
solid-phase enzyme-linked immunospot
ELISPOT assay
Elixicon
elixir
Bromaline E.
Bromanate E.
Bromphen E.
Dimaphen E.
Dimetapp E.
Genatap E.
K-G E.
Lortab E.
Tylenol and Codeine E.
Elixomin
Elixophyllin
ellipsis
elliptocyte
elliptocytosis
hereditary e. (HE)
spherocytic hereditary e.
Ellis-van Creveld syndrome
ELM
early language milestone
ELM scale
ELN
elastin
Elocon

elongation
rete ridge e.
urethral e.
ELP
exogenous lipoid pneumonia
Elspar
ELT
euglobulin lysis time
Eltroxin
EM
erythema multiforme
EMA
endomysium antibody
emaciated
Emadine
emancipated minor
EMB
ethambutol
embarrassment
respiratory e.
Embden-Meyerhof pathway
embolectomy
Fogarty arterial e. (FAE)
embolic abscess
embolism (*See also* embolus)
air e.
cerebral e.
fat e.
pulmonary e. (PE)
pulmonary fat e.
embolization
aortopulmonary collateral coil e.
arterial e.
catheter e.
patent ductus arteriosis coil e.
transcatheter coil e.
transvenous coil e.
embolus (*See also* embolism)
air e.
massive pulmonary e.
pulmonary e.
septic e.
embrace reflex
embryo
gastrulating e.
embryogenesis
embryogenic induction disorder
embryology
embryonal
e. carcinoma
e. RMS

NOTES

183

embryonic
- e. branchial system
- e. development
- e. hemoglobin
- e. neural retina
- e. noxae
- e. organ culture study
- e. renomedullary interstitial cell
- e. tissue

embryopathy
- diabetic e.
- retinoic acid e.
- thalidomide e.
- warfarin e.

embryoscopy

embryotoxon
- posterior e.

EMD
- electromechanical dissociation

emedastine

emergency
- e. contraceptive pill
- e. medical services for children (EMS-C)
- e. medicine

Emery-Dreifuss
- E.-D. muscular dystrophy
- E.-D. syndrome

emesis
- bile-stained e.
- bilious e.
- coffee-ground e.
- posttussive e.

emetic agent

EMG
- electromyogram
- electromyography
- EMG syndrome

Emgel

eminence
- malar e.

emission
- evoked otoacoustic e. (EOAE)
- nasal air e.
- otoacoustic e. (OAE)
- transient evoked otoacoustic e. (TEOAE)

EMIT
- enzyme-multiplied immunoassay technique

Emitrip

EMLA
- eutectic mixture of local anesthetic
- EMLA anesthetic disc
- EMLA cream
- EMLA disc topical anesthetic adhesive system
- EMLA patch

emmetropia

emollient cream

emotional
- e. abuse
- e. disorder
- e. lability
- e. response
- e. state

Emotionality Activity Sociability Scale (EAS)

emotionally
- e. disturbed
- e. impaired

empathy

emphysema
- congenital lobar e.
- lobar e.
- pulmonary interstitial e. (PIE)
- subcutaneous e.

empirical

empiric therapy

Empirin

emprosthotonos

emptying
- delayed gastric e.

empty sella syndrome

empyema
- encapsulated e.
- epidural e.
- intracranial e.
- e. necessitatis
- subdural e.
- symptomatic chronic e.

EMRN
- encephalomyeloradiculoneuropathy

EMS
- encephalomyosynangiosis

EMSA
- electrophoretic mobility shift assay

EMS-C
- emergency medical services for children

EM/TEN
- erythema multiforme/toxic epidermal necrolysis

emulsion
- Dizac Injectable E.
- fat e.

Emulsoil

E-Mycin

E-Mycin-E

enalapril

enalaprilat

enamel
- e. hypoplasia
- mottled e.

enamelogenesis

enanthem
  hemorrhagic e.
  oral e.
en bloc resection
Enbrel
encainide
encapsulated empyema
encelitis, enceliitis
encephalitide
encephalitis, pl. **encephalitides**
  acute chagasic e.
  acute influenza A e.
  allergic e.
  arboviral e.
  brainstem e.
  California e.
  cerebellar e.
  chagasic e.
  chronic focal e.
  chronic granulomatous amebic e.
  chronic mumps e.
  chronic progressive e.
  Dawson e.
  diffuse periaxial e.
  eastern equine e. (EEE)
  enterovirus e.
  epidemic e.
  equine e.
  focal postviral e.
  giant cell e.
  hemorrhagic e.
  herpes simplex e. (HSE)
  herpes simplex virus e.
  herpesvirus e.
  influenza A e.
  Japanese e.
  La Crosse e.
  e. lethargica
  Marie-Strümpell e.
  measles inclusion body e. (MIBE)
  multinucleated cell e.
  mumps e.
  periaxial e.
  e. periaxialis concentrica
  postinfectious e.
  postinfluenza vaccination e.
  postmeasles e.
  postviral e.
  Powassan e.
  progressive e.
  Rasmussen e.
  Russian spring-summer e.

  Schilder e.
  septic e.
  St. Louis e. (SLE)
  subacute e.
  tick-borne e. (TBE)
  Toxoplasma e.
  toxoplasmic e.
  varicella e.
  Venezuelan equine e. (VEE)
  viral e.
  western equine e. (WEE)
encephalitogenic cell
encephaloarteriosynangiosis
encephalocele
  cranial e.
  frontal e.
  nasal e.
  parietal e.
  transalar sphenoidal e.
encephaloclastic
encephaloduroarteriosynangios (EDAS)
encephalofacial angiomatosis
encephalomalacia
  cystic e.
  multicystic e.
  periventricular e.
  polycystic e.
encephalomeningocele
encephalomyelitis
  acute disseminated e. (ADEM)
  allergic e.
  experimental allergic e. (EAE)
  fatal e.
  immune-mediated disseminated e.
  inflammatory demyelinating e.
  postinfectious e.
  postrabies vaccine e.
  varicella-zoster e.
encephalomyelopathy
  Leigh necrotizing e.
encephalomyeloradiculoneuropathy (EMRN)
encephalomyopathy
  mitochondrial e.
  subacute necrotizing e.
encephalomyosynangiosis (EMS)
encephalopathic crisis
encephalopathy
  AIDS e.
  bilirubin e.
  bovine spongiform e.
  Brett epileptogenic e.

E

NOTES

encephalopathy *(continued)*
    burn e.
    childhood epileptic e.
    chronic spongiform e.
    demyelinating e.
    early infantile epileptic e.
    epileptic e.
    epileptogenic e.
    fatal neonatal hyperammonemic e.
    hepatic e. (HE)
    human immunodeficiency virus e.
    hypertensive e.
    hypoxic e.
    hypoxic-ischemic e. (HIE)
    infantile epileptic e.
    infantile subacute necrotizing e.
    late radiation e.
    lead e.
    Leigh subacute necrotizing e.
    myoclonic e.
    necrotizing e.
    neonatal e. (NE)
    neonatal hypoxic-ischemic e.
    nonspecific e.
    overt bilirubin e.
    phenytoin e.
    plateau e.
    postasphyxial e.
    postvaccinal e.
    progressive e.
    radiation e.
    Reye hepatic e.
    Sarnat e.
    spongiform e.
    static e.
    subacute necrotizing e.
    transient bilirubin e.
    transmissible spongiform e. (TSE)
    uremic e.
    Wernicke e. (WE)
encephalotrigeminal angiomatosis
enchondral ossification
enchondroma, pl. **enchondromata**
    multiple bone enchondromata
enchondromatosis
encoding
encopresis
Endantadine
endarterectomy
endarteritis
    infective e.
    obliterative e.
end-diastolic
    e.-d. velocity (EDV)
    e.-d. volume (EDV)
endemic
    e. Burkitt lymphoma
    e. cretinism
    malaria e.
    e. syphilis
    e. Tyrolean infantile cirrhosis
endemicity
Endep
Enders Edmonston measles strain
end-expiratory lung volume (EELV)
end ileostomy
end-inspiratory airway occlusion
endobronchial tuberculosis
endocardial
    e. cushion
    e. cushion defect
    e. fibroelastosis (EFE)
    e. fibrosis
    e. sclerosis
    e. thrombus
endocarditis
    acute bacterial e.
    bacterial e.
    enterococcal e.
    fetal e.
    fungal e.
    infectious e. (IE)
    infective e. (IE)
    Libman-Sacks e.
    marantic e.
    nonbacterial thrombotic e.
    subacute bacterial e.
    thrombotic e.
    verrucous e.
endocardium
    mural e.
endocholecystitis
    cryptosporidial e.
endochondral ossification
endocrine
    e. disorder
    e. gland
    e. nonfunctional testis
    e. pancreatic dysfunction
endocrinologist
endocrinology
    pediatric e. (PdE)
endocrinopathy
endocytosis
    receptor-mediated e.
endodermal
    e. sinus
    e. sinus tumor
endoesophageal pH
endogenicity/melancholia
endogenous
    e. fat
    e. opioid
endoglin

endoluminal
>   e. stent
>   e. stenting

endomesenchymal tract

endometriosis

endometritis

endomyocardial
>   e. biopsy
>   e. fibrosis

endomysial staining

endomysium antibody (EMA)

endoneurial fibrosis

endonuclease

endopeptidase

endophthalmitis
>   nematode e.

endophytic

endoplasm

endorectal pull-through

endoreduplication

end-organ complication

endoscope
>   Olympus GIF-XP10 video e.
>   Pentax EG-2430 video e.
>   Pentax FG 24-x video e.
>   rigid open-tube e.

endoscopic
>   e. cautery
>   e. choroid plexus extirpation
>   e. correction
>   e. elastic band ligation
>   e. elastic band ligation of varix
>   e. ethmoidectomy
>   e. incision
>   e. incision with flap
>   e. retrograde
>   cholangiopancreatography
>   e. sclerotherapy
>   e. sinus surgery
>   e. strip craniectomy
>   e. unroofing
>   e. variceal ligation (EVL)
>   e. variceal sclerotherapy (EVS)

endoscopy
>   flexible fiberoptic e.

endothelial
>   e. cell
>   e. cell lysate
>   e. dystrophy
>   e. nitric oxide synthetase

endothelin-1

endothelium
>   fenestrated vascular e.
>   vascular e.

endotoxemia

endotoxic shock

endotoxin
>   gram-negative e.
>   meningococcal e.

endotracheal (ET)
>   e. intubation (ETI)
>   e. intubation and mechanical
>   ventilation (EI/MV)
>   e. tube

endovascular hemolytic-uremic syndrome

end-point dilution method

Endrate

Endrin

end-stage
>   e.-s. cirrhosis
>   e.-s. heart failure
>   e.-s. liver disease
>   e.-s. renal disease (ESRD)

end-systolic
>   e.-s. stress (ESS)
>   e.-s. volume (ESV)
>   e.-s. wall stress

end-tidal
>   e.-t. breath carbon monoxide
>   e.-t. carbon dioxide (E_TCO_2)
>   e.-t. CO
>   e.-t. CO_2
>   e.-t. CO_2 tension

end-to-side
>   e.-t.-s. anastomosis
>   e.-t.-s. portocaval shunt

enema
>   air e.
>   air-contrast barium e.
>   antegrade continence e. (ACE)
>   barium e.
>   Fleet Mineral Oil E.
>   Gastrografin e.
>   hydrogen peroxide e.
>   phosphate e.
>   e. procedure
>   rectocolonic saline e.
>   water e.
>   water-soluble contrast e.

Ener-B

energy
>   e. healing
>   e. metabolism

E

NOTES

EnfaCare formula
Enfamil
    E. AR formula
    E. 22, 24 formula
    E. Human Milk Fortifier
    E. Human Milk Fortifier formula
    E. Low Iron formula
    E. NextStep toddler formula
    E. Premature 20 Formula
    E. with Iron
    E. with Iron formula
enflurane
ENG
    electronystagmography
Engerix-B
    E.-B immunization
    E.-B vaccine
English
    manual E.
    signed E. (SE)
    signed exact E. (SEE)
engorgement
    e. of intussusceptum
    venous e.
enhanced
    e. inactivated polio vaccine (eIPV)
    e. urinalysis
enhancement
    rapid acquisition with resolution e. (RARE)
enhancer
    surfactant-associated protein C e.
enlarged liver
enlargement
    areolar e.
    breast e.
    corneal e.
    lymph node e.
    muscle e.
Enlon
enmeshment
ENNAS
    Einstein Neonatal Neurobehavioral Assessment Scale
enolase
    neuron-specific e.
Enomine
enophthalmos
Enovil
enoxaparin
Enseals
    Potassium Iodide E.
Ensure
    E. High Protein
    E. High Protein formula
    E. Plus
    E. Plus HN formula
    E. with Fiber formula

EN-tabs
    Azulfidine EN-t.
Entamoeba
    E. dispar
    E. histolytica
Entera formula
enteral feeding
enteric
    e. adenovirus
    e. cytopathogenic human orphan (ECHO)
    e. cytopathogenic human orphan virus
    e. fever
    e. gentamicin
    e. gram-negative bacillary (EGNB)
    e. hyperoxaluria
    e. infection
    e. neuropeptide
enteritidis
    Salmonella e.
enteritis
    bacterial e.
    Campylobacter e.
    CMV e.
    inflammatory bacterial e.
    regional e.
    rotavirus e.
    tuberculous e.
    viral e.
Enterobacter
    E. cloacae
    E. pneumonia
Enterobacteriaceae
enterobiasis
Enterobius vermicularis
enterochromaffin
    e. cell
    e. cell stimulation
enterococcal endocarditis
Enterococcus
    E. casseliflavus
    E. faecalis
    E. faecium
enterococcus, pl. **enterococci**
    glycopeptide-resistant e. (GRE)
    vancomycin-resistant e. (VRE)
    viridans e.
enterocolic fistula
enterocolitica
    Yersinia e.
enterocolitis
    allergic e.
    dietary protein e.
    Hirschsprung e.
    necrotizing e. (NEC)
    e. syndrome
enterocutaneous fistula

enterocyte
Enterocytozoon
> *E. bieneusi*
> *E. intestinalis*

enteroenteric fistula
enterogenous cyst
enteroglycagon
enterohemorrhagic *Escherichia coli*
(EHEC)
enterohepatic
> e. shunt
> e. shunting

enterokinase deficiency
enteropathica
> acrodermatitis e.
> dermatitis e.

enteropathogenic *Escherichia coli*
(EPEC)
enteropathy
> autoimmune e. (AIE)
> dermatitis herpetiformis-associated
>   gluten-sensitive e.
> gluten e.
> gluten-induced e.
> gluten-sensitive e.
> protein-losing e.

enteroscopy
> small bowel e.

enterostomy
> diverting e.
> proximal e.
> Santulli e.
> Santulli-Blanc e.

Entero-Test
enterotoxigenic *Escherichia coli* (ETEC)
enterotoxin
> sporulation e.

enterovaginal fistula
enterovesical fistula
enteroviral
> e. infection
> e. meningitis
> e. meningoencephalitis
> e. myocarditis

enterovirus
> e. 71
> e. encephalitis
> nonpolio e.

Entex
enthesis
> tender e.

enthesitis

enthesopathy
entitled demander
Entozyme
Entralife HN30 formula
entrapment
> penile zipper e.
> saphenous nerve e.

EntriStar
> E. Gastrostomy System
> E. Skin Level Tube
> E. Skin Level Tube for
>   gastrostomy

entropy
enucleation
> surgical e.

Enulose
enunciate
enuresis
> diurnal e.
> head banding e.
> nocturnal e.
> primary nocturnal e.
> secondary e.

enuretic episode
envelope
> lipid e.

envenomation
> arachnid e.
> snakebite e.

environment
> Home Observation for Measurement
>   of the E. (HOME)
> least restrictive e. (LRE)
> natural e.
> thermal neutral e.

environmental
> e. risk
> e. teratogen
> c. tobacco smoke (ETS)

enzygotic twin
enzymatic block
enzyme
> angiotensin-converting e. (ACE)
> antioxidant e.
> e. assay
> e. CoA
> cytochrome-*c* oxidative e.
> e. defect
> e. deficiency
> human recombinant antioxidant e.
> e. immunoassay (EIA)
> e. immunosorbent assay (EIA)

E

NOTES

enzyme *(continued)*
> peroxidative e.
> recombinant e.
> e. replacement therapy
> e. supplement
> *Taq* I e.

enzyme-linked
> e.-l. immunofiltration assay (ELIFA)
> e.-l. immunosorbent assay (ELISA)
> e.-l. immunotransfer blot (EITB)

enzyme-multiplied immunoassay technique (EMIT)
enzymic acid hydrolysis
enzymopathy
EOAE
> evoked otoacoustic emission

EOIT
> ego-oriented individual therapy

EOM
> equal ocular movement
> extraocular movement

Eoprotin
EOS
> early-onset schizophrenia

eosin
> hematoxylin and e. (H&E)
> e. stain

eosinopenia
eosinophil
> e. cell
> e. peroxidase

eosinophilia
> nonallergenic rhinitis with e.
> peripheral e.
> pulmonary e.
> pulmonary infiltrate with e. (PIE)
> sputum e.

eosinophilia-myalgia syndrome
eosinophilic
> e. adenoma
> e. allergic colitis
> e. ascites
> e. cationic protein (ECP)
> e. cystitis
> e. esophagitis
> e. fasciitis
> e. gastroenteritis
> e. gastroenteropathy
> e. granuloma
> e. infiltrate
> e. leukemia
> e. meningitis
> e. meningoencephalitis
> e. myositis
> e. nonallergic rhinitis
> e. pleocytosis

> e. pneumonia
> e. pustular folliculitis (EPF)

EPDS
> Edinburgh Postnatal Depression Scale

EPEC
> enteropathogenic *Escherichia coli*

ependyma
ependymitis
> granular e.

ependymoblastoma
ependymoma
> posterior fossa anaplastic e.
> supratentorial anaplastic e.

eperezolid
EPF
> eosinophilic pustular folliculitis

ephaptic interaction
ephebiatrics
ephebic
ephebogenesis
ephebogenic
ephebology
ephedrine
ephelides
> nevi, atrial myxomas, myxoid neurofibromas, e. (NAME)

ephelis
ephemeral
> e. fever
> e. temperature

EPI
> extremely premature infant

Epi
> E. E-Z Pen
> E. E-Z Pen-Jr

epiblast
epiblepharon
epibulbar dermoid
epicanthal fold
epicanthus
epicardial pacing
epicardium
epicomus syndrome
epicondyle
> traction apophysitis of medial e.

epicondylitis
> lateral e.

epicranial aponeurosis
Epics XL flow cytometer
epicutaneous test
epidemic
> e. encephalitis
> e. keratoconjunctivitis (EKC)
> e. keratoconjunctivitis herpes simplex
> e. motor polyradiculoneuritis
> e. parotitis
> e. pleurodynia

e. relapsing fever
e. vertigo

epidemica
myalgia cruris e.

epidemiologic
E. Catchment Program

epidemiological study
epidemiology
epidermal
e. covering
e. growth factor (EGF)
e. growth factor receptor (EGFR)
e. hyperkeratosis
e. inclusion cyst
e. nevus
e. nevus syndrome

epidermidis
Staphylococcus e.

epidermis, pl. **epidermides**
Staphylococcus e.

epidermodysplasia verruciformis
epidermoid cyst
epidermolysis
e. bullosa (EB)
e. bullosa acquisita
e. bullosa letalis
e. bullosa simplex
e. bullosa simplex of feet
e. bullosa simplex of hands

epidermolytic
e. hyperkeratosis
e. toxin

Epidermophyton floccosum
epidermophytosis
epididymal
e. sperm aspiration
e. vessel vasculitis

epididymis
epididymitis
epidural
e. abscess
e. analgesia
e. empyema
e. hematoma
e. hemorrhage

Epifrin
epigastric
e. hernia
e. tenderness

epiglottic surface culture
epiglottis
omega-shaped e.

epiglottitis
acute e.

epilepsia partialis continua
epilepsy
abdominal e.
absence e.
benign childhood e.
benign myoclonic e.
benign partial e.
benign rolandic e. (BRE)
centrencephalic e.
childhood absence e.
complex myoclonic e.
complex partial e.
fictitious e.
focal e.
E. Foundation
grand mal e.
idiopathic e.
infantile e.
International League Against E.
(ILAE)
jacksonian e.
juvenile absence e.
juvenile myoclonic e.
midtemporal e.
myoclonic e.
myoclonus e.
nocturnal e.
partial complex e.
petit mal e.
photosensitive e.
posttraumatic e.
primary generalized e.
progressive bulbar palsy with e.
progressive myoclonic e.
psychomotor e.
reactive e.
reflex e.
rolandic e.
secondary e.
e. seizure
severe myoclonic e.
startle e.
sylvian e.
symptomatic e.
television e.
temporal lobe e.
typical absence e.
vestibulogenic e.
video game e.
visual reflex e.

E

NOTES

epileptic
    e. aura
    e. convulsion
    e. encephalopathy
    e. idiocy
    e. myoclonus
    e. syndrome
epilepticus
    absence status e.
    complex partial status e.
    convulsive status e.
    febrile status e.
    idiopathic status e.
    limbic status e.
    nonconvulsive status e. (NCSE)
    partial status e.
    refractory status e. (RSE)
    status e. (SE)
    symptomatic status e.
epileptiform
    e. activity
    e. discharge
epileptogenesis
epileptogenic
    e. encephalopathy
    e. lesion
epileptogenicity
epileptologist
epileptology
epiloia
epimyoepithelial island
epinephrine
    aerosolized racemic e.
    e. deficiency
    higher-dose therapy with e. (HDE)
    lidocaine and e.
    e. provocation
    racemic e.
    self-injectable e.
    Xylocaine With E.
epineurium
EpiPen
    E. Jr.
    E. Sr.
epipericardial connective tissue
epiphora
epiphyseal
    e. dysplasia
    e. growth
    e. growth plate
    e. plate injury
    e. stapling
    e. syndrome
epiphyses (*pl. of* epiphysis)
epiphysiodesis
epiphysiolysis
epiphysis, pl. **epiphyses**
    capital femoral e.

    capitellar e.
    congenital stippled e.
    double epiphyses
    femoral e.
    intraarticular e.
    proximal femoral e.
    proximal tibial e.
    radial e.
    slipped e.
    slipped capital femoral e. (SCFE)
    slipped upper femoral e. (SUFE)
    stippled e.
    stippling of epiphyses
    tibial e.
    upper humeral e.
epiplocele
episcleritis
episode
    enuretic e.
    hyperammonemic e.
    hypomanic e.
    mitochondrial myopathy, encephalopathy, lactic acidosis, strokelike e.'s (MELAS)
    myopathy, encephalopathy, lactic acidosis, strokelike e.'s (MELAS)
    present e.
    protracted depressive e.
    Schedule for Affective Disorders and Schizophrenia for School-Age Children-Present E. (K-SADS-P)
    syncopal e.
    vasoocclusive e.
episodic
    e. angioedema
    e. ataxia (1, 2)
    e. blanching
    e. dyscontrol
    e. dyscontrol syndrome
    e. flushing
    e. memory
epispadias
    female e.
    simple e.
epispadias-exstrophy complex
epistaxis
    recurrent e.
    refractory e.
epitaxy
epithelial
    e. bud
    e. cell
    e. cell proliferation
    e. keratitis
    e. lining fluid (ELF)
    e. liver tumor
    e. pearl
    e. tuft

epithelial-mesenchymal interaction
epithelioid
    e. cell nevus
    e. leiomyosarcoma
epithelioma
    e. adenoides cysticum
    basal cell e.
    calcifying e.
epithelium
    airway e.
    artificial vaginal e.
    circumferential eversion of
      urethral e.
    infarction of oral e.
    oral e.
    respiratory e.
    retinal pigment e. (RPE)
    urethral e.
Epitol
epitope
epitopic
epituberculosis
epitympanic recess
Epivir
EPO
    erythropoietin
    evening primrose oil
epoch
    growth e.
    sleep e.
epoetin alfa
Epogen
EPP
    erythropoietic protoporphyria
epsilon-aminocaproic acid
epsilon toxin
Epstein-Barr
    E.-B. nuclear antigen
    E.-B. virus (EBV)
Epstein pearl
epulis
equal
    e. conjoined twin
    e. ocular movement (EOM)
equalization
    pressure e. (PE)
equation
    Henderson-Hasselbalch e.
    Schofield weight-based resting
      energy expenditure prediction e.

    Schofield weight- and height-based
      resting energy expenditure
      prediction e.
    Weir e.
equatorial plane
equi
    Rhodococcus e.
Equilet
equilibration
equilibrium
    Donnan e.
    e. reaction
equina
    cauda e.
equine
    e. antitoxin
    e. encephalitis
    e. estrogen
equinovalgus
    talipes e.
equinovarus
    idiopathic talipes e.
    neurogenic talipes e.
    pes e.
    e. pes deformity
    talipes e. (TEV)
equinus
    ankle e.
    e. clubfoot
    e. deformity
    e. gait
    e. position
equivalent
    genome e. (GE)
E-R
    Betachron E-R
ERA
    evoked response audiometry
eradication therapy
Erb
    E. juvenile muscular dystrophy
    E. palsy
Erb-Duchenne
    E.-D. palsy
    E.-D. paralysis
Erb-Goldflam syndrome
Erb-Klumpke palsy
Ercaf
Erdheim disease
erectile dysfunction (ED)
erection
    penile e.

E

NOTES

erethism
ERG
  electroretinogram
  electroretinography
ergocalciferol
ergogenic
Ergomar
ergometer
    bicycle e.
    Rodby Electronik AB braked
    cycle e.
ergosterol
ergotamine
Ergotamine Tartrate and Caffeine
  Cafatine
Erhardt developmental prehension
  assessment
Erlenmeyer flask appearance
E-R-O Ear Drops
erosion
    bony e.
erosive
    e. esophagitis
    e. rhinitis
ERP
  event-related potential
erratic
    e. blood pressure
    e. temperature
error
    Garrodian inborn e.
    inborn e.
    refractive e.
erucic acid
eructation
    flatus e.
eructio nervosa
eruption
    bullous drug e.
    Christmas tree distribution e.
    creeping e.
    delayed tooth e.
    Kaposi varicelliform e.
    maculopapular e.
    monomorphous papular e.
    papular e.
    papulosquamous e.
    polymorphous light e.
    pruritic vesiculopapular e.
    purpuric light e.
    scarlatiniform e.
    seabather's e.
    vesicobullous e.
    vesiculopapular e.
    violaceous e.
eruptive
    e. fever
    e. hidradenoma

    e. lichen planus
    e. nevus
    e. syringoma
    e. temperature
    e. vellus hair cyst
    e. xanthoma
ERV
  expiratory reserve volume
Eryc
Erycette
EryDerm
Erygel
Erymax
EryPed
erysipelas
    necrotizing e.
Erysipelothrix rhusiopathiae
Ery-Tab
erythema
    e. chronicum migrans (ECM)
    e. chronicum migrans rash
    fixed e.
    gingival e.
    heliotropic e.
    e. induration of Bazin (EIB)
    e. infectiosum
    Jacquet e.
    linear gingival e.
    e. marginatum
    e. migrans
    e. multiforme (EM)
    e. multiforme exudativum
    e. multiforme/toxic epidermal
    necrolysis (EM/TEN)
    e. neonatorum toxicum
    e. nodosum
    e. nodosum leprosum
    palmar e.
    periorbital violaceous e.
    periungual e.
    scarlatiniform e.
    e. streptogene
    toxic e.
    e. toxicum
    e. toxicum neonatorum
    vasculitic e.
    violaceous e.
erythematosus
    discoid lupus e.
    disseminated lupus e.
    lupus e.
    neonatal lupus e. (NLE)
    systemic lupus e. (SLE)
erythematous
    e. blush
    e. confluent plaque
    e. halo
    e. macule

e. papule
e. rash
e. satellite lesion
erythrasma
erythredema polyneuropathy
erythroblastic
e. anemia
e. anemia of childhood
erythroblastopenia
transient e.
erythroblastosis
fetal e. (FE)
e. fetalis
e. neonatorum
Erythrocin
erythrocyte
e. acquired defect
burr-shaped e.
dysmorphic e.
e. glutathione peroxidase deficiency
e. mosaicism
e. pyruvate kinase deficiency
e. sedimentation rate (ESR)
erythrocytopoiesis
erythrocytosis
familial e.
stress e.
erythroderma
atopic e.
bullous congenital ichthyosiform e.
congenital ichthyosiform e.
e. desquamativum
exfoliative e.
generalized e.
ichthyosiform e.
nonbullous congenital
ichthyosiform e.
erythrodermic
erythrohepatic protoporphyria
erythroid
e. hyperplasia
e. hypoplasia
myeloid to e. (M:E)
e. progenitor
e. progenitor cell
erythrokeratoderma
symmetric progressive e.
e. variabilis
erythroleukoblastosis
erythromelalgia
erythromycin
e. estolate

e. ethylsuccinate (EES)
e. lactobionate
e. and sulfisoxazole
erythromycin-sulfisoxazole
erythrophagocytic
erythropoiesis
compensatory e.
dermal e.
e. failure
megaloblastic e.
stress e.
erythropoietic
e. porphyria
e. porphyria congenita
e. protoporphyria (EPP)
erythropoietin (EPO)
human e.
recombinant human e. (r-EPO,
rHuEPO, rHuEpo)
serum e.
Erythroxylum coca
Eryzole
ES
Pertussin ES
Vicodin ES, HP
ESA Coulochem multi-electrode
escape rhythm
escharotomy
Escherichia
E. coli
E. coli sepsis
E-selectin
Eserine
Isopto E.
Esidrix
ESIMS
electrospray ionization mass spectrometry
Eskalith
esmolol
esodeviation
E-Solve-2
esophageal
e. anastomosis
e. atresia (EA)
e. candidiasis
e. coin
e. dilation
e. hiatus
e. manometry
e. perforation
e. reflux
e. replacement

E

NOTES

esophageal *(continued)*
   e. spasm
   e. sphincter
   e. stenosis
   e. stricture
   e. transection
   e. ulceration
   e. varix (EV)
   e. web
esophagectomy
esophagitis
   allergic e.
   eosinophilic e.
   erosive e.
   infectious e.
   monilial e.
   peptic e.
   reflux e.
   tetracycline-induced e.
   viral e.
esophagogastroduodenoscopy (EGD)
esophagogram
   barium e.
   contrast e.
esophagography
   barium e.
esophagoscopy
esophagostomy
   cervical e.
esophagotracheal primordium
esophagram
   barium e.
   Gastrografin e.
esophagus
   cervical e.
   nutcracker e.
   stenosis of e.
EsopHogram software
esophoria
esotropia
   accommodative e.
   congenital e.
ESPGHAN
   European Society of Paediatric
   Gastroenterology, Hepatology, and
   Nutrition
espundia
ESR
   erythrocyte sedimentation rate
ESRD
   end-stage renal disease
ESS
   end-systolic stress
essential
   e. amino acid
   e. benign pentosuria
   e. fatty acid (EFA)
   e. fatty acid deficiency

   e. fructosuria
   e. hypertension
   e. myoclonus
   e. thrombocythemia (ET)
   e. tremor
Essiac
established
   e. medical diagnosis
   e. risk
Estar
ester
   cholesterol e.
   tosylarginine methyl e. (TAME)
esterase
   tosylarginine methyl ester e.
esthesioneuroblastoma
Estivin II Ophthalmic
estolate
   erythromycin e.
Estrace
Estraderm
estradiol
Estratest HS
Estren-Damashek subtype
estriol
   unconjugated e. (uE3)
Estro-Cyp
estrogen
   conjugated equine e.
   equine e.
   fetal e.
Estroject-L.A.
estrone
Estronol-LA
Estrostep
ESV
   end-systolic volume
ET
   endotracheal
   essential thrombocythemia
     K+ Care ET
     ET tube
etanercept
E-tank wrench
ETEC
   enterotoxigenic *Escherichia coli*
E-test
   E.-t. technique
ETF
   electron transfer flavoprotein
ETF-DH
   electron transfer flavoprotein
    dehydrogenase
ETH
   ethionamide
ethacrynic acid
ethambutol (EMB)

ethane
    exhaled e.
ethanol
ethionamide (ETH)
ethmocephaly
ethmoid
    e. bone
    e. sinus
ethmoidectomy
    endoscopic e.
ethnic
ethologic
ethosuximide
ethyl
    e. alcohol (EtOH)
    e. chloride
ethylenediamine
ethylenediaminetetraacetic acid (EDTA)
ethylene glycol
ethylester
    tryptophan e.
ethylmalonic-adipic aciduria
ethylsuccinate
    erythromycin e. (EES)
Ethyol
ETI
    endotracheal intubation
etidronate disodium
etiology
    fever of unknown e.
    opsoclonus-myoclonus e.
etiopathogenesis
EtOH
    ethyl alcohol
etomidate
etoposide (VP-16)
    Ara-C, Platinol, e. (APE)
etretinate
ETS
    environmental tobacco smoke
ETS-2% Topical
eucapnia
Eucerin
    E. cream
    E. Plus Creme
Euclidean distance
euglobulin
    e. clot lysis time (ECLT)
    e. lysis time (ELT)
euglycemia
eugonadal
eugonadotropic oligospermia

eukaryotic cell
EULAR
    European League Against Rheumatism
        EULAR classification
Eulenburg disease
Euler and Byrne score
eumelanin
eunuchoid
    e. gigantism
    e. habitus
euphoria
euphoriant
Eurax
European
    E. League Against Rheumatism
        (EULAR)
    E. League Against Rheumatism
        classification
    E. Society of Paediatric
        Gastroenterology, Hepatology, and
        Nutrition (ESPGHAN)
eustachian
    e. tube
    e. tube defect
    e. tube dysfunction
eutectic mixture of local anesthetic
    (EMLA)
euthymic
euthyroid sick syndrome
eutopic congenital hypothyroidism
EV
    esophageal varix
Evac-Q-Mag
evacuation proctography
Evalose
evaluation
    Acute Physiology and Chronic
        Health E. (APACHE)
    audiometric e.
    Collaborative Home Infant
        Monitoring E. (CHIME)
    genetic e.
    longitudinal interval followup e.
        (LIFE)
evanescent
    e. maculopapular rash
Evans
    E. calcaneal lengthening
    E. syndrome
evaporated milk formula
evening primrose oil (EPO)

E

NOTES

197

event
  acute life-threatening e. (ALTE)
  apneic e.
  apparent life-threatening e. (ALTE)
  asphyxial e.
  idiopathic apparent life-
    threatening e.
  intracellular e.
  e. monitor
  thromboembolic e. (TE)
  unexplained apparent life-
    threatening e. (UALTE)
eventration
  congenital e.
  e. of diaphragm
  diaphragmatic e.
event-related potential (ERP)
Everone Injection
eversion
  circumferential e.
  e. injury
every (q., q.q.)
  quaque horo (e. hour) (q.h.)
E-Vitamin
EVL
  endoscopic variceal ligation
EVLW
  extravascular lung water
evoked
  e. otoacoustic emission (EOAE)
  e. potential
  e. response
  e. response audiometry (ERA)
EVS
  endoscopic variceal sclerotherapy
Ewing
  E. sarcoma
  E. sarcoma gene
  E. tumor
EX
  Diabetic Tussin EX
  Naldecon Senior EX
Ex
  Touro Ex
exacerbation
  asthma e.
Exacta-Med oral dispenser
Exact Cream
ExacTech glucose measuring device
examination
  Allen and Capute neonatal
    neurodevelopmental e.
  audiometric e.
  buffy-coat e.
  colposcopic e.
  darkfield e.
  Dubowitz e.
  eating disorders e. (EDE)

  Pediatric Early Elemental E.
    (PEEX)
  personality disorder e. (PDE)
  preparticipation sports e. (PSE)
  rectal e.
  roentgenographic e.
  serial neurologic e.
  slit-lamp e.
  speculum e.
exanthem
  Boston e.
  laterothoracic e.
  maculopapular e.
  measles e.
  papular e.
  polymorphous e.
  scarlet fever e.
  toxin-induced scarlet fever e.
  unilateral laterothoracic e. (ULE)
  vesicular e.
  viral e.
exanthema
  e. multiforme exudativum
  rheumatic e.
exanthematous disease
exanthum subitum
excavatum
  pectus e.
Excedrin IB
excess
  adrenal e.
  apparent mineralocorticoid e.
    (AME)
  glucocorticoid e.
  hyponatremia of water e.
  sodium e.
  TBG e.
excessive
  e. acid secretion
  e. hoarseness
  e. insulin action
  e. insulin secretion
  e. penile curvature
  e. pulmonary arterial flow
  e. sleeping
  e. sweating
exchange
  perfluorocarbon-assisted gas e.
  plasma e.
  regional gas e. (R_{AW})
  e. transfusion (EXT)
excision
  atrial septum e.
  diathermy loop e.
  thyroglossal duct cyst e.
  wide e.
excitotoxic
  e. amino acid (EAA)

e. injury
e. mechanism
e. necrosis
excitotoxicity
exclamation-mark hair
excoriation
excreta
excrete
excretion
coproporphyrin e.
fractional e.
urinary e.
urobilinogen e.
excretory urogram
excursion
thoracic wall e.
excyst
metacercaria e.
executive
e. cognitive functioning (ECF)
e. function
exencephaly
exenteration
exercise
e. bronchial challenge
eccentric e.
e. intolerance
isometric quadriceps e.
visual training e.
exercise-induced
e.-i. asthma (EIA)
e.-i. bronchospasm (EIB)
exertional reactive airway disease
exertion-induced dyskinesia
exfoliation failure
exfoliative
e. dermatitis
e. erythroderma
exhaled
e. ethane
e. pentane
exhibitionism
Exidine Scrub
EXIT
ex utero intrapartum treatment
exocervix
exocrine
e. pancreatic dysfunction
e. pancreatic hypoplasia
e. pancreatic insufficiency
exodeviation

exogenous
e. lipoid pneumonia (ELP)
e. medication
e. obesity
e. surfactant
e. surfactant therapy
exomphalos
e., macroglossia, gigantism
e., macroglossia, gigantism syndrome
Exophiala werneckii
exophoria
exophthalmos
apparent e.
pulsating e.
exophytic
e. lesion
e. mass
e. wart
exostosis, pl. exostoses
calcified e.
multiple cartilaginous e.
subungual e.
Exosurf Neonatal
exotoxemia
exotoxin-A
streptococcal e.-A (SPEA)
exotropia
constant e.
intermittent e.
expandable esophageal stent (EES)
expander
tissue e.
volume e.
expansion
GAA trinucleotide e.
palatal e.
expectorant
Anti-Tuss E.
Benylin E.
GuiaCough E.
Triaminic E.
expectorate
expenditure
resting energy e. (REE)
total daily energy e. (TDEE)
total energy e.
experience
appropriate learning e.
separation-reunion e.
experimental
e. allergic encephalomyelitis (EAE)

E

NOTES

experimental *(continued)*
  e. lymphocytic choriomeningitis
  e. pneumococcal meningitis
expiration
expiratory
  e. apnea
  e. flow volume
  e. grunting
  e. to inspiratory ratio
  e. reserve volume (ERV)
  e. scan
expire
explanted
exploration
  oral e.
explosive watery diarrhea
exponential
exposed
  chemically e.
exposure
  airway, breathing, circulation and
    control bleeding, disability, e.
    (ABCDE)
  intrauterine e.
  lead e.
  radiation e.
  teratogenic e.
  in utero drug e. (IUDE)
expression
  facial e.
expressionless face
expressive
  e. aphasia
  e. language
  e. language development
  E. One-Word Picture Vocabulary
    Test
expulsion
Exsel shampoo
exstrophic
  e. cecum
  e. vagina
exstrophy
  bladder e.
  cloacal e.
EXT
  exchange transfusion
Extencaps
  Micro-K 10 E.
extended
  e. end-to-end anastomosis
  e. family
  e. internal dosing
extended-release methylphenidate
extension
  medial hip rotation in e.
  protective e.

Score for Neonatal Acute
    Physiology-Perinatal E.
extensive support
extensor
  e. fit
  e. hypertonus
  e. leg posture
  e. thrust pattern
Extentabs
  Dimetane E.
  Quinidex E.
externa
  malignant otitis e.
  otitis e. (OE)
external
  e. anal sphincter
  e. anal thrombosis
  e. auditory canal
  e. auditory meatus
  e. beam radiation therapy
  e. branchial sinus
  e. ear
  e. femoral torsion
  e. hemorrhage
  e. hordeolum
  e. hydrocephalus
  e. jugular venipuncture
  e. male genitalia
  e. ophthalmoplegia
  e. otitis
  e. rotation
  e. sphincter muscle
  e. tibial torsion
  e. urethral meatus
  e. virilization
externalizing
  e. behavior
  E. Behavior Scale
  e. score
extinction
extirpation
  endoscopic choroid plexus e.
extraabdominal organ system disease
Extra Action Cough Syrup
extraaxial
  e. arachnoid cyst
  e. fluid
extracardiac
  e. abnormality
  e. anomaly
  e. conduit cavopulmonary
    anastomosis
  e. malformation
  e. shunt
extracellular
  e. fluid (ECF)
  e. fluid compartment
  e. matrix signal

e. plasma potassium
e. volume (ECV)
extracorporeal
e. circulation
e. life support (ECLS)
e. membrane oxygenation (ECMO)
e. rewarming
extracranial foreign body
extract
calf lung surfactant e. (CLSE)
malt soup e.
modified bovine surfactant e.
pyrethrum e.
extraction
peripheral fractional oxygen e.
(PFOE)
testicular sperm e. (TESE)
vacuum e.
extractor
comedones e.
extracutaneous sporotrichosis
extradural
e. abscess
e. hematoma
extrafamily offender
extraglomerular
extragonadal germ cell tumor
extrahepatic
e. bile duct resection
e. biliary atresia
e. biliary tree
e. portal vein obstruction
e. presinusoidal obstruction
extraintestinal manifestation (EIM)
extralobar sequestration
extraluminal
e. fluid
e. gas bubble
extramedullary hematopoiesis
extranodal
e. marginal zone
e. marginal zone B-cell lymphoma
extraocular
e. movement (EOM)
e. muscle
e. muscle surgery
extraordinary urinary frequency
syndrome
extraosseous Ewing sarcoma
extra ossification
extraplacental membrane
extrapolate

extrapolation
extrapulmonary
e. cryptococcosis
e. extravasation
e. extravasation of air
e. tuberculosis
extrapyramidal
e. cerebral palsy
e. lesion
e. manifestation
e. movement
e. nervous system
e. sign
e. tract
extrapyramidal-pyramidal syndrome
extrarenal
e. rhabdoid tumor
e. saline
extrasystole
extrathoracic
e. tuberculosis
e. ventilator
extrauterine life
extravasation
blood e.
extrapulmonary e.
extravascular lung water (EVLW)
extraventricular
extravesical
e. mass
e. ureteral reimplantation
extreme
e. benign hyperbilirubinemia
e. leukocytosis
extremely
e. low birth weight (ELBW)
e. low birth weight infant
e. premature infant (EPI)
extremis
extremity
long thin e.
lower e. (LE)
e. lymphedema
upper e. (UE)
extrinsic
e. alveolar alveolitis
e. compression of airway
e. dyssomnia
e. extravesical mass
extrophy
cloacal e.

E

NOTES

extrusion
dental e.
e. reflex
extrusion/lateral luxation
extrusive luxation
extubate
extubation
exudate
alveolar fibrinous e.
cheesy e.
cotton-ball e.
fibrinopurulent e.
fibrinous e.
inflammatory e.
opaque white e.
peritoneal e.
subretinal e.
tonsillar e.
tonsillopharyngeal e.
exudative
e. ascites
e. conjunctivitis
e. meningitis
e. pharyngitis
e. retinal detachment
e. tonsillitis
exudativum
erythema multiforme e.
exanthema multiforme e.
ex utero intrapartum treatment (EXIT)
Eyberg Child Behavior Inventory
eye
amblyopic e.
Clear E.'s
dancing e.'s

deep set e.'s
e. deviation
e. dominance
downslanting e.'s
dry e.
e.'s, ears, nose, throat (EENT)
lazy e.
e. movement
muscle, liver, brain, e. (Mulibrey)
nonfixing e.
ox's e.
e. popping
raccoon e.'s
e. retraction with adduction
e. salvage therapy
e. slant
sunset e.'s
sunsetting e.'s
widely spaced e.'s
eyebrow
confluent e.'s
eyeground
eye-hand coordination
eyelash trichomegaly
eyelid
Dennie lines of lower e.'s
heliotrope e.
e. muscle
e. squeezing
e. tumor
eye-of-the-tiger sign
E-Z Heat hot pack
Ezide
E-Z-On Vest

FA
Fanconi anemia
femoral anteversion
FA screening
FAB
French-American-British
FAB classification
fab
digoxin immune f.
FABP
finger arterial blood pressure
fabric
Solumbra 30+ SPF f.
Fabry
F. crisis
F. disease
FACE
fluorophore-assisted carbohydrate
electrophoresis
FACE kit
face
abnormal f.
dysmorphic f.
ectodermal dysplasia of f.
expressionless f.
f., legs, activity, cry, consolability
(FLACC)
f. mask
f. presentation
round moon f.
f. tent
f. underdevelopment
face-near-straight-down (FNSD)
face-out, whole-body plethysmograph
FACES
Family Adaptability and Cohesion
Evaluation Scale
face-straight-down (FSD)
facet
f. dislocation
jumped f.
locked f.
medial talocalcaneal f.
subtalar f.
f. syndrome
face-to-side (FTS)
facial
f. affect recognition
f. angioma
f. buttress
f. diplegia
f. dysmorphia syndrome
f. dysmorphism
f. expression
f. expression and sleeplessness

f. nerve palsy
f. pain
f. paralysis
facialis
herpes f.
faciei
lupus miliaris disseminatum f.
facies
abnormal f.
asymmetric crying f.
birdlike f.
Campbell Soup kid f.
cushingoid f.
elfinlike f.
flat f.
moon f.
moon-shaped f.
peculiar f.
Potter f.
progeroid f.
seborrheic-like f.
soup kid f.
thalassemia f.
triangular f.
facilitated communication (F/C)
facility
intermediate care f. (ICF)
facioauriculovertebral spectrum (FAVS)
faciodigitogenital syndrome
faciolingual-masticatory diplegia
facioscapulohumeral (FSH)
**facioscapulohumeral muscular dystrophy
(FSHD)**
faciotelencephalopathy
Facit polyp forceps
factitial panniculitis
factitious
f. disorder
f. disorder by proxy (FDP)
factor
f. I deficiency
f. II deficiency
f. IV
f. V
f. V deficiency
f. V Leiden
f. V Leiden mutation
f. VII
f. VIII deficiency
f. VIII hemophilia
f. VIII inhibitor
f. IX
f. X
f. Xa inhibition assay
f. X deficiency

F

203

factor *(continued)*
f. XI deficiency
f. XII
f. XIIIa
f. XIII deficiency
activated clotting f. X
antihemophilic f. (AHF)
atrial natriuretic f. (ANF)
autocrine-acting growth f.
autocrine/paracrine-acting growth f.
basic fibroblast growth f. (bFGF)
binding protein-2 insulinlike
    growth f.
binding protein-3 insulinlike
    growth f.
biomedical f.
biotin f.
brain-derived neurotrophic f.
    (BDNF)
chemotactic f.
Christmas f.
ciliary neurotrophic f. (CNTF)
colony-stimulating f.
complement chemotactic f.
contact f.
contagion f.
f. D deficiency
decay-accelerating f.
deficiency of f. B, D
DNAse B f.
epidermal growth f. (EGF)
fibrin-stabilizing f.
fibroblast growth f. (FGF)
glial cell line derived
    neurotrophic f. (GDNF)
gonadotropin-releasing f. (GRF)
granulocyte colony-stimulating f.
    (G-CSF)
granulocyte-macrophage colony-
    stimulating f. (GM-CSF)
growth control f.
H f.
Hageman f.
f. H deficiency
hepatocyte nuclear f. (HNF)
hidden rheumatoid f.
highly purified f. IX
high molecular weight kininogen f.
HMWK f.
hyaluronic acid f.
hyaluronidase f.
insulinlike growth f. (IGF)
insulinlike growth f. 1 (IGF-1)
insulinlike growth f. 2 (IGF-2)
intrinsic f. (IF)
labile f.
f. M

migration inhibitory f. (MIF)
M protein f.
müllerian inhibiting f. (MIF)
necrotizing f.
paracrine-acting growth f.
perinatal risk f.
perisphincteric f.
PK f.
plasma f.
plasma coagulation f. VIII, IX
postnatal f.
prenatal f.
properdin f. B
prostacyclin-stimulating f. (PSF)
proteinase f.
pyrogenic exotoxin A, B, C f.
pyruvate kinase f.
recombinant f. VIIA (rFVIIa)
Rh f.
Rhesus f.
rheumatoid f. (RF)
Service Utilization and Risk F.'s
    (SURF)
specific transcription f.
spreading f.
stable f.
streptokinase f.
Stuart-Prower f.
tissue f.
tumor necrosis f. (TNF)
vascular endothelial growth f.
    (VEGF)
vascular permeability f.
von Willebrand f. (vWF)
f. Z

factor-1
recombinant human insulin-like
    growth f.-1 (rhIGF-1)
steroidogenic f.-1 (SF-1)
thyroid transcription f.-1 (TTF-1)
transforming growth f.-1 (TGF-1)

factor-alpha
tumor necrosis f.-a. (TNF-alpha)

Factrel

facultative scotoma

FAD
flavin adenine dinucleotide

fading

FAE
fetal alcohol effect
Fogarty arterial embolectomy
    FAE catheter

faecalis
Enterococcus f.

faecium
Enterococcus f.

Fagan
    F. test
    F. Test of Infant Intelligence
FAH
    fumarylacetoacetate hydrolase
Fahr disease
failed
    f. breastfeeding
    f. Fontan circuit
    f. reduction
failure
    acute renal f. (ARF)
    bilateral gonadal f.
    cardiac f.
    chronic renal f. (CRF)
    congestive heart f. (CHF)
    end-stage heart f.
    erythropoiesis f.
    exfoliation f.
    fulminant hepatic f. (FHF)
    growth f.
    heart f.
    high-output f.
    hypoxic respiratory f.
    impending renal f.
    kidney f.
    left ventricular f.
    multiorgan system f.
    multiple organ system f. (MOSF)
    neurogenic respiratory f.
    primary testicular f.
    progressive central nervous system f.
    progressive renal f.
    renal f.
    respiratory f.
    right-sided heart f.
    severe growth f.
    f. to thrive (FTT)
    ventilatory f.
failure-to-thrive syndrome
faint
    vasovagal f.
Fairbank skeletal abnormality
falciparum
    f. malaria
    Plasmodium f.
fall-away response
falling sickness
Fallot
    acyanotic tetralogy of F.
    F. pentalogy

    pink tetralogy of F.
    tetralogy of F. (TOF)
    F. trilogy
Falope ring
false
    f. fontanelle
    f. localizing sign
    f. negative
    f. positive
    f. vocal cord
falx
    cerebral f.
    f. sign
famciclovir
familial
    f. achalasia
    f. adenomatous polyposis
    f. adenomatous polyposis coli
    f. APOA-I deficiency
    f. atypical multiple mole melanoma syndrome
    f. cardiac myxoma
    f. chylomicronemia syndrome
    f. combined hyperlipidemia (FCHL)
    f. Creutzfeldt-Jakob disease
    f. defective apolipoprotein B-100
    f. disorder
    f. dominant thrombocytopenia
    f. dysautonomia
    f. erythroblastic anemia
    f. erythrocytosis
    f. erythrophagocytic lymphohistiocytosis (FEL)
    f. exudative vitreoretinopathy (FEV)
    f. glomerulonephritis
    f. glycinuria
    f. hemiplegic migraine (FHM)
    f. hemophagocytic lymphohistiocytosis (FHLH)
    f. Hibernian fever
    f. hypercalcemia
    f. hypercalcemia with hypocalciuria (FHH)
    f. hypercholesterolemia
    f. hyperinsulinemic hypoglycemia
    f. hyperinsulinism of infancy
    f. hyperlipidemia
    f. hyperlysinemia
    f. hypertriglyceridemia (FHTG)
    f. hypoalphalipoproteinemia
    f. hypobetalipoproteinemia

F

NOTES

familial *(continued)*
    f. hypocalciuric hypercalcemia (FHH)
    f. hypokalemic periodic paralysis
    f. hypomagnesemia
    f. hypophosphatemia (FHR)
    f. hypophosphatemic rickets
    f. iminoglycinuria
    f. insomnia syndrome
    f. intrahepatic cholestasis
    f. juvenile gout
    f. juvenile hyperuricemic nephropathy
    f. juvenile nephrophthisis
    f. lecithin:cholesterol acyltransferase deficiency
    f. loading
    f. lumbosacral syringomyelia
    f. lymphedema praecox
    f. macrocephaly
    f. male precocious puberty
    f. Mediterranean fever (FMF)
    f. multiple lipomatosis
    f. muscular atrophy
    f. neonatal seizure
    f. neuroblastoma
    f. osteochondrodystrophy
    f. panhypopituitarism
    f. protein intolerance
    f. pure gonadal dysgenesis
    f. pyridoxine-dependency syndrome
    f. recurrent hematuria
    f. short stature
    f. spastic paraplegia (FSP)
    f. spinal neurofibromatosis
    f. tremor
    f. visceral myopathy
    f. visceral neuropathy
family
    F. Adaptability and Cohesion Evaluation Scale (FACES)
    F. Adaptability and Cohesion Scale-III
    f. APGAR
    F. APGAR questionnaire
    f. dynamics
    f. dysfunction
    dysfunctional f.
    F. Environment Scale
    extended f.
    f. history research diagnostic criteria (FH-RDC)
    F. Inventory of Resources for Management (FIRM)
    F. Medical Leave Act (FMLA)
    f. member presence (FMP)
    Poxviridae f.
    f. therapy

famotidine
Famvir
Fanconi
    F. anemia (FA)
    F. aplastic anemia
    F. pancytopenia
    F. pancytopenia syndrome
Fanconi-Bickel syndrome
fanning
fan-shaped hemorrhagic infarct
Fansidar
fantasy
    revenge f.
FAO
    fatty acid oxidation
Farber
    F. disease
    F. lipogranulomatosis
    F. syndrome
    F. test
farcinica
    Nocardia f.
farmeri
    Citrobacter f.
farmer's lung
Farr test
farsightedness
FAS
    fetal alcohol syndrome
fascia, pl. **fasciae**
    f. adherens
    plantar f.
    presacral f.
fascicle
fasciculation
    muscle f.
    tongue f.
fasciculus, pl. **fasciculi**
    syndrome of median longitudinal f.
fasciitis, fascitis
    cranial f.
    diffuse f.
    eosinophilic f.
    gas gangrene f.
    necrotizing myositis f.
    nodular f.
    plantar f.
Fasciola hepatica
fascioliasis
fascitis *(var. of* fasciitis)
FAST
    Focused Assessment by Sonography for Trauma
    FAST blood test
fast
    fast channel syndrome
    protein-sparing modified fast (PSMF)

fasting
    f. blood sugar
    f. plasma cholecystokinin
FAT
  female athlete triad
fat
    f. absorption
    f. analysis
    f. deposition
    f. distribution pattern
    f. embolism
    f. emulsion
    endogenous f.
    f. flexor hallucis longus tendon
    f. herniation
    f. malabsorption
    f. mass (FM)
    microscopic f.
    f. necrosis
    percent body f. (PBF)
    f. plane
fatal
    f. cutaneous aspergillosis
    f. encephalomyelitis
    f. familial insomnia
    f. infantile myopathy
    f. neonatal hyperammonemic
      encephalopathy
fat-free mass (FFM)
fatigability
    easy f.
    increased f.
fatigue
    f. fracture
    f. syndrome
fat-induced infarct
fatty
    f. acid
    f. acid content
    f. acid oxidation (FAO)
    f. acid oxidation disorder
    f. acid profile
    f. liver
fava
    f. bean
    f. bean ingestion
favism
FAVS
  facioauriculovertebral spectrum
Fazio-Londe
    F.-L. atrophy
    F.-L. disease

FBEP
  Fort Bragg evaluation project
FBM
  fetal bone marrow
5-FC
  5-fluorocytosine
F/C
  facilitated communication
  fevers and chills
FCHL
  familial combined hyperlipidemia
FDA
  Food and Drug Administration
FDP
  factitious disorder by proxy
  fibrinogen degradation product
FE
  fetal erythroblastosis
    Slow FE
fear
    social-evaluative f.
feasible
feature
    coarse facial f.'s
    f. matching
    mood-congruent psychotic f.
    sharp facial f.'s
febrile
    f. baby
    f. convulsion
    f. nonhemolytic transfusion reaction
    f. paroxysm
    f. seizure
    f. status epilepticus
    f. UTI
fecal
    f. acidity
    f. bolus
    f. hoarding
    f. impaction
    f. microflora
    f. shedding
    f. shedding of virus
fecalith
    appendiceal f.
    calcified f.
fecaloma
feces
feed
    full enteral f.
    full nipple f.

F

NOTES

feed *(continued)*
    trophic f.
    tube f.
feedback
    tubuloglomerular f.
feeding
    bolus tube f.
    f. bradycardia
    coercive f.
    complex enteral f.
    continuous tube f.
    cup f.
    f. difficulty
    f. disturbance
    D-tube f.
    enteral f.
    finger f.
    gavage f.
    hydrolyzed f.
    f. intolerance
    intragastric f.
    intravenous f.
    liquid f.
    by mouth f.
    nasogastric drip f.
    nasogastric tube f.
    nipple f.
    p.o. f.
    poor f.
    f. problem
    transpyloric tube f.
    f. tube
Feer disease
feet *(See also* foot)
    dancing f.
    epidermolysis bullosa simplex of f.
FEF
    forced expiratory flow
FEL
    familial erythrophagocytic
    lymphohistiocytosis
felbamate
Felbatol
Feldene
felis
    Afipia f.
    Rickettsia f.
Felix-Weil reaction
felon drainage
Felty syndrome
female
    f. athlete triad (FAT)
    f. epispadias
    f. genital mutilation
    phenotypic f.
    f. pseudohermaphroditism
FemCap
feminine

feminization
    testicular f.
Femiron
femora
    biologically plastic f.
femoral
    f. antetorsion
    f. anteversion (FA)
    f. artery
    f. bulb
    f. deficiency
    f. epiphysis
    f. head dislocation
    f. hernia
    f. length
    f. neck
    f. osteosarcoma
    f. osteotomy
    f. retroversion
    f. testis
    f. torsion
femoral-tibial angle
femoris
    rectus f.
femur
    metaphyseal lesion of distal f.
    NSA of f.
FeNa
    fractional excretion of sodium
fencing position
Fenesin DM
fenestrated vascular endothelium
fenestration
    Fontan f.
    third ventricle f.
fenfluramine
fenoterol
fentanyl
    f. citrate
    droperidol and f.
    f. lollipop
    F. Oralet
    f. patch
    therapeutic transdermal f. (TTS-fentanyl)
Fentendo clip
Feosol
Feostat
FEP
    free erythrocyte protoporphyrin
Feratab
ferberizing
Ferber method
Fergon
Fer-In-Sol
Fer-Iron
fermentans
    Mycoplasma f.

fermentum
    Lactobacillus f.
Fero-Gradumet
Ferospace
Ferralet
Ferralyn Lanacaps
Ferra-TD
ferric
    f. chloride reaction
    f. chloride test
ferritin
    F. IRMA kit
    serum f.
Ferro-Sequels
ferrous
    f. chloride
    f. fumarate
    f. gluconate
    f. sulfate
Fertil-A-Chron
fertilization
    microassisted f.
Fertinex
fetal
    f. acidosis
    f. alcohol effect (FAE)
    f. alcohol effects syndrome
    f. alcohol syndrome (FAS)
    f. anemia
    f. arterial velocimetry
    f. ascites
    f. asphyxia
    f. bone marrow (FBM)
    f. brain sparing
    f. cerebral oxygenation
    f. cord blood
    f. crowding
    f. cytokinemia
    f. death
    f. demise
    f. Dilantin syndrome
    f. echocardiography
    f. endocarditis
    f. erythroblastosis (FE)
    f. estrogen
    f. fibronectin
    f. growth restriction (FGR)
    f. heart frequency (FHF)
    f. hemoglobin (HbF)
    f. histocompatibility antigen
    f. hydantoin syndrome (FHS)
    f. hydronephrosis

    f. hydrostatic pressure
    f. hyperinsulinism
    f. inflammatory response
    f. leptin concentration
    f. liver
    f. lobectomy
    f. loss
    f. lung fluid
    f. malnutrition
    f. monitor
    f. nonimmune hydrops
    f. nutritional deprivation syndrome
    f. organogenesis
    f. overgrowth syndrome
    f. parathyroid suppression
    f. presentation
    f. pulmonary circulation
    f. pulmonary vascular resistance
    f. red cell
    f. reentrant supraventricular tachycardia
    f. rubella syndrome
    f. scalp blood sampling
    f. scalp monitoring
    f. spleen
    f. stem cell transplantation
    f. surgery
    f. surgical procedure
    f. thrombopoietin concentration
    f. tracheal occlusion
    f. transfusion syndrome
    f. urine
    f. vascular conduit
    f. vasculitis
fetalis
    erythroblastosis f.
    hydrops f.
    immune hydrops f.
    nonimmune hydrops f. (NIHF)
fetal-placental circulation
fetid breath
fetofetal
    f. transfusion
    f. transfusion syndrome
fetomaternal
    f. alloimmune thrombocytopenia (FMAIT)
    f. bleed
    f. transfusion
    f. transfusion reaction
fetometry
    ultrasound f.

NOTES

F

fetopathy
    diabetic f. (DF)
fetoplacental
fetoprotein
    alpha f. (AFP)
    amniotic fluid alpha f. (AFAFP)
    maternal serum alpha f. (MSAFP)
fetor
    f. hepaticus
    f. oris
fetoscopy
fetus
    acardiac f.
    Campylobacter f.
    harlequin f.
    nonhydropic f.
    postmature f.
Feuerstein-Mimms syndrome
FEV
    familial exudative vitreoretinopathy
    forced expiratory volume
FEV$_1$
    forced expiratory volume in 1 second
fever
    acute rheumatic f. (ARF)
    African tick bite f.
    Argentine hemorrhagic f.
    arthritis of rheumatic f.
    artificial f.
    aseptic f.
    biphasic f.
    blackwater f.
    f. blister
    Bolivian hemorrhagic f.
    boutonneuse f.
    cat-scratch f.
    childbed f.
    f.'s and chills (F/C)
    Colorado tick f.
    Crimean-Congo hemorrhagic f.
    dehydration f.
    dengue f.
    dengue hemorrhagic f.
    diquotidian f.
    drug f.
    Ebola hemorrhagic f.
    enteric f.
    ephemeral f.
    epidemic relapsing f.
    eruptive f.
    familial Hibernian f.
    familial Mediterranean f. (FMF)
    Flinders Island spotted f.
    glandular f.
    Haverhill f.
    hay f.
    hemorrhagic f.
    inanition f.

    intermittent f.
    intrapartum maternal f.
    Katayama f.
    Korean hemorrhagic f.
    Lassa f.
    louse-borne f.
    Omsk hemorrhagic f.
    Oriental spotted f.
    Oroya f.
    paratyphoid f.
    parrot f.
    PediaCare F.
    Pel-Ebstein f.
    pharyngoconjunctival f.
    phlebotomus f.
    f. phobia
    Pontiac f.
    Q f.
    query f.
    quotidian f.
    rat-bite f.
    recrudescence of f.
    relapsing f.
    revised Jones criteria for diagnosis of acute rheumatic f.
    rheumatic f.
    Rift Valley f.
    Rocky Mountain spotted f. (RMSF)
    saddleback f.
    San Joaquin f.
    scarlet f.
    South African tick f.
    spirillary rat-bite f.
    spotted f.
    staphylococcal scarlet f.
    surgical scarlet f.
    tactile f.
    three-day f.
    tick f.
    tick-borne relapsing f.
    transitory f.
    trench f.
    tsutsugamushi f.
    typhoid f.
    f. of undetermined origin (FUO)
    undulant f.
    unexplained f.
    f. of unknown etiology
    f. of unknown origin (FUO)
    uveoparotid f.
    Valley f.
    yellow f.
    yellow f. 17D
Feverall
FEV$_1$/FVC ratio
fexofenadine
FF
    flatfoot

FFM
    fat-free mass
FFP
    fresh frozen plasma
FGF
    fibroblast growth factor
FGFR
    fibroblast growth factor receptor
FGR
    fetal growth restriction
FG syndrome
FHF
    fetal heart frequency
    fulminant hepatic failure
FHH
    familial hypercalcemia with hypocalciuria
    familial hypocalciuric hypercalcemia
FHLH
    familial hemophagocytic
     lymphohistiocytosis
FHM
    familial hemiplegic migraine
FHR
    familial hypophosphatemia
FH-RDC
    family history research diagnostic criteria
FHS
    fetal hydantoin syndrome
FHTG
    familial hypertriglyceridemia
fiber
    f. bone
    myoclonus, epilepsy, ragged
     red f.'s (MERRF)
    myoclonus epilepsy with ragged
     red f.'s (MERRF)
    parasympathetic f.
    Perdiem F.
    postsynaptic f.
    Purkinje f.
    ragged red f. (RRF)
    Rosenthal f.
Fiberall
    F. Powder
    F. Wafer
fiberglass jacket
fiberoptic
    f. bronchoscopy
    f. headband
    f. phototherapy (FO-PT)
FiberSource HN formula
fiber-type disproportion

fibril
    anchoring f.
fibrillary
    f. astrocytoma
    f. gliosis
    f. tangle
fibrillation
    atrial f.
    f. potential
fibrillatory wave
fibrin
    basal perivillous f.
    f. degradation product
    f. deposition
    f. split product (FSP)
    f. thrombus
fibrinogen
    f. deficiency
    f. degradation product (FDP)
    f. fibrin degradation product
    radiolabeled f.
    f. split product
fibrinoid necrosis
fibrinolytic therapy
fibrinopurulent exudate
fibrinous
    f. coalition
    f. exudate
    f. pericarditis
fibrin-stabilizing factor
fibroadenoma
    juvenile f.
fibroblast
    f. culture
    cultured skin f.
    genital skin f.
    f. growth factor (FGF)
    f. growth factor-10 null phenotype
    f. growth factor receptor (FGFR)
fibroblastic osteosarcoma
fibroblastoid synoviocyte
fibrocortical defect
fibrocystic disease
**fibrodysplasia ossificans progressiva
(FOP)**
fibroelastosis
    endocardial f. (EFE)
    prenatal f.
fibrogenesis
fibrolamellar hepatocellular carcinoma
fibroma
    benign nasopharyngeal f.

F

NOTES

fibroma *(continued)*
    chondromyxoid f.
    digital f.
    histiocytic f.
    infantile digital f.
    nasopharyngeal f.
    nonossifying f.
    ossifying f.
    periungual f.
    sternocleidomastoid f.
    subungual f.
fibromatosis
    infantile f.
fibromuscular dysplasia
fibromyalgia
    childhood f.
fibromyxoid stroma
fibronectin
    fetal f.
    f. receptor
fibroplasia
    retrolental f. (RLF)
fibropurulent
fibrosa
    osteitis f.
fibrosarcoma
    congenital f.
fibrosing
    f. colonopathy
    f. inflammation
    f. mediastinitis
fibrosis
    cavernosal f.
    cerebellar vermis hypoplasia, oligophrenia, congenital ataxia, coloboma, hepatic f. (COACH)
    chronic interstitial f.
    congenital hepatic f.
    cutaneous f.
    cystic f. (CF)
    endocardial f.
    endomyocardial f.
    endoneurial f.
    gum f.
    hepatic f.
    idiopathic diffuse interstitial f.
    interstitial f.
    meningeal f.
    neoplastic f.
    peribronchial f.
    peritoneal f.
    peritubular f.
    portal f.
    pulmonary interstitial f.
    retroperitoneal f.
    tubular interstitial f.
fibrosum
    pedunculated molluscum f.

fibrotic
fibrous
    f. anlage
    f. cortical defect
    f. dysplasia
    f. tissue
fibroxanthoma
fibula
    congenital longitudinal deficiency of f.
fibular
    f. hemimelia
    f. osteotomy
    f. shaft fracture
Fick principle
Ficoll-Hypaque centrifugation
Ficoll separation
fictitious epilepsy
fidget
fidgety
Fiedler myocarditis
field
    f. block
    central visual f.
    involved f. (IF)
    f. of view
    f. of vision
    visual f.
fifth-day fit
fifth disease
fight-and-flight response
fighter
    Flimm F.
FIGLU
    formiminoglutamic acid
figure
    matching familiar f.'s (MFF)
    f. 3 sign
figure-of-eight
    f.-o.-e. apparatus
    f.-o.-e. clavicle strap
    f.-o.-e. harness
    f.-o.-e. strapping
figure-of-four test
filament
    sarcomeric f.
filamentous hemagglutinin
filariasis
Filatov-Dukes disease
filgrastim
filiform
    f. papule
    f. plaque
    f. wart
Fillauer night splint
filling
    ventricular f.

film
> cross-table lateral f.
> scoliosis f.
> tear f.
> tibial f.
> upright chest f.

Filmtab
> Rondec F.

Filshie clip

filter
> HEPA f.
> high-efficiency particulate air f.
> leukocyte-depletion f.
> leukocyte-removal f.
> leukodepletion f.
> Millipore f.
> f. paper (FP)
> f. paper blood lead testing

filtration
> f. fraction
> glomerular f.
> hemodia, f.

filum terminale

fimbria, pl. **fimbriae**

fimbrial adhesion

Finapres
> F. blood pressure monitor
> F. device

find
> Child F.

finding
> congenital familial lymphedema
>   with ocular f.'s

fine
> f. inspiratory crackle
> f. lens opacity
> f. motor
> f. motor development
> f. motor domain
> f. motor index
> f. motor total DMQ

fine-needle aspiration biopsy (FNAB)

finger
> f. agnosia
> f. arterial blood pressure (FABP)
> baseball f.
> bent f.
> boutonniere f.
> coach's f.
> curved f.
> f. feeding
> f. gnosis

> index f.
> mallet f.
> middle f.
> f. opposition
> overriding f.
> f. plethysmography
> pollicization of index f.
> ring f.

fingernail

finger-nose-finger test

fingerprint

fingerspelling

finger-tapping test

fingertip number writing test

finger-to-nose test

Finnish
> congenital nephrotic syndrome, F.
>   (CNF)
> F. type

Finnish-type congenital nephrotic syndrome

FIO₂, FiO₂

FIO_2, FiO_2
> fraction of inspired oxygen

Fioricet With Codeine

fire
> f. setting
> St. Anthony's f.

fire-setting behavior

FIRM
> Family Inventory of Resources for
>   Management

firm hepatomegaly

first
> f. arch syndrome
> f. bicuspid
> f. disease
> f. heart sound
> f. Korotkoff sound
> f. permanent molar
> f. primary molar

first-degree
> f.-d. atrioventricular block
> f.-d. burn
> f.-d. hypospadias

first-generation cephalosporin

first-morning
> f.-m. gastric washing
> f.-m. urine collection

first-pass effect

FISCA
> Functional Impairment Scale for Children
>   and Adolescents

F

NOTES

FISH
    fluorescent in situ hybridization
        FISH analysis
fish
    f. oil
    f. poisoning
Fisher
    F. correlation
    F. exact test
fishmouth
    f. abnormality
    f. meatus
    f. vertebra
fish-shaped mouth
fish-tank granuloma
fissure
    abnormal palpebral f.
    anal f.
    f. in ano
    downslanting palpebral f.
    mild downslant to palpebral f.
    palpebral f.
    rectal f.
    f. of sternum
    superior vesical f.
    upslanting palpebral f.
fissured
    f. lips
    f. tongue
fissuring
fisting
fistula, pl. **fistulae, fistulas**
    anterior rectoperineal f.
    arterioportal f.
    arteriovenous f.
    branchial cleft f.
    bronchobiliary f.
    bronchoesophageal f.
    bronchopleural f.
    bronchopulmonary f. (BPF)
    carotid artery-cavernous sinus f.
    carotid-cavernous f.
    congenital perilymphatic f.
    coronary arteriovenous f.
    coronary artery f. (CAF)
    coronary-cameral f.
    enterocolic f.
    enterocutaneous f.
    enteroenteric f.
    enterovaginal f.
    enterovesical f.
    hepatic arteriovenous f.
    H-type tracheoesophageal f.
    H-type transesophageal f.
    intracranial arteriovenous f.
    intrahepatic arterioportal f.
    palatal f.

    perianal f.
    perilymphatic f. (PLF)
    perineal f.
    peripheral arteriovenous f.
    rectal-fourchette f.
    rectourethral f.
    sinus f.
    spit f.
    tracheocutaneous f.
    tracheoesophageal f. (TEF, TOF)
    transesophageal f.
    urethrocutaneous f.
    vesicocutaneous f.
    vestibular f.
fistulotomy
fistulous vascular communication
fit
    arrest/akinetic f.
    extensor f.
    fifth-day f.
    flexor f.
    mixed flexor/extensor f.
    uncinate f.
five-component vaccine
five-hop test
five-word sentence
fixation
    buttonpexy f.
    complement f.
    flexible intramedullary f.
    intramedullary rod f.
    f. nystagmus
    percutaneous pin f.
fixative
    Carnoy f.
fixator
    Ilizarov external f.
fixed
    f. erythema
    f. flexion deformity
    f. pulmonary hypertension
fixed-wing transport
FK-506
    tacrolimus
FK binding protein (FKBP)
FLACC
    face, legs, activity, cry, consolability
        FLACC scale
flaccid
    f. contracture
    f. lesion
    f. paralysis
    f. paraparesis
    f. paraplegia
    f. paresis
    f. quadriparesis

f. tetraplegia
f. tone
flaccidity
penile f.
flag sign
Flagyl Oral
flail
f. chest
f. mitral leaflet (FML)
FLAIR
fluid-attenuated inversion recovery
flaking
periungual f.
flame burn
flammeus
nevus f.
flange
tracheostomy tube f.
flank
bluish discoloration of f.
bulging f.
f. dullness
f. mass
f. pain
flap
butterfly f.
double-onlay preputial f.
Duckett transverse preputial
island f.
endoscopic incision with f.
foreskin f.
island f.
liver f.
onlay island f.
preputial f.
f. tracheostomy
vein f.
flare
cell and f.
Flarex
flaring
f. of alae nasi
alar f.
metaphyseal f.
nasal f.
flashback
flashlamp-pulsed
f.-p. dye laser
f.-p. laser therapy
Flashtab
flash VEP

flat
f. abdominal radiograph
f. acetabular roof
f. affect
f. back
f. facies
f. fontanelle
f. frontal bone
f. nasal bridge
f. nose
f. red-black telangiectasia
f. T wave
f. wart
flatfeet
flatfoot (FF)
calcaneovalgus f.
developmental f.
flexible f.
hypermobile f.
peroneal spastic f.
physiologic f.
flatness to percussion
flattened
f. occiput
f. T wave
f. villus
flatulence
Flatulex
flatus eructation
flavimaculatus
fundus f.
flavin adenine dinucleotide (FAD)
Flaviviridae
Flavobacterium
flavoprotein
electron transfer f. (ETF)
Flavorcee
flavus
Aspergillus f.
flecainide
Fleet
F. Babylax Rectal
F. Flavored Castor Oil
F. Laxative
F. Mineral Oil Enema
F. Phospho-Soda
F. Relief
fleeting paralysis
flesh-colored papule
Flexaphen
flexible
f. fiberoptic bronchoscopy

F

NOTES

flexible *(continued)*
    f. fiberoptic endoscopy
    f. flatfoot
    f. intramedullary fixation
    f. kyphosis
    f. pes planovalgus
    f. Teflon catheter
flexion
    f. contracture
    f. reflex
flexion-distraction injury
flexion-extension
flexneri
    Shigella f.
    Shigella f. 2b
flexor
    f. fit
    f. hallucis longus tendon
    f. tone
flexural
    f. area
    f. crease
flexure
    splenic f.
flight
    f. of color
    f. of ideas
Flimm Fighter
Flinders Island spotted fever
Flint Infant Security Scale
floating
    f. great toe
    f. thumb
floccosum
    Epidermophyton f.
flocculation
Flonase
floor
    decidual f.
    orbital f.
Flo-Pack
floppy
    f. infant
    f. infant syndrome
    f. larynx
flora
    skin f.
Florical
florid pulmonary valvular incompetence
Florinef Acetate
flottant
    pouce f.
flour
    carob seed f.
Flovent Rotadisk
flow
    aboral f.
    f. angulation

    bulk f.
    carotid blood f. (CaBF)
    cerebral blood f. (CBF)
    coaxial f.
    f. cytometric analysis
    f. cytometry
    f. cytometry analysis
    duct-dependent pulmonary blood f.
    excessive pulmonary arterial f.
    forced expiratory f. (FEF)
    hyperemic cerebral blood f.
    f. murmur
    f. pattern
    placental blood f.
    pulmonary arterial f.
    pulmonary blood f.
    renal blood f. (RBF)
    retrograde axoplasmic f.
    systemic f.
    to-and-fro f.
    torrential pulmonary f.
    umbilical venous f.
    f. velocity dynamic
    venous f.
    f. void
flow-volume
    f.-v. curve
    f.-v. loop
Floxin Otic
flu
    influenza
flucloxacillin
fluconazole
fluctuance
fluctuant
fluctuating tone
5-flucytosine
Fludara
fludarabine
fludrocortisone
fluency
    cross-modal f.
    verbal f.
fluid
    amniotic f. (AF)
    ascitic f.
    BAL f.
    f. bolus
    bronchoalveolar f.
    cerebrospinal f. (CSF)
    f. diet
    duodenal f.
    epithelial lining f. (ELF)
    extraaxial f.
    extracellular f. (ECF)
    extraluminal f.
    fetal lung f.
    hydrocele f.

interstitial f.
intracellular f. (ICF)
isotonic f.
meconium-stained amniotic f.
  (MSAF)
middle ear f. (MEF)
milky f.
negative balance of body f.
proteinaceous subretinal f.
pseudochylous milky f.
f. restriction
f. resuscitation
retained fetal lung f. (RFLF)
f. sift
subretinal f.
synovial f.
third spacing of f.
tracheobronchial aspirate f. (TAF)
ventricular f.
viscous f.
f. wave
xanthochromic f.
fluid-attenuated inversion recovery
  (FLAIR)
fluke
lung f.
flulike syndrome
Flumadine Oral
flumazenil
flumecinol
FluMist
flunisolide
flunitrazepam
fluocinolone
fluocinonide
Fluonid Topical
fluorangiography
fluorescein
f. fundus angiography
f. isothiocyanate
f. stain
fluorescence spot test
fluorescens
Pseudomonas f.
fluorescent
f. polarization immunoassay (FPIA)
f. in situ hybridization (FISH)
f. treponemal antibody
f. treponemal antibody absorption
  test (FTA-ABS)
f. treponemal antibody test (FTA)
fluoridation

fluoride
Listermint with F.
polyvinylidene f. (PVDF)
Fluorigard
Fluori-Methane
fluorine
Fluorinse
Fluoritab
FluoroCare Neutral
5-fluorocytosine (5-FC)
fluoroimmunoassay
time-resolved f.
fluorometholone (FML)
fluorophore-assisted carbohydrate
  electrophoresis (FACE)
Fluoroplex Topical
fluoroquinolone
fluoroscope
fluoroscopy
airway f.
image intensification f.
5-fluorouracil (5-FU)
fluoxetine hydrochloride
fluoxymesterone
fluphenazine
Flura
Flura-Drops
Flura-Loz
flurandrenolide
flurazepam
flurbiprofen
Flurobate
Fluro-Op
Flurosyn Topical
flush
ciliary f.
cyanotic f.
heparin lock f.
malar f.
f. method
flushing
episodic f.
flutamide
Flutex Topical
fluticasone
f. propionate
f. propionate dry powder inhaler
f. propionate inhalation powder
flutter
atrial f.
f. device

F

NOTES

flutter *(continued)*
   ocular f.
   f. wave
flutterlike oscillation
fluvoxamine
flux
   bile acid f.
Fluzone
fly
   tsetse f.
flying squirrel typhus
FM
   fat mass
FMAIT
   fetomaternal alloimmune
    thrombocytopenia
FMF
   familial Mediterranean fever
FML
   flail mitral leaflet
   fluorometholone
    FML Forte
FMLA
   Family Medical Leave Act
FMP
   family member presence
FMR1 gene
fMRI
   functional MRI
FMRP
   fragile X mental retardation protein
FNAB
   fine-needle aspiration biopsy
FNSD
   face-near-straight-down
FO
   foot orthosis
foam
   f. cell
   f. stability test (FST)
focal
   f. atrophy
   f. axonal swelling
   f. brainstem glioma
   f. cerebral edema
   f. convulsion
   f. cortical dysplasia
   f. dermal hypoplasia
   f. dermal hypoplasia syndrome
   f. dystonia
   f. epilepsy
   f. facial ectodermal dysplasia
   f. glomerulosclerosis
   f. hemorrhage
   f. heterotopia
   f. lupus nephritis
   f. motor seizure
   f. neurologic deficit

   f. nodular hyperplasia
   f. pontine leukoencephalopathy
   f. postviral encephalitis
   f. scleroderma
   f. segmental glomerular sclerosis
   f. and segmental glomerular
    sclerosis-hyalinosis
   f. segmental glomerulosclerosis
    (FSGS)
   f. segmental lupus
    glomerulonephritis
focus, pl. foci
   echogenic f.
   Simon f.
focused
   F. Assessment by Sonography for
    Trauma (FAST)
   f. computed tomography
Fogarty
   F. arterial embolectomy (FAE)
   F. arterial embolectomy catheter
   F. atrioseptostomy catheter
Fogo selvagem
Foille Medicated First Aid
folacin
folate
   f. antagonist
   f. folic acid deficiency
   f. level
fold
   absent antihelical f.
   antihelical f.
   aryepiglottic f.
   Dennie-Morgan f.
   epicanthal f.
   gluteal f.
   pleuroperitoneal f.
   skin f.
Foley
   F. catheter
   F. tube
folia
   cerebellar f.
foliaceus
   pemphigus f.
folic
   f. acid
   f. acid deficiency
folinic acid
follicle
   primordial f.
follicle-stimulating hormone (FSH)
follicular
   f. bronchitis
   f. conjunctivitis
   f. dermatitis
   f. desquamation
   f. duct

f. hyperplasia
f. ostium
f. plugging
f. tonsillitis
follicularis
keratosis f.
folliculitis
eosinophilic pustular f. (EPF)
fungal f.
hot tube f.
Staphylococcus epidermidis f.
follicurum
Demodex f.
Folling disease
follistatin
Follow-Up
Carnation F.-U.
F.-U. Soy formula
Follutein
Folvite
folyl polyglutamate
fomepizole
fomite
Fontan
F. fenestration
F. operation
F. principle
F. procedure
fontanelle, fontanel
anterior f.
bulging f.
depressed f.
false f.
flat f.
posterior f.
pulsatile f.
sunken anterior f.
fonticulus, pl. **fonticuli**
food
F. and Drug Administration (FDA)
f. foraging
f. impaction
f. poisoning
f. seeking
thermic effect of f. (TEF)
food-antigen sensitization
food-induced
f.-i. enterocolitis syndrome
f.-i. pulmonary hemosiderosis
foot (*See also* feet)
athlete's f.
calcaneovalgus f.

cavovarus f.
cavus f.
congenital rocker-bottom f.
f. drop
high arch f.
hyperdorsiflexed f.
Madura f.
narrow f.
f. orthosis (FO)
pronated f.
rocker-bottom f.
Z f.
footballer migraine
football-shaped vesicle
footplate
astrocyte f.
foot-progression angle (FPA)
FOP
fibrodysplasia ossificans progressiva
FO-PT
fiberoptic phototherapy
foraging
food f.
foramen, pl. **foramina**
bulboventricular f.
f. of Luschka
f. of Magendie
f. magnum
f. of Monro
f. of Morgagni
f. of Morgagni hernia
outlet foramina
f. ovale
f. ovale persistence
parietal foramina
f. primum
f. secundum
sternomastoid f.
stylomastoid f.
Forbes-Albright syndrome
force
acceleration-deceleration f.
oncotic f.
shearing f.
Starling f.
forced
f. bowel training
f. choice
f. expiratory flow (FEF)
f. expiratory volume (FEV)
f. expiratory volume in 1 second (FEV$_1$)

F

NOTES

forced *(continued)*
    f. grasp reflex
    f. vital capacity (FVC)
forced-air blanket
forceps
    alligator f.
    bayonet f.
    f. birth trauma
    Facit polyp f.
    McGill f.
Forchheimer spot
Fordyce
    F. disease
    F. granule
    F. spot
forefoot
    f. abduction
    f. adduction
    adductus of f.
    f. adductus
    f. valgus
    f. varus
foregut
    f. duplication
    f. malformation
forehead
    broad f.
foreign
    f. body
    f. body aspiration
forelock
    white f.
foreskin
    f. flap
    large f.
forest
    conidial f.
forking
    aqueductal f.
form
    balsa vaginal f.
    child behavior rating f. (CBRF)
    connatal f.
    lucite f.
    MedWatch f.
    parenchymatous f.
    phosphorylated drug f.
    racemose f.
    serous f.
    Teacher Rating F. (TRF)
    Teacher Report F. (TRF)
    Vineland Adaptive Behavior Scales, Survey F.
formaldehyde
formalin
formation
    alveolar saccule f.
    cataract f.

    chylomicron f.
    colostomy f.
    crescent f.
    Dandy-Walker f.
    kerion f.
    macular star f.
    neoaorta f.
    onion bulb f.
    perivascular pseudorosette f.
    pneumatocele f.
    popcorn f.
    primary lung bud f.
    recurrent hernia f.
    sequestrum f.
    terminal blush f.
Forma water-jacketed incubator
formazan dye
formboard
formic acid
formiminoglutamic acid (FIGLU)
formiminotransferase deficiency
formula
    Accupep f.
    Advance f.
    Advera f.
    AL 110 f.
    Alcare f.
    Alimentum f.
    Alitra Q f.
    Alprem f.
    Alsoy f.
    Aptamil f.
    Bazett f.
    BC Cold Powder Non-Drowsy F.
    Bebelac #1 f.
    Bebelac FL f.
    Bonamil with Iron f.
    Byrne and Euler f. (BEF)
    20-calorie f.
    24-calorie f.
    Carnation Follow-Up soy f.
    Carnation Good Start f.
    Carvajal f.
    Casec f.
    casein hydrolysate f.
    Compleat Modified f.
    Compleat Pediatric f.
    Comply f.
    Comtrex Cough F.
    Criticare H f.
    Deliver f.
    dextro f.
    diluted f.
    Dumex Infant F.
    Dutch Baby Food f.
    EleCare f.
    electrodialyzed whey f.
    EnfaCare f.

Enfamil 22, 24 f.
Enfamil AR f.
Enfamil Human Milk Fortifier f.
Enfamil Low Iron f.
Enfamil NextStep toddler f.
Enfamil Premature 20 F.
Enfamil with Iron f.
Ensure High Protein f.
Ensure Plus HN f.
Ensure with Fiber f.
Entera f.
Entralife HN30 f.
evaporated milk f.
FiberSource HN f.
Follow-Up Soy f.
fortified f.
Frisolac f.
Frisopep 1 f.
Frisosoy f.
full-strength f.
Gerber Baby F.
Gerber Soy f.
Glucerna f.
goat's milk f.
Good Start HA f.
Gorlin f.
half-strength f.
high-caloric density f.
high-calorie f.
high-fructose f.
high-glucose f.
hydrolysate f.
hydrolyzed premature f.
hypercaloric f.
Infalyte f.
Intralipid f.
Isocal HN f.
Isomil DE, DF, SF f.
Isomil with Iron f.
IsoSource 1.5 Cal f.
IsoSource HN f.
IsoSource Standard f.
I-Soyalac f.
Jevity Plus f.
Kaopectate Advanced F.
Kindercal f.
Lactofree f.
Lactogen FP f.
lactose-containing f.
lactose-free f.
Liposyn f.
Lonalac f.

Lytren f.
Magnacal f.
Mamex f.
MCT oil f.
Mepro f.
Meritene f.
Microlipid f.
milk-based f.
Milupa f.
Moducal f.
Mollifene Ear Wax Removing F.
Nan 2 f.
Nan 1 LP f.
Nativa f.
NeoCare f.
Neocate One+ f.
Nestac f.
Newtrition Isofiber f.
Newtrition Isotonic f.
NextStep Soy Toddler f.
nucleotide-fortified f.
Nursoy f.
Nutramigen f.
Nutrapak f.
Nutren 1.0, 1,5, 2.0 f.
Nutren Junior f.
Nutren Junior with Fiber f.
Nutricia f.
Osmolite HN Plus f.
Oxepa f.
Parent's Choice f.
Parkland f.
PC f.
Pedialyte f.
PediaSure with Fiber f.
Pelargon f.
Peptamen Jr. f.
Perative f.
PM-60/40 f.
Polycose liquid f.
Polycose powder f.
Portagen f.
powdered milk f.
predigested f.
Pregestimil f.
Prematil f.
preterm f.
prethickened f.
Profiber f.
Promil f.
Pro-Mix f.
ProMod f.

F

NOTES

formula *(continued)*
    Promote with Fiber f.
    Propac f.
    ProSobee f.
    protein hydrolysate f.
    Pulmocare f.
    quarter-strength f.
    rapid dissolution f. (RDF)
    RCF f.
    Rehydralyte f.
    Resource Just for Kids f.
    Resource Plus f.
    Resource Standard f.
    Ross carbohydrate-free f.
    S-14 f.
    S-26 f.
    S-29 f.
    S-44 f.
    semielemental casein hydrolysate f.
    Similac 24 f.
    Similac Natural Care f.
    Similac NeoCare f.
    Similac PM 60/40 Low Iron f.
    Similac Special Care with Iron 20 f.
    Similac Special Care with Iron 24 f.
    Sim SC-20 f.
    Sim SC-24 f.
    Sim SC-40 f.
    S-26 LBW f.
    S-M-A f.
    sodium-free f.
    Soyalac f.
    soy-based protein isolate f.
    Sumacal f.
    Suplena f.
    Sustacal Plus f.
    Sustagen f.
    Tolerex f.
    Traumacal f.
    Triaminic AM Decongestant F.
    TwoCal HN f.
    vegetable oil fat-based f.
    Vicks F. 44
    Vicks F. 44D
    Vicks F. 44 Pediatric F.
    Vital HN f.
    Vitaneed f.
    Vivonex Pediatric f.
    Vivonex Plus f.
    Vivonex Ten f.
    WHO f.
Forssman titer
Fortaz
Fort Bragg evaluation project (FBEP)
Forte
    Biotin F.

    FML F.
    Robinul F.
fortified formula
fortifier
    Enfamil Human Milk F.
    human milk f. (HMF)
    Similac Human Milk F. (SHMF)
Fortovase
fortuitum
    Mycobacterium f.
forward
    f. chaining
    f. tandem gait
forward-bending test
foscarnet
Foscavir
fosphenytoin
fossa
    iliac f.
    ischiorectal f.
    f. navicularis
    olecranon f.
    f. ovalis
    posterior cranial f.
foster care
Fostex
    F. Bar
    F. 10% BPO Gel
Fototar
foul-smelling discharge
foundation
    Children's Digestive Health and Nutrition F. (CDHNF)
    Epilepsy F.
    Medic-Alert F.
four-chamber view
fourchette
    posterior f.
four-point position
fourth heart sound
fowleri
    Naegleria f.
Fowler-Stephens orchiopexy
Fox-Fordyce disease
FP
    filter paper
    FP blood lead testing
FPA
    foot-progression angle
FPIA
    fluorescent polarization immunoassay
fraction
    cardiac ejection f.
    filtration f.
    increased globulin f.
    f. of inspired oxygen (FIO_2, FiO_2)
    intrapulmonary shunt f. (Qs/Qt)
    left ventricular ejection f. (LVEF)

regurgitant f.
shortening f.

fractional
f. excretion
f. excretion of sodium (FeNa)
f. shortening

fractionated sterotactic radiotherapy
fracture
avulsion f.
basal skull f.
bend f.
blowout f.
bowing f.
boxer's f.
bucket-handle pattern of f.
buckle f.
bursting f.
calcaneal f.
Chance f.
clavicular f.
coccygeal f.
comminuted f.
complete f.
compression f.
corner f.
cribriform f.
depressed skull f.
diaphyseal f.
diastatic f.
direct orbital floor f.
distal humeral physeal f.
fatigue f.
fibular shaft f.
Galeazzi f.
greenstick f.
growing f.
hangman's f.
hindfoot f.
indirect orbital floor f.
intertrochanteric f.
Jefferson f.
Jones stress f.
juvenile Tillaux f.
laryngeal f.
lateral condylar f.
Le Fort f.
linear skull f.
Maisonneuve f.
Malgaigne f.
mastoid bone f.
medial epicondylar f.
metacarpal f.

metaphyseal f.
Monteggia f.
NOE f.
nonaccidental spiral tibial f.
nonpathologic f.
olecranon f.
open f.
orbital blowout f.
orbital wall f.
osteochondral f.
patellar f.
pathologic f.
f. pattern
f. of penis
physeal f.
ping-pong f.
plastic deformation f.
plate f.
pond f.
proximal humeral stress f.
pubic ramus stress f.
radial head f.
radial neck f.
f. reduction
f. remodeling
Salter-Harris classification of f.
Salter-Harris epiphyseal f.
Salter-Harris f. (type I–V)
scapular f.
shear f.
sleeve f.
spiral tibial f.
sternal f.
stress f.
supracondylar humeral f.
talar dome f.
tibial shaft f.
tibial stress f.
f. of Tillaux
Tillaux f.
toddler's f.
torus f.
triplane f.
ulnar styloid f.
zygomaticomaxillary f.

fragile
medically f.
f. tissue
f. X
f. X analysis
f. X chromosome

NOTES

F

fragile *(continued)*
>   f. X mental retardation protein (FMRP)
>   f. X mental retardation syndrome
>   f. X type A (FRAXA)

fragilis
>   *Bacteroides f.*
>   *Dientamoeba f.*

fragilitas ossium
fragmentation of necrotic bone
fragmented poikilocyte
Franceschetti-Klein syndrome
Franceschetti syndrome
Francisella
>   *F. tularensis*
>   *F. tularensis holarctica*

Francois syndrome
Frank-Starling mechanism
Frank vaginal construction
Frantz tumor
Fraser syndrome
FRAST
>   Free Running Asthma Test

frataxin
fraternal twin
FRAXA
>   fragile X type A

Frazier suction tip
FRC
>   functional residual capacity

freckling
>   axillary f.
>   inguinal f.

free
>   f. beta test
>   Breathe F.
>   f. choline
>   f. erythrocyte protoporphyrin (FEP)
>   f. fatty acid
>   f. iron
>   f. peritoneal air
>   f. radial generation
>   f. radical
>   F. Running Asthma Test (FRAST)
>   f. testosterone
>   thimerosal f.
>   f. thyroxine
>   f. tracheal autograft
>   f. triiodothyronine

freebase cocaine
free-flow oxygen
Freeman-Sheldon syndrome
freeze-thaw-freeze
Freezone Solution
Freiberg
>   F. disease
>   F. infraction

Freidman splint

Frejka pillow splint
fremitus
>   diminished f.
>   tactile f.
>   vocal f.

frena
French-American-British (FAB)
>   F.-A.-B. classification

7-French sheath
frenulum, pl. frenula
>   lingual f.
>   multiple oral frenula

Frenzel maneuver
frequency
>   f. dysuria syndrome
>   fetal heart f. (FHF)
>   high f. (HF)
>   low f. (LF)
>   spectral edge f. (SEF)

fresh frozen plasma (FFP)
fresh-packed RBCs
freshwater near drowning
freundii
>   *Citrobacter f.*
>   *Clostridium f.*

friable
>   f. clot
>   f. hair

fricative
>   glottal f.

friction
>   f. dermatitis
>   f. diaper rash
>   f. rub

Friedman Splint brace
Friedreich ataxia
Fried syndrome
Frigiderm
Frisolac formula
Frisopep 1 formula
Frisosoy formula
frogleg
>   f. lateral radiograph
>   f. posture
>   f. view

Fröhlich syndrome
frontal
>   f. baldness
>   f. bossing
>   f. encephalocele
>   f. plagiocephaly
>   f. pole area

frontometaphyseal dysplasia
frontoparietal sensorimotor cortex
frontostriatal
frontotemporal cortical atrophy
frostbite
frothy discharge

frottage
frozen biopsy
fructokinase
fructose
f. galactokinase deficiency
f. intolerance
f. intolerance test
fructosemia
fructosuria
benign f.
essential f.
fruity breath odor
Fryn syndrome
FSD
face-straight-down
FSGS
focal segmental glomerulosclerosis
FSH
facioscapulohumeral
follicle-stimulating hormone
FSH muscular dystrophy
FSHD
facioscapulohumeral muscular dystrophy
FSP
familial spastic paraplegia
fibrin split product
FS Shampoo Topical
FST
foam stability test
FT
full term
FTA
fluorescent treponemal antibody test
FTA test
FTA-ABS
fluorescent treponemal antibody
absorption test
F test
FTS
face-to-side
FTT
failure to thrive
5-FU
5-fluorouracil
Fucidin
fucosidase
fucosidosis
fugax
amaurosis f.
Fukuyama
F. CMD

F. congenital muscular dystrophy
F. disease
full
f. enteral feed
f. inclusion
f. lepromatous leprosy
f. mutation
f. nipple feed
f. term (FT)
f. tuberculoid leprosy
fullness
periorbital f.
full-strength formula
full-syndrome eating disorder
full-term
f.-t. infant
f.-t. newborn
full-thickness burn
fulminans
acne f.
neonatal purpura f.
purpura f.
fulminant
f. disease
f. early-onset neonatal pneumonia
f. hepatic failure (FHF)
f. hepatitis
f. sepsis
f. ulcerative colitis
fulminating meningitis
Fulvicin
F. P/G
F. U/F
fumarate
ferrous f.
quetiapine f.
fumarylacetoacetate hydrolase (FAH)
Fumasorb
fume
Fumerin
fumigatus
Aspergillus f.
function
atrioventricular node f.
binocular f.
brain f.
brainstem f.
ciliary f.
executive f.
global assessment of f. (GAF)
impaired cognitive f.
mucociliary f.

F

NOTES

function *(continued)*
    peroneal nerve f.
    pituitary-adrenal f.
    pulmonary f.
    serotonergic f.
    sinus node f.
functional
    f. abdominal pain
    f. age
    f. alveolus
    f. asplenia
    F. Assessment Scale
    f. behavior
    f. brain imaging
    f. cloning
    f. constipation
    f. impairment
    F. Impairment Scale for Children
      and Adolescents (FISCA)
    F. Independence Measure for
      Children (WeeFIM)
    f. MRI (fMRI)
    f. murmur
    f. outlet obstruction
    f. posterior rhizotomy
    f. prepubertal castrate syndrome
    f. pulmonary atresia
    f. residual capacity (FRC)
functioning
    executive cognitive f. (ECF)
    global level of f. (GLOF)
fundal plication
Fundamentals-Preschool
    Clinical Evaluation of
      Language F.-P.
fundi *(pl. of* fundus)
fundic gland polyp
fundoplication
    laparoscopic f. (LF)
    Nissen f.
    Thal f.
fundus, pl. **fundi**
    f. flavimaculatus
    red f.
funduscopic
funduscopy
fungal
    f. ball
    f. endocarditis
    f. folliculitis
    f. id reaction
    f. meningitis
    f. oil
fungemia
fungi *(pl. of* fungus)
fungiform papilla

Fungizone
Fungoid
    F. Creme
    F. Tincture
    F. Topical Solution
fungoides
    mycosis f.
fungus, pl. **fungi**
    f. ball
    lipophilic f.
funisitis
funnel chest
FUO
    fever of undetermined origin
    fever of unknown origin
Furadantin
Furalan
Furan
Furanite
furazolidone
furfur
    Malassezia f.
furoate
    mometasone f.
furosemide
Furoxone
furrow
furrowing
    surface f.
furuncle
    staphylococcal f.
furunculosis
    staphylococcal f.
Fusarium
fused raphe
fusiform
    f. aneurysm
    f. dilation
    f. dilation of urethra
    f. nerve thickening
fusion
    anterior spinal f.
    calcaneonavicular f.
    joint f.
    labial f.
    labioscrotal f.
    spinal f.
    talocalcaneal f.
    thought action f.
fusobacteria
Fusobacterium necrophorum
fusospirillary gangrenous stomatitis
fusospirochetal gingivitis
FVC
    forced vital capacity

G

G protein
G syndrome

g

gram

GA

gestational age

GAA

gossypol acetic acid
GAA trinucleotide expansion

GABA

gamma-aminobutyric acid
gamma-aminobutyric acidemia
GABA transaminase deficiency

gabapentin

GABHS

group A beta-hemolytic streptococcus
GABHS pharyngitis

Gabitril

GAD

generalized anxiety disorder
glutamic acid decarboxylase

gadolinium

chelated g.

gadopentetate dimeglumine

GAF

global assessment of function

Gaffney joint

GAG

glycosaminoglycan

Gage sign

gag reflex

gain

absolute length g.
absolute weight g.
poor weight g.
weight g.

gait

antalgic g.
g. apraxia
g. ataxia
broad-based g.
circumduction g.
crouch g.
g. dysfunction
equinus g.
forward tandem g.
heel-toe g.
g. laboratory
nonreciprocal g.
outtoe g.
reciprocating g.
slapping storklike g.
teddy-bear g.
toe-in g.

toe-out g.
Trendelenburg g.
waddling g.
wide-based shuffling g.

galactitol

galactokinase deficiency

galactolipid

galactosamine

galactose

g. breath test
g. uridine diphosphate

galactose-free diet

galactosemia

hereditary g.
transferase deficient g.

galactose-1-phosphate

g.-1-p. uridyltransferase (GALT)
g.-1-p. uridyl transferase deficiency

galactosialidosis

galactosidase

ceramide trihexoside alpha g.

galactosuria

Galant reflex

Galarina

Galeazzi

G. fracture
G. fracture dislocation
G. sign

Galen

aneurysm of vein of G.
vein of G.

gallbladder

atretic g.
g. disease
duplication of g.
hydropic g.
g. resection
g. stasis

gallium

g. scan
g. scintography

gallium-67 scan

gallop

protodiastolic g.
g. rhythm
summation g.

gallstone

cholesterol g.
g. pancreatitis

GALT

galactose-1-phosphate uridyltransferase
gastrointestinal-associated lymphoid tissue
gut-associated lymphoid tissue

Gamastan

G

Gambian
    G. disease
    G. trypanosomiasis
gamble
    Procter and G. (P&G)
gamekeeper's thumb
gamete
    overmature g.
gametogenesis
Gamimune N
gamma
    g. globulin (GG)
    g. globulin replacement
    g. glutamyl transpeptidase
    interferon g. (IFN-gamma)
    g. interferon
    g. knife surgery
gamma-aminobutyric
    g.-a. acid (GABA)
    g.-a. acidemia (GABA)
    g.-a. acidemia transaminase
    deficiency
Gammagard S/D
**gamma-irradiated cellular products
    transfusion**
Gammar
Gammar-IV
Gammar-P IV
ganciclovir
ganglia (*pl. of* ganglion)
gangliocytoma
    dysplastic g.
ganglioglioma
ganglion, pl. **ganglia**
    basal g.
    g. cell
    gasserian g.
    herpes zoster of geniculate g.
    sympathetic g.
    volar g.
ganglioneuroblastoma
ganglioneuroma
ganglioneuromatosis
ganglionic differentiation
ganglioside
    g. degradation
    GM_2 g.
gangliosidosis
    GM_1 g.
    GM_2 g.
    juvenile GM_2 g.
    Sandhoff GM_2 g. (type I, II)
gangrene
    acute streptococcal g.
    gas g.
    Meleney synergistic g.
    streptococcal g.
    synergistic g.

gangrenosa
    ecthyma g.
    varicella g.
gangrenosum
    ecthyma g.
    pyoderma g.
gangrenous
    g. appendicitis
    g. stomatitis
GANT
    gastrointestinal autonomic nerve tumor
Gantanol
Gantrisin
gap
    anion g.
    g. junction
    osmotic g.
gape
    allergic g.
Garamycin
Gardner
    G. Expressive One-Word
        Vocabulary Test-Revised
    G. syndrome
Gardnerella vaginalis
Gardner-Wells tongs
gargoylism
garinii
    Borrelia g.
Garrodian inborn error
Gartner duct
gas
    arterial blood g. (ABG)
    g. bloat
    blood g.
    g. chromatography
    g. chromatography-mass
        spectrometry
    g. chromatography-mass
        spectroscopy (GC-MS)
    g. gangrene
    g. gangrene fasciitis
    intramural g.
    Mylanta G.
    partial pressure of carbon dioxide
        in arterial g. ($PaCO_2$)
    paucity of g.
GASA
    growth-adjusted sonographic age
gaseous distention
gasping respiration
gasseri
    Lactobacillus g.
gasserian ganglion
Gasser syndrome
gastric
    g. acid hypersecretion
    g. acid hyposecretion

g. atony
g. atrophy
g. balloon
g. dilation
g. duplication
g. dysmotility
g. inhibitory polypeptide (GIP)
g. irrigation
g. lavage
g. mobilization
g. mucosa
oral g. (OG)
g. perforation
g. peristaltic wave
g. pull-up
g. regurgitation
g. residual volume (GRV)
g. stapling
g. tonometry
g. volvulus
g. wash
g. washing
g. web

gastrinoma

gastritis
antral g.
infectious g.
lymphocytic g.
micronodular g.
nodular g.
peptic g.

gastrocnemius
g. aponeurosis
g. contracture
g. muscle

gastrocnemius-semimembranosus bursa

gastrocolic reflex

Gastrocrom

gastrocystoplasty

gastroduodenoscopy

gastroenteritis, pl. **gastroenteritides**
allergic eosinophilic g.
Campylobacter g.
eosinophilic g.
parasitic gastroenteritides
rotavirus g.
Salmonella g.

gastroenterologist

gastroenteropathy
allergic g.
eosinophilic g.

gastroepiploic artery (GEA)

gastroesophageal (GE)
g. angle of His
g. balloon tamponade
g. incompetence
g. junction
g. reflux (GER)
g. reflux disease (GERD)
g. reflux-reflex apnea recording

Gastrografin
G. enema
G. esophagram

gastrointestinal (GI)
g. anaphylaxis
g. atresia
g. autonomic nerve tumor (GANT)
g. decontamination
g. disorder
g. dysmotility
g. hemorrhage
g. loss
g. polyp
g. priming
g. reflux
g. syndrome
g. tract
g. tube
g. tuberculosis
upper g.

gastrointestinal-associated lymphoid tissue (GALT)

gastrojejunostomy

gastroparesis

gastropathy
AIDS g.
congestive g.
hypertrophic g.

gastrophrenic ligament

gastroschisis

Gastrosed

gastrostomy
g. button
EntriStar Skin Level Tube for g.
percutaneous endoscopic g. (PEG)
Stamm g.
g. tube
g. tube placement

gastrulating embryo

Gas-X

G

NOTES

gate-control hypothesis
gated blood pool scanning
gateway drug
Gaucher
    G. cell
    G. disease (type 1–3)
Gaucher-type histiocyte
21-gauge hypodermic needle
gaussian distribution
gauze
    iodoform g.
    Oxycel g.
    Vaseline-impregnated g.
gavage feeding
Gaviscon
gay
    g. bowel disease
    g., lesbian, bisexual (GLB)
    g., lesbian, bisexual youths
gaze
    conjugate upward g.
    downward g.
    eccentric g.
    g. palsy
    paralysis of conjugate upward g.
    upward g.
gaze-evoked nystagmus
gaze-paretic nystagmus
G-banded karyotype
GBM
    glomerular basement membrane
GBS
    group B streptococcus
    Guillain-Barré syndrome
    GBS meningitis
    GBS screening culture
    GBS (type Ia, Ib, Ic, II, III)
    GBS vaccine
GBV-C
    GB virus C
GB virus C (GBV-C)
GCDAS
    Gesell Child Development Age Scale
GC-MS
    gas chromatography-mass spectroscopy
GCS
    Glasgow Coma Scale
G-CSF
    granulocyte colony-stimulating factor
G-CSF-R
    granulocyte colony-stimulating factor
    receptor
GDNF
    glial cell line derived neurotrophic factor
GDS
    Gesell Developmental Scale
    Gordon diagnostic system

GE
    gastroesophageal
    genome equivalent
GEA
    gastroepiploic artery
    GEA graft
Gebauer ethyl chloride
gel
    ACTH g.
    Acthar g.
    Advanced Formula Oxy
      Sensitive G.
    amethocaine g.
    Ametop g.
    Aquatar g.
    Benzac AC G.
    Benzac W G.
    Del Aqua-5 G.
    Del Aqua-10 G.
    Desquam-E G.
    Desquam-X G.
    Differin g.
    Dryox G.
    Fostex 10% BPO G.
    H.P. Acthar G.
    Itch-X g.
    miconazole g.
    Orabase g.
    Perfectoderm G.
    RID g.
    Vergogel G.
gelastic convulsion
gelatin-encapsulated microbubble
gelatinosa
    substantia g.
Gelfoam
Gel-Kam
gelling
Gel-Tin
Gemella
    G. bergeriae
    G. haemolysans
    G. morbillorum
    G. sanguinis
gemeprost
Gemini red reflex
gemistocyte
Genabid
Genac
Genagesic
Genahist Oral
Genapap
Genasoft Plus
Genaspor
Genatap Elixir
Genatuss DM
Gencalc 600

gender
- g. assignment
- g. difference
- g. dysphoria syndrome
- g. identity disorder (GID)

gene
- adhalin g.
- allelic g.
- apoB g.
- autosomal g.
- Bruton/B-cell tyrosine kinase g.
- candidate g.
- cell interaction g.
- COL7A1 g.
- g. complex
- CTNS g.
- DAX1 g.
- derepressed g.
- DMD/BMD g.
- dominant g.
- Ewing sarcoma g.
- FMR1 g.
- glucose transporter g. 1 (GLUT1)
- glucose transporter g. 3 (GLUT3)
- H g.
- histocompatibility g.
- human jagged-1 g. (JAG1)
- immune response g.
- immune suppressor g.
- immunoglobulin g.
- imprinted g.
- Ir g.
- Is g.
- g. mutation
- PAX3 g.
- recessive g.
- recombinase activating g.
- SGLT1 g.
- sodium/glucose co-transporter g.
- SOX9 g.
- g. study
- g. therapy

GeneAmp PCR test
Genebs
Genentech
- G. biosynthetic human growth hormone
- G. growth chart

general
- g. anesthesia
- g. practitioner

- g. reading backwardness (GRB)
- g. triceps contracture

generalization
generalized
- g. albinism
- g. alopecia
- g. aminoaciduria
- g. anxiety disorder (GAD)
- g. atrophic benign epidermolysis bullosa
- g. bilaterally synchronous sharp-wave and slow-wave complexes
- g. convulsion
- g. dystonia
- g. elastolysis
- g. epileptogenic discharge
- g. erythroderma
- g. gray matter atrophy
- g. lipodystrophy
- g. obstructive overinflation
- g. phlebectasia
- g. pustular psoriasis
- g. slowing
- g. tetanus
- g. tonic-clonic seizure
- g. vigilance
- g. white matter atrophy

generation
- free radial g.

genetic
- g. counselor
- g. disorder
- g. evaluation
- g. heterogeneity
- g. isolated CD59 deficiency
- g. linkage analysis
- g. polymorphism
- reverse g.'s
- g. testing
- g. thrombophilia

geneticist
genetotrophic disease
genetous idiocy
Genex
geniculate
- g. herpes
- lateral g.

geniculostriate
genioglossus muscle
genital
- g. aphthous ulcer
- g. mucosa

NOTES

genital *(continued)*
  g. papule
  g. skin fibroblast
  g. ulceration
  g. wart
genitalia
  ambiguous external g.
  external male g.
genitalium
  Mycoplasma g.
genitofemoral nerve
genitogram
  g. with IVP
  g. without IVP
genitopalatocardiac syndrome
genitoplasty
genitourinary (GU)
  g. tract
Gen-K
genocide
genocopy
genodermatosis, pl. genodermatoses
genome equivalent (GE)
genomic imprinting
genomovar (I–VI)
Genoptic
Genotonorm
Genotropin Injection
genotype
genotypic assay
genotyping
  CYP21 g.
Genpril
Gentacidin
Gent-AK
gentamicin
  g. cream
  enteric g.
  prednisolone and g.
  g. sulfate
gentian violet
Gentran
Gentrasul
genu
  g. recurvatum
  g. valgum
  g. varum
  g. varum deformity
Gen-XENE
10-Genzagel
Geocillin
geographic tongue
geohelminth
geometric
  g. design test
  g. mean titer (GMT)
geophagia

georgiae
  Actinomyces g.
GER
  gastroesophageal reflux
Gerber
  G. Baby Formula
  G. Soy formula
GERD
  gastroesophageal reflux disease
Geref
gerencseriae
  Actinomyces g.
Geridium
germ
  g. cell
  g. cell mosaicism
  g. cell neoplasm
  g. cell teratoma
  g. cell testicular tumor
German measles
germ-cell depletion
germinal
  g. cell tumor
  g. center
  g. matrix
  g. matrix hemorrhage
  g. zone
germinolysis
  subependymal g.
germinoma
  pineal g.
Gerstmann-Sträussler-Scheinker
  syndrome
Gerstmann syndrome
Gesell
  G. Adaptive and Personal Behavior
    Domain, Revised
  G. Child Development Age Scale
    (GCDAS)
  G. Developmental Model
  G. Developmental Scale (GDS)
  G. Developmental Schedules
  G. Developmental Schedules,
    Revised
  G. Gross Motor Domain, Revised
  G. Infant Scale
  G. Preschool Test
  G. School Readiness Test
Gestalt closure
gestation
  multiple g.
  stuck twin g.
gestational
  g. age (GA)
  g. age assessment
  g. chickenpox
  g. diabetes

g. diabetes mellitus
g. trophoblastic disease
gestationis
herpes g.
gesturing
GFAP
glial fibrillary acidic protein
GFD
gluten-free diet
GFR
glomerular filtration rate
GG
gamma globulin
Lactobacillus GG
Lactobacillus rhamnosus strain GG
(L-GG)
GG-Cen
GH
growth hormone
GHBP
growth hormone-binding protein
GHD
growth hormone deficiency
GHI
growth hormone insensitivity
Ghon
G. complex
G. tubercle
ghost
peroxisomal g.
g. vessel
GHR
growth hormone receptor
GHRD
growth hormone receptor deficiency
GI
gastrointestinal
GI bleeding
GI tract venous malformation
Gianotti-Crosti syndrome
Gianotti disease
giant
g. axonal neuropathy
g. cell
g. cell arteritis
g. cell encephalitis
g. cell hepatitis
g. cell myocarditis
g. cell pneumonia
g. colon
g. congenital pigmented nevus
g. coronary artery aneurysm

g. hemangioma
g. metamyelocyte
g. neuroaxonal dystrophy
g. platelet alpha-granule
g. platelet granulation
Gianturco-Grifka vascular occlusion device
Giardia lamblia
giardiasis
gibbus
lumbar g.
Gibson-Coke method
Gibson murmur
GID
gender identity disorder
giddiness
Giemsa stain
GIFT
granulocyte immunofluorescence test
gigantism
cerebral g.
eunuchoid g.
exomphalos, macroglossia, g.
hyperpituitary g.
pituitary g.
gigantocellularis
nucleus reticularis g.
giggle incontinence
Gilbert
G. disease
G. syndrome
Gilbert-Dreyfus syndrome
Gilles
G. de la Tourette
G. de la Tourette syndrome
Gillespe-Numerof Burnout Inventory
Gillette joint
Gilmore Oral Reading Test (GORT)
gingiva
gingival
g. cyst
g. cyst of newborn
g. erythema
g. hyperplasia
g. lesion
g. overgrowth
gingivitis
acute necrotizing ulcerative g. (ANUG)
fusospirochetal g.
herpetic g.
necrotizing g.

NOTES

G

233

gingivitis *(continued)*
    necrotizing ulcerating g. (NUG)
    Vincent g.
gingivostomatitis
    herpetic g.
    primary herpetic g.
ginkgo biloba
ginseng
GIP
    gastric inhibitory polypeptide
girdle weakness
girl
    premenarchal g.
Gitelman
    G. disease
    G. syndrome
GITUP
    glanduloplasty and in situ tubularization
      of urethral plate
    GITUP procedure
glabella
glabellar response
glabrata
    Torulopsis g.
gladiatorum
    herpes g.
    tinea g.
gladioli
    Burkholderia g.
gland
    adrenal g.
    Bartholin g.
    Brunner g.
    endocrine g.
    hypoplastic parathyroid g.
    g. infection
    lacrimal g.
    late-onset congenital large
      ectopic g.
    meibomian g.
    Moll g.
    parathyroid g.
    parotid g.
    Philip g.
    pilosebaceous g.
    pituitary g.
    salivary g.
    sebaceous g.
    sublingual g.
    submaxillary g.
    sweat g.
    thymus g.
    thyroid g.
glanders
glandular
    g. disease
    g. disk

    g. fever
    g. tularemia
**glanduloplasty and in situ
  tubularization of urethral plate
  (GITUP)**
glans-cavernosal procedure
glans clitoris
glanular urethral meatus
Glanzmann
    G. disease
    G. syndrome
    G. thrombasthenia
Glasgow Coma Scale (GCS)
glass
    Polaroid g.'s
glatiramer acetate
glaucoma
    acute angle closure g.
    congenital g.
    infantile g.
    primary congenital g.
    traumatic g.
Glaucon
GLB
    gay, lesbian, bisexual
    GLB youths
Glenn
    G. anastomosis
    G. operation
    G. shunt
Glenn-Anderson technique
glenohumeral
    g. instability
    g. joint
glenoid dysplasia
glia
gliadin
glial
    g. cell line derived neurotrophic
      factor (GDNF)
    g. fibrillary acidic protein (GFAP)
glide consonant
gliding movement
**gli family zinc-finger transcriptional
  activators**
glioblastoma multiforme
glioma
    brainstem g.
    cervicomedullary brainstem g.
    chiasmal g.
    chiasmatic-hypothalamic g.
    cystic brainstem g.
    focal brainstem g.
    g. of optic nerve
    optic nerve g.
    optic pathway g.
    spinal cord g.
    tectal brainstem g.

gliosis
>aqueductal g.
>astrocytic g.
>compensatory g.
>fibrillary g.

gliotic reaction
Glisson capsule
glistening dot
global
>g. aphasia
>g. assessment of function (GAF)
>g. brain hypoxia
>g. brain swelling
>g. developmental delay
>g. glomerulosclerosis
>g. hypertonia
>g. hypoplasia
>g. level of functioning (GLOF)
>g. neurologic dysfunction
>g. seasonality score
>G. Severity Index of Brief Symptom Inventory (GSI-BSI)

globe
>g. cell anemia
>ruptured g.

globiformis
>*Arthobacter g.*

globin chain
globoid cell leukodystrophy
globoside
globule
>milk fat g. (MFG)

globulin
>antilymphocyte g.
>antithymocyte gamma g. (ATGAM, ATG)
>botulinum immune g.
>cortisol-binding g.
>cytomegalovirus immune g. (CMVIG)
>gamma g. (GG)
>hepatitis B immune g. (HBIG, H-BIG, HBIg)
>human immune g.
>human rabies immune g. (HRIG)
>immune g.
>intravenous gamma g. (IVGG)
>intravenous immune g. (IVIG, IVIg)
>lymphocyte immune g.
>purified gamma g.
>rabies immune g. (RIG)

regular immune g.
respiratory syncytial virus immune g. (RSVIG, RSV-IG)
Rho(D) immune g.
sex hormone-binding g. (SHBG)
specific immune g.
tetanus immune g.
thyroid-binding g. (TBG)
thyroxine-binding g. (TBG)
varicella-zoster immune g. (VZIG)

globus
>g. hystericus
>g. pallidus

GLOF
>global level of functioning

glomerular
>g. basement membrane (GBM)
>g. disorder
>g. filtration
>g. filtration rate (GFR)
>g. insufficiency
>g. proteinuria
>g. renal disease
>g. sclerosis
>g. sialoglycoprotein
>g. tuft

glomeruli (*pl. of* glomerulus)
glomerulocystic disease
glomerulonephritis
>acute g.
>acute postinfectious g. (APGN)
>acute poststreptococcal g. (APSGN)
>autoimmune g.
>chronic g.
>crescentic g.
>diffuse proliferative g.
>familial g.
>focal segmental lupus g.
>hemorrhagic cystitis g.
>hypocomplementemic g.
>idiopathic rapidly progressive g.
>immune complex-mediated g.
>membranoproliferative g. (MPGN)
>membranous g.
>mesangial proliferative g.
>mesangiocapillary g. (type I, II) (MPGN)
>necrotizing g.
>Pauci-immune g.
>postinfectious g.
>poststreptococcal g.

NOTES

glomerulonephritis *(continued)*
    proliferative g.
    rapidly progressive g.
glomerulopathy
glomerulosclerosis
    focal g.
    focal segmental g. (FSGS)
    global g.
glomerulotubular
glomerulus, pl. **glomeruli**
glomus tumor
GLORIA
    gold-labeled optical rapid immunoassay
glossa
glossitis
    benign migratory g.
    candidal g.
glossodynia
glossopalatine ankylosis syndrome
glossopharyngeal
glossoptosis
glottal
    g. fricative
    g. obstruction
glottic
    g. opening
    g. spasm
glottis
glove
    Mylar g.
    sheepskin g.
    g.'s and socks syndrome
glubionate
    calcium g.
glucagon
Glucerna formula
glucoamylase deficiency
glucocerebrosidase
    macrophage-targeted g.
glucocorticoid
    g. deficiency
    g. excess
    g. insufficiency
glucogenesis
glucoglycinuria
glucokinase
gluconate
    calcium g.
    chlorhexidine g.
    ferrous g.
    quinidine g.
gluconeogenesis
    hepatic g.
glucosamine
glucose
    g. challenge test
    g. concentration
    g. intolerance

    g. oxidase test tape
    g. plus insulin
    g. production rate (GPR)
    serum g.
    g. tolerance
    g. tolerance test (GTT)
    g. transporter (GLUT)
    g. transporter gene 1 (GLUT1)
    g. transporter gene 3 (GLUT3)
glucose-dependent insulinotropic peptide
glucose-galactose malabsorption
glucose-6-phosphate
    g.-6-p. dehydrogenase (G6PD)
    g.-6-p. dehydrogenase enzyme deficiency
glucosuria
glucuronidation
glucuronide
    isovaleryl g.
glucuronosyltransferse
glucuronyl
    g. transferase deficiency
    g. transferase inactivity
glue
    airplane g.
    g. ear
glue-sniffing neuropathy
Glukor
GLUT
    glucose transporter
GLUT1
    glucose transporter gene 1
GLUT3
    glucose transporter gene 3
glutamate formiminotransferase deficiency
glutamic
    g. acid
    g. acid decarboxylase (GAD)
    g. acid decarboxylase antibody
glutamic-oxalacetic
    serum g.-o.
glutamic-pyruvic transaminase
glutamine
glutamine-supplemented diet
glutamyltransferase
glutaric
    g. acidemia (type I, II)
    g. aciduria (type I, II)
    g. aciduria syndrome (type I, II)
glutathione
    g. peroxidase
    g. synthetase deficiency
glutathionemia
gluteal
    g. fold
    g. muscle

gluten
- g. allergy
- g. challenge
- g. enteropathy
- g. intolerance
- g. sensitivity

gluten-free diet (GFD)
gluten-induced enteropathy
gluten-sensitive enteropathy
glutethimide
gluteus
- g. maximus muscle
- g. medius muscle
- g. minimus muscle

Glyate
glycemic
- g. index
- g. index diet

glycerin suppository
glycerophosphorylcholine
glycine
- blood g.
- CSF g.

glycinuria
- familial g.

glycocorticoid
glycogen
- g. accumulation
- g. storage disease (type Ia, Ib, II–VII) (GSD)
- g. synthetase deficiency

glycogenesis
- hepatic g.
- g. (type I, II)

glycogenolysis
glycol
- ethylene g.
- polyethylene g.
- propylene g.

glycol-ADA
- polyethylene g.-ADA (PEG-ADA)

glycolic
- Aqua G.

glycolipid metabolism
glycolysis
glycopeptide-resistant enterococcus (GRE)
glycophorin
- g. C

glycoprotein
- g. degradation
- KL-6 mucinous g.

glycoproteinosis
glycopyrrolate
glycosaminoglycan (GAG)
- urinary g.

glycoside
- cardiac g.

glycosphingolipid
glycosuria
glycosuric diuresis
glycosylated hemoglobin (HgA$_{1c}$)
glycosylation
Glycotuss
Glycotuss-dM
Glylorin
Gly-Oxide Oral
Glytuss
GM$_2$
- GM$_2$ ganglioside
- GM$_2$ gangliosidosis

GM-CSF
- granulocyte-macrophage colony-stimulating factor

GMDS
- Griffiths Mental Developmental Scale

GM$_1$ gangliosidosis
GMT
- geometric mean titer

G-myticin
gnashing
Gnathostoma spinigerum
gnathostomiasis
gnosis
- finger g.

GNR
- gram-negative rod

GnRH
- gonadotropin-releasing hormone

goal
- annual g.

goat's milk formula
Go-Evac
goiter
- drug-induced neonatal g.

goitrogen ingestion
goitrous
- g. hypothyroidism
- g. hypothyroidism with deafness

gold
- g. salt
- g. sodium thiomalate

Goldberg syndrome

NOTES

G

Goldenhar
  G. microphthalmia syndrome
  G. oculoauricular vertebra
gold-labeled optical rapid immunoassay (GLORIA)
Goldmann perimeter visual field test
Goldstein disease
Golgi
  G. apparatus
  G. stain
Goltz
  G. focal dermal hypoplasia
  G. syndrome
Goltz-Gorlin syndrome
GoLYTELY
Gomco clamp
Gomori
  G. methenamine-silver stain
  G. trichrome reaction
  G. trichrome stain
gonad
  dysgenetic g.
  palpable g.
  streak g.
gonadal
  g. agenesis
  g. agenesis syndrome
  g. aplasia
  g. dysfunction
  g. dysgenesis
  g. dysplasia
  g. germ cell neoplasm
  g. mosaicism
  g. steroid
gonadarche
gonadectomy
gonadoblastoma
gonadometer
  Prader g.
gonadorelin
gonadotropic deficiency
gonadotropin
  beta-human chorionic g. (beta-hCG)
  chorionic g.
  human chorionic g. (hCG)
  human menopausal g. (hMG, HMG)
gonadotropin-releasing
  g.-r. factor (GRF)
  g.-r. hormone (GnRH, GRH)
Gonal-F
gondii
  Toxoplasma g.
Gonic
goniometer
goniometry
gonioscopy

gonococcal
  g. arthritis
  g. arthritis of newborn
  g. conjunctivitis
  g. infection
  g. ophthalmia neonatorum
  g. perihepatitis
  g. septicemia
  g. urethritis
gonococcus, pl. **gonococci**
  penicillinase-producing g.
gonorrhea
  g. culture
  disseminated g.
  pharyngeal g.
gonorrhoeae
  Neisseria g.
Goodell sign
Goodenough-Harris Drawing Test
Goodman syndrome
Goodpasture syndrome
Good Start HA formula
gooseflesh
gooseneck
  g. deformity
  g. deformity of left ventricular outflow tract
Gordofilm Liquid
Gordon
  G. diagnostic system (GDS)
  G. Distractibility Test
  G. reflex
  G. syndrome
Gorlin
  G. formula
  G. syndrome
GORT
  Gilmore Oral Reading Test
GORT-R
  Gray Oral Reading Test-Revised
gossypol acetic acid (GAA)
Gottron papule
gout
  familial juvenile g.
gouty arthritis
Gower
  G. maneuver
  G. sign
  G. sign C
Gower-1, -2 hemoglobin
gp41
  transmembrane glycoprotein gp41
gp120 viral protein
G6PD
  glucose-6-phosphate dehydrogenase
  G6PD deficiency
GPR
  glucose production rate

gracilis
    Campylobacter g.
    g. muscle
grade
    Roenigk g.
graded compression ultrasonography
Gradenigo syndrome
gradient
    A-a g.
    alveolar-arterial oxygen g.
    alveolar-arterial pressure g.
    arterial-alveolar g.
    arterial-ascitic fluid pH g.
    blood pressure g.
    diastolic g.
    echo Doppler g.
    hepatic venous wedge pressure g.
    peak instantaneous g.
    pressure g.
    sucrose g.
    transtubular potassium
      concentration g. (TTKG)
    tympanometric g.
grading
    Papile g.
graevenitzii
    Actinomyces g.
graft
    bone g.
    buccal mucosa g.
    donor venous g.
    GEA g.
    IILA-identical marrow g.
    oral mucous membrane g.
    skin g.
    T-cell-depleted g.
graft-versus-host disease (GVHD)
graft-versus-leukemia (GVL)
    graft-versus-leukemia reaction
Graham Steell murmur
gram (g)
    G. stain
grammar
gram-negative
    g.-n. acne
    g.-n. bacillus
    g.-n. endotoxic shock
    g.-n. endotoxin
    g.-n. endotoxin-induced shock
    g.-n. pneumonia
    g.-n. rod (GNR)
    g.-n. ventriculitis

gram-positive diplococcus
grand
    g. mal
    g. mal attack
    g. mal epilepsy
    g. mal seizure
grandiose delusion
grandiosity
granisetron
granular
    g. ependymitis
    g. osmiophilic deposit
granulation
    arachnoid g.
    giant platelet g.
    pacchionian g.
granule
    Birbeck g.
    g. deficiency
    E.E.S. G.'s
    Fordyce g.
    large lysosome-like g.
    Nissl g.
    Reilly g.
granulocyte
    g. colony-stimulating factor (G-CSF)
    g. colony-stimulating factor receptor (G-CSF-R)
    g. count
    g. immunofluorescence test (GIFT)
    g. transfusion
granulocyte-macrophage colony-stimulating factor (GM-CSF)
granulocytic
    g. ehrlichiosis
    g. leukemia
    g. leukocytosis
    g. sarcoma
granulocytopenia
granulocytopoiesis
granuloma, pl. **granulomata**
    g. annulare
    cholesterol g.
    coccidioidal g.
    disseminated g.
    eosinophilic g.
    fish-tank g.
    g. gluteal infantum
    g. gravidarum
    g. inguinale
    Majocchi g.

G

NOTES

granuloma *(continued)*
  mediastinal g.
  noncaseating sarcoidlike g.
  palisading g.
  progressive g.
  pyogenic g.
  rheumatoid g.
  swimming pool g.
  telangiectatic g.
  umbilical g.
granulomatis
  Calymmatobacterium g.
granulomatosis
  g. infantiseptica
  juvenile systemic g.
  larval g.
  Wegener g. (WG)
granulomatous
  g. amebic meningoencephalitis
  g. angiitis
  g. colitis
  g. disease
  g. lymphadenitis
  g. perivasculitis
  g. vasculitis
granuloplasty
granulopoiesis
  neutrophil g.
granulosa cell tumor
granulosa-theca cell tumor
granulosus
  Echinococcus g.
graphesthesia
grasp
  inferior pincer g.
  neat pincer g.
  palmar g.
  pincer g.
  radial digital g.
  radial palmar g.
  g. reflex
  toe g.
  ulnar palmar g.
grass
  perennial rye g.
  g. pollen
  timothy g.
Graves disease
gravida
gravidarum
  granuloma g.
  hyperemesis g.
gravis
  autoimmune myasthenia g.
  congenital myasthenia g.
  g. Ehlers-Danlos syndrome
  myasthenia g.

neonatal myasthenia g.
  transient neonatal myasthenia g.
gray
  g. baby
  g. baby syndrome
  g. matter
  g. matter heterotopia
  G. Oral Reading Test
  G. Oral Reading Test-Revised
    (GORT-R)
  g. platelet syndrome
  g. scale
gray-white junction
GRB
  general reading backwardness
GRE
  glycopeptide-resistant enterococcus
greasy stool
great
  G. Smoky Mountains Study of
    Youth (GSMS)
  g. toe
  g. vessel
  g. vessel of thorax
greater
  g. saphenous vein
  g. saphenous vein cutdown
  g. trochanter
  g. trochanteric bursa
green
  g. clay
  indocyanine g.
  g. light
Greenspan approach
greenstick
  g. fracture
  g. injury
Greig
  G. cephalopolysyndactyly syndrome
grepafloxacin
Grey scale imaging
Grey-Turner sign
GRF
  gonadotropin-releasing factor
GRH
  gonadotropin-releasing hormone
gridiron incision
grief
  anticipatory g.
Grieg cephalopolysyndactyly anomaly
grieving process
Griffith General Quotient
Griffiths
  G. Mental Developmental Scale
    (GMDS)
  G. Scale of Mental Development
Grifulvin V
grimacing

grip
    milkmaid's g.
    g. myotonia
grippotyphosa
    Leptospira g.
Grisactin Ultra
Griscelli syndrome
Grisel syndrome
griseofulvin microcrystalline
griseus
    Streptomyces g.
Gris-PEG
groin ringworm
groove
    Harrison g.
    intercondylar g.
    transverse nail g.
    vomerian g.
Groover Pegboard
gross
    g. motor
    g. motor development
    g. motor domain
    g. motor function measure
    g. motor index
    g. motor total DMQ
grossly bloody stool
ground-glass osteopenia
ground itch
group
    g. A beta-hemolytic streptococcal
    g. A beta-hemolytic streptococcal
      infection
    g. A beta-hemolytic streptococcus
      (GABHS)
    AIDS Clinical Trials G. (ACTG)
    g. A streptococcal impetigo
    blood g.
    g. B streptococcal infection
    g. B streptococcal meningitis
    g. B streptococcal pneumonia
    g. B streptococcal sepsis
    g. B streptococcus (GBS)
    g. B streptococcus disease
    Children's Cancer G. (CCG)
    Children's Cancer Study G.
      (CCSG)
    g. C pharyngitis
    g. C streptococcus
    g. G streptococcus
    Lucarelli risk g.

    National Wilms Tumor Study G.
      (NWTS)
    Pediatric Oncology G.
    polyarteritis nodosa g.
    g. problem-solving therapy
    spotted fever g.
    streptococcal g.
    typhus g.
grouping
    clinical g.
growing fracture
growth
    g. arrest
    g. control factor
    g. curve
    g. and deafness
    g. delay
    g. disturbance
    epiphyseal g.
    g. epoch
    g. failure
    g. hormone (GH)
    g. hormone-binding protein (GHBP)
    g. hormone deficiency (GHD)
    g. hormone immunoassay
    g. hormone insensitivity (GHI)
    g. hormone receptor (GHR)
    g. hormone receptor deficiency
      (GHRD)
    g. hormone-releasing hormone
    g. hormone stimulation test
    g. index
    linear g.
    g. parameter
    g. plate
    poor linear g.
    g. rate
    g. retardation
    slow g.
    g. spurt
    g. stunting
    g. velocity (GV)
    g. zone
growth-adjusted sonographic age
  (GASA)
growth-remaining method
Gruelich and Pyle atlas
grunting
    expiratory g.
    g. respiration
GRV
    gastric residual volume

G

NOTES

GSD
    glycogen storage disease (type Ia, Ib, II–VII)
GSH pathway disorder
GSI-BSI
    Global Severity Index of Brief Symptom Inventory
GSMS
    Great Smoky Mountains Study of Youth
GTP
    guanosine triphosphate
GTT
    glucose tolerance test
GU
    genitourinary
guaiac-negative stool
guaiac-positive stool
guaiac test
guaifenesin
    g. and codeine
    g. and dextromethorphan
    g., phenylpropanolamine, phenylephrine (ULR)
Guaifenex
    G. DM
    G. LA
Guaituss AC
guanfacine hydrochloride
guanidine salt
guanidinoacetate
guanine
    9-13-dihydroxypropoxymethyl g.
    g. nucleotide
guanosine
    g. triphosphate (GTP)
    g. triphosphate cyclohydrolase
guard
    high g.
    mouth g.
guardian ad litem
gubernacular attachment
gubernaculum
GuiaCough Expectorant
Guiatex
Guiatuss DM
Guiatussin With Codeine
guidance
    hand-over-hand g.
    g. officer
    pictorial anticipatory g. (PAG)
guidewire
Guillain-Barré-Landry syndrome
Guillain-Barré syndrome (GBS)
guilliermondi
    Candida g.
guilt
    survivor g.
guinea worm infection

gum
    g. arabic rehydration solution
    bean g.
    g. bleeding
    carob g.
    g. fibrosis
    g. hyperplasia
gumma, pl. **gummata**
    pituitary gland g.
    tuberculous g.
gum-tooth interface
gunstock deformity
Günther disease
gurgling
gustatory
gut
    g. motility
    g. rest
    g. tonometry
    torsion of g.
    g. vasculitis
gut-associated lymphoid tissue (GALT)
Guthrie
    bacterial inhibition assay method of G.
    G. count
    G. test
guttate psoriasis
GV
    growth velocity
GVHD
    graft-versus-host disease
GVL
    graft-versus-leukemia
    GVL reaction
G-well
gym
    jungle g.
gymnastics
gymnast's wrist
gynecoid fat distribution pattern
gynecomastia
    benign transient g.
    drug-induced g.
    involutional g.
    neonatal g.
    pathological g.
    physiological g.
    pubertal g.
Gynecort Topical
Gyne-Lotrimin Vaginal
Gynogen L.A. 20
gyral
    g. abnormality
    g. anomaly
    g. atrophy
    g. pattern

gyrata
    cutis verticis g.
gyrate atrophy
Gyrocaps
    Slo-bid G.
    Slo-Phyllin G.
gyrus, pl. **gyri**

    cingulate g.
    mushroom g.
    orbitofrontal gyri

NOTES

G

H
 H factor
 H gene
 H and Lewis blood group activity
 H protein
H₂
 histamine 2
H-7000 electron microscope
HA
 hyperalimentation
Haab stria
HAART
 highly active antiretroviral therapy
habit
 h. cough
 mentalis h.
 h. tic deformity
habitual
 h. shoulder dislocation
 h. shoulder subluxation
 h. snoring
habituation
habitus
 body h.
 craniosynostosis-marfanoid h.
 cushingoid body h.
 eunuchoid h.
HACEK
 Haemophilus aphrophilus, Actinobacillus
 actinomycetemcomitans,
 Cardiobacterium hominis, Eikenella
 corrodens, Kingella kingae
 HACEK coccobacillus
haematobium
 Schistosoma h.
haem iron
haemolysans
 Gemella h.
haemolyticum
 Arcanobacterium h.
 Corynebacterium h.
Haemophilus
 H. aphrophilus
 H. aphrophilus, Actinobacillus
 actinomycetemcomitans,
 Cardiobacterium hominis,
 Eikenella corrodens, Kingella
 kingae (HACEK)
 H. ducreyi
 H. influenzae
 H. influenzae cellulitis
 H. influenzae meningitis

H. influenzae type b (Hib)
H. influenzae type b conjugate
 vaccine
H. influenzae type b immunization
Hageman factor
hair
 axillary h.
 bamboo h.
 brittle h.
 h. bulb incubation test
 h. cotinine analysis
 exclamation-mark h.
 friable h.
 lanugo h.
 lumbosacral tuft of h.
 Menkes kinky h.
 h. patch
 h. pulling
 sparse h.
 h. spray
 spun glass h.
 h. tourniquet
 h. tourniquet injury
 tuft of h.
 twisted h.
 vellus h.
 h. whorl
 wispy h.
HAIR-AN
 hirsutism, androgen excess, insulin
 resistance, acanthosis nigricans
 HAIR-AN syndrome
hairlike tumor
hairline
 low occipital h.
hair-on-end appearance
hairy
 h. leukoplakia
 h. patch
 h. tongue
Hakim syndrome
halcinonide
Halcion
Haldol Decanoate
Haley's M-O
half-desmosome
**half-Fourier acquisition single-shot turbo
 spin-echo (HASTE)**
half-kneeling position
half-life
Halfprin

H

half-strength formula
halitosis
Haller cell
Hallermann-Streiff syndrome
Hallervorden-Spatz
    H.-S. disease
    H.-S. syndrome
Hallopeau-Siemens syndrome
Hall-Pallister syndrome
hallucal
hallucination
    hypnagogic h.
    olfactory h.
    visual h.
    visual phobic h.
hallucinogen
hallucis
    spastic abductor h.
hallux
    purple h.
    h. rigidus
    h. valgus
halo
    h. effect
    erythematous h.
    h. nevus
    H. Sleep System
    h. test
    h. traction
halobetasol
halofantrine
Halog
halogen
    h. acne
    h. lamp
    h. spotlight phototherapy
halogenated hydrocarbon
haloperidol
haloprogin
Halotestin
Halotex
halothane
Halotussin DM
Haltia-Santavuori neural ceroid
  lipofuscinosis
Haltran
HAM
    HTLV-I associated myelopathy
    human T-cell lymphotrophic virus type I
    associated myelopathy
hamartin
hamartoma
    iris h.
    mesenchymal h.
    smooth muscle h.
hamartomatous
    h. malformation
    h. mass

HAMD
    Hamilton Depression Scale
Ham F10 media
Hamilton Depression Scale (HAMD)
Hamman-Rich syndrome
hammer
Hammersmith
    hemoglobin H.
hammertoe
hammock
hamstring
    lengthening of h.
    h. lengthening
HAM/TSP
    HTLV-I associated myelopathy/tropical
    spastic paraparesis
hand
    choreic h.
    cleft h.
    dominant h.
    epidermolysis bullosa simplex
     of h.'s
    mechanic's h.
    milkmaid's h.
    narrow h.
    h. preference
    h. wringing
hand-bagging
handbook
    Harriet Lane H.
hand-eye coordination
hand-foot-and-mouth disease (HFMD)
hand-foot-genital syndrome
hand-foot-mouth syndrome
hand-foot-uterus syndrome
handheld flutter device
handicap
    mental h.
handle
    laryngoscope h.
handling
hand-over-hand guidance
Hand-Schüller-Christian
    H.-S.-C. disease
    H.-S.-C. syndrome
hands-feet position
hand-to-mouth movement
handwashing
hand-wringing movement
hand-wrist bone age
hangman's fracture
hangover
Hanhart syndrome
Hanks balanced salt solution (HBSS)
Hansel stain
Hantaan virus
hantavirus
    h. antigen**

h. cardiopulmonary syndrome (HCPS)
h. immunoglobulin M antibody
h. pulmonary syndrome

HAPE
high-altitude pulmonary edema
haploid cell
haploidentical bone marrow transplant
haploinsufficiency
haplotype relative risk (HRR)
happy
h. puppet syndrome
h. wheezer
hapten
hapten-antibody
hypersensitive h.-a.
haptoglobin
harassing cough
hard hepatomegaly
harelip
harlequin
h. color change
h. fetus
harmony
harness
figure-of-eight h.
Kicker Pavlik h.
Pavlik h.
Wheaton Pavlik h.
HARP
hypobetalipoproteinemia, acanthocytosis, retinitis pigmentosa, and pallidal degeneration
HARP syndrome
Harpenden stadiometer
Harriet Lane Handbook
Harrington rod
Harris
H. growth arrest line
H. view
Harrison
H. groove
H. sulcus
harsh pansystolic murmur
Harter self-esteem questionnaire
Hartnup
H. defect
H. disease
H. disorder
HAS
hospitalized attempted suicide
Hashimoto thyroiditis

hashish
Hassall corpuscle
HASTE
half-Fourier acquisition single-shot turbo spin-echo
HAstV-1
human astrovirus type 1
hat
silver thermal h.
thermal h.
hatchet face appearance
Hausman test
HAV
hepatitis A vaccine
hepatitis A virus
Haverhill fever
haversian system
Havrix vaccine
Hawaii
H. agent
H. Early Learning Profile (HELP)
hawkinsinuria
Haw River syndrome
hay fever
hazard
Cox proportional h.
Weibull h.
haze
corneal h.
HB
hepatitis B
Recombivax IIB
HB vaccine
Hb, hgb
hemoglobin
Hb E beta-thalassemia
HBcAb
hepatitis B core antibody
HBeAb
hepatitis B early antibody
HbF
fetal hemoglobin
HBIG, H-BIG, HBIg
hepatitis B immune globulin
HBIR
Hering-Breuer inflation reflex
HBL
hepatoblastoma
H₂ blocker
HBLP
hyperbetalipoproteinemia

NOTES

H

HbOC
hepatitis B oligosaccharide-CRM197 vaccine

HBQ
human health and behavior questionnaire

HBs
hepatitis B surface

HBsAb
hepatitis B surface antibody

HBsAg
hepatitis B surface antigen

HBSS
Hanks balanced salt solution

HbSS
homozygosity for hemoglobin S

HBV
hepatitis B virus
HBV vaccine

HC
head circumference
Bancap HC

HCC
hepatocellular carcinoma

H(c)ELISA
hemagglutinin enzyme-linked immunosorbent assay

hCG
human chorionic gonadotropin

HCII
heparin cofactor II
HCII coagulation inhibitor

HCl
hydrochloride

HCO₃
bicarbonate

HCP
hereditary coproporphyria

HCPS
hantavirus cardiopulmonary syndrome

HCRM
home cardiorespiratory monitor

HCS
holocarboxylase synthetase
HCS deficiency

hct
hematocrit

HCTZ
hydrochlorothiazide

HCV
hepatitis C virus

HCW
healthcare worker

HD
Huntington disease

HDCV
human diploid cell rabies vaccine

HDE
higher-dose therapy with epinephrine

HDL
high-density lipoprotein

HDN
hemorrhagic disease of newborn

HDS
hematuria-dysuria syndrome

HDV
hepatitis D virus

HE
hepatic encephalopathy
hereditary elliptocytosis
spherocytic HE

H&E
hematoxylin and eosin
H&E stain

head
h. banding enuresis
h. banging
h. bobbing
h. box
h. circumference (HC)
h. control
cracked-pot h.
cupping of optic nerve h.
h. drop
h. growth velocity
h. lag
h. louse
malformed radial h.
h. positioner
h. righting
h. size
H. Start
h. tilt
h. trauma
h. ultrasound
zygomatic h.

headache
acute h.
chronic h.
classic migraine h.
cluster h.
common migraine h.
complicated migraine h.
h. diary
migraine h.
migraine-type h.
migrainous h.
nonmigrainous h.
postlumbar puncture h.
primary h.
recurrent h.
secondary h.
sleep-related h.
vascular h.

headband
fiberoptic h.

imaging h.
plagiocephaly h.

head-righting
lateral h.-r.

head-sparing intrauterine growth retardation

head-up tilt (HUT)

healing
energy h.

health
mental h.
National Institute of Mental H. (NIMH)
National Institutes of H. (NIH)
pediatric public h.
H. Scan Assess Plus peak flow meter
H. Utilities Index Mark 2 (HUIZ)
World Association for Infant Mental H.

healthcare
h. worker (HCW)

health-related
h.-r. quality-of-life (HRQOL)
h.-r. quality-of-life assessment
h.-r. quality-of-life questionnaire

hearing
h. aid
h. loss
residual h.

heart
air filled h.
h. block
boot-shaped h.
h. defect
h. defect syndrome
h. disease
h. failure
hole in h.
Holmes h.
hypoplastic left h.
h. lesion
h. massage
h. murmur
h. rate (HR)
h. rate power spectral analysis (HRSA)
h. rate variability (HRV)
h. shadow
h. sound
h. transplant

h. transplantation
upstairs-downstairs h.

heart-hand syndrome

heat
prickly h.

heater probe thermal contact

heatstroke

Heat-Treated
Profilnine H.-T.

heave
apical h.

heavy metal poisoning

hebdomadis

hebephrenia

hebephrenic silliness

hebetic

hedgehog
Sonic h.

heel
h. cord
h. cord lengthening
h. cup
h. lance (HL)
h. pain
h. stick
h. strike
Thomas h.
h. valgus

heel-cord contracture

heel-shin test

heel-stick
h.-s. hematocrit
h.-s. procedure

heel-toe gait

heel-to-shin test

Heerfordt syndrome

Hegar sign

Hegman procedure

heidelberg
Salmonella h.

height
minimal acceptable h. (MAH)
sitting h. (SH)
h. velocity (HV)
h. velocity z-score

heilmannii
Helicobacter h.

Heimlich
H. maneuver
H. valve

Heineke-Mikulicz pyloroplasty

Heiner syndrome

NOTES

H

249

Heinz body
Hektoen agar
helical scan
helices (*pl. of* helix)
Helicobacter
    H. *heilmannii*
    H. *pylori*
heliotrope
    h. eyelid
    h. pattern
    h. rash
heliotropic
    h. discoloration
    h. erythema
heliox
    helium and oxygen
helium and oxygen (heliox)
helix, pl. **helices**
Heller
    H. dementia
    H. myotomy
Heller-Nissen operation
HELLP
    hemolysis, elevated liver enzymes, low
      platelet count
      HELLP syndrome
helmet
    cranial molding h.
    plagiocephaly h.
helmet-molding therapy
helminth
helminthic disease
HELP
    Hawaii Early Learning Profile
helper
    T h.
    h. T cell
helplessness
hemagglutination
    indirect h. (IHA)
    h. inhibition (HI)
    h. inhibition antibody (HIA)
    h. test
hemagglutinin
    h. enzyme-linked immunosorbent
      assay (H(c)ELISA)
    filamentous h.
hemangiectatic hypertrophy
hemangioblastoma
    cerebellar h.
hemangioendothelioma
    kaposiform h.
hemangioma, pl. **hemangiomata**
    bone h.
    capillary h.
    cardiac h.
    cavernous h.
    cryptic h.

    cutaneous h.
    giant h.
    hepatic h.
    infantile h.
    Kaposi-like form of infantile h.
    lobular capillary h.
    macular h.
    proliferating h.
    strawberry h.
hemangiomatosis
    diffuse neonatal h.
    disseminated h.
    pulmonary h.
hemangiopericytoma
    infantile h.
hemapoiesis
hemapoietic
hemarthrosis
    acute h.
hematemesis
    coffee-ground h.
Hematest test
hematobilia
hematochezia
hematocolpometra
hematocolpos
hematocrit (hct)
    automated h.
    heel-stick h.
    spun h.
hematogenous
    h. infection
    h. metastasis
    h. osteomyelitis
    h. primary tuberculosis
    h. seeding
    h. septic arthritis
hematology
hematoma
    acute subdural h.
    adrenal h.
    auricular h.
    epidural h.
    extradural h.
    interhemispheric subdural h.
    intracerebral h.
    intracranial h.
    intraparenchymal h.
    retroplacental h.
    secondary h.
    subcapsular hepatic h.
    subdural h. (SDH)
    subgaleal h. (SGH)
    sublingual h.
    submental h.
    testicular h.
    traumatic h.
hematometra

hematometrocolpos
hematometry
hematophagocytic syndrome
hematopoiesis
    extramedullary h.
hematopoietic
    h. differentiation
    h. stem cell transplantation
    h. syndrome
    h. system
hematosalpinx
hematotympanum
hematoxylin
    h. and eosin (H&E)
    h. and eosin stain
hematuria
    benign recurrent h.
    familial recurrent h.
    macroscopic h.
    painless h.
    recurrent gross h. (RGH)
hematuria-dysuria syndrome (HDS)
heme
    h. oxygenase (HO)
    h. oxygenase inhibitor
heme-negative stool
heme-positive stool
Hemet Rectal
hemianopia, hemianopsia
    bitemporal h.
    homonymous h.
    transient h.
hemiatrophy
    progressive facial h.
hemiatrophy-hemihypertrophy
hemiblock
    left anterior h.
hemichorea
hemicord
hemicortectomy
hemicrania
    migraine sine h.
hemidesmosome
hemidystonia
hemiepiphysiodesis
hemifacial
    h. microsomia
    h. spasm
hemi-Fontan procedure
hemifusion
hemigland thyroid
hemihyperplasia

hemihypertrophy
hemihypoplasia
hemihysterectomy
hemimegalencephaly
    unilateral h.
hemimelia
    congenital fibular h.
    congenital tibial h.
    dysplasia epiphysealis h.
    fibular h.
    paraxial fibular h.
    paraxial tibial h.
    tibial h.
hemimelus
hemineural plate
hemiparesis
    congenital h.
    postconvulsive h.
    spastic h.
hemiparetic
    h. cerebral palsy
    h. posture
hemiplegia
    acute infantile h.
    alternating h.
    congenital h.
    double h.
    infantile h.
    postmigrainous stroke h.
    spastic h.
    syndrome of acute h.
hemiplegic
    h. cerebral palsy
    h. migraine
hemisection of cord
hemisensory deficit
hemisphere
    cerebral h.
hemispherectomy
    total h.
hemisyndrome
    left h.
hemivagina
hemivertebra
hemizygosity
hemizygous
hemoblastic leukemia
Hemocaine
Hemoccult test
hemochromatosis
    neonatal h. (NH)
hemoconcentration

NOTES

H

HemoCue AB hemoglobin measurement device
Hemocyte
hemocytometer
hemodia filtration
hemodialysis
    continuous venovenous h. (CVVHD)
hemodynamic
    h. data
    h. instability
Hemofil M
hemofiltration
    continuous arteriovenous h. (CAVH)
    continuous venovenous h. (CVVH)
hemoglobin (Hb, hgb)
    h. A1c
    h. C
    h. CC
    h. Chesapeake
    h. concentration
    cord blood h.
    h. E
    h. electrophoresis
    elevated fetal h.
    embryonic h.
    h. F
    fetal h. (HbF)
    glycosylated h. (HgA$_{1c}$)
    Gower-1, -2 h.
    h. Hammersmith
    hereditary persistence of fetal h. (HPFH)
    high-affinity h.
    homozygous h. E
    h. Kempsey
    Lepore h.
    h. Malmö
    mean corpuscular h. (MCH)
    h. M Hyde Park
    h. M Saskatoon
    Portland h.
    h. S
    h. SC
    h. SC, SS phenotype
    sickle h.
    h. sickle cell disease
    h. SS
    h. S solubility test
    h. SS phenotype
    h. S-Thal phenotype
    h. subtype method
hemoglobinopathy
    sickle cell h.
hemoglobin-oxygen dissociation curve

hemoglobinuria
    march h.
    paroxysmal nocturnal h. (PNH)
hemoglobulinopathy
hemolymphatic stage
hemolysin
    Donath-Landsteiner cold h.
hemolysis
    chronic intravascular h.
    h., elevated liver enzymes, low platelet count (HELLP)
    h., elevated liver enzymes, low platelet count syndrome
    immune h.
    massive intravascular h.
    nonimmune h.
hemolytic
    h. anemia
    h. complement (CH$_{50}$)
    h. crisis
    h. disease
    h. disease of newborn
    h. uremia syndrome associated with pregnancy
    h. uremic syndrome (HUS)
hemopericardium
hemoperitoneum
hemophagocytic
    h. lymphohistiocytosis
    h. syndrome
hemophilia
    h. A, B, C
    acquired h.
    factor VIII h.
hemophiliac
hemophilic arthropathy
hemopneumothorax
hemopoiesis
hemopoietic
hemoptysis
hemorrhage
    adrenal h.
    cerebellar h.
    CNS h.
    epidural h.
    external h.
    focal h.
    gastrointestinal h.
    germinal matrix h.
    idiopathic pulmonary h. (IPH)
    iliopsoas h.
    interhemispheric subarachnoid h.
    intracerebellar h.
    intracranial h. (ICH)
    intraparenchymal h.
    intraretinal h. (IH)
    intraventricular h. (grade I–IV) (IVH)

maternal-fetal h.
orbital h.
perinatal cerebral h.
periventricular h. (PVH)
periventricular-intraventricular h.
  (PIVH)
petechial h.
pinpoint h.
posterior fossa h.
pulmonary h.
retinal h.
splinter h.
subarachnoid h.
subconjunctival h.
subdural h.
subependymal germinal matrix h.
subgaleal h.
subhyaloid h.
hemorrhagic
  h. colitis
  h. cystitis
  h. cystitis glomerulonephritis
  h. diathesis
  h. disease
  h. disease of newborn (HDN)
  h. edema of infancy
  h. enanthem
  h. encephalitis
  h. *Escherichia coli*
  h. fever
  h. fever with renal syndrome
    (HFRS)
  h. pleural effusion
  h. scurvy
  h. shock
  h. shock and encephalopathy
    syndrome (HSES)
  h. shock-encephalopathy system
  h. shock syndrome
  h. telangiectasia
hemorrhagica
  purpura h.
hemorrhoid
  Pazo H.
hemorrhoidal preparation
hemosiderin deposition
hemosiderinuria
hemosiderosis
  food-induced pulmonary h.
  primary pulmonary h.
  pulmonary h.
  transfusion-induced h.

hemostasis
  surgical h.
hemostat
hemothorax
hemotympanum
HEMPAS
  hereditary erythroblastic multinuclearity
    with positive acidified serum
  HEMPAS test
Hem-Prep
Henderson-Hasselbalch equation
Henle
  loop of H.
Hennebert sign
Henoch-Schönlein purpura (HSP)
henselae
  Bartonella h.
  Rochalimaea h.
Hensen node
HEP
  hepatoerythropoietic porphyria
HEPA
  high-efficiency particulate air
  HEPA filter
hepadnavirus
heparin
  h. cofactor II (HCII)
  h. cofactor II deficiency
  h. cofactor II inhibitor
  low molecular weight h. (LMWH)
  h. sodium
  h. sulfate
  h. sulfate accumulation
heparinized saline
heparin-lock flush
hepatectomy
  left h.
  partial h.
  right h.
  total h.
hepatic
  h. amebiasis
  h. arteriovenous fistula
  h. capillariasis
  h. capsular calcification
  h. cirrhosis
  h. coma
  h. copper
  h. copper overload syndrome
  h. crisis
  h. encephalopathy (HE)
  h. fibrosis

NOTES

H

hepatic *(continued)*
  h. gluconeogenesis
  h. glycogenesis
  h. glycogen storage disease
  h. hemangioma
  h. iron concentration (HIC)
  h. lipase deficiency
  h. lobe
  h. necrosis
  h. parenchymal disorder
  h. porphyria
  h. sinusoid
  h. transaminase
  h. transplantation
  h. venous wedge pressure gradient
  h. wedged venography
hepatica
  Fasciola h.
hepaticojejunostomy
hepaticus
  fetor h.
hepatis
  bacillary peliosis h.
  peliosis h.
  porta h.
hepatitis
  h. A
  anicteric h.
  autoimmune h.
  h. A vaccine (HAV)
  h. A virus (HAV)
  h. B (HB)
  h. B antigen
  h. B arthritis-dermatitis syndrome
  h. B core antibody (HBcAb)
  h. B early antibody (HBeAb)
  h. B immune globulin (HBIG, H-
    BIG, HBIg)
  h. B immunization
  h. B oligosaccharide-CRM197
    vaccine (HbOC)
  h. B surface (HBs)
  h. B surface antibody (HBsAb)
  h. B surface antigen (HBsAg)
  h. B vaccine
  h. B virus (HBV)
  h. C
  chronic active h.
  chronic cryptogenic h. (CCH)
  chronic non-A-E h.
  cryptogenic h.
  h. C virus (HCV, HVC)
  h. D
  h. D virus (HDV)
  h. E
  h. E virus (HEV)
  fulminant h.
  h. F virus (HFV)

  h. G
  giant cell h.
  h. G virus (HGV)
  icteric h.
  idiopathic neonatal giant-cell h.
  infectious h.
  neonatal h.
  non-A h.
  non-ABCDE h.
  non-A, non-B h. (NANBH)
  non-B h.
  serum h.
  toxic h.
  viral h.
hepatobiliary
  h. disease
  h. scintigraphy
hepatoblastoma (HBL)
hepatocellular
  h. carcinoma (HCC)
  h. disease
  h. injury
  h. lysome
hepatoclavicular
hepatocyte
  h. nuclear factor (HNF)
  pleomorphism of h.
hepatocyte
hepatoerythropoietic porphyria (HEP)
hepatolenticular degeneration
hepatoma
hepatomegaly
  firm h.
  hard h.
hepatopathy
  sickle h.
hepatoportoenterostomy
hepatopulmonary syndrome (HPS)
hepatorenal
  h. syndrome
  h. tyrosinemia
hepatosplenic candidiasis
hepatosplenomegaly
hepatotoxicity
  nutritional h.
hepatotoxic syndrome
hepatotoxin
hepatotropic virus
Hep-B-Gammagee
Hep-Lock
Heptalac
heptavalent
Heptavax-B
Heptest Xa assay
herald patch
herb
  moxa h.

herbal
    h. medicine
    h. tea
hereditaria
    adynamia episodica h.
    atrophia bulborum h.
hereditary
    h. angioedema (type I)
    h. areflexic dystasia
    h. arthroophthalmopathy
    h. autonomic neuropathy
    h. benign intraepithelial dyskeratosis syndrome
    h. bone dysplasia
    h. chin trembling
    h. coproporphyria (HCP)
    h. dentatorubral-pallidoluysian atrophy
    h. disease
    h. dysplastic nevus syndrome
    h. ectodermal dysplasia
    h. ectodermal polydysplasia
    h. edema
    h. elliptocytosis (HE)
    h. erythroblastic multinuclearity
    h. erythroblastic multinuclearity associated with positive acidified serum lysis test
    h. erythroblastic multinuclearity with positive acidified serum (HEMPAS)
    h. fructose intolerance
    h. galactosemia
    h. hemorrhagic telangiectasia (HHT)
    h. lymphedema
    h. methemoglobinemia
    h. motor-sensory neuropathy
    h. motor-sensory neuropathy (type IA, III–VII) (HMSN)
    h. nephritis
    h. neuropathy with liability to pressure palsy (HNPP)
    h. nonpolyposis colorectal cancer
    h. optic neuron atrophy
    h. osteoarthrophthalmopathy
    h. pancreatitis
    h. paroxysmal ataxia
    h. persistence of fetal hemoglobin (HPFH)
    h. pyropoikilocytosis (HPP)
    h. renal adysplasia
    h. renal agenesis

    h. retinoblastoma
    h. retinoschisis
    h. sensory and autonomic neuropathy
    h. sensory radicular neuropathy
    h. spastic paraplegia
    h. spherocytosis
    h. spinal muscular atrophy
    h. stomatocytosis
    h. thrombophilia
    h. trait
    h. tremor
    h. trichodysplasia
    h. tyrosinemia
    h. urogenital adysplasia
heredity
    autosomal h.
heredoataxia
heredodegenerative
    h. disease
    h. disorder
heredofamilial
heredopathia atactica polyneuritiformis
heredosyphilis
Hering-Breuer inflation reflex (HBIR)
heritability
heritable
Herlitz epidermolysis bullosa letalis
Hermansky-Pudlak syndrome
hermaphroditism
Hermed catheter
hernia
    Bochdalek h.
    complete h.
    congenital diaphragmatic h. (CDH)
    contralateral h.
    diaphragmatic h.
    epigastric h.
    femoral h.
    foramen of Morgagni h.
    hiatal h.
    incarcerated h.
    incomplete h.
    indirect inguinal h.
    inguinal h.
    internal h.
    lung h.
    Morgagni h.
    ovary in inguinal h.
    paraduodenal h.
    paraesophageal hiatal h.
    peritoneal h.

NOTES

H

hernia *(continued)*
    retrocecal h.
    retrosternal h.
    Richter h.
    sliding hiatal h.
    transmesenteric h.
    umbilical h.
    uncomplicated h.
herniated
    h. disk
    h. stomach
    h. viscera
herniation
    brain h.
    brainstem h.
    cerebral h.
    chronic tonsillar h.
    disk h.
    fat h.
    muscle h.
    transtentorial h.
    uncal h.
herniorrhaphy
heroin
herpangina
herpes
    h. aseptic meningitis
    cervical h.
    congenital h.
    h. facialis
    geniculate h.
    h. gestationis
    h. gladiatorum
    h. keratitis
    h. labialis
    ophthalmic h.
    orolabial h.
    perinatal h.
    h. simplex (HS)
    h. simplex encephalitis (HSE)
    h. simplex labialis
    h. simplex pneumonia
    h. simplex virus (HSV)
    h. simplex virus 1 (HSV1, HSV-1)
    h. simplex virus 2 (HSV2, HSV-2)
    h. simplex virus encephalitis
    h. stomatitis
    toxoplasmosis, other agents, rubella, cytomegalovirus, h. (TORCH)
    h. virus
    h. zoster
    h. zoster of geniculate ganglion
    h. zoster meningitis
    h. zoster ophthalmicus (HZO)
    h. zoster oticus
Herpesviridae
herpesvirus
    Cercopithecine h. 1

    h. encephalitis
    h. hominis
    Kaposi sarcoma-associated h.
herpetic
    h. corneal infection
    h. gingivitis
    h. gingivostomatitis
    h. keratopathy
    h. stomatitis
    h. whitlow
herpeticum
    eczema h.
herpetiform
    h. aphthous ulcer
    h. corneal ulcer
herpetiformis
    dermatitis h. (DH)
    h. epidermolysis bullosa simplex
Herplex
herringbone pattern
Hers disease
Herson-Todd score
Hertoghe sign
hertz (Hz)
hesitancy
Hespan
hetastarch
heterochromatin
heterochromia
    congenital h.
    h. of inner canthus
    h. iridis
    h. of iris
heterocyclic antidepressant
heterodimer
heterodimeric
heteroduplex
heterogeneity
    genetic h.
heterogeneous
heterogenic
heterograft
heteroinoculation
heterologous
    h. surfactant
    h. twin
heteroovular twin
heterophil antibody
heterophile test
heteroplasmy
heterosexual
heterosomal aberration
heterotaxia
heterotaxy
    abdominal h.
    h. syndrome
    visceral h.

heterotopia
 band h.
 bilateral periventricular nodular h.
 focal h.
 gray matter h.
 leptomeningeal h.
 mesodermal h.
 neuroglial h.
 periventricular h.
 subcortical laminar h.
 subependymal h.
heterotopic
 h. gray matter
 h. liver transplantation
heterotypical chromosome
heterozygosity
heterozygote
heterozygous familial hypercholesterolemia
HEV
 hepatitis E virus
hexacetonide
 triamcinolone h.
hexachlorophene
 h. bath
 h. wash
hexadactyly
 postaxial h.
Hexadrol
 H. Phosphate Injection
 H. Tablet
hexamethyldislazane (IIMDS)
hexamethyl propylene amine oxime leukocyte (HMPAO)
hexoprenaline sulfate
hexosamine
hexosaminidase
 h. Λ, B
 serum h. A
hexosaminidase-A deficiency
hexose
Heyer-Schulte valve
Heyman-Herndon clubfoot procedure
HF
 high frequency
HFA
 high-functioning autism
 Proventil HFA
HFD
 human figure drawing
 HFD test

HFFI
 high-frequency flow interruption
HFJV
 high-frequency jet ventilation
HFMD
 hand-foot-and-mouth disease
HFO
 high-frequency oscillation
HFOV
 high-frequency oscillatory ventilation
HFPPV
 high-frequency positive-pressure ventilation
HFRS
 hemorrhagic fever with renal syndrome
HFV
 hepatitis F virus
 high-frequency ventilation
HgA$_{1c}$
 glycosylated hemoglobin
hgb (*var. of* Hb)
HGE
 human granulocytic ehrlichiosis
HGH, hGH
 human growth hormone
HGV
 hepatitis G virus
HHH
 hyperammonemia, hyperornithinemia, homocitrullinuria
 HHH syndrome
HHS
 Hoyeraal-Hreidarsson syndrome
HHT
 hereditary hemorrhagic telangiectasia
HHV-6
 human herpesvirus 6
HHV-7
 human herpesvirus 7
HHV-8
 human herpesvirus 8
HI
 hemagglutination inhibition
 HI antibody
 HI titer
HIA
 hemagglutination inhibition antibody
hiatal hernia
hiatus
 diaphragmatic h.
 esophageal h.
 h. leukemicus

NOTES

257

HIB
> hypoxia, intussusception, brain mass

Hib
> *Haemophilus influenzae* type b
> Hib conjugate vaccine
> Hib polysaccharide vaccine

HibDT-Vaccinol
Hibiclens
Hibistat
HibTITER
> Acel-Imune H.
> H. vaccine

HIC
> hepatic iron concentration

hiccups
hickey
Hickman catheter
Hi-Cor-1.0 Topical
Hi-Cor-2.5 Topical
hidden
> h. penis
> h. rheumatoid factor
> h. testis

hidradenitis suppurativa
hidradenoma
> eruptive h.

hidrotic ectodermal dysplasia
HIE
> hypoxic-ischemic encephalopathy

HIFT
> high-frequency ventilation trial

high
> h. airway obstruction syndrome
> h. annular testis
> h. arch foot
> h. bladder pressure
> h. frequency (HF)
> h. frontal bone
> h. gastrin level
> h. guard
> h. imperforate anus
> h. molecular weight kininogen (HMWK)
> h. molecular weight kininogen deficiency
> h. molecular weight kininogen factor
> h. myopia
> h. output
> h. oxygen percentage (HOPE)
> h. oxygen percentage in retinopathy of prematurity (HOPE-ROP)
> h. oxygen percentage in retinopathy of prematurity study
> h. pain threshold
> h. risk
> h. scrotal testis

> h. tone
> h. urogenital sinus

high-affinity hemoglobin
high-altitude pulmonary edema (HAPE)
high-arched palate
high-caloric density formula
high-calorie
> h.-c. diet
> h.-c. formula

high-density lipoprotein (HDL)
high-efficiency
> h.-e. particulate air (HEPA)
> h.-e. particulate air filter

higher-dose
> h.-d. therapy
> h.-d. therapy with epinephrine (HDE)

high-flow
> h.-f. nasal cannula
> h.-f. nonrebreather

high-frequency
> h.-f. flow interruption (HFFI)
> h.-f. hearing loss
> h.-f. jet ventilation (HFJV)
> h.-f. oscillation (HFO)
> h.-f. oscillator
> h.-f. oscillatory
> h.-f. oscillatory ventilation (HFOV)
> h.-f. positive-pressure ventilation (HFPPV)
> h.-f. ventilation (HFV)
> h.-f. ventilation trial (HIFT)
> h.-f. ventilator

high-fructose formula
high-functioning autism (HFA)
high-glucose formula
high-intensity click stimulus
highly
> h. active antiretroviral therapy (HAART)
> h. purified factor IX

high-oscillation ventilator
high-output failure
high-performance
> h.-p. capillary electrophoresis (HPCE)
> h.-p. liquid chromatography (HPLC)

high-phosphate diet
high-pitched
> h.-p. bowel sound
> h.-p. voice
> h.-p. wheeze
> h.-p. wheezing

high-power liquid chromatography (HPLC)
high-pressure liquid chromatography (HPLC)

high-resolution
    h.-r. chest computed tomography
    h.-r. computed tomography (HRCT)
high-riding prostate
high-risk register (HRR)
high-tone hearing loss
high-voltage slow activity (HVSA)
Higoumenakis sign
hilar
    h. dance
    h. lymphadenopathy
    h. region
Hilgenreiner line
hindfoot
    h. fracture
    h. valgus
    h. valgus deformity
hindgut
hinge
    knee h.
Hinman syndrome
hip
    h. adduction release
    h. click
    h. clunk
    congenital dislocation of h. (CDH)
    developmental dysplasia of h.
      (DDH)
    dislocated h.
    h. dysplasia
    incongruent h.
    irritable h.
    neurogenic dysplasia of h. (NDH)
    nonspherical congruent h.'s
    observation h.
    h. pointer
    h. rotation
    h. rotation test
    snapping h.
    spherical congruent h.'s
    h. spica cast
    subluxed h.
hip-knee-ankle angle
hip-knee-ankle-foot orthosis (HKAFO)
hippocampal
    h. neuron
    h. pathologic injury
    h. sclerosis
hippocampus
hippocratic nail
hippurate
    methenamine h.

Hiprex
Hirschberg
    H. corneal reflex test
    H. light reflex test
hirschfeldii
    Salmonella h.
Hirschsprung
    H. colitis
    H. disease
    H. enterocolitis
hirsutism
    h., androgen excess, insulin
      resistance, acanthosis nigricans
      (HAIR-AN)
    h., androgen excess, insulin
      resistance, acanthosis nigricans
      syndrome
    moderate h.
hirudin
his
    angle of H.
    H. bundle
    bundle of H.
    gastroesophageal angle of H.
Hismanal
Hispanic
His-Purkinje system
Histadyl
histamine
    h. 2 (H$_2$)
    h. fish poisoning
    h. H$_2$ receptor antagonist
    h. interleukin
histamine-1 antihistamine
Histerone Injection
histidase
histidine
histidinemia
histidinuria
histiocyte
    Gaucher-type h.
    sea-blue h.
histiocytic
    h. disorder
    h. fibroma
    h. lymphoma
histiocytoid cardiomyopathy
histiocytoma
    malignant fibrous h. (MFH)
histiocytosis
    acute disseminated h.
    Langerhans cell h. (LCH)

NOTES

H

histiocytosis *(continued)*
    malignant h.
    sinus h.
    h. X
histochemical
histocompatibility
    h. gene
    h. leukocyte antigen (HLA)
    maternal-fetal h.
histocytic necrotizing lymphadenitis
Histofreezer
histology
    Shimada-Chatten h.
histolytica
    Entamoeba h.
histone antigen
Histoplasma capsulatum
histoplasmosis
    chronic pulmonary h.
    disseminated h.
    infantile disseminated h.
    pulmonary h.
history
    prenatal h.
    h. of present illness (HPI)
    sudden infant death unexplained
      by h.
histrelin acetate
Hitachi 717
hitchhiker's thumb
HIV
    human immunodeficiency virus
    HIV classification
    HIV Classification for Children
      (P0, P1, P2)
    HIV infected
    HIV infection
    HIV microangiopathy
    HIV test
HIV-1
    human immunodeficiency virus-1
    HIV-1 RNA PCR assay
Hivagen test
HIV-associated nephropathy
Hi-Vegi-Lip
hives
Hivid
HIVIG
    human immunodeficiency virus
      immunoglobulin
hiving
HKAFO
    hip-knee-ankle-foot orthosis
    Rochester HKAFO
HL
    heel lance
HLA
    histocompatibility leukocyte antigen

    human leukocyte antigen
    HLA typing
HLA-A10
HLA-B5/B51
HLA-B27 antigen
HLA-B27-positive
HLA-DR7
HLA-DRw11
HLA-DRw53
HLA-identical
    HLA-i. haploidentical bone marrow
      stem cell
    HLA-i. marrow graft
HLA-mismatch
HLHS
    hypoplastic left heart syndrome
HLP
    hyperlipoproteinemia
HMB
    hydroxy beta methylbutyrate
HMD
    hyaline membrane disease
HMDS
    hexamethyldislazane
HME
    human monocytic ehrlichiosis
HMF
    human milk fortifier
hMG, HMG
    human menopausal gonadotropin
    HMG aciduria
HMPAO
    hexamethyl propylene amine oxime
    leukocyte
HMS Liquifilm
HMSN
    hereditary motor-sensory neuropathy
      (type IA, III–VII)
HMWK
    high molecular weight kininogen
    HMWK factor
HNF
    hepatocyte nuclear factor
HNPP
    hereditary neuropathy with liability to
      pressure palsy
HO
    heme oxygenase
    HO inhibitor
HOA
    hypertrophic osteoarthropathy
hoarding
    fecal h.
hoarse
    h. cry
    h. voice
hoarseness
    excessive h.

HOBT
   hyperbaric oxygen therapy
Hodgkin
   H. disease
   H. lymphoma
Hoffer procedure
Hoffmann
   H. clamp
   H. reflex
holarctica
   Francisella tularensis h.
hold
   Children's H.
   H. DM
holder
   Cameco syringe h.
   needle h.
holding
   breath h.
   h. chamber
hole in heart
Hollingshead 5-factor index
hollow viscera
Holmes heart
holoacranial
holocarboxylase
   h. synthetase (HCS)
   h. synthetase deficiency
holophrase
holoprosencephaly (HPE)
   alobar h.
   semilobar h.
holosystolic murmur
holovisceral myopathy
Holtain height stadiometer
Holter
   H. monitor
   II. valve
Holt-Oram syndrome
Homans sign
HOME
   Home Observation for Measurement of
   the Environment
      HOME scale
home
   h. antibiotic infusion therapy
   h. blood glucose monitoring
   h. cardiorespiratory monitor
   (HCRM)
   h. cognitive score
   H. Observation for Measurement of
   the Environment (HOME)
   H. Observation for Measurement of
   the Environment scale
   h. parenteral nutrition (HPN)
   h. uterine activity monitoring
   (HUAM)
homeobox
   short stature h. (SHOX)
homeopathy
homeostasis
   body h.
   copper h.
homeothermy
   servocontrolled h.
Homer Wright rosette
homicide
hominis
   Blastocystis h.
   herpesvirus h.
   Mycoplasma h.
   poliovirus h.
homocitrullinemia
homocysteine loading test
homocysteinuria
homocystine
homocystinemia
homocystinuria
homogeneity
homogeneous
homogenize
homograft conduit
homolateral weakness
homolog
homologous surfactant
homology
homonymous hemianopia
homoplasmy
   mutant h.
homosexuality
homothermic
homovanillic acid (HVA)
homozygosity for hemoglobin S (HbSS)
homozygote
homozygous
   h. achondroplasia
   h. familial hypercholesterolemia
   h. hemoglobin E
   h. hyperlipidemia (type I, II)
   h. sickle cell anemia
   h. thalassemia
honei
   Rickettsia h.
honeycombed appearance

NOTES

H

honeycomb lung
honey-crusted plaque
hood
> dorsal h.
> h. O$_2$
> oxygen h.

hookworm
> h. disease
> h. infection

HOP
> hypothyroxinemia of prematurity

HOPE
> high oxygen percentage

hopelessness
HOPE-ROP
> high oxygen percentage in retinopathy of prematurity
> HOPE-ROP study

Hopkins
> H. symptom checklist
> H. syndrome

hopping
> bunny h.

hora somni (at bedtime) (h.s.)
hordeolum
> external h.
> internal h.

Horizon 2000
horizontal
> h. nystagmus
> h. supranuclear gaze palsy
> h. suspension
> h. suspension in newborn
> h. transmission

Hormodendrum
hormone
> adrenal androgen-stimulating h. (AASH)
> adrenocorticotropic h. (ACTH)
> antidiuretic h. (ADH)
> cortical androgen-stimulating h. (CASH)
> corticotropin-releasing h. (CRH)
> follicle-stimulating h. (FSH)
> Genentech biosynthetic human growth h.
> gonadotropin-releasing h. (GnRH, GRH)
> growth h. (GH)
> growth hormone-releasing h.
> human growth h. (HGH, hGH)
> inappropriate antidiuretic h. (IADH)
> LATS h.
> luteinizing h. (LH)
> luteotropic h.
> parathyroid h. (PTH)

> peptide h.
> recombinant follicle-stimulating h. (rFSH)
> recombinant human growth h. (rhGH)
> syndrome of inappropriate antidiuretic h. (SIADH)
> syndrome of inappropriate secretion of antidiuretic h. (SIADH)
> thyroid-stimulating h. (TSH)
> thyrotropin-releasing h. (TRH)

hormone-secreting tumor
hormonosynthetic
horn
> h. cell disease
> iliac h.
> uterine h.

Horner syndrome
horse-riding stance
horseshoe kidney
HOS
> hypoosmotic swelling

hospice care
hospital
> H. for Sick Children (HSC)
> St. Jude Research H.
> Texas Scottish Rite H. (TSRH)

hospitalization
hospitalized attempted suicide (HAS)
hot
> h. nodule
> h. potato voice
> h. tube folliculitis

Hotelling test
hotline center
hour
> quaque horo (every h.) (q.h.)
> Sudafed 12 H.

hourglass configuration
hour-specific total serum bilirubin
house dust mite
housemaid's knee
Howell-Jolly body
Hoxa-5 null mutant
Hoyeraal-Hreidarsson syndrome (HHS)
HP
> Ku-Zyme HP
> Profasi HP

HPA
> human pancreatic amylase
> hypothalamic-pituitary-adrenal axis
> hypothalamic-pituitary axis

H.P. Acthar Gel
HPCE
> high-performance capillary electrophoresis

HPE
   holoprosencephaly
HPFH
   hereditary persistence of fetal
     hemoglobin
HPH
   hypoxia-induced pulmonary hypertension
HPI
   history of present illness
HPLC
   high-performance liquid chromatography
   high-power liquid chromatography
   high-pressure liquid chromatography
HPN
   home parenteral nutrition
HPP
   hereditary pyropoikilocytosis
HPS
   hepatopulmonary syndrome
   hypertrophic pyloric stenosis
HPV
   human papillomavirus
   human parvovirus
     HPV B19
HR
   heart rate
HRCT
   high-resolution computed tomography
H_1 receptor
HRIG
   human rabies immune globulin
HRQOL
   health-related quality-of-life
     HRQOL assessment
     HRQOL questionnaire
HRR
   haplotype relative risk
   high-risk register
HRSA
   heart rate power spectral analysis
HRV
   heart rate variability
HS
   herpes simplex
     Estratest HS
h.s.
   hora somni (at bedtime)
HSC
   Hospital for Sick Children
     HSC Scale
HSD2
   hydroxysteroid dehydrogenase type 2

HSE
   herpes simplex encephalitis
HSES
   hemorrhagic shock and encephalopathy
     syndrome
HSP
   Henoch-Schönlein purpura
HS-tk gene therapy
HSV
   herpes simplex virus
     syphilis, toxoplasmosis, other
      agents, rubella, cytomegalovirus,
      HSV
     toxoplasmosis, other agents, rubella,
      CMV, HSV
     HSV type 1
HSV1, HSV-1
   herpes simplex virus 1
HSV2, HSV-2
   herpes simplex virus 2
     HSV2 proctitis
HTLV-I
   human T-cell lymphotropic virus type I
     HTLV-I associated myelopathy
     (HAM)
     HTLV-I associated
      myelopathy/tropical spastic
      paraparesis (HAM/TSP)
     human T-cell lymphotrophic virus
      type I associated myelopathy
      (HAM)
HTLV-II
   human T-cell lymphotropic virus type II
HTP
   hypothalamic, pituitary, thyroid
5-HTT
   serotonin transporter 5-HTT
H-type
     H-t. tracheoesophageal fistula
     H-t. transesophageal fistula
HUAM
   home uterine activity monitoring
huang
     ma h.
HuCV
   human calicivirus
Hudson
     H. prongs
     H. T Up-Draft II disposable
      nebulizer
hue
     blue scleral h.

NOTES

H

hue *(continued)*
> purple h.
> violaceous h.
> white scleral h.

huffing

HUIZ
> Health Utilities Index Mark 2

Hulka clip

hum
> benign venous h.
> venous h.

Humalog

human
> h. calicivirus (HuCV)
> h. chorionic gonadotropin (hCG)
> h. diploid cell rabies vaccine (HDCV)
> h. diploid cell vaccine
> h. erythropoietin
> h. factor IX complex
> h. figure drawing (HFD)
> H. Figure Drawing Test
> h. granulocytic ehrlichiosis (HGE)
> h. growth hormone (HGH, hGH)
> h. health and behavior questionnaire (HBQ)
> h. immune globulin
> h. immunodeficiency virus (HIV)
> h. immunodeficiency virus-1 (HIV-1)
> h. immunodeficiency virus encephalopathy
> h. immunodeficiency virus immunoglobulin (HIVIG)
> h. immunodeficiency virus infected children
> h. immunodeficiency virus infection
> h. immunodeficiency virus test
> h. jagged-1 gene (JAG1)
> h. leukocyte antigen (HLA)
> h. leukocyte antigen-associated disorder
> h. menopausal gonadotropin (hMG, HMG)
> h. milk
> h. milk-fed
> h. milk fortifier (HMF)
> h. monocytic ehrlichiosis (HME)
> h. pancreatic amylase (HPA)
> h. papillomavirus (HPV)
> h. parvovirus (HPV)
> h. parvovirus arthropathy
> h. parvovirus B19
> h. rabies immune globulin (HRIG)
> h. recombinant antioxidant enzyme
> h. recombinant DNase
> h. scabies
> h. T-cell lymphotropic virus 1 tropic meloneuropathy
> h. T-cell lymphotropic virus type I (HTLV-I)
> h. T-cell lymphotropic virus type II (HTLV-II)
> h. T-lymphotropic virus (type I, II)
> Velosulin H.

human astrovirus type 1 (HAstV-1)

human herpesvirus 6 (HHV-6)

human herpesvirus 7 (HHV-7)

human herpesvirus 8 (HHV-8)

humanus
> *Pediculus h.*

Humate-P

Humatin

Humatrope Injection

humeroperoneal muscular dystrophy

humerus

Humibid
> H. L.A.
> H. Sprinkle

humidified
> h. air
> h. isolette

humidifier
> bubbler h.
> cool-mist h.

HuMist Nasal Mist

humor
> aqueous h.
> vitreous h.

humoral
> h. antibody
> h. antibody deficiency
> h. immune system
> h. immunity
> h. immunodeficiency

hump
> buffalo h.
> rib h.

Humulin
> H. 50/50
> H. 70/30
> H. L, N R, U
> H. U Ultralente

Hünermann-Happle syndrome

hunger
> air h.
> unusual h.

Hunter
> H. canal
> H. syndrome

Hunter-Hurler phenotype

Huntington
> H. chorea
> H. disease (HD)
> polyglutamine-expanded H.

Hurler-like facial appearance
Hurler-Scheie syndrome
Hurler syndrome
HUS
    hemolytic uremic syndrome
husband
        therapeutic insemination, h. (THI,
        TIH)
HUT
    head-up tilt
Hutchinson
        H. incisor
        H. syndrome
        H. teeth
        H. triad
Hutchinson-Gilford syndrome
hutchinsonian molar
HUVS
    hypocomplementemic urticarial vasculitis
    syndrome
HV
    height velocity
HVA
    homovanillic acid
HVC
    hepatitis C virus
HVSA
    high-voltage slow activity
hyaline
        h. body
        h. eosinophilic inclusion
        h. membrane disease (HMD)
        h. membrane syndrome
hyalinosis cutis et mucosae
hyaluronic acid factor
hyaluronidase factor
hybridization
        allele-specific oligonucleotide h.
        DNA h.
        fluorescent in situ h. (FISH)
        multispectral fluorescent in situ h.
        (M-FISH)
        nucleic acid h.
        in situ h.
hyclate
        doxycycline h.
Hycort Topical
hydantoin
hydatid
        h. cyst
        h. disease

hydatidosis
        alveolar h.
hydralazine
hydramnios
        maternal h.
Hydramyn Syrup
hydranencephaly
hydrate
        chloral h.
        H. Injection
hydration
hydrazide
        isonicotinic acid h. (INH)
hydrazine sulfate
Hydrea
        Droxia H.
hydroa
        h. aestivale
        h. puerorum
        h. vacciniforme
hydrocarbon
        aliphatic h.
        halogenated h.
        h. pneumonia
hydrocele
        abdominoscrotal h.
        h. fluid
        owl's eyes view of h.
        transitory h.
hydrocelectomy
hydrocephalic idiocy
hydrocephalocele
hydrocephaloid disease
hydrocephalus
        acute h.
        arrested h.
        benign external h.
        chronic h.
        communicating h.
        compensated h.
        corpus callosum hypoplasia,
        retardation, adducted thumbs,
        spastic paraplegia, h. (CRASH)
        external h.
        h. ex vacuo
        new-onset h.
        noncommunicating h.
        normal-pressure h.
        obstructive h.
        otitic h.
        permanent posthemorrhagic h.
        posthemorrhagic h. (PHH)

NOTES

H

hydrocephalus *(continued)*
  shunt-dependent h.
  shunted h.
  symptomatic progressive h.
  uncompensated h.
  X-linked h.
hydrocephaly
Hydrocet
hydrochloride (HCl)
  arginine h.
  Aventyl H.
  betaine h.
  bupropion h.
  buspirone h.
  cetirizine h.
  ciprofloxacin h.
  clomipramine h.
  clonidine h.
  cyclopentolate h.
  cysteine h.
  dicyclomine h.
  dobutamine h.
  dopamine h.
  doxapram h.
  fluoxetine h.
  guanfacine h.
  imipramine h.
  levalbuterol h.
  loperamide h.
  mefloquine h.
  meperidine h.
  mepivacaine h.
  methylphenidate h.
  Mustargen H.
  naloxone h.
  nortriptyline h.
  olopatadine h.
  OROS methylphenidate h.
  proguanil h.
  promethazine h.
  propranolol h.
  sertraline h.
  thioridazine h.
  tolazoline h.
  trimethobenzamide h.
  vancomycin h.
  venlafaxine h.
hydrochlorothiazide (HCTZ)
  h. and spironolactone
Hydrocil
hydrocodone and acetaminophen
hydrocolloid
hydrocolpos
hydrocortisone
  h. base
  h. butyrate
  h. cypionate

  neomycin, (bacitracin) polymyxin
    B, h.
  h. sodium succinate
  h. valerate
  Vioform h.
Hydrocortone
  H. Acetate Injection
  H. Oral
  H. Phosphate Injection
Hydrocort Topical
hydrodensitometry
HydroDIURIL
hydrogen
  h. in concentration (pH)
  h. peroxide
  h. peroxide enema
  h. pump inhibitor
Hydrogesic
hydrolase
  fumarylacetoacetate h. (FAH)
hydrolysate
  casein h.
  h. formula
  milk protein h. (MPH)
  protein h.
hydrolysis
  enzymic acid h.
hydrolyzed
  h. feeding
  h. premature formula
  h. protein
  h. whey
hydrometrocolpos
hydromorphone
hydromucocolpos
hydromyelia
hydronephrosis
  congenital h.
  fetal h.
  intermittent h.
  perinatal h.
  prenatal h.
  progressive h.
  unilateral neonatal h.
hydronephrotic kidney
Hydro-Par
hydroperoxide
  total h. (TH)
hydrophila
  Aeromonas h.
hydrophilic ointment
hydrophobia
hydrophobic
  short h. (SH)
hydrophthalmos
hydropic
  h. gallbladder
  h. infant

hydrops
    h. fetalis
    fetal nonimmune h.
    intrauterine h.
    nonimmune h.
hydropslike cholecystitis
hydrostatic
    h. pressure
    h. reduction
hydrosyringomyelia
Hydro-Tex Topical
hydrotherapy
hydrothorax
hydroureter
hydroureteronephrosis
hydroxide
    aluminum h.
    magnesium h.
    potassium h. (KOH)
    sodium h.
hydroxocobalamin
3-hydroxy-3-methylglutaric aciduria
hydroxy beta methylbutyrate (HMB)
hydroxybutyrate
hydroxychloroquine sulfate
25-hydroxycholecalciferol
hydroxyeicosatetraenoic acid
5-hydroxyindoleacetic assay
hydroxylase
    h. enzyme defect
    phenylalanine h. (PAH)
21-hydroxylase deficiency
11-hydroxylase deficiency
17-hydroxylase deficiency syndrome
hydroxylation
    kynurenine h.
hydroxyl radical (OH)
17-hydroxypregnenolone
    ACTH-stimulated 17-h.
17-hydroxyprogesterone
hydroxyproline
    proline h.
hydroxyprolinemia
hydroxysteroid dehydrogenase type 2 (HSD2)
hydroxyurea
25-hydroxy vitamin D
hydroxyzine
hygiene
    poor dental h.
    sleep h.

hygroma
    cystic h.
hymen
    cribriform h.
    imperforate h.
    stenotic h.
hymeneal tag
hymenectomy
Hymenoptera venom
hyoid bone
hyointestinalis
    Campylobacter h.
hyos
hyoscine
    Isopto H.
hyoscyamine, atropine, scopolamine, phenobarbital
Hyosophen
Hy-Pam Oral
hyperabduction
    thumb h.
hyperacidity
hyperactive
    h. distractible
    dominantly h.
    h. impulsivity
hyperactive/impulsive dimension
hyperactivity
    central serotonergic h.
    motor h.
hyperactivity/impulsivity domain
hyperacusis
hyperacute
    h. infarction
    h. rejection
hyperaeration
hyperaldosteronism
hyperalimentation (HA)
hyperalimentation-associated cholestasis
hyperalphalipoproteinemia
hyperammonemia
    h., hyperornithinemia, homocitrullinuria (HHH)
    h., hyperornithinemia, homocitrullinuria syndrome
    transient h.
    h. variant
hyperammonemic
    h. episode
    h. hepatic coma
    h. state
hyperamylasemia

NOTES

H

hyperandrogenemia
hyperandrogenism
    ovarian h.
hyperargininemia
hyperarousal
hyperbaric
    h. oxygen
    h. oxygen therapy (HOBT)
hyperbetalipoproteinemia (HBLP)
hyperbilirubinemia
    congenital nonhemolytic
      unconjugated h.
    conjugated h.
    direct h.
    extreme benign h.
    indirect h.
    neonatal h.
    prolonged indirect h.
    prolonged unconjugated h.
    transient familial neonatal h.
    unconjugated h.
hyperbilirubinemic
hypercalcemia
    h. elfin-facies syndrome
    familial h.
    familial hypocalciuric h. (FHH)
    hypocalciuric h.
    idiopathic infantile h.
    infantile h.
    maternal h.
hypercalcemic
hypercalciuria
    absorptive h.
    autosomal recessive renal proximal
      tubulopathy and h. (ARPTH)
    renal h.
hypercaloric formula
hypercapnia
    permissive h.
hypercarbia
hypercarotenemia
hypercellular
hypercellularity
    mesangial h.
    segmental mesangial h.
hyperchloremia
hyperchloremic
    h. metabolic acidosis
    h. renal acidosis
hypercholesterolemia
    familial h.
    heterozygous familial h.
    homozygous familial h.
hyperchromic acidosis
hypercoagulable state
hypercoagulation
hypercortisolism
hypercyanotic spell

hyperdibasic aminoaciduria
hyperdorsiflexed foot
hyperdynamic
    h. precordium
    h. ventricle
    h. ventricle with high output
hyperekplexia
hyperelastica
    cutis h.
hyperemesis gravidarum
hyperemia
    conjunctival h.
    optic disk h.
    posttraumatic h.
hyperemic cerebral blood flow
hypereosinophilic
    h. mucoid cast
    h. syndrome
hyperesthesia
hyperexcitability
hyperextensibility
    knee joint h.
hyperextensible joint
hyperextensile skin
hyperextension
    h. deformity
    dystonic h.
hyperferritinemia
hyperfiltration
hyperfractionated
    h. radiation therapy
    h. radiotherapy
hypergammaglobulinemia
    polyclonal h.
hypergastrinemia
    infant h.
hyperglycemia
hyperglycemic clamp technique
hyperglycinemia
    ketotic h.
    nonketotic h. (NKH)
hypergonadotropic hypogonadism
hyperhemolysis
HyperHep
hyperhidrosis
    volar h.
hyperhomocystinemia
hyperhydroxyprolinemia
hyper-IgD syndrome
hyper-IgE syndrome
hyper IgM
hyper-IgM syndrome
hyperimmune
    h. Ig
    h. immunoglobulin
hyperimmunoglobulin
    h. E
    h. E syndrome

hyperimmunoglobulinemia
hyperinflation
hyperinsulinemia
hyperinsulinemic
    h. hypoglycemia
    h. infant
hyperinsulinism
    fetal h.
    h. with hyperammonemia variant
hyperinsulinism/hyperammonemia
  syndrome
hyperintensity
hyperirritable stage
hyperkalemia
hyperkalemic
    h. periodic paralysis
    h. RTA
hyperkeratosis
    epidermal h.
    epidermolytic h.
    palmar and plantar punctate h.
    punctate h.
    striate h.
hyperkeratotic
    h. dry skin
    h. ridge
hyperkinesis
hyperkinetic
    h. behavior pattern
    h. child syndrome
    h. disorder
    h. pulmonary hypertension
hyperkyphosis
hyperlacticacidemia
hyperlaxity
    skin h.
hyperleukocytosis
hyperlexia
hyperlinearity
    palmar h.
hyperlipemia
    triglyceride h.
hyperlipidemia
    familial h.
    familial combined h. (FCHL)
    homozygous h. (type I, II)
    mixed h.
hyperlipoproteinemia (HLP)
hyperlordosis
hyperlucent
    h. lung
    h. lung syndrome

hyperlysinemia
    familial h.
hypermagnesemia
    iatrogenic acute h.
hypermenorrhea
hypermetabolism
hypermethioninemia
hypermobile
    h. Ehlers-Danlos syndrome
    h. flatfoot
    h. joint
    h. pes planus
hypermobility
    posterior occipitoatlantal h. (POAH)
    h. syndrome
hypermyelination
hypernasality
hypernasal speech
hypernatremia
hypernatremic dehydration
hypernitrosopnea
hyperopia
    asymmetric h.
hyperornithinemia
hyperosmolality
hyperosmolar
    h. coma
    h. dehydration
    h. state
hyperostosis
    cortical h.
    infantile cortical h.
hyperoxaluria
    enteric h.
    primary h.
    primary h. type 1 (PH-1)
    secondary h.
hyperoxia test
hyperoxygenation
hyperparasitemia
hyperparathyroidism
hyperperfusion
    ictal h.
hyperphagia
hyperphagic
hyperphenylalaninemia (MHP)
    benign h.
    malignant h.
hyperphosphatemia
hyperphosphaturic syndrome
hyperpigmentation
    diffuse h.

NOTES

H

hyperpigmentation *(continued)*
    periorbital h.
    reticulated h.
    whorled macular h.
hyperpigmented lichenified plaque
hyperpipecolic acidemia
hyperpituitary gigantism
hyperplasia
    adrenal h.
    adrenocortical h.
    angiofollicular lymph node h.
    benign lymphoid h.
    h. of beta cell
    congenital adrenal h. (CAH)
    congenital adrenal lipoid h.
    crypt h.
    elastic tissue h.
    erythroid h.
    focal nodular h.
    follicular h.
    gingival h.
    gum h.
    intimal h.
    Kupffer cell h.
    Leydig cell h.
    lymphoid h.
    lymphonodular h.
    neonatal breast h.
    nodular adrenal h.
    nodular lymphoid h.
    nonclassical adrenal h. (NCAH)
    21-OH nonclassical adrenal h.
    parietal cell h.
    pigmented nodular adrenal h.
    pseudoepitheliomatous h.
    pulmonary lymphoid h. (PLH)
    sebacceous h.
hyperplastic
    h. joint
    h. lymphoid tissue
    h. polyp
    h. right heart syndrome
hyperpnea
hyperpolarization
hyperprolactinemia
hyperprolinemia
hyperpronate
hyperpronation
hyperprostaglandin E$_2$ syndrome
hyperprostaglandinuric tubular syndrome
hyperpyrexia
    malignant h.
hyperreflexia
    detrusor h.
hyperreninemia
    chronic h.
hyperreninemic hypertension
hyperresonance to percussion

hyperresonant calvarial percussion note
hyperresponsive
hyperriboflavinemia
hypersecretion
    gastric acid h.
hypersegmentation
hypersegmented neutrophil
hypersensitive hapten-antibody
hypersensitivity
    h. angiitis
    delayed-type h. (DTH)
    h. pneumonitis
    h. reaction
    h. vasculitis
hypersensitization
hypersensitize
hypersexual behavior
hypersexuality
hypersomnia
    menstrual-associated periodic h.
    primary h.
hypersomnolence
hypersplenism
Hyperstat I.V.
hypersynchronization
hypersynchronous discharge
hypersynchrony of neural discharges
hypertelorism
    ocular h.
hypertelorism-hypospadias syndrome
hypertension
    accelerated h.
    benign intracranial h.
    essential h.
    fixed pulmonary h.
    hyperkinetic pulmonary h.
    hyperreninemic h.
    hypoxia-induced pulmonary h.
     (HPH)
    iatrogenic h.
    idiopathic intracranial h. (IIH)
    infantile h.
    intracranial h.
    malignant h.
    maternal h.
    pediatric h.
    persistent pulmonary h. (PPH)
    portal h.
    pregnancy-induced h. (PIH)
    presinusoidal h.
    pulmonary h.
    rebound h.
    white-coat h.
hypertensive
    h. crisis
    h. encephalopathy
hyperthermia
    malignant h. (MH)

neonatal h.
h. in newborn
hyperthermic rhabdomyolysis
hyperthyroidism
hypertonia
axial h.
global h.
hypertonic
h. dehydration
h. saline solution
hypertonicity
hypertonus
extensor h.
hypertransaminasemia
hypertransfusion regimen
hypertrichosis
h. lanuginosa
vellus h.
hypertriglyceridemia
familial h. (FHTG)
hypertrophic
h. cardiomyopathy
h. gastropathy
h. growth zone
h. interstitial neuropathy of infancy
h. nail
h. osteoarthropathy (HOA)
h. pyloric stenosis (HPS)
h. scar
h. stenosis
h. zone (HZ)
hypertrophied tissue
hypertrophy
adenoidal h.
adenotonsillar h.
atrial h.
biventricular h.
cerebellar h.
clitoral h.
congenital thyroid deficiency with
muscular h.
contralateral h.
hemangiectatic h.
juxtaglomerular apparatus h.
labial h.
left atrial h.
left ventricular h.
myocytic h.
pontile h.
right atrial h.
right ventricular h.
synovial h.

trigonal h.
ventricular h.
Viard h.
hypertropia
ipsilateral h.
hypertrypsinemia
hypertryptophanemia
hypertyrosinemia
hyperuricemia
hyperuricosuria
hypervalinemia
hyperventilation
central neurogenic h.
h. provocative test
h. syndrome
hypervigilance
hyperviscosity syndrome
hypervitaminosis
h. A
chronic h. A
hypervolemia
hyphema
eight-ball h.
traumatic h.
Hy-Phen
hypnagogic hallucination
hypnotherapeutic
hypnotherapy
hypnotic
hypoactivity
**hypoadrenalism neural ceroid
lipofuscinosis**
hypoalbuminemia
hypoalbuminemic
hypoaldosteronism
hypoallergenic
hypoalphalipoproteinemia
familial h.
primary h.
hypoarousal
sustained autonomic h.
hypobetalipoproteinemia
h., acanthocytosis, retinitis
pigmentosa, and pallidal
degeneration (HARP)
familial h.
hypocalcemia
cardiac abnormality, abnormal
facies, thymic hypoplasia, cleft
palate, h. (CATCH 22)
cardiac abnormality, T-cell deficit,
clefting, h. (CATCH)

NOTES

H

hypocalcemia (*continued*)
    late h.
    late neonatal h.
    h. and microdeletion 22q11
      syndrome
    neonatal h.
hypocalcemic
    h. seizure
    h. tetany
hypocalcification
    linear h.
hypocalciuria
    familial hypercalcemia with h.
    (FHH)
hypocalciuric hypercalcemia
hypocapnia
hypocarbia
hypocarnitinemia
hypocellularity
hypochloremia
hypochloremic metabolic alkalosis
hypochlorhydria
hypochlorous acid
hypochondriasis
    primary h.
    secondary h.
hypochondrogenesis
hypochondroplasia syndrome
hypochromic anemia
hypocitraturia
hypocoagulability
hypocomplementemia
hypocomplementemic
    h. glomerulonephritis
    h. urticarial vasculitis syndrome
    (HUVS)
hypodense
hypodermoclysis
hypodontia
hypodysplasia
    renal h.
hypoesthesia
    corneal h.
hypoesthesic skin lesion
hypoestrogenism
hypoferremia
hypofibrinogenemia
hypofluorescent
hypogammaglobulinemia,
  hypogammaglobinemia
    acquired h.
    adult-onset h.
    common variable h.
    congenital h.
    late-onset h.
    physiologic h.
    transient h.
    X-linked h.

hypoganglionic segment of Aldrich
hypoganglionosis
hypoglossia-hypodactyly syndrome
hypoglycemia
    familial hyperinsulinemic h.
    hyperinsulinemic h.
    hypoketotic h.
    insulin-induced h.
    ketotic h.
    neonatal h.
    nonfamilial hyperinsulinemic h.
    nonhyperinsulinemic h.
    nonketotic h.
    refractory h.
    severe refractory h.
    transient h.
hypoglycemic seizure
hypoglycin
hypoglycorrhachia
hypoglycosylation
hypogonadism
    congenital hypogonadotropic h.
    hypergonadotropic h.
    hypogonadotropic h.
    isolated hypogonadotropic h. (IHH)
hypogonadotropic hypogonadism
hypogonadotropism
hypohidrotic
    h. ectodermal dysplasia
    h. sweating
hypokalemia
hypokalemic
    h. acidosis
    h. periodic paralysis
    h. salt-losing tubulopathy
hypoketotic hypoglycemia
hypokinesia
hypokinetic
hypokyphosis
hypolordosis
hypomagnesemia
    congenital h.
    familial h.
    ionized h.
    primary h.
hypomagnesemic tetany
hypomania
    pharmacologically induced h.
hypomanic episode
hypomelanosis of Ito
hypomelanotic
hypomelia, hypotrichosis, facial
  hemangioma syndrome
hypomentia
hypometabolic
hypometabolism
    caudate h.
hypomyelination

hyponasality
hyponasal speech
hyponatremia of water excess
hyponatremic
    h. dehydration
    h. seizure
hypoosmotic swelling (HOS)
hypoparathyroidism
    idiopathic h.
    physiologic transient h.
hypoperfusion
    cerebral h.
    interictal h.
hypoperistalsis
    megacystis, microcolon, intestinal h.
      (MMIH)
hypopharyngeal-glottal obstruction
hypopharynx
hypophosphatasia
    congenital lethal h.
    h. tarda
hypophosphatemia
    familial h. (FHR)
    X-linked h.
hypophosphatemic
    h. bone disease
    h. rickets
hypophysis
hypopigmentation
    perianal h.
    vulvar h.
hypopigmented
    h. macule
    h. mycosis
hypopituitarism
    congenital h.
hypoplasia
    bilateral lung h.
    biliary h.
    cartilage hair h. (CHH)
    cerebellar h.
    congenital h.
    crypt h.
    dental enamel h.
    enamel h.
    erythroid h.
    exocrine pancreatic h.
    focal dermal h.
    global h.
    Goltz focal dermal h.
    ipsilateral lung h.
    iris h.

    linear h.
    h. of lung
    mandibular h.
    maxillary h.
    midface h.
    midfacial h.
    odontoid process h.
    optic nerve h.
    orbital bone h.
    pontocerebellar h.
    pulmonary h.
    right lung h.
    secondary adrenal h.
    segmental h.
    h. syndrome
    thymic h.
    transverse arch h.
    tubular h.
    vermis h.
    h. of vermis
hypoplastic
    h. anemia
    h. congenital anemia syndrome
    h. dens
    h. digit
    h. kidney
    h. left heart
    h. left heart syndrome (HLHS)
    h. left ventricle
    h. lung
    h. mandible
    h. nail
    h. parathyroid gland
    h. patella
    h. philtrum
    h. prostate
    h. pulmonary vascular bed
    h. radius
    h. superior cerebellar vermis
    h. teeth
    h. thumb
    h. tongue
    h. uterus
    h. zygomatic arch
hypopnea
hypopotassemia
hypoproteinemia
    idiopathic h.
hypoprothrombinemia
hypopyon
hyporeflexia

NOTES

H

273

hyposecretion
    gastric acid h.
hyposegmentation
hyposensitization
hyposmia
hyposomatotropism
    obesity-related h.
hypospadias
    first-degree h.
    penoscrotal h.
    perineoscrotal h.
    proximal h.
    pseudovaginal perineoscrotal h.
     (PPSH)
    h. repair
    second-degree h.
    subcoronal h.
    third-degree h.
hyposplenia
hyposplenism
hypostatic pneumonia
hyposthenuria
hyposulfite
    sodium h.
hypotelorism
    orbital h.
hypotension
    instantaneous orthostatic h. (INOH)
    neurally mediated h.
    orthostatic h.
hypotensive anesthesia
hypothalamic
    h. dysfunction
    h. lesion
    h., pituitary, thyroid (HTP)
    h. set point
    h. tumor
hypothalamic-hypophyseal destruction
hypothalamic-hypopituitary
   hypothyroidism
hypothalamic-pituitary
    h.-p. axis (HPA)
    h.-p. dysfunction
hypothalamic-pituitary-adrenal
    h.-p.-a. axis (HPA)
    h.-p.-a. axis dysregulation
hypothalamic-pituitary-ovarian axis
hypothalamus
hypothenar
hypothermia
    cerebral h.
    cranial h.
    deep systemic h.
hypothesis, pl. **hypotheses**
    differential detection h.
    differential treatment h.
    dormant basket cell h.
    gate-control h.

    Lyon h.
    school failure h.
    serotonin h.
    susceptibility h.
hypothesize
hypothyroidism
    acquired h.
    athyrotic h.
    central h.
    congenital h. (CH)
    congenital goitrous h.
    eutopic congenital h.
    goitrous h.
    hypothalamic-hypopituitary h.
    maternal h.
    maternal thyrotropin receptor
     blocking antibody-induced
     congenital h.
    mixed h.
    neonatal nongoitrous h.
    primary h.
    h. syndrome
    tertiary h.
hypothyroid myopathy
hypothyroxinemia
    h. of prematurity (HOP)
    transient h.
hypotonia
    benign congenital h.
    benign infantile h.
    congenital h.
    infantile h.
    muscular h.
    nonparalytic h.
    Oppenheim congenital h.
    paralytic h.
    transient h.
hypotonic
    h. cerebral palsy
    h. dehydration
    h. saline
    h. weakness
hypotonicity
hypotony
    ocular h.
hypotransferrinemia
hypotrichosis
    Matie-Unna h.
hypotropia
hypouricemia
hypoventilation
    central alveolar h.
    congenital central h.
    h. syndrome
hypovitaminosis
hypovolemia
hypovolemic shock
hypoxanthine/creatinine ratio

hypoxemia
  perinatal h.
hypoxemic
hypoxia
  alveolar h.
  cellular h.
  centrizonal h.
  global brain h.
  intestinal h.
  intrauterine h.
  h., intussusception, brain mass
    (HIB)
  subacute fetal h.
  in utero h.
hypoxia-induced pulmonary hypertension
  (HPH)
hypoxia-ischemia
hypoxic
  h. encephalopathy
  h. respiratory failure
  h. spell
  h. vasoconstriction
hypoxic-ischemic
  h.-i. brain injury
  h.-i. cerebral injury
  h.-i. encephalopathy (HIE)
HypRho-D Mini-Dose
hypsarrhythmia

hypsarrhythmic pattern
Hyrexin-50 Injection
hysteria
hysteric
  h. convulsion
  h. seizure
hysterical
  h. amnesia
  h. glottic closure
  h. paralysis
  h. seizure
  h. visual loss
hystericus
  globus h.
hysterotomy
hystrix
  ichthyosis h.
Hytakerol
Hytone Topical
Hytuss
Hytuss-2X
Hyzine-50 Injection
HZ
  hypertrophic zone
Hz
  hertz
HZO
  herpes zoster ophthalmicus

NOTES

I₂
> prostaglandin I_2

I-20
> pulse oximeter sensor N-25 and I-20

IAA
> ileoanal anastomosis

IAC
> indwelling arterial catheter
> interatrial communication

IADH
> inappropriate antidiuretic hormone
> IADH syndrome

IAHS
> infection-associated hemophagocytic syndrome

IAI
> intraabdominal infection
> intraamniotic infection

I antigen score

IAP
> intrapartum antibiotic prophylaxis

IART
> intraatrial reentrant tachycardia

IASA
> idiopathic acquired sideroblastic anemia

iatrogenic
> i. acute hypermagnesemia
> i. airway injury
> i. anemia
> i. bladder
> i. CJD
> i. complete heart block
> i. Creutzfeldt-Jakob disease
> i. effect
> i. hypertension
> i. pneumothorax
> i. pyopneumothorax

IB
> infantile botulism
> Excedrin IB
> Midol IB
> Motrin IB
> Pamprin IB

ibandronate

IBD
> identical by descent
> inflammatory bowel disease

IBDQ
> Inflammatory Bowel Disease Questionnaire

IBR
> Infant Behavior Record

IBS
> irritable bowel syndrome

IBT
> immunobead test

Ibuprin

ibuprofen

Ibuprohm

Ibu-Tab Junior Strength Motrin

ibutilide

IC
> immune complex
> inspiratory capacity
> Babytherm IC

iC3b receptor

ICA
> islet cell antibody

ICAM-1
> intercellular adhesion molecule 1

ICC
> Indian childhood cirrhosis
> Interagency Coordinating Council

ICD
> immune complex dissociation
> International Classification of Diseases

ICD-p24 test

iced
> i. saline
> i. saline submersion

I-cell
> inclusion cell
> I-cell disease

ICF
> intermediate care facility
> intracellular fluid

ICFM
> isolated congenital folate malabsorption

ICH
> intracranial hemorrhage

ichthyosiform
> congenital i.
> i. dermatosis
> i. erythroderma

ichthyosis
> congenital i.
> i. hystrix
> lamellar i.
> i. linearis circumflexa
> i. vulgaris
> i. with keratitis and deafness syndrome
> X-linked i.

ICI
> intracranial injury

ICN
> intensive care nursery

icosahedral triple-shelled virus

ICP
    intracranial pressure
        ICP monitoring
ICS
    inhaled corticosteroid
ICSD
    International Classification of Sleep
    Disorders
        ICSD criteria
ICSI
    intracytoplasmic sperm injection
ictal hyperperfusion
icteric
        i. hepatitis
        i. leptospirosis
        i. phase
icterogenic breast milk
icterohaemorrhagiae
        Leptospira i.
icterometer
icterus
        i. gravis neonatorum
        scleral i.
I&D
    incision and drainage
IDA
    iron-deficiency anemia
Idamycin
idarubicin
IDC
    intervertebral disk calcification
IDDM
    insulin-dependent diabetes mellitus
IDEA
    Individuals with Disabilities Education
    Act
idea
        flight of i.'s
ideation
        paranoid i.
        suicidal i.
identical
        i. by descent (IBD)
        i. twin
identification
IDI
    intractable diarrhea of infancy
idiocy
        amaurotic familial i.
        Batten-Bielschowsky type of late
          infantile and juvenile amaurotic i.
        cretinism i.
        i. by deprivation
        eclamptic i.
        epileptic i.
        genetous i.
        hydrocephalic i.
        inflammatory i.

        juvenile amaurotic i.
        late infantile amaurotic i.
        microcephalic i.
        paralytic i.
        Spielmeyer-Vogt type of late
          infantile and juvenile amaurotic i.
        traumatic i.
idioglossia
idiolalia
idiopathic
        i. acquired sideroblastic anemia
        (IASA)
        i. apnea
        i. apnea of prematurity
        i. apparent life-threatening event
        i. cavernous sinusitis
        i. chronic arthritis
        i. clubfoot
        i. constipation
        i. copper toxicosis
        i. dermatosis
        i. diffuse interstitial fibrosis
        i. diffuse interstitial fibrosis of
        lung
        i. epilepsy
        i. facial paralysis
        i. growth hormone deficiency
        i. heel-cord tightness
        i. hemolytic uremia syndrome
        i. hypertrophic subaortic stenosis
        (IHSS)
        i. hypoparathyroidism
        i. hypoproteinemia
        i. infantile hypercalcemia
        i. intracranial hypertension (IIH)
        i. intussusception
        i. juvenile avascular necrosis
        i. long Q-T syndrome
        i. low molecular weight proteinuria
        i. minimal lesion nephrotic
        syndrome (IMLNS)
        i. neonatal giant-cell hepatitis
        i. nephrotic syndrome (INS)
        i. neutropenia
        i. peptic ulcer disease
        i. polyserositis
        i. precocious puberty
        i. pulmonary hemorrhage (IPH)
        i. rapidly progressive
        glomerulonephritis
        i. respiratory distress syndrome
        i. scoliosis
        i. scrotal edema
        i. seizure
        i. short stature (ISS)
        i. status epilepticus
        i. steatorrhea

i. steroid-resistant
  proteinuria/nephrotic syndrome
i. talipes equinovarus
i. thrombocytopenic purpura (ITP)
i. tibia vara
i. toe walking (ITW)
i. torsion dystonia
i. torticollis
i. ulcer
i. urticaria
idiopathy priapism
idiosyncratic marrow aplasia
IDM
infant of diabetic mother
intensive diabetes management
IDMS
isolated diffuse mesangial sclerosis
idoxuridine
id reaction
IDS
iduronate sulfatase
IDU
intravenous drug use
5-iodo-2'-deoxyuridine
iduronate sulfatase (IDS)
iduronic acid
IDV
indinavir
IE
infectious endocarditis
infective endocarditis
I/E, I:E
inspiratory to expiratory ratio
  I/E ratio
IEM
inborn error of metabolism
IEP
Individualized Education Program
IF
intrinsic factor
involved field
  IF radiation
IFA
immunofluorescent antibody
immunofluorescent assay
indirect fluorescent antibody
ifenprodil
Ifex
IFI
intrafollicular insemination
IFN-gamma
interferon gamma

ifosfamide
IFSP
Individualized Family Service Plan
Ig
immunoglobulin
  hyperimmune Ig
IgA
immunoglobulin A
  IgA AGA test
  IgA antiendomysial
  IgA antiendomysium antibody
  IgA antigliadin
  IgA antireticulin antibody
  IgA deficiency
  IgA mesangial deposition
IgA1
immunoglobulin A subclass 1
IgA2
immunoglobulin A subclass 2
IgE
immunoglobulin E
  IgE antibody
  antistaphylococcal IgE
  IgE syndrome
IGF
insulinlike growth factor
IGF-1
insulinlike growth factor 1
IGF-2
insulinlike growth factor 2
IGFBP
insulinlike growth factor-binding protein
IGFBP-3
insulinlike growth factor-binding protein-3
IgG
immunoglobulin G
  IgG antibody titer
  IgG anti-HAV
  IgG2 deficiency
  IgG-IFA test
  IgG indirect fluorescent antibody test
IgG2
immunoglobulin G2
IgG4
immunoglobulin G4
  IgG4 deficiency
IGHD
isolated growth hormone deficiency
IGIV
immunoglobulin, intravenous

NOTES

IgM
  immunoglobulin M
    IgM antibody
    IgM antibody titer
    IgM deficiency
    hyper IgM
    IgM-IFA test
    IgM indirect fluorescent antibody
     test
    IgM titer
    X-linked immunodeficiency with
     hyper IgM
ignoring
  active i.
IGT
  impaired glucose tolerance
IH
  intraretinal hemorrhage
    mucopolysaccharidosis IH
IHA
  indirect hemagglutination
    IHA test
IHD
  ischemic heart disease
IHH
  isolated hypogonadotropic hypogonadism
IHPS
  infantile hypertrophic pyloric stenosis
IHSS
  idiopathic hypertrophic subaortic stenosis
IIF
  indirect immunofluorescence
IIH
  idiopathic intracranial hypertension
IL
  interleukin
    IL 2R
     interleukin-2 receptor
IL-1
  interleukin-1
IL-2
  interleukin-2
IL-3
  interleukin-3
IL-4
  interleukin-4
IL-5
  interleukin-5
IL-6
  interleukin-6
IL-7
  interleukin-7
IL-8
  interleukin-8
IL-9
  interleukin-9
IL-10
  interleukin-10
IL-11
  interleukin-11
IL-12
  interleukin-12
IL-13
  interleukin-13

IL-14
  interleukin-14
IL-15
  interleukin-15
ILAE
  International League Against Epilepsy
ILAR
  International League Against
   Rheumatism
    ILAR peripheral arthritis
     classification
ILD
  interstitial lung disease
ileal
  i. atresia
  i. conduit
  i. interposition
  i. limb
  i. loop
  i. loop diversion
  i. pouch-anal anastomosis (IPAA)
  i. reservoir
  i. stoma
  i. ureter
ileitis
  backwash i.
  nonspecific i.
  regional i.
  terminal i.
ileoanal
  i. anastomosis (IAA)
  i. pull-through
ileocecal conduit diversion
ileocolic intussusception
ileocolitis
ileoileal
  i. anastomosis
  i. intussusception
ileoileocolic intussusception
ileostomy
  Bishop-Koop i.
  end i.
Iletin
  Lente I. I, II
  NPH I. I, II
  Pork Regular I. II
  Regular I. I, II
ileum
  distal i.
  duplication of i.
  native i.
ileus
  adynamic i.
  complicated meconium i.
  duodenal i.
  meconium i. (MI)
  paralytic i.
  simple meconium i.
iliac
  i. apophysis maturation index
  i. crest
  i. crest apophysitis

i. crest contusion
i. fossa
i. horn
i. spine
iliofemoral artery
iliopectineal bursa
iliopsoas hemorrhage
iliotibial
i. band
i. band friction syndrome
ilium
Ilizarov
I. device
I. external fixator
I. limb-lengthening procedure
illegal substance
Illinois Test of Psycholinguistic Abilities (IPTA)
illness
acute i.
childhood severity of psychiatric i. (CSPI)
chronic i.
communicable i.
history of present i. (HPI)
Integrated Management of Childhood I. (IMCI)
leptospiral i.
lower respiratory i. (LRI)
manic-depressive i.
mental i.
nonthyroidal i. (NTI)
present i. (PI)
prodromal i.
roseola-like i.
seroconversion i.
upper respiratory i.
illocutionary stage
iloprost
Ilosone Pulvules
Ilotycin
Ilozyme
IL-7R deficiency
IM
infectious mononucleosis
intestinal malrotation
intramuscular
image
body i.
i. intensification fluoroscopy
i. intensifier
image-degradation amblyopia

imagery
traumatic i.
imaginal desensitization
imaging
chemical shift i. (CSI)
cine magnetic resonance i. (cine-MRI)
color Doppler flow i. (CDFI)
diffusion-weighted i. (DWI)
diffusion-weighted magnetic resonance i.
dynamic pulmonary i. (DPI)
echoplanar functional magnetic resonance i.
functional brain i.
Grey scale i.
i. headband
magnetic resonance i. (MRI)
magnetic source i. (MSI)
medical optimal i. (MOI)
MIGB i.
neuraxis tumor i.
OPS i.
orthogonal polarization spectral i.
phosphorus magnetic resonance i. (^{31}P MRI)
plantar i.
radionuclide i.
thallium i.
tissue Doppler i. (TDI)
imbalance
neuromuscular i.
ventilation-perfusion i.
IMCI
Integrated Management of Childhood Illness
Imerslünd
I.-Gräsbeck syndrome
I. syndrome
imidazole
i. carboxamide (DTIC)
topical i.
imino acid
iminoacidura
iminoglycinuria
familial i.
imipenem and cilastatin
imipramine hydrochloride
imiquimod
imitative play
Imitrex Injection

NOTES

IMLNS
idiopathic minimal lesion nephrotic
    syndrome
immanent justice
immature teratoma (grade 0–3)
immaturity
parathyroid gland i.
pulmonary i.
immediate
i. extrauterine adaptation
i. hypersensitivity reaction
immersion
i. burn
i. oil
immitis
Coccidioides i.
Dirofilaria i.
immobile
immobilization
cervical spine i.
Treponema pallidum i. (TPI)
immobilizer
straight-leg i.
immotile
i. cilia syndrome
i. cilium
Immulite
immune
i. complex (IC)
i. complex disease
i. complex dissociation (ICD)
i. complex-mediated
    glomerulonephritis
i. complex-mediated pericarditis
i. complex-mediated vasculitis
i. complex vasculitis
i. deficiency
i. globulin
i. hemolysis
i. hydrops fetalis
i. neutropenia
i. phase
i. response
i. response gene
i. suppressor gene
i. system
i. thrombocytopenia
i. thrombocytopenic purpura (ITP)
immune-competent children
immune-mediated
i.-m. disseminated encephalomyelitis
i.-m. neutropenia
i.-m. thrombocytopenia
immunity
cell-mediated i. (CMI)
humoral i.
immunization
active i.

diphtheria-tetanus-pertussis i.
Engerix-B i.
Haemophilus influenzae type b i.
hepatitis B i.
measles, mumps, rubella i.
passive i.
polio i.
Recombivax HB i.
tetanus-diphtheria i.
varicella i.
immunizing unit (IU)
immunoassay
Biostar Flu optical i.
enzyme i. (EIA)
fluorescent polarization i. (FPIA)
gold-labeled optical rapid i.
    (GLORIA)
growth hormone i.
optical i. (OIA)
Premier Platinum HpSA enzyme i.,
    The
immunobead test (IBT)
immunobiologic
immunoblastic
i. lymphoma
i. sarcoma
immunoblot
i. assay
Western i.
immunocompetence
immunocompetent
immunocompromised
immunocytochemistry
immunodeficiency
acquired i.
cellular i.
combined i. (CID)
common variable i. (CVI, CVID)
humoral i.
primary i.
severe combined i. (SCID)
i. syndrome
X-linked severe combined i. (X-
    SCID)
immunodeficient
immunodilator
immunoelectrophoresis
immunofluorescence
3-color i.
direct i. (DIF)
indirect i. (IIF)
i. study
immunofluorescent
i. antibody (IFA)
i. assay (IFA)
immunofunctional assay
immunogenic

immunogenicity
immunoglobulin (Ig)
    i. A (IgA)
    i. A deficiency
    i. A nephropathy
    i. antibody
    antihepatitis A virus i. G
    i. A subclass 1 (IgA1)
    i. A subclass 2 (IgA2)
    cluster of differentiation 4 i. G
      (CD4-IgG)
    i. deposition
    i. E (IgE)
    i. E level
    i. G (IgG)
    i. G2 (IgG2)
    i. G4 (IgG4)
    i. gene
    i. G subclass deficiency
    human immunodeficiency virus i.
      (HIVIG)
    hyperimmune i.
    i., intravenous (IGIV)
    intravenous i. (IVIG, IVIg)
    i. M (IgM)
    quantitative i.
    respiratory syncytial virus i.
      (RSVIG, RSV-IG)
    respiratory syncytial virus
      intravenous i. (RSV-IVIG)
    RhD i.
    tetanus i. (TIG)
    varicella-zoster i. (VZIG)
    Venilon human i.
immunohistochemical
immunologic disturbance
immunology
    nutritional i.
immunomodulation
immunomodulator
immunomodulatory treatment
immunoosseous dysplasia
immunoperoxidase stain
immunoproliferative small intestinal
  disease
immunoprophylaxis
immunoreactive trypsinogen (IRT)
immunosorbent agglutination assay
  (ISAGA)
immunosuppression
    pharmacologic i.
immunosuppressive therapy

immunotherapy
    rush i.
Imodium
    I. A-D
    I. Advanced
impacted
    i. bowel
    i. twin
impaction
    fecal i.
    food i.
impaired
    i. cognitive function
    emotionally i.
    i. glucose tolerance (IGT)
    i. rectal sensation
    i. taste
    i. vision
impairment
    auditory i.
    bilateral hearing i.
    conductive hearing i.
    cortical visual i. (CVI)
    functional i.
    mixed hearing i.
    neurocognitive i.
    neurosensory i. (NSI)
    sensorineural hearing i.
    sensory i.
    somatosensory i.
    unilateral hearing i.
impedance
    i. audiometry
    bioelectrical i.
    i. cardiogram
    i. tympanometry
impending renal failure
imperfecta
    amelogenesis i.
    dentinogenesis i.
    osteogenesis i. (OI)
    perinatal lethal osteogenesis i.
    progressive deforming
      osteogenesis i.
    Sillence classification of
      osteogenesis i. (type I, IA, IB,
      II, III, IV, IVA, IVB)
imperforate
    i. anus
    i. anus repair
    i. hymen
    i. vagina

NOTES

impetigo
>Bockhart i.
>bullous i.
>i. contagiosa
>group A streptococcal i.
>i. neonatorum
>nonbullous i.
>staphylococcal i.
>i. strain

impingement
>i. syndrome
>i. test

Implanon
implant
>Clarion hearing i.
>cochlear i.

implantation
>bilateral PC-IOL i.
>prosthetic graft i.

impotence
impression
>basilar i.
>Clinical Global I.'s (CGI)

imprinted gene
imprinting
>genomic i.

improper formula preparation
impulse
>apical i.
>point of maximum i. (PMI)
>i. spectrum disorder

impulsive
impulsivity
>hyperactive i.

Imuran
IMV
>intermittent mandatory ventilation

in
>rooming i.
>i. situ
>i. situ hybridization
>i. situ pinning
>i. situ tubularization
>toeing i.
>i. utero (IU)
>i. utero drainage
>i. utero drainage of fetal bladder
>i. utero drug exposure (IUDE)
>i. utero hypoxia
>i. utero reduction
>i. utero reduction of herniated
> viscera
>i. utero resection
>i. utero stem cell therapy
>i. utero transplantation
>i. vitro
>i. vitro antibody production (IVAP)

>i. vitro antibody production assay
>i. vivo

inactivated
>i. poliomyelitis vaccine
>i. polio vaccine
>i. poliovirus
>i. poliovirus vaccine (IPV)
>i. virus vaccine
>i. X chromosome

inactivation
>random X i.

inactivity
>alert i.
>glucuronyl transferase i.

inadequate body awareness
inanition fever
I-Naphline Ophthalmic
inapparent poliomyelitis
inappropriate
>i. antidiuretic hormone (IADH)
>i. antidiuretic hormone secretion

Inapsine
inattention
>i. dimension
>i. domain

inattention-overactivity with aggression (IOWA)
inattentive
inborn
>i. error
>i. error of bile acid biosynthesis
>i. error of bile acid synthesis
>i. error of metabolism (IEM)

INCA
>infant nasal cannula assembly

incadronate
incarcerated hernia
incarceration
incidence
incipient
incision
>abdominal i.
>bilateral subcostal i.'s
>i. and drainage (I&D)
>endoscopic i.
>gridiron i.
>Lanz i.
>McBurney i.
>Pfannenstiel i.
>rooftop i.
>subcostal i.
>transverse i.

incisional neuroma
incisor
>barrel-shaped upper central i.
>central i.
>Hutchinson i.
>intruded i.

lateral i.
peg-shaped upper central i.
prominent maxillary i.
single central maxillary i. (SCMI)
incisure
Schmidt-Lantermann i.
incline
inclusion
i. body
i. body of chlamydial conjunctivitis
i. cell (I-cell)
i. cell disease
i. cyst
full i.
hyaline eosinophilic i.
intracytoplasmic i.
lipid i.
Paneth cell i.
paracrystalline i.
incognito
tinea i.
incoherence
income
Supplemental Security I. (SSI)
incomitant strabismus
incompatibility
ABO i.
blood group i.
minor group antigen i.
platelet-antigen i.
Rh i.
incompetence
cervical i.
congenital palatopharyngeal i. (CPI)
florid pulmonary valvular i.
gastroesophageal i.
organic tricuspid i.
pharyngeal i.
sphincteric i.
velopharyngeal i. (VPI)
incompetent
i. cervix
i. lower esophageal sphincter
incomplete
i. bowel obstruction
i. cleft
i. conjoined twin
i. hernia
i. rectal prolapse
incongruent hip
inconsequential occurrence
inconspicuous penis

incontinence
giggle i.
stress i.
incontinentia
i. pigmenti
i. pigmenti achromians
i. pigmenti syndrome
increased
i. anteroposterior chest diameter
i. bone density
i. fatigability
i. femoral anteversion
i. globulin fraction
i. intracranial pressure
i. renin release
i. tear meniscus
i. vascular resistance
incubate
incubation period
incubator
Air Shields i.
convection-warmed i.
double-insulated i.
double-walled i.
Forma water-jacketed i.
single-walled i.
incus
independent
Inderal LA
indeterminate
i. leprosy
i. sleep
indeterminus
situs i.
index, pl. **indices**
acetabular i. (AI)
amniotic fluid i. (AFI)
anal i. (AI)
anxiety sensitivity i. (ASI)
axial acetabular i. (AAI)
Bayley mental developmental i.
Bayley Psychomotor
Developmental I.
body mass i. (BMI)
Clinical Colitis Activity I. (CCAI)
clinical global i. (CGI)
Conners Hyperactivity indices
Doppler myocardial performance i.
fine motor i.
i. finger
glycemic i.
gross motor i.

NOTES

index *(continued)*
    growth i.
    Hollingshead 5-factor i.
    iliac apophysis maturation i.
    left ventricular stroke work i.
      (LVSWI)
    Lloyd-Still i.
    McGoon i.
    mental development i. (MDI)
    mental developmental i. (MDI)
    migration i. (MI)
    mixed obstructive apnea/hypopnea i.
      (MOAHI)
    neural i.
    nonverbal developmental i.
    oxygenation i. (OI)
    Paediatric Crohn Disease
      Activity I. (PCDAI)
    Parental Stress I. (PSI)
    Parenting Stress I. (PSI)
    Physiologic Stability I. (PSI)
    placental maturity i.
    ponderal i. (PI)
    Pourcelot i.
    Prehospital I. (PHI)
    psychomotor development i. (PDI)
    pulsatility i.
    Quetelet body mass i.
    radiographic bone strength i.
      (RBSI)
    Rohrer i.
    weight/height i.
    W/H i.

India
    I. ink stain
    I. ink test

Indian childhood cirrhosis (ICC)
indican
indicanuria
indicator
    Bioself fertility i.
indices *(pl. of* index)
indifference
    la belle i.
indinavir (IDV)
    i. calculi
    i. crystal
indirect
    i. calorimetry
    i. Coombs test
    i. cystography
    i. fluorescent antibody (IFA)
    i. hemagglutination (IHA)
    i. hemagglutination test
    i. hyperbilirubinemia
    i. immunofluorescence (IIF)
    i. immunofluorescence assay
    i. inguinal hernia

    i. laryngoscopy
    i. laser ophthalmoscope
    i. ophthalmoscope
    i. ophthalmoscopy
    i. orbital floor fracture
    i. visualization
indium 111
indium-labeled leukocyte scan
individualized
    I. Education Program (IEP)
    I. Family Service Plan (IFSP)
individuals
    I. with Disabilities Act
    I. with Disabilities Education Act
      (IDEA)
Indocin
    I. I.V.
    I. I.V. Injection
    I. SR
    I. SR Oral
indocyanine green
indolent
    i. carditis
    i. granular CMV retinitis
indomethacin
indrawing
    intercostal i.
    supraclavicular i.
induced
    i. abortion
    i. sputum analysis (ISA)
induction
    rapid sequence i.
    i. therapy
induration
    nonpitting i.
indurative edema
indwelling
    i. arterial catheter (IAC)
    i. catheter
    i. optode
    i. thumb
    i. venous catheter (IVC)
    i. venous line (IVL)
ineffective myelopoiesis
inequality
    limb length i.
Infalyte formula
infancy
    acropustulosis of i.
    acute hemorrhagic edema of i.
      (AHEI)
    anaclitic depression of i.
    apnea of i.
    autoimmune neutropenia of i.
      (ANI)
    benign myoclonus of i.
    benign paroxysmal torticollis of i.

chronic nonspecific diarrhea of i.
chronic pneumonitis of i. (CPI)
cricopharyngeal incoordination of i.
diencephalic syndrome of i.
familial hyperinsulinism of i.
hemorrhagic edema of i.
hypertrophic interstitial neuropathy
  of i.
intractable diarrhea of i. (IDI)
nonfamilial hyperinsulinism of i.
normal gastroesophageal reflux
  of i.
protracted diarrhea of i.
severe myoclonic epilepsy in i.
  (SMEI)
transient hypogammaglobulinemia
  of i. (THI)

Infanrix vaccine
infant
at-risk i.
I. Behavior Record (IBR)
i. development
i. development program
i. development specialist
i. of diabetic mother (IDM)
i. dietary supplement
dysmature i.
i. dyssomnia
i. educator
ELBW i.
extremely low birth weight i.
extremely premature i. (EPI)
floppy i.
full-term i.
hydropic i.
i. hypergastrinemia
hyperinsulinemic i.
LBW i.
low birth weight i.
i. nasal cannula assembly (INCA)
Neurodevelopmental Assessment of
  Preterm I.'s (NAPI)
Neurodevelopmental Assessment
  Procedure for Preterm I.'s
periodic breathing in i.'s
postmature i.
premature i.
preterm i.
i. respiratory distress syndrome
  (IRDS)
i. size (IS)
small premature i.

I. Star 8000 oscillator
I. Star ventilator
i. stimulation program
i. subdural tap
i. of substance-abusing mother
  (ISAM)
i. suffocation
i. teacher
term i.
very low birth weight i.
vigorous i.
VLBW i.

infantile
i. acquired aphasia
i. acropustulosis
i. agranulocytosis
i. Alexander disease
i. anorexia
i. arteriosclerosis
i. asthma
i. autism
i. beriberi
i. botulism (IB)
i. celiac disease
i. cerebral sphingolipidosis
i. colic
i. corneal clouding
i. cortical hyperostosis
i. diarrhea
i. diarrhea rotavirus
i. digital fibroma
i. diplegia
i. disseminated histoplasmosis
i. eczema
i. epilepsy
i. epileptic encephalopathy
i. fibromatosis
i. Gaucher disease
i. glaucoma
i. hemangioma
i. hemangiopericytoma
i. hemiplegia
i. hypercalcemia
i. hypertension
i. hypertrophic pyloric stenosis
  (IHPS)
i. hypotonia
i. idiopathic scoliosis
i. monoclonic seizure
i. motor neuron disease
i. muscular torticollis
i. myoclonic jerk

NOTES

infantile *(continued)*
- i. myoclonic seizure
- i. myofibrillar myopathy
- i. myofibromatosis
- i. myxedema
- i. NCL
- i. neural ceroid lipofuscinosis
- i. neuroaxonal dystrophy
- i. neuronal degeneration
- i. neuropathic cystinosis
- i. obstructive cholangiopathy
- i. onset
- i. paralysis
- i. periarteritis nodosa
- i. PKD
- i. poikiloderma
- i. polyarteritis nodosa (IPN)
- i. polycystic disease
- i. polyneuritis
- i. pustulosis
- i. pyknocytosis
- i. Refsum disease
- i. Refsum disease continuum
- i. respiratory distress syndrome
- i. scurvy
- i. seborrhea
- i. spasm
- i. spinal muscular atrophy
- i. subacute necrotizing encephalopathy
- i. tetany
- i. tibia vara
- i. tremor syndrome

infantile-onset spinocerebellar ataxia
infantilism
- sexual i.

infantis
- *Bifidobacterium i.*

infantiseptica
- granulomatosis i.

infantum
- cholera i.
- dermatitis exfoliativa i.
- dermatitis gangrenosa i.
- granuloma gluteal i.
- *Leishmania i.*
- roseola i.
- tabes i.

infarct
- bilirubin i.
- fan-shaped hemorrhagic i.
- fat-induced i.
- multiple villous i.'s
- uric acid i.

infarction
- acute myocardial i. (AMI)
- bowel i.
- cavernosal i.

CFE i.
CNS i.
- i. of herniated stomach
- hyperacute i.
- myocardial i. (MI)
- i. of oral epithelium
- parasagittal cortical i.
- periventricular i.
- pulmonary i.
- i. of skinfold

Infasurf intratracheal suspension
Infatab
infected
- HIV i.
- vertically i.

infection
- acute lower respiratory i. (ALRI)
- acute lower respiratory tract i. (ALRTI)
- acute respiratory i. (ARI)
- adenovirus i.
- *Bartonella henselae* i.
- bloodstream i. (BSI)
- *Campylobacter* i.
- chorioamniotic i.
- chronic conjunctival i.
- chronic parvoviral i.
- congenital rubella i.
- congenital syphilitic i.
- conjunctival i.
- Coxsackie A16 i.
- Coxsackievirus i.
- cytomegalovirus i.
- dermatophyte i.
- droplet i.
- enteric i.
- enteroviral i.
- gland i.
- gonococcal i.
- group A beta-hemolytic streptococcal i.
- group B streptococcal i.
- guinea worm i.
- hematogenous i.
- herpetic corneal i.
- HIV i.
- hookworm i.
- human immunodeficiency virus i.
- intraabdominal i. (IAI)
- intraamniotic i. (IAI)
- intraarticular i.
- intrauterine i. (IUI)
- intrauterine parvovirus B19 i.
- latent i.
- lower respiratory i. (LRI)
- lower respiratory tract i. (LRTI)
- lytic i.
- MAI i.

middle ear i.
multiple opportunistic pathogen i.
multiplicity of i. (MOI)
nail-fold i.
neisserial i.
neonatal herpes simplex virus i.
nontuberculous mycobacterial i.
nosocomial i.
nosocomial bacterial i. (NBI)
opportunistic i.
overwhelming i.
parameningeal i.
parvoviral i.
pediatric gonococcal i.
perinatally acquired HIV i.
i. point
prenatal i.
primary i.
pyogenic i.
recurrent staphylococcal i.
respiratory tract i.
rhinocerebral i.
rickettsial i.
rubella i.
SEM i.
Serratia marcescens i.
simplex i.
sinopulmonary tract i.
skin, eye, or mucocutaneous i.
spirochetal i.
stage A, B, C, N i.
staphylococcal i.
Stenotrophomonas maltophilia i.
streptococcal i.
suppurative i.
syphilitic i.
TORCH i.
transplacental i.
trichomonal i.
upper respiratory i. (URI)
upper respiratory tract i. (URTI)
upper urinary tract i.
urinary tract i. (UTI)
Vincent i.
viral upper respiratory tract i.
yersinial i.
infection-associated hemophagocytic
syndrome (IAHS)
infectiosum
erythema i.
infectious
i. colitis

i. eczematoid dermatitis
i. endocarditis (IE)
i. esophagitis
i. gastritis
i. hepatitis
i. lymphocytosis
i. mononucleosis (IM)
i. myocarditis
i. pancreatitis
i. pericarditis
i. peritonitis
i. polyneuritis
i. pulmonary tuberculosis
i. rhinitis
infective
i. dermatitis
i. endarteritis
i. endocarditis (IE)
i. phlebitis
Infectrol Ophthalmic
InFeD
inferior
i. clivus
i. colliculus
i. mesenteric vein
i. olivary nucleus
i. peduncle
i. pincer grasp
i. turbinate surgery
i. vena cava (IVC)
i. vena cava disruption
infertility
infestation
louse i.
pinworm i.
infibulation
infiltrate
cellular i.
eosinophilic i.
inflammatory i.
interstitial i.
leukemia i.
liver i.
lung i.
miliary i.
perihilar i.
perivascular eosinophilic i.
perivascular inflammatory i.
perivascular polymorphonuclear i.
plasma cell i.
pleomorphic cellular i.
polymorphonuclear i.

NOTES

infiltrate *(continued)*
> pulmonary i.
> retinal i.
> white retinal i.
> xanthogranulomatous i.
> yellow retinal i.

infiltration
> leukocyte i.
> lymphohistiocytic i.
> nodular i.
> patchy i.
> peribronchial i.

Inflamase
> I. Forte Ophthalmic
> I. Mild Ophthalmic

inflamed

inflammation
> acute renal parenchymal i.
> chronic synovial i.
> fibrosing i.
> orbital i.
> portal i.
> transmural i.

inflammatory
> i. arteritis
> i. bacterial enteritis
> i. bowel disease (IBD)
> I. Bowel Disease Questionnaire (IBDQ)
> i. Brown syndrome
> i. colitis
> i. demyelinating encephalomyelitis
> i. demyelination
> i. exudate
> i. idiocy
> i. infiltrate
> i. myositis
> i. polyp
> i. process
> i. pseudotumor (IPT)
> i. response

inflection
> voice i.

infliximab

influenza (flu)
> i. A, B
> i. a/b
> i. A encephalitis
> i. A virus
> i. vaccine

influenzae
> *Haemophilus* i.

influenza-like syndrome

influenzal meningitis

information
> integrate sensory i.
> pediatric dosing i.
> sensory i.

infraclavicular area

infraction
> Freiberg i.

infraorbital nerve

infrared thermographic calorimetry (ITC)

Infrasurf surfactant

infratentorial
> i. tuberculoma
> i. tumor

infravesical obstruction

infundibular
> i. chamber
> i. stenosis

infundibulum
> right ventricular i.

Infuse-A-Port catheter

infusion
> alkali i.
> apotransferrin i.
> bicarbonate i.
> continuous milk i.
> insulin i.
> intraosseous i. (IOI)
> IO i.
> i. pump

ingestion
> accidental i.
> caustic i.
> copper sulfate i.
> fava bean i.
> goitrogen i.
> iron i.
> lead i.
> organophosphate i.
> paraquat i.

ingrown toenail

inguinal
> i. adenitis
> i. adenopathy
> i. area
> i. freckling
> i. hernia
> i. ligament
> i. lymphadenitis

inguinale
> granuloma i.
> lymphogranuloma i.

INH
> isoniazid
> isonicotinic acid hydrazide

inhalation
> Atrovent Aerosol I.
> i. bronchial challenge testing
> INOmax for i.
> intrapulmonary i.
> NebuPent I.
> nitrogen dioxide i.

i. suspension
tobramycin solution for i. (TOBI)
inhaled
i. beta-2 agonist
i. bronchodilator
i. corticosteroid (ICS)
i. nitric oxide (iNO, I-NO)
i. steroid
inhaler
AeroBid-M Oral Aerosol I.
AeroBid Oral Aerosol I.
Azmacort Oral I.
Beclovent Oral I.
Beconase AQ Nasal I.
Dexacort Phosphate Respihaler
Oral I.
Diskhaler metered-dose i.
Diskus i.
dry powder i. (DPI)
fluticasone propionate dry
powder i.
metered-dose i. (MDI)
Nasalide Nasal I.
Serevent Diskus i.
steroid i.
Vancenase AQ I.
Vancenase Nasal I.
Vanceril Oral I.
inheritance
autosomal dominant i.
dominant i.
mitochondrial i.
recessive i.
X-linked recessive i.
inherited
i. bleeding disorder
i. hemolytic uremia syndrome
inhibin A, B
inhibition
behavioral i.
callosal i.
hemagglutination i. (HI)
response i.
vagal i.
inhibitive casting
inhibitor
a-2AP coagulation i.
a-2AT coagulation i.
ACE i.
alpha-1 proteinase i. (A1PI)
a-2M coagulation i.
angiotensin-converting enzyme i.

a-2 antiplasmin coagulation i.
antithrombin III coagulation i.
a-2 antitrypsin i.
AT-III coagulation i.
calcineurin i.
carbonic anhydrase i.
C1 esterase i.
C1INH coagulation i.
COX-2 i.
cyclooxygenase-2 i.
factor VIII i.
HCII coagulation i.
heme oxygenase i.
heparin cofactor II i.
HO i.
hydrogen pump i.
leukotriene i.
lupus i.
M2 i.
a-2 macroglobulin coagulation i.
monoamine oxidase i. (MAOI,
MOA)
neuraminidase i.
nonnucleoside reverse
transcriptase i. (NNRTI)
nucleoside reverse transcriptase i.
(NRTI)
phosphodiesterase i. (PDI)
plasminogen activator i. (PAI)
protease i. (PI, Pi)
protein C coagulation i.
protein S coagulation i.
proton pump i. (PPI)
reverse transcriptase i. (RTI)
selective serotonin reuptake i.
(SSRI)
serotonin reuptake i. (SRI)
scrum protease i.
initial apnea
inject
Dekasol-L.A. I.
injectable
Cardizem I.
injection
Adlone I.
Adrucil I.
Aerosporin I.
A-hydroCort I.
Amcort I.
A-methaPred I.
Andro-L.A. I.
Andropository I.

NOTES

injection *(continued)*
    Anergan I.
    Antilirium I.
    Antispas I.
    Apresoline I.
    Arfonad I.
    Aristocort Forte I.
    Aristocort Intralesional I.
    Aristospan Intra-articular I.
    Aristospan Intralesional I.
    Arrestin I.
    Articulose-50 I.
    Astramorph PF I.
    Baci-IM I.
    Bena-D I.
    Benadryl I.
    Ben-Allergin-50 I.
    Bentyl Hydrochloride I.
    bulbar conjunctival i.
    Byclomine I.
    Celestone Phosphate I.
    Cel-U-Jec I.
    Chlor-Pro I.
    Chlor-Trimeton I.
    Cipro I.
    conjunctival i.
    Dalalone D.P. I.
    Dalalone L.A. I.
    Decadron-LA I.
    Decadron Phosphate I.
    Decaject I.
    Decaject-LA I.
    Dekasol I.
    Delatest I.
    Delatestryl I.
    Demadex I.
    depAndro I.
    depMedalone I.
    Depoject I.
    Depo-Medrol I.
    Depopred I.
    Depo-Provera I.
    Depotest I.
    Depo-Testosterone I.
    Dexasone L.A. I.
    Dexone LA I.
    Diazemuls I.
    Dibent I.
    Dihyrex I.
    Dilaudid I.
    Dilaudid-HP I.
    Dilocaine I.
    Dilomine I.
    Dinate I.
    Diphenacen-50 I.
    Diprivan I.
    direct egg i.
    Di-Spaz I.

D-Med I.
Dramilin I.
Dramoject I.
Duo-Trach I.
Duraclon I.
Duralone I.
Duramorph I.
Duratest I.
Durathate I.
Dymenate I.
Edecrin Sodium I.
Everone I.
Genotropin I.
Hexadrol Phosphate I.
Histerone I.
Humatrope I.
Hydrate I.
Hydrocortone Acetate I.
Hydrocortone Phosphate I.
Hyrexin-50 I.
Hyzine-50 I.
Imitrex I.
Indocin I.V. I.
intracardiac i.
intracytoplasmic sperm i. (ICSI)
Isuprel I.
Kefurox I.
Kenaject I.
Kenalog I.
Key-Pred I.
Key-Pred-SP I.
Kytril I.
Lasix I.
Levothroid I.
Lyphocin I.
Marmine I.
Medralone I.
medroxyprogesterone i.
Mestinon I.
Metro I.V. I.
Monistat I.V. I.
M-Prednisol I.
Nafcil I.
Nallpen I.
Nebcin I.
Nervocaine I.
Neut I.
Nitro-Bid I.V. I.
nonexudative conjunctival i.
Norditropin I.
Nordryl I.
Nuromax I.
Nutropin AQ I.
Nydrazid I.
Octocaine I.
Or-Tyl I.
Osmitrol I.
Pentam-300 I.

Phenazine I.
Phenergan I.
Predalone 50 I.
Prednisol TBA I.
Prometh I.
Prorex I.
Protropin I.
Quiess I.
Regonol I.
Romazicon I.
round spermatid nuclei i. (ROSNI)
Saizen I.
i. sclerotherapy
Selestoject I.
Serostim I.
Solu-Cortef I.
Solu-Medrol I.
Solurex LA I.
somatropin (rDNA origin) for i.
Spasmoject I.
Sublimaze I.
subtrigonal i.
subureteric Teflon i.
subzonal i. (SUZI)
Sufenta I.
Synthroid I.
Tac-3 I.
Tac-40 I.
Tesamone I.
Ticon I.
Tigan I.
Toradol I.
Triam-A I.
Triam Forte I.
Triamonide I.
Tridil I.
Tri-Kort I.
Trilog I.
Trilone I.
Triostat I.
Trisoject I.
Unipen I.
Valium I.
Vancocin I.
Vancoled I.
Vistacon-50 I.
Vistaquel I.
Vistaril I.
Vistazine I.
Zinacef I.

injector
INJEX jet i.
MadaJet XL needle-free i.
INJEX jet injector
injury
AAST Organ Injury Scaling of vulva, vagina, bladder, urethral, rectal i. (grade I–V)
acceleration i.
acute i.
airbag i.
asphyxial birth i.
asphyxial brain i.
axonal i.
blowout i.
blunt cardiac i. (BCI)
brain i.
caustic i.
cerebral i.
clavicular i.
clenched fist i.
closed head i. (CHI)
compression i.
contrecoup i.
coup i.
deceleration i.
degloving i.
diaphragmatic i.
diffuse axonal i. (DAI)
epiphyseal plate i.
eversion i.
excitotoxic i.
flexion-distraction i.
greenstick i.
hair tourniquet i.
hepatocellular i.
hippocampal pathologic i.
hypoxic-ischemic brain i.
hypoxic-ischemic cerebral i.
iatrogenic airway i.
intracranial i. (ICI)
intrapleural i.
Lauge-Hansen mechanism of i.
ligamentous i. (grade I–III)
mechanical birth i.
meniscal i.
mitochondrial i.
neonatal brain i.
neonatal cold i.
nerve i.
oxidative brain i.
parasagittal cerebral i.

NOTES

injury *(continued)*
    penetrating brain i.
    peripheral nerve i.
    physeal i.
    popsicle i.
    radiation-induced physeal i.
    reperfusion i.
    Salter-Harris classification of
      epiphyseal plate i.
    Salter i. (type I–IV)
    scalding i.
    i. severity score (ISS)
    straddle i.
    stress i.
    submersion i.
    The I. Prevention Program (TIPP)
    thermal i.
    traction i.
    transfusion-associated lung i.
      (TRALI)
    traumatic brain i. (TBI)
    ventilator-induced lung i. (VILI)
    ventilatory-associated lung i.
      (VALI)
    whiplash i.
inlet
in-line probe
innate
inner
    i. canthus
    i. canthus displacement
    i. ear
innervated
innervation
    sympathetic i.
innocent murmur
innocuous
innominate
    i. artery
    i. osteotomy
    i. vein
Innovar
iNO, I-NO
    inhaled nitric oxide
Inocor
inoculata
inoculate
inoculation
inoculum
    intranasal i.
INOH
    instantaneous orthostatic hypotension
INOmax for inhalation
inorganic mercury salt
inosiplex
inotropic
    i. effect
    i. support

inotropy
Inoue-Melnick virus
INOvent delivery system
inpatient
input
    abnormal cortical visual i.
    labyrinthine afferent i.
    proprioceptive i.
    unequal visual i.
    vestibular i.
INR
    international normalized ratio
INS
    idiopathic nephrotic syndrome
insecticide
    organophosphate i.
insect sting reaction
insemination
    direct intraperitoneal i. (DIPI)
    intrafollicular i. (IFI)
    intravaginal i. (IVI)
    therapeutic donor i. (TDI)
insensible
    i. water loss
insensitivity
    congenital i.
    growth hormone i. (GHI)
    partial (incomplete) androgen i.
      (PAI)
insert
    Cookie I.
Inser-Tape
insertion
    Achilles tendon i.
    deltoid i.
    marginal i.
    i. potential
    subzonal i.
    velamentous i.
insipidus
    central diabetes i.
    diabetes i. (DI)
    nephrogenic diabetes i.
    X-linked recessive-type diabetes i.
insomnia
    fatal familial i.
    primary i.
    i. syndrome
insonnation
inspiration
    i. time
inspiratory
    i. capacity (IC)
    i. to expiratory ratio (I/E, I:E)
    i. pressure
    i. reserve volume (IRV)
    i. stridor

i. time (IT)
i. whoop
inspire
inspired oxygen
inspissated
i. bile
i. bile syndrome
i. milk syndrome
inspissation
mucous i.
INSS
International Neuroblastoma Staging
System
instability
atlantoaxial i.
glenohumeral i.
hemodynamic i.
occipitoatlantal i.
instantaneous orthostatic hypotension (INOH)
Institute of Personality and Ability Testing (IPAT)
institutionalize
instruction
adult-directed i.
child-directed i.
instrument
Lusk i.
Primedic-Mobicard-type ECG i.
Welch Allyn AudioPath Platform
hearing acuity i.
instrumentation
anterior spinal i.
bladder i.
Cotrel-Dubousset i. (CDI)
Miami Moss i.
posterior segmental fixation i.
segmental spinal i.
Texas Scottish Rite i.
insufficiency
adrenal i.
adrenocortical i.
adrenocorticotropic hormone i.
alacrima, achalasia, adrenal i.
aortic i.
chronic adrenal i.
chronic mitral i.
chronic pulmonary i.
chronic renal i.
exocrine pancreatic i.
glomerular i.
glucocorticoid i.

mitral i.
pancreatic exocrine i.
placental i.
prerenal i.
primary adrenal i.
pulmonary i.
renal i.
respiratory i.
tricuspid i.
uteroplacental i. (UI)
valvular i.
insufflation
continuous tracheal gas i.
insulin
i. deficiency
glucose plus i.
i. infusion
i. lipoatrophy
i. lispro
NPH I.
Regular Purified Pork I.
i. resistance
i. response
i. secretion
i. shock
insulin-dependent
i.-d. diabetes
i.-d. diabetes mellitus (IDDM)
insulin-induced hypoglycemia
Insulin Lente L
insulinlike
i. growth factor (IGF)
i. growth factor 1 (IGF-1)
i. growth factor 2 (IGF-2)
i. growth factor-binding protein (IGFBP)
i. growth factor-binding protein-3 (IGFBP-3)
insulinopenia
insulinotropic peptide
insulin-secreting pancreatic tumor
insulitis
insult
perinatal i.
insurance
Social Security Disability I. (SSDI)
intake
caloric i.
maximal oxygen i. (MOI)
oral i.
poor caloric i.
poor oral i.

NOTES

Intal
Integra
integrate
    i. sensation
    i. sensory information
integrated
    I. Management of Childhood
      Illness (IMCI)
    i. visual and auditory (IVA)
integration
    Developmental Test of Visual-
      Motor I.
    sensorimotor i.
    sensory i.
    structural i.
    visual-motor i. (VMI)
    visuomotor i.
integrin
integrity
intellectual disability
intelligence
    borderline i.
    Fagan Test of Infant I.
    normal i.
    i. quotient (IQ)
    subaverage i.
    i. test
    Wechsler Preschool and Primary
      Scale of I. (WPPSI)
Intelligence-Revised
    Wechsler Preschool and Primary
      Scale of I.-R. (WPPSI-R)
intense emotional state
intensifier
    image i.
intensity
intensity/time (I/T)
intensive
    i. care nursery (ICN)
    i. diabetes management (IDM)
    i. phototherapy
    i. special care nursery (ISCN)
    i. special care unit (ISCU)
intensivist
Intensol
    Diazepam I.
intention
    i. myoclonus
    secondary i.
    i. tremor
interaction
    ephaptic i.
    epithelial-mesenchymal i.
    Interview Schedule for Social I.
    mother-child i.
    poor feeding i.

interactive play therapy
Interagency Coordinating Council (ICC)
interarticularis
    pars i.
interarytenoid notch
interatrial communication (IAC)
interbody ankylosis
intercalary
    i. defect
    i. defect of pollical ray
intercalatum
    Schistosoma i.
intercellular
    i. adhesion molecule 1 (ICAM-1)
    i. edema
intercondylar
    i. groove
    i. notch
    i. radiograph
intercostal
    i. indrawing
    i. retraction
    i. space
intercourse
    interfemoral i.
    sexual i.
    vulvar i.
interdigital
    i. candidosis
    i. web
interdigitation
interdisciplinary team
interest
    atypical i.
interface
    gum-tooth i.
    tendon-bone i.
interfemoral intercourse
interferon
    i. alpha
    i. alpha-2a
    i. alpha-2b
    gamma i.
    i. gamma (IFN-gamma)
    interstitial positive-pressure i. alpha
    i. therapy
interferon-alpha
intergluteal cleft
interhemispheric
    i. subarachnoid hemorrhage
    i. subdural hematoma
interictal
    i. discharge
    i. EEG
    i. hypoperfusion

i. myokymia
i. spike
interleukin (IL)
histamine i.
interleukin-1 (IL-1)
interleukin-2 (IL-2)
i. receptor (IL 2R)
i. receptor alpha chain mutation
interleukin-3 (IL-3)
interleukin-4 (IL-4)
interleukin-5 (IL-5)
interleukin-6 (IL-6)
interleukin-7 (IL-7)
interleukin-8 (IL-8)
interleukin-9 (IL-9)
interleukin-10 (IL-10)
interleukin-11 (IL-11)
interleukin-12 (IL-12)
interleukin-13 (IL-13)
interleukin-14 (IL-14)
interleukin-15 (IL-15)
interlobar
intermaxillary narrowness
InterMed Bear
intermedia
thalassemia i.
intermediate
i. care facility (ICF)
i. dystonic stage
intermedius
Staphylococcus i.
intermittent
i. exotropia
i. fever
i. hydronephrosis
i. mandatory ventilation (IMV)
i. mechanical ventilation
i. porphyria
i. positive-pressure breathing (IPPB)
i. positive-pressure ventilation
(IPPV)
i. strabismus
i. support
intermuscular abscess
intern
internal
i. branchial sinus
i. derangement
i. femoral torsion
i. hernia
i. hordeolum
i. jugular vein
i. ophthalmoplegia
i. representation
i. tibial torsion

internalization
internalize
internalizing
I. Behavior Scale
i. problem
i. score
international
I. Classification of Diseases (ICD)
I. Classification of Sleep Disorders
(ICSD)
I. Classification of Sleep Disorders
criteria
I. League Against Epilepsy (ILAE)
I. League Against Rheumatism
(ILAR)
I. League Against Rheumatism
peripheral arthritis classification
I. Neuroblastoma Staging System
(INSS)
i. normalized ratio (INR)
I. Society for Heart Transplantation
(ISHT)
I. Staging System
I. Unit (IU)
interneuron
aspiny i.
internist
internuclear ophthalmoplegia
internus
obturator i.
interobserver variability
interpeak latency
interposition
antiperistaltic intestinal i.
cartilage i.
colonic i.
costal cartilage i.
ileal i.
intestinal i.
isoperistaltic intestinal i.
interpretation
interrogans
Leptospira i.
interrogation
continuous wave Doppler i.
interrupted
i. aortic arch (type A, B)
interruption
high-frequency flow i. (HFFI)
intersex disorder
intersexuality
intersphincteric
i. abscess
i. space

NOTES

interstitial
 i. deletion
 i. edema
 i. fibrosis
 i. fluid
 i. infiltrate
 i. keratitis
 i. lung disease (ILD)
 i. myocarditis
 i. nephritis
 i. pneumonitis
 i. positive-pressure interferon alpha
interstitium
 renal i.
intertriginous
 i. area
 i. candidiasis
 i. candidosis
intertrigo
intertrochanteric fracture
interval
 atlantodens i. (ADI)
 PR i.
 prolonged QT i.
 pulse i.
 QRS i.
 QT i.
 R-R i.
 short PR i.
intervention
 antiinflammatory i.
 early i.
 psychopharmacological i.
 pulsed i.
 school-based i.
interventionist
 early i.
interventricular septum
intervertebral
 i. disk (IVD)
 i. disk calcification (IDC)
 i. diskitis
interview
 autism diagnostic i. (ADI)
 Brown and Harris i.
 Life Events and Difficulty
  Schedule I.
 psychiatric diagnostic i. (PDI)
 I. Schedule for Children and
  Adolescents (ISCA)
 I. Schedule for Social Interaction
 semistructured psychiatric i. (SSI)
Interview-Revised
 Autism Diagnostic I.-R. (ADI-R)
interweaving pattern
intestinal
 i. atresia
 i. bladder augmentation

 i. disorder
 i. duplication
 i. hypoxia
 i. interposition
 i. ischemia
 i. malrotation (IM)
 i. metaplasia
 i. motility
 i. mucosa
 i. neuronal dysplasia
 i. obstruction
 i. ostomy
 i. permeability (IP)
 i. polyp
 i. polyposis
 i. pseudoobstruction
 i. telangiectasia
 i. transplantation
 i. villous atrophy
 i. volvulus
intestinalis
 Campylobacter fetus i.
 Enterocytozoon i.
 pneumatosis i.
 Septata i.
intestine
 large i.
 small i.
intestine-associated lymphoid tissue
intima
intimal
 i. hyperplasia
 i. thickening
intoeing
intolerance
 cold i.
 delayed orthostatic i.
 disaccharide i.
 exercise i.
 familial protein i.
 feeding i.
 fructose i.
 glucose i.
 gluten i.
 hereditary fructose i.
 lactose i.
 lysinuric protein i.
 milk protein i.
 orthostatic i.
 primary lactose i.
 protein i.
 transient protein i.
intoxicate
intoxication
 acute scombroid i.
 aluminum i.
 anticonvulsant i.
 barbiturate i.

I

botulinus i.
chronic vitamin A i.
ciguatera i.
lead i.
manganese i.
mepivacaine i.
metal i.
methylmercury i.
phenothiazine i.
salicylate i.
scombroid i.
sugar i.
thallium i.
vitamin A, D i.
water i.
intraabdominal
   i. abscess
   i. cyst
   i. infection (IAI)
   i. testis
intraamniotic infection (IAI)
intraaortic balloon counterpulsation
intraarterial chemotherapy
intraarticular
   i. epiphysis
   i. infection
intraatrial
   i. redirection
   i. redirection of venous return
   i. reentrant tachycardia (IART)
   i. repair
intrabronchial obstruction
intrabronchiolar obstruction
intracardiac
   i. dcfcct
   i. injection
   i. shunt
   i. tunnel
intracellular
   i. event
   i. fluid (ICF)
   i. hydrogen ion concentration (pHi)
   i. pH
intracerebellar hemorrhage
intracerebral
   i. aneurysm
   i. hematoma
   i. seeding of bacteria
intracisternal therapy
intraclass correlation coefficient
intracoronary ultrasound

intracranial
   i. arterial aneurysm
   i. arteriovenous fistula
   i. calcification
   i. cystic space
   i. empyema
   i. foreign body
   i. hematoma
   i. hemorrhage (ICH)
   i. hypertension
   i. injury (ICI)
   i. pressure (ICP)
   i. suppuration
   i. venous sinus thrombosis
   i. volume
intractable diarrhea of infancy (IDI)
intracytoplasmic
   i. inclusion
   i. sperm injection (ICSI)
intradermal
   i. nevus
   i. test
intraepidermal
   i. blister
   i. vesiculation
intraepithelial dyskeratosis syndrome
intrafamilial genoidentical donor
intrafamily offender
intrafollicular insemination (IFI)
intragastric
   i. feeding
   i. pH
intrahepatic
   i. arterioportal fistula
   i. bile duct
   i. bile duct paucity
   i. biliary atresia
   i. cholestasis
intralesional
   i. steroid therapy
Intralipid formula
intralobar
   i. rest
   i. sequestration
intraluminal
   i. electrical impedance technique
   i. nutrient
   i. obstruction
   i. plug
   i. pressure
   i. web

NOTES

intramedullary
    i. rod
    i. rod fixation
intramural gas
intramuscular (IM)
intranasal
    i. desmopressin
    i. influenza vaccine
    i. inoculum
    i. spray
intranuclear
    i. hyaline inclusion disease
    i. inclusion body
intraocular
    i. lymphoma
    i. malignancy
    i. optic neuritis
    i. pressure (IOP)
    i. tumor
intraosseous (IO)
    i. infusion (IOI)
    i. line placement
    i. needle
intraparenchymal
    i. bleed
    i. hematoma
    i. hemorrhage
intrapartum
    i. antibiotic prophylaxis (IAP)
    i. asphyxia
    i. maternal fever
intrapleural injury
intrapsychic phenomenon
intrapulmonary
    i. inhalation
    i. shunt
    i. shunt fraction (Qs/Qt)
    i. shunting
    i. shunt ratio (Qs/Qt)
intrarenal
    i. anastomosis
    i. reflux
    i. venous radical
intraretinal hemorrhage (IH)
intraspinous vascular anomaly
intrathecal
    i. anti-HIV antibody
    i. medication
    i. methotrexate
intrathoracic
    i. tracheomalacia
    i. tuberculosis
intratonsillar
intratracheal
    i. magnesium (ITMg)
    i. pulmonary ventilation (ITPV)
intratumoral desmoplasia
intrauterine (IU)

    i. acquisition
    i. asphyxia
    i. compression
    i. device (IUD)
    i. exposure
    i. growth restriction (IUGR)
    i. growth retardation (IUGR)
    i. hydrops
    i. hypoxia
    i. infection (IUI)
    i. intussusception
    i. involvement
    i. lymphedema
    i. maternofetal transfusion
    i. parvovirus B19 infection
    i. position
    i. positional defect
    i. ureteral obstruction
    i. viral myositis
intravaginal
    i. foreign body use
    i. insemination (IVI)
    i. suppository
intravascular
    i. oncotic pressure
    i. sickling
    i. ultrasonography
    i. ultrasound (IVUS)
    i. volume
    i. volume depletion
intravenous (IV)
    cytomegalovirus immune globulin i. (CMV-IGIV)
    i. drip (IVD)
    i. drug use (IDU)
    i. feeding
    i. gamma globulin (IVGG)
    i. immune globulin (IVIG, IVIg)
    i. immunoglobulin (IVIG, IVIg)
    i. line
    peripheral i. (PIV)
    i. pyelogram (IVP)
    i. pyelography
    scalp i.
    i. urography (IVU)
intraventricular
    i. bleed
    i. fibrinolytic therapy
    i. hemorrhage (grade I–IV) (IVH)
    i. neurocysticercosis
    i. ribavirin
intrinsic
    i. asthma
    i. dyssomnia
    i. factor (IF)
    i. flow resistance (R_{int})
    i. tumor

introducer
> P.D. Access with Peel-Away
> needle i.

introitus
> vaginal i.

Intron A

Intropin

intruded incisor

intrusion
> dental i.
> i. symptom

intrusive luxation

intubated

intubation
> controlled i.
> endotracheal i. (ETI)
> nasotracheal i.
> orotracheal i.
> rapid sequence i. (RSI)
> Silastic tube i.
> stenosis post i.

intussusception
> apex of i.
> appendiceal i.
> cecocolic i.
> colocolic i.
> idiopathic i.
> ileocolic i.
> ileoileal i.
> ileoileocolic i.
> intrauterine i.
> prolapsing apex of i.

intussusceptum
> engorgement of i.

invaginata
> trichorrhexis i.

invaginated bowel

invagination
> basilar i.

invagination

invasive
> i. candidiasis
> i. sinusitis

invecta
> *Solenopsis i.*

inventory
> Battelle Developmental I. (BDI)
> Beck Depression I. (BDI)
> Children's Depression I. (CDI)
> Child Sexual Behavior I. (CSBI)
> communal traumatic experiences i. (CTEI)

communicative development i.
Eating Disorders I.
Eyberg Child Behavior I.
Gillespe-Numerof Burnout I.
Global Severity Index of Brief
> Symptom I. (GSI-BSI)
18-item Birleson Depression I.
Leyton Obsessional I.
Maslach Burnout I.
Minnesota Multiphasic
> Personality I. (MMPI)
Neonatal Perception I. (NPI)
Neonatal Withdrawal I. (NWI)
Pediatric Evaluation of Disability I.
> (PEDI)
peer conformity i.
Spielberger State-Trait I.
Spielberger State-Trait Anxiety I.
> (STAI)
standardized reading i.
State-Trait Anxiety I. (STAI)
Weinberger Adjustment I. (WAI)

Inventory-Adolescent
> Minnesota Multiphasic
> Personality I.-A. (MMPI-A)

inverse
> i. cerebellum
> i. ratio ventilation (IRV)

inversion
> appendiceal i.
> i. deformity
> i. stress tilt test
> T-wave i.
> ventricular i.

inversion-ligation appendectomy

inversus
> situs i.
> visceroatrial situs i.

inverted appendiceal stump

inverted-V mouth

inverted-Y detrusor dissection

invertogram

Invirase

involucrum, pl. **involucra**

involuntary movement

involuting nevus

involution
> spontaneous thymic i.

involutional gynecomastia

involved field (IF)

involved-field radiation

NOTES

involvement
  intrauterine i.
  pleuropulmonary i.
INVOS 3100 cerebral oximeter
IO
  intraosseous
  IO infusion
iodide
  cesium i. (CsI)
  potassium i.
  saturated solution of potassium i.
    (SSKI)
iodine
  i. povidone solution
  tincture of i.
  urinary i.
5-iodo-2′-deoxyuridine (IDU)
iodoform gauze
Iodopen
iodoquinol
iohexol
IOI
  intraosseous infusion
ionic contrast media
Ionil-T shampoo
ionized
  i. hypomagnesemia
  i. magnesium
Iontocaine
iontophoresis
  pilocarpine i.
ion trapping
IOP
  intraocular pressure
IOWA
  inattention-overactivity with aggression
IP
  intestinal permeability
IPAA
  ileal pouch-anal anastomosis
I-Paracaine
IPAT
  Institute of Personality and Ability
    Testing
IPAT Depression Scale
ipecac
  i. cardiomyopathy
  syrup of i.
  i. syrup
I-Pentolate
IPH
  idiopathic pulmonary hemorrhage
I-Phrine Ophthalmic Solution
I-Picamide
IPN
  infantile polyarteritis nodosa
IPOL poliovirus vaccine

IPPB
  intermittent positive-pressure breathing
IPPV
  intermittent positive-pressure ventilation
ipratropium
  i. bromide
  i. nebulization
ipsilateral
  i. anhidrosis
  i. anisocoria
  i. hypertropia
  i. lateral rectus muscle
  i. lung hypoplasia
  i. miosis
IPT
  inflammatory pseudotumor
IPTA
  Illinois Test of Psycholinguistic Abilities
IPV
  inactivated poliovirus vaccine
  Salk IPV
  IPV vaccine
IQ
  intelligence quotient
  Raven IQ
Ircon
IRDS
  infant respiratory distress syndrome
Ir gene
iridectomy
irides (*pl. of* iris)
iridis
  heterochromia i.
iridocyclitis
  acute i.
  chronic i.
  relapsing i.
iridodonesis
iris, pl. **irides**
  i. dilator
  i. hamartoma
  heterochromia of i.
  i. hypoplasia
  i. lesion
  i. Lisch nodule
  stellate i.
  i. vessel
iritis
  photophobic i.
iron
  i. chelation
  i. chelator
  i. deficiency
  i. dextran complex
  Enfamil with I.
  free i.
  haem i.
  i. ingestion

nonhaem i.
i. overload
plasma-free i.
i. poisoning
Similac with I.
i. supplement
total body i.
i. toxicity
unbound i.
iron-binding
i.-b. capacity
i.-b. protein
iron-catalyzed pseudoperoxidation
iron-deficiency anemia (IDA)
irradiated
irradiation
low-dose involved-field i.
low-dose splenic i.
total body i. (TBI)
irrational
irregular
i. cortex
i. menses
i. stereotyped movement
i. stereotyped vocalization
i. tooth placement
irrigant
Neosporin G.U. I.
irrigation
gastric i.
whole-bowel i. (WBI)
irritability
early morning i.
irritable
i. bowel syndrome (IBS)
i. hip
irritant
i. contact dermatitis
i. diaper dermatitis
i. receptor
irritation
i. diaper rash
meningeal i.
perineal i.
irritative vulvovaginitis
IRT
immunoreactive trypsinogen
IRV
inspiratory reserve volume
inverse ratio ventilation

IS
infant size
mucopolysaccharidosis IS
ISA
induced sputum analysis
Isaacs syndrome
ISAGA
immunosorbent agglutination assay
ISAM
infant of substance-abusing mother
ISCA
Interview Schedule for Children and
Adolescents
ischemia
cerebral i.
intestinal i.
myocardial i.
penile i.
ischemic
i. edema
i. exercise test
i. heart disease (IHD)
i. necrosis
ischiorectal
i. abscess
i. fossa
ischium, pl. **ischia**
ISCN
intensive special care nursery
ISCU
intensive special care unit
ISDN
isosorbide dinitrate
isethionate
pentamidine i.
Is gene
ISHT
International Society for Heart
Transplantation
island
epimyoepithelial i.
i. flap
islander
Pacific I.
islet
i. cell adenoma
i. cell adenomatosis
i. cell antibody (ICA)
i. cell tumor
isoametropic amblyopia
isobutyric acid
Isocal HN formula

NOTES

isochromatic
isochromosome Xq
isodense lesion
isodisomy
> paternal uniparenteral i.

isoenzyme
> MB i.
> muscle-brain i.
> myocardial muscle creatine
> kinase i. (CK-MB)

isoetharine
> I. Bronkometer Aerosol
> Dey-Lute I.

isoflurane
isohemagglutinin
> anti-A i.
> anti-B i.

isoimmune
> i. hemolytic disease
> i. thrombocytopenia

isoimmunization
> blood group i.
> Rh i.

Isojima test
isolate
isolated
> i. cleft palate
> i. congenital folate malabsorption
> (ICFM)
> i. diffuse mesangial sclerosis
> (IDMS)
> i. gonadotropin deficiency
> i. growth hormone deficiency
> (IGHD)
> i. hypogonadotropic hypogonadism
> (IHH)
> i. TGA

isolating
isolation
> social i.

isolette
> humidified i.
> temperature-controlled i.

isoleucine
isomerase
> triose phosphate i. (TPI)

isomerism
isometric
> i. quadriceps exercise

Isomil
> I. DE, DF, SF formula
> I. with Iron formula

isomorphic presentation
isonatremia
isonatremic dehydration
isoniazid (INH)
isonicotinic acid hydrazide (INH)
isoperistaltic intestinal interposition

Isoprinosine
isopropanol
isopropyl alcohol
isoproterenol
> Arm-a-Med I.
> Dey-Dose I.
> Dispos-a-Med I.

Isoptin SR
Isopto
> I. Atropine Ophthalmic
> I. Carpine Ophthalmic
> I. Eserine
> I. Frin Ophthalmic Solution
> I. Hyoscine

isosexual
> i. precocious puberty
> i. precocity

isosorbide dinitrate (ISDN)
IsoSource
> I. 1.5 Cal formula
> I. HN formula
> I. Standard formula

Isospora belli
isosporiasis
isosthenuria
isothiocyanate
> fluorescein i.

isotonic
> i. bolus
> i. dehydration
> i. electrolyte solution
> i. fluid
> i. saline
> i. sodium chloride

isotope scanning
isotretinoin
Isotrex
isovaleric
> i. acid
> i. acidemia
> i. aciduria

isovalericacidemia
isovaleryl-CoA dehydrogenase
isovaleryl glucuronide
isovolumic relaxation time (IVRT)
isoxsuprine
I-Soyalac formula
israelii
> *Actinomyces i.*

ISS
> idiopathic short stature
> injury severity score

isthmus
I-Sulfacet
Isuprel Injection
IT
> inspiratory time

I/T
> intensity/time
>> I/T ratio

ITC
> infrared thermographic calorimetry

itch
> Absorbine Jock I.
> ground i.
> swimmer's i.

itchiness
itching
> perineal i.

itch-scratch cycle
Itch-X
> I.-X gel
> I.-X spray

ITMg
> intratracheal magnesium

Ito
> hypomelanosis of I.
> nevus of I.
> I. nevus

ITP
> idiopathic thrombocytopenic purpura
> immune thrombocytopenic purpura
>> acute childhood ITP
>> chronic ITP
>> recurrent ITP

ITPV
> intratracheal pulmonary ventilation

itraconazole
I-Tropine Ophthalmic
ITW
> idiopathic toe walking

IU
> immunizing unit
> International Unit
> intrauterine
> in utero

IUD
> intrauterine device

IUDE
> in utero drug exposure

IUGR
> intrauterine growth restriction
> intrauterine growth retardation
>> asymmetric IUGR
>> symmetric IUGR

IUI
> intrauterine infection

IV
> intravenous
> IV anti-D therapy
> astrocytoma (grade I–IV)
> factor IV
> scalp IV

I.V.
> Hyperstat I.V.
> Indocin I.V.
> Vasotec I.V.

IVA
> integrated visual and auditory
>> IVA visual consistency test

IVAP
> in vitro antibody production

IVC
> indwelling venous catheter
> inferior vena cava

IVD
> intervertebral disk
> intravenous drip
>> Quantikine IVD

Iveegam
Ivemark syndrome
ivermectin
IVGG
> intravenous gamma globulin

IVH
> intraventricular hemorrhage (grade I–IV)

IVI
> intravaginal insemination

IVIG, IVIg
> intravenous immune globulin
> intravenous immunoglobulin

IVL
> indwelling venous line

IVP
> intravenous pyelogram
>> genitogram with IVP
>> genitogram without IVP

IVRT
> isovolumic relaxation time

IVU
> intravenous urography

IVUS
> intravascular ultrasound

Ixodes
> *I. pacificus*
> *I. persulcatus*
> *I. ricinus*
> *I. scapularis*

NOTES

JA
    juvenile arthritis
jabbering
Jaccoud deformity
jacket
    body j.
    fiberglass j.
    Orthoplast j.
    yellow j.'s
jackknife seizure
jacksonian
    j. epilepsy
    j. march
    j. seizure
Jackson-Weiss syndrome
Jacobsen syndrome
Jacquet
    J. erosive diaper dermatitis
    J. erythema
Jadassohn
    nevus of J.
Jadassohn-Lewandowski syndrome
Jaffe-Lichtenstein syndrome
JAG1
    human jagged-1 gene
Jag Tycker Jag Ar self-esteem questionnaire
Jakob-Creutzfeldt (JC)
    J.-C. syndrome
Jamaican vomiting sickness
jamais vu
James syndrome
Janeway lesion
Janimine
Jansen
    J. metaphyseal chondrodysplasia
    J. syndrome
Jansky-Bielschowsky
    J.-B. disease
    J.-B. neural ceroid lipofuscinosis
    J.-B. syndrome
Janus syndrome
Janz syndrome
Japanese
    J. B encephalitis virus
    J. encephalitis
japonica
    Rickettsia j.
japonicum
    Schistosoma j.
Jarcho-Levin syndrome
jargon
Jarisch-Herxheimer reaction
JAS
    juvenile ankylosing spondylitis

Jatene
    J. arterial switch procedure
    J. operation
    J. valve
jaundice
    benign j.
    breastfeeding j.
    breast-milk j.
    cholestatic j.
    neonatal cholestatic j.
    physiologic j.
    prolonged j.
javanica
jaw
    j. deformity
    j. deviation
    j. jerk
    lumpy j.
    j. myoclonus
    small j.
    j. thrust
    j. thrust-spine stabilization maneuver
JC
    Jakob-Creutzfeldt
    joint contracture
    polyomavirus JC
    JC syndrome
    JC virus
JDM
    juvenile dermatomyositis
    juvenile-onset diabetes mellitus
    amyopathic JDM
    new-onset JDM
JDMS
    juvenile dermatomyositis
Jefferson fracture
jejunal
    j. atresia
    j. biopsy
    j. ulcer
jejuni
    Campylobacter fetus j.
jejunitis
    necrotizing j.
jejunoileal
    j. atresia
    j. bypass
jejunojejunal anastomosis
jejunostomy
jejunum
    distal j.
    proximal j.
    villous atrophy of j.

J

jelly
    petroleum j.
    Wharton j.
Jenamicin
Jensen syndrome
jerk
    infantile myoclonic j.
    jaw j.
    myoclonic j.
    j. nystagmus
Jervell-Lange-Nielsen syndrome
Jervell syndrome
Jeryl Lynn mumps strain
JET
    junctional ectopic tachycardia
jet
    j. nebulizer
    pulsatile air j.
    j. ventilation
    j. ventilator
Jeune
    J. syndrome
    J. thoracic dystrophy
Jevity Plus formula
Jew
    Ashkenazi J.
    Sephardic J.
JGCT
    juvenile granulosa cell tumor
    juxtaglomerular cell tumor
JIA
    juvenile idiopathic arthritis
jitteriness
jitters
jittery baby
JMML
    juvenile myelomonocytic leukemia
Jo-1 antibody
Job syndrome
JODM
    juvenile-onset diabetes mellitus
jogger's ankle
Johanson-Blizzard syndrome
joint
    AC j.
    acromioclavicular j.
    j. attention
    j. bleed
    j. capsule
    Charcot j.
    Clutton j.
    j. compression
    j. contracture (JC)
    cricoarytenoid j.
    j. degeneration
    diarthrodial j.
    j. fusion
    Gaffney j.
    Gillette j.
    glenohumeral j.
    hyperextensible j.
    hypermobile j.
    hyperplastic j.
    lax j.
    j. laxity
    j. line tenderness
    metacarpophalangeal j.
    metatarsophalangeal j.
    naviculocuneiform j.
    neural arch j.
    Oklahoma ankle j.
    painful j.
    Select j.
    septic j.
    j. stability
    j. suppuration
    swollen j.
    synovial j.
    temporomandibular j. (TMJ)
JOMID
    juvenile-onset multisystem inflammatory disease
Jones
    J. procedure
    J. rheumatic fever diagnostic criteria
    J. stress fracture
    J. wedge metroplasty
Josephs-Diamond-Blackfan syndrome
Joshi criteria
Joubert syndrome (type B)
J-pouch
JR
    Aerolate JR
Jr.
    Caltrate, Jr.
    EpiPen Jr.
    Nutren Jr.
    Peptamen Jr.
JRA
    juvenile rheumatoid arthritis (type I, II)
    pauciarticular-onset JRA
    polyarticular JRA
J-shaped sella
J tracking
Juberg-Marsidi syndrome
Judkins catheter
jughandle view
jugular
    j. bulb catheter
    j. bulb catheterization
    j. bulb monitoring
    j. shunt
    j. vein
    j. vein thrombosis
    j. venous A wave

j. venous cannulation
j. venous pulse
jugulovenous distention (JVD)
jumped facet
jumper's knee
junction
cervicomedullary j.
corticomedullary j.
costochondral j.
dermoepidermal j.
dioesophageal j.
gap j.
gastroesophageal j.
gray-white j.
lumbosacral j.
mesencephalic-diencephalic j.
mucocutaneous j.
neuromuscular j. (NMJ)
pontomedullary j.
sternochondral j.
striatothalamic j.
ureteropelvic j. (UPJ)
junctional
j. ectopic tachycardia (JET)
j. epidermolysis bullosa
j. nevus
j. rhythm
j. tachycardia
jungle gym
Junin virus
justice
distributive j.
immanent j.
juvenile
j. absence epilepsy
j. aldosteronism
j. Alexander disease
j. amaurotic idiocy
j. amyotrophic lateral sclerosis
j. ankylosing spondylitis (JAS)
j. arthritis (JA)
j. avascular necrosis
j. cataract
j. chronic arthritis
j. colonic polyp
j. dermatomyositis (JDM, JDMS)
j. dystonic lipidosis
j. fibroadenoma
j. GM$_2$ gangliosidosis
j. granulosa cell tumor (JGCT)
j. granulosa cell tumor of ovary
j. hereditary motor neuron disease

j. idiopathic arthritis (JIA)
j. idiopathic polyarticular arthritis
j. idiopathic scoliosis
j. melanoma
j. metachromatic leukodystrophy
j. MLD
j. muscular dystrophy
j. muscular torticollis
j. myasthenia
j. myelomonocytic leukemia (JMML)
j. myoclonic epilepsy
j. myotonic dystrophy
j. nasopharyngeal angiofibroma
j. NCL
j. neural ceroid lipofuscinosis
j. neuronopathic Gaucher disease
j. onset
j. osteomalacia
j. osteoporosis
j. Paget disease
j. Parkinson disease
j. periodontitis
j. pernicious anemia
j. pilocytic astrocytoma
j. plantar dermatitis
j. plantar dermatosis
j. polymyositis
j. psoriatic arthritis
j. rheumatoid arthritis (type I, II) (JRA)
j. spinal muscular atrophy
j. systemic granulomatosis
j. tabes
j. tibia vara
j. Tillaux fracture
J. Wellness and Health Survey (JWHS)
j. xanthogranuloma (JXG)
j. X-linked retinoschisis
juvenile-onset
j.-o. diabetes
j.-o. diabetes mellitus (JDM, JODM)
j.-o. inflammatory bowel disease
j.-o. multisystem inflammatory disease (JOMID)
juvenilis
arcus j.
kyphoscoliosis dorsalis j.
kyphosis dorsalis j.
osteochondritis deformans j.

NOTES

J

juvenilis *(continued)*
    osteodystrophia j.
    verruca plana j.
juxtaarticular osteopenia
juxtacardiac
juxtaductal aortic coarctation
juxtaglomerular
    j. apparatus hypertrophy
    j. cell tumor (JGCT)

juxtamedullary
juxtapleural inflammatory lesion
juxtapose
JVD
    jugulovenous distention
JWHS
    Juvenile Wellness and Health Survey
JXG
    juvenile xanthogranuloma

K
  potassium
    K coefficient
    K diet
    K values
K+ 8
K+ 10
K+2 diet
KABC
  Kaufman Assessment Battery for
  Children
Kabikinase
Kabuki make-up syndrome
Kahn
    K. approach
    K. test
kala azar
Kalcinate Cal Plus
kaliuresis
kallikrein
kallikrein-kinin system
Kallmann syndrome
kanamycin
kangaroo
    k. care
    k. contact
    K. enteral feeding pump
Kanner syndrome
kansasii
    Mycobacterium k.
Kaochlor
Kaochlor-Eff
Kaodene
Kao Lectrolyte
kaolin and pectin
Kaon
    S-F K.
Kaon-Cl
Kaopectate
    K. Advanced Formula
    Children's K.
    K. II
    K. Maximum Strength
Kao-Spen
Kapectolin
Kaplan-Meier
    K.-M. method
    K.-M. survival curve
Kaposi
    K. sarcoma (KS)
    K. sarcoma-associated herpesvirus
    K. varicelliform eruption
    K. varicelliform sarcoma
kaposiform hemangioendothelioma

Kaposi-like form of infantile
  hemangioma
kappa coefficient
Karidium
Karigel
Karigel-N
Karo syrup
Kartagener syndrome
karyorrhexis
karyotype
    chromosomal k.
    G-banded k.
    XO k.
    XXY k.
    46 XY k.
karyotyping
    spectral k. (SKY)
Kasabach-Merritt
    K.-M. phenomenon
    K.-M. syndrome
Kasai
    K. operation
    K. peritoneal venous shunt
    K. portoenterostomy
    K. procedure
Kashin-Beck disease
Kasof
Katayama fever
Kato
Katoxin
Katz-Wachtel criterion
Kaufman
    K. Assessment Battery for Children
    (KABC)
    K. Factor Score
    K. Survey of Early Academic and
    Language Skills (K-SEALS)
    K. syndrome
    K. Test of Educational
    Achievement (K-TEA)
kava kava
Kawasaki
    K. disease
    K. syndrome (KS)
Kaybovite-1000
Kay Ciel
Kayexalate
Kaylixir
Kayser-Fleischer ring
Kaznelson syndrome
kcal
    kilocalorie
K+ Care ET
K-cell

KCl
 potassium chloride
kDNA
 kinetoplast deoxyribonucleic acid
K-Dur
Kearns-Sayre syndrome (KSS)
keel chest
Keflex
Keflin
Keftab
Kefurox Injection
Kefzol
Keipert syndrome
Keith-Wagener retinopathy
K-Electrolyte
Kell
 K. antigen
 K. series
Kelley-Seegmiller syndrome
keloid
Kempsey
 hemoglobin K.
Kenacort Oral
Kenaject Injection
Kenalog
 K. Injection
 K. in Orabase
 K. Topical
Kendall
 K. coefficient
 K. double-lumen catheter
Kenny-Caffey syndrome
Kenny syndrome
Kenonel Topical
Kent Infant Development Scale
keratan sulfate
keratinization
keratinized cyst
keratinizing nasopharyngeal carcinoma
keratinocyte growth factor receptor (KGFR)
keratinous
 k. debris
 k. plug
keratitis
 Acanthamoeba k.
 bacterial k.
 dendritic k.
 disciform k.
 epithelial k.
 herpes k.
 k., ichthyosis, deafness (KID)
 k., ichthyosis, deafness syndrome
 interstitial k.
 neurotrophic k.
 punctate epithelial k.
 k. sicca

 syphilitic k.
 transient k.
keratoconjunctivitis
 epidemic k. (EKC)
 microsporidial k.
 k. sicca
 tuberculous k.
keratoconus
keratocyst
 odontogenic k.
keratocyte
keratoderma
 k. blennorrhagicum
 mutilating k.
 palmoplantar k.
 k. palmoplantaris transgrediens
keratolysis
 k. neonatorum
 pitted k.
keratoma hereditarium mutilans
keratomalacia
keratopathy
 band k.
 herpetic k.
keratosis
 crusting telangiectasia k.
 k. follicularis
 k. palmaris
 k. palmaris et plantaris
 k. pilaris
keratotic
 k. debris
 k. papule
 k. scaling
kerion formation
Kerley B lines
kernicterus
Kernig sign
Kernohan sign
Keshan disease
Ketalar
ketamine sedation
ketanserin
ketoacid
 k. accumulation
 branched chain k.
 serum k.
 urine k.
ketoacidosis
 diabetic k. (DKA)
 severe k.
ketoaciduria
 branched-chain k.
ketoconazole
ketogenic diet
ketone
 k. body
 k. production

ketonemia
ketonuria
 branched-chain k.
ketorolac tromethamine
ketosis
 starvation k.
ketosis-prone diabetes
ketosis-resistant diabetes
ketotic
 k. hyperglycinemia
 k. hypoglycemia
ketotifen
keyhole pupil
Key-Pred Injection
Key-Pred-SP Injection
kg
 kilogram
K-G Elixir
K-Gen
KGFR
 keratinocyte growth factor receptor
KHD
 kinky-hair disease
Kibrick method
Kibuchi histocytic necrotizing lymphadenitis
Kicker Pavlik harness
KID
 keratitis, ichthyosis, deafness
 KID syndrome
kid
 Caladryl for K.'s
 K.'s Eating Disorder Survey
Kid-EXB 2 child's chair for bus transport
Kid-EXO 2 child's chair
Kid-Kart
kidney
 Ask-Upmark k.
 duplex k.
 dysplastic k.
 k. failure
 horseshoe k.
 hydronephrotic k.
 hypoplastic k.
 k. internal splint/stent (KISS)
 medullary sponge k.
 multicystic k.
 multicystic dysplastic k. (MDK)
 palpable k.
 palpably enlarged k.
 pelvic k.

 k. pole
 polycystic k.
 solitary k.
 k. stone
 supernumerary k.
 k. transplantation
 k.'s, ureters, bladder (KUB)
Kienböck disease
Kiesselbach
 K. area
 K. plexus
Kikuchi disease
killed virus vaccine
killer
 k. cell
 natural k. (NK)
kilocalorie (kcal)
kilogram (kg)
kilohms
kilovolt (kV)
kilowatt (kW)
Kimmelstiel-Wilson
 K.-W. disease
 K.-W. syndrome
Kimura procedure
kinase
 creatine k. (CK)
 phosphoglycerate k. (PGK)
 protein k. C
 pyruvate k. (PK)
 tyrosine k.
 viral thymidine k.
Kindercal formula
kindergarten
kindling
Kinesed
kinesigenic paroxysmal dyskinesia
kinesthesia
kinesthetic learner
kinetic
kinetoplast
 k. deoxyribonucleic acid (kDNA)
 k. DNA
King
 K. classification
 K. operation
kingae
 Haemophilus aphrophilus,
 Actinobacillus
 actinomycetemcomitans,
 Cardiobacterium hominis,

K

NOTES

kingae (continued)
    Eikenella corrodens, Kingella
        kingae (HACEK)
    Kingella k.
Kingella kingae
kinin
kininogen
    high molecular weight k. (HMWK)
kinky-hair
    k.-h. disease (KHD)
    k.-h. syndrome
Kinney Sticks
Kinsbourne syndrome
Kinyoun
    K. acid-fast stain
    K. acid-fast staining test
    K. carbol fuchsin stain
Kionex
Kirby-Bauer method
Kirner disease
Kirschner wire
KISS
    kidney internal splint/stent
kiss
    angel's k.
kissing
    k. disease
    k. patella
kit
    Coat-a-Count neonatal 17
        hydroxyprogesterone k.
    FACE k.
    Ferritin IRMA k.
    Ovudate fertility test k.
    Perkin Elmer rhodamine dye
        terminator k.
    PNEUMOTEST k.
KL-6 mucinous glycoprotein
K-Lease
Klebsiella pneumoniae
kleeblattschädel
    k. deformity
    k. syndrome
Kleihauer-Betke
    K.-B. stain
    K.-B. test
Kleihauer stain
Kleine-Levin syndrome
Klein-Waardenburg syndrome
kleptomania
Klinefelter syndrome
Klippel-Feil syndrome
Klippel-Trenaunay syndrome
Klippel-Trenaunay-Weber syndrome
Klonopin
K-Lor
Klor-Con
Klor-Con/25

Kloromint Oral
Klorvess
Klotrix
Klumpke
    K. brachial palsy
    K. paralysis
K-Lyte/Cl
K-Lyte DS
knee
    k. angle
    anterior translation of k.
    breaststroker's k.
    k. height measuring device
    k. hinge
    housemaid's k.
    k. jerk reflex
    k. joint hyperextensibility
    jumper's k.
knee-ankle-foot orthosis
knee-chest position
kneel-stand position
knemometry
Kniest
    K. dwarfism
    K. dysplasia
    K. syndrome
knob
    aortic k.
knock
    pericardial k.
knock-knee
knockout
    alpha k.
K-Norm
Koate-HP
Koate-HS
Kobberling-Dunnigan
Köbner phenomenon
Kocher-Debré-Sémélaigne syndrome
Koch pouch diversion
Koebner
    K. epidermolysis bullosa simplex
    K. reaction
    K. response
Koenen tumor
Koerber-Salus-Elschnig syndrome
Koffex DM
KOH
    potassium hydroxide
Köhler bone disease
Kohn canal
koilonychia
Kolobow membrane lung
Kolyum K-Tab
Konakion
Kondremul
Konsyl

Konsyl-D
Konyne 80
konzo
Koplik spot
Korean hemorrhagic fever
Korotkoff
    K. phase
    K. sound
koseri
    Citrobacter k.
Kostmann
    K. disease
    K. neutropenia
    K. syndrome
Koyanagi procedure
Kozlowski spondylometaphyseal dysplasia
K-Phos
    K-P. M.F.
    K-P. Neutral
    K-P. Original
Krabbe
    K. disease
    K. leukodystrophy
Krebs cycle
Kreiselman unit
Kremer test
Kristalose
krusei
    Candida k.
Kruskal-Wallis (KW)
    K.-W. test
KS
    Kaposi sarcoma
    Kawasaki syndrome
K-SADS
    Schedule for Affective Disorders and
    Schizophrenia for School-Age Children
K-SADS-E
    Schedule for Affective Disorders and
    Schizophrenia for School-Age Children-
    Epidemiologic Version
K-SADS-P
    Schedule for Affective Disorders and
    Schizophrenia for School-Age Children-
    Present Episode
K-SEALS
    Kaufman Survey of Early Academic and
    Language Skills

KSS
    Kearns-Sayre syndrome
K-Tab
    Kolyum K-T.
K-TEA
    Kaufman Test of Educational
    Achievement
KUB
    kidneys, ureters, bladder
Kufs disease
Kugelberg-Welander (KW)
    K.-W. disease
Küntscher rod
Kupffer
    K. cell
    K. cell hyperplasia
kuru
    k. disease
Kurzrok-Miller test
Kussmaul
    K. respiration
    K. sign
Ku-Zyme HP
kV
    kilovolt
KW
    Kruskal-Wallis
    Kugelberg-Welander
    KW disease
    KW test
kW
    kilowatt
kwashiorkor
    dermatosis of k.
    k. disease
Kwell shampoo
Kyasanur Forest disease
kynurenine hydroxylation
kyphoscoliosis dorsalis juvenilis
kyphosis
    congenital k.
    dorsal k.
    k. dorsalis juvenilis
    flexible k.
    Scheuermann juvenile k.
    thoracic k.
    thoracolumbar k.
Kytril Injection

K

NOTES

L-A
    Bicillin L-A
LA
  latex agglutination
    Guaifenex LA
    Inderal LA
    Zephrex LA
L.A.
    Humibid L.A.
    Theoclear L.A.
la
    la belle indifference
    La Crosse encephalitis
    La Crosse virus
    La Leche League
LA:Ao
  left atrial to aortic
    LA:Ao ratio
labeling
labetalol
labia (*pl. of* labium)
labial
    l. adhesion
    l. fusion
    l. hypertrophy
    l. traction technique
labialis
    herpes l.
    herpes simplex l.
labile
    l. asthma
    l. factor
lability
    emotional l.
    mood l.
labiodental speech sound
labioscrotal
    l. fusion
    l. Y-V plasty
labium, pl. labia
    labia majora
    l. majus
    l. minus, pl. labia minora
labor
    precipitous l.
    premature l.
laboratory
    gait l.
    Venereal Disease Research L.
      (VDRL)
labrum
    acetabular l.
labyrinth
labyrinthine
    l. afferent input

    l. concussion
    l. reflex
    l. stimulation
labyrinthitis
    acute l.
    bacterial l.
    progressive l.
    suppurative l.
    traumatic l.
LAC
  La Crosse
laceration
    cerebral l.
    posterior pharyngeal l.
    suture penile l.
    tentorial l.
Lachman test
Lac-Hydrin
lack of natural killer cell
Lacri-Lube SOP
lacrima
lacrimal
    l. bone
    l. duct
    l. duct obstruction
    l. duct stenosis
    l. gland
    l. sac distention
    l. sac massage
lacrimation
lacrimoauriculodentodigital syndrome
La Crosse (LAC)
lactacidemia
lactacidosis
LactAid
    L. device
    L. STARTrainer Nursing System
lactalbumin
    alpha l. (ALA)
lactamase
    beta l.
lactase
    congenital absence of l.
    l. deficiency
lactate
    ammonium l.
    amrinone l.
    arterial l.
    blood l.
    l. dehydrogenase (LDH)
    l. dehydrogenase deficiency
    plasma l.
    Ringer's l.
lactating
lactation

L

lacteal
> crusta l.

lactic
> l. acid
> l. acidemia
> l. acidosis

Lacticare
LactiCare-HC Topical
lactiferous duct
Lactina Select breast pump
Lactinex
Lactobacillus
> *L. acidophilus*
> *L. bifidus*
> *L. bulgaricus*
> *L. fermentum*
> *L. gasseri*
> *L. plantarum*
> *L. rhamnosus*
> *L. rhamnosus* strain GG (L-GG)

lactobacillus
> *l.* GG

lactobezoar
lactobionate
> erythromycin l.

lactoferrin
> plasma l.

Lactofree
> L. formula

Lactogen FP formula
lactoovovegetarian
lactose
> l. breath hydrogen test
> l. deficiency
> l. intolerance
> l. malabsorption
> l. monohydrate
> l. tolerance test

lactose-containing formula
lactose-free formula
Lactosorb
lactovegetarian
lactulose
> L. PSE

lacunar
LAD
> left anterior descending
> leukocyte adhesion deficiency

LAD-1
> leukocyte adhesion deficiency-1

LAD-2
> leukocyte adhesion deficiency-2

Ladd
> L. band
> L. monitor
> L. operation
> L. procedure
> L. syndrome

Laerdal mask (0–2)
lafaxine
Lafora
> L. body
> L. body disease

laforin
lag
> head l.
> lid l.

lagophthalmos
LA-HFOV
> liquid-assisted high-frequency oscillatory ventilation

lait
lake
> venous l.

lallation
LALT
> larynx-associated lymphoid tissue

LAM
> laser-assisted myringotomy

LAMB
> lentigines, atrial myxomas, cutaneous papular myxomas, blue nevi
> LAMB syndrome

lambdoid synostosis
Lambert canal
Lambert-Eaton syndrome
lamblia
> *Giardia l.*

lamellar
> l. body (LB)
> l. body number density
> l. bone
> l. ichthyosis
> l. inclusion body

lamellated appearance
Lamictal
lamina, pl. **laminae**
> basal l.
> l. cribrosa
> duplicated elastic l.
> elastic l.
> l. lucida
> l. propria
> l. terminalis

laminar airflow
Lamisil
lamivudine (3TC)
lamotrigine
lamp
> halogen l.
> Wood ultraviolet l.

Lamprene
Lanacane
Lanacaps
> Ferralyn L.

Lanacort Topical

lance
  heel l. (HL)
Lancefield typing system
lancet
  Quikheel l.
Landau
  L. reflex
  L. response
  L. test
Landau-Kleffner
  L.-K. syndrome (LKS)
  L.-K. syndrome variant
Landmark catheter
Landouzy-Dejerine muscular dystrophy
Landouzy dystrophy
Landry
  L. type
  L. type of paralysis
Landry-Guillain-Barré syndrome
Lange-Nielsen syndrome
Langer
  L. mesomelic dwarfism
  L. mesomelic dysplasia
Langer-Giedion syndrome
Langerhans
  L. cell
  L. cell histiocytosis (LCH)
Langhans giant cell
language
  American Sign L. (ASL)
  body l.
  l. delay
  l. development
  l. disorder
  l. domain
  expressive l.
  receptive l.
  sign l.
Laniazid Oral
lanolin
Lanophyllin
Lanoxicaps
Lanoxin
lansoprazole
lanuginosa
  hypertrichosis l.
lanuginous
lanugo hair
Lanz incision
LAO
  left anterior oblique

laparoscopic
  l. fundoplication (LF)
  l. laser-assisted autoaugmentation
laparoscopically assisted anorectoplasty
laparoscopy
laparotomy
  salvage l.
lap belt complex
LAR
  laryngeal adductor reflex
  late asthmatic response
large
  l. B-cell lymphoma
  l. bowel stasis
  l. cell anaplastic Ki-1 lymphoma
  l. cell immunoblastic lymphoma
  l. foreskin
  l. for gestational age (LGA)
  l. intestine
  l. lysosome-like granule
  l. tongue
large-bore catheter
large-volume
  l.-v. blood study
  l.-v. nonobstruction
L-arginine
lari
  Campylobacter l.
Larodopa
Laron syndrome
Laron-type dwarfism
Larsen syndrome
larval granulomatosis
larvicide
laryngeal
  l. adductor reflex (LAR)
  l. atresia
  l. atresia syndrome
  l. chemoreflex
  l. cleft
  l. closure
  l. diphtheria
  l. edema
  l. fracture
  l. mask airway (LMA)
  l. nerve
  l. nerve paralysis
  l. papilloma
  l. papillomatosis
  l. paresis
  l. spasm
  l. stenosis

NOTES

laryngeal *(continued)*
  l. stridor
  l. vagal reflex
  l. wart
  l. web
larynges (*pl. of* larynx)
laryngitis
  acute spasmodic l.
  viral l.
laryngologist
laryngomalacia
laryngopharyngeal
  l. sensory stimulation (LPSS)
  l. sensory stimulation testing
laryngopharynx
laryngoscope
  l. blade
  l. handle
  Pentax l.
  Siker l.
laryngoscopy
  direct l.
  indirect l.
  mirror l.
laryngospasm
laryngotracheal
  l. reconstruction
  l. stenosis (LTS)
laryngotracheitis
laryngotracheobronchitis
  bacterial l.
  membranous l.
  viral l.
laryngotracheoesophageal cleft
larynx, pl. **larynges**
  atresia of l.
  floppy l.
larynx-associated lymphoid tissue (LALT)
laser
  l. ablation
  carbon dioxide l.
  flashlamp-pulsed dye l.
  l. myringotomy
  l. office ventilation of ears (LOVE)
  l. office ventilation of ears with insertion of tubes (LOVE IT)
  l. photocoagulation
  l. surgery
laser-assisted myringotomy (LAM)
Lasix
  L. Injection
  L. Oral
L-asparaginase
Lassa
  L. fever
  L. virus

La/SSB antigen
last menstrual period (LMP)
LAT
  lateral atrial tunnel
  lidocaine, adrenaline, tetracaine
lata (*pl. of* latum)
latching-on process
late
  l. apnea
  l. arrhythmia
  l. asthmatic response (LAR)
  l. complication
  l. complication of transfusion
  l. congenital syphilis
  l. deceleration
  l. hemorrhagic disease
  l. hypocalcemia
  l. infantile amaurotic idiocy
  l. infantile MLD
  l. infantile NCL
  l. infantile neural ceroid lipofuscinosis (LINCL)
  l. luteal phase syndrome
  l. mature
  l. neonatal hypocalcemia
  l. phase
  l. radiation encephalopathy
latency
  interpeak l.
  REM l.
  response l.
  sleep l.
latent
  l. celiac disease
  l. class analysis (LCA)
  l. diabetes
  l. infection
  l. nystagmus
late-onset
  l.-o. congenital large ectopic gland
  l.-o. hypogammaglobulinemia
  l.-o. SED
  l.-o. sepsis
lateral
  l. atrial tunnel (LAT)
  l. atrial tunnel cavopulmonary anastomosis
  l. collateral ligament complex
  l. compartment
  l. condylar fracture
  l. condyle
  l. curvature
  l. curvature of spine
  l. displacement of inner canthus
  l. epicondylitis
  l. femoral torsion (LFT)
  l. geniculate
  l. geniculate body

l. head-righting
l. head tilt
l. hip rotation
l. incisor
l. lemniscus
l. luxation
l. malleolus
l. radiograph
l. rectus muscle
l. rectus palsy
l. rotation (LR)
l. shoulder sway
l. sinus thrombosis
l. tibial bowing
l. tibial torsion (LTT)
l. view

lateralis
vastus l.

laterality
l. defect
l. disorder

lateralization process
lateralizing sign
laterothoracic exanthem
latex
l. agglutination (LA)
l. agglutination assay
l. fixation test
l. particle agglutination
l. particle agglutination test
l. test for *Pneumococcus*

lathyrism
lato
Borrelia burgdorferi sensu l.

latrodectism
LATS
long-acting thyroid stimulator
LATS hormone

latum, pl. **lata**
condylomata lata
Diphyllobothrium l.

Laudanum
Lauenstein
L. lateral radiograph
L. pelvic x-ray

Lauge-Hansen mechanism of injury
Laugier-Hunziker syndrome
Launois-Cléret syndrome
Laurell rocket immune electrophoresis
Laurence-Moon-Bardet-Biedl syndrome
Laurence-Moon-Biedl (LMB)
L.-M.-B. syndrome

lavage
alveolar l.
antral l.
bronchoalveolar l. (BAL)
bronchopulmonary l.
diagnostic peritoneal l. (DPL)
gastric l.
nasal l.
nonbronchoscopic bronchoalveolar l.
oral colonic l. (OCL)
pulmonary l.
saline l.
surfactant l.
therapeutic pulmonary l.
tracheal l.

law
Collins l.
Public L. 93-247
Public L. 94-142
Public L. 99-457
Public L. 101-336

Lawrence-Seip syndrome
lax
l. joint
l. ligament

laxa
acquired cutis l.
cutis l.

laxative
Fleet L.

laxity
anteroposterior l.
joint l.
ligamentous l.
suspensory ligament l.

layer
Bowman l.
l. of Brun
buffy-coat l.

LazerSporin-C Otic
lazy
l. bladder syndrome
l. eye
l. leukocyte syndrome

LB
lamellar body

LBM
lean body mass

LBW
low birth weight
LBW infant

NOTES

LBWC
   limb-body wall complex
LCA
   latent class analysis
LCAD
   long-chain acyl-CoA dehydrogenase
LCAD/MCAD
   long- and medium-chain fatty acid
    coenzyme-A dehydrogenase deficiency
LCAD/VLCAD
   long- and very-long-chain acyl-CoA
    dehydrogenase
     LCAD/VLCAD deficiency
L-carnitine
LCD
   liquor carbonis detergens
    LCD cream
    LCD ointment
LCH
   Langerhans cell histiocytosis
LCHAD
   long-chain 3-hydroxyacyl-CoA
    dehydrogenase
   long-chain hydroxyacyl-coenzyme A
    dehydrogenase
     LCHAD deficiency
LCL
   localized cutaneous leishmaniasis
LCMV
   lymphocytic choriomeningitis virus
    LCMV syndrome
LCP
   Legg-Calvé-Perthes
LCPD
   Legg-Calvé-Perthes disease
LCPUFA
   long-chain polyunsaturated fatty acid
LCR
   ligase-chain reaction
    LCR assay
LD
   learning disability
LDH
   lactate dehydrogenase
LDL
   low-density lipoprotein
    LDL apheresis
L-dopa
LE
   lower extremity
    LE cell preparation
Le
   L. Fort fracture
   L. Fort fracture pattern
LEA
   local education agency
lead
   l. agency

augmented voltage unipolar left arm l. (aVL)
augmented voltage unipolar left foot l. (aVF)
augmented voltage unipolar right arm l. (aVR)
blood l.
l. bra
l. encephalopathy
l. exposure
l. II, III
l. ingestion
l. intoxication
limb l.
l. line
organic l.
l. pipe stiffness
l. point
l. poisoning
tetraethyl l.
l. triphosphate
l. wire
Leadcare handheld blood lead analyzer
leaf
leaflet
   flail mitral l. (FML)
league
   La Leche L.
leak
   air l.
   capillary l.
   cerebrospinal fluid l.
lean body mass (LBM)
learner
   active l.
   auditory l.
   kinesthetic l.
   visual l.
learning
   l. disability (LD)
   discrete-trial l.
   l. disorder
   Mullen Scales of Early L. (MSEL)
   situated l.
   slow rate of l.
   l. style
   wide range assessment of memory and l. (WRAML)
Lea shield
least restrictive environment (LRE)
Leber
   L. congenital retinal amaurosis
   L. disease
   L. hereditary atrophy
   L. hereditary optic neuropathy (LHON)
   L. optic neuropathy

LEC
    life events checklist
lecithin
    l. to sphingomyelin (L/S)
    l. to sphingomyelin ratio
Lectrolyte
    Kao L.
Ledercillin VK
LEDS
    life events and difficulties schedule
Lee-White clotting time
left
    l. anterior descending (LAD)
    l. anterior hemiblock
    l. anterior oblique (LAO)
    l. arterial pressure
    l. atrial to aortic (LA:Ao)
    l. atrial hypertrophy
    l. atrium
    l. axis deviation
    l. bundle branch block
    l. common carotid
    l. costovertebral angle
    l. ear
    l. hemisyndrome
    l. hepatectomy
    l. lateral decubitus position (LLDP)
    l. lower quadrant (LLQ)
    l. main coronary artery
    l. renal vein
    l. upper quadrant (LUQ)
    l. ventricle (LV)
    l. ventricular (LV)
    l. ventricular apical aneurysm
    l. ventricular dysfunction (LVD)
    l. ventricular ejection fraction (LVEF)
    l. ventricular end-diastolic dimension
    l. ventricular end-systolic dimension
    l. ventricular failure
    l. ventricular hypertrophy
    l. ventricular outflow tract (LVOT)
    l. ventricular outflow tract obstruction (LVOTO)
    l. ventricular outlet obstruction
    l. ventricular paced beat
    l. ventricular stroke work index (LVSWI)
    l. vertical vein

left/right
    l./r. asymmetry
    l./r. dynein
left-sided lesion
left-to-right
    l.-t.-r. shunt
    l.-t.-r. shunting
    l.-t.-r. shunt lesion
Lefty-1, -2
leg
    l. atrophy
    l. length discrepancy (LLD)
    W position of l.'s
legally blind
Legatrin
Legg-Calvé-Perthes (LCP)
    L.-C.-P. disease (LCPD)
Legg-Perthes disease
Legionella
    L. micdadei
    L. pneumophila
legionellosis
Legionnaires disease
Leiden
    factor V L.
Leigh
    L. disease
    L. necrotizing encephalomyelopathy
    L. subacute necrotizing encephalopathy
    L. syndrome
Leiner
    L. disease
    L. syndrome
leiomyoblastoma
leiomyoma
leiomyosarcoma
    epithelioid l.
Leishmania
    L. braziliensis
    L. infantum
    L. major
    L. mexicana
    L. panamensis
    L. tropica
leishmaniasis
    cutaneous l.
    diffuse cutaneous l. (DCL)
    localized cutaneous l. (LCL)
    mucosal l.
    post-kala azar dermal l. (PKDL)
    visceral l.

L

NOTES

Leiter
> L. International Performance Scale
> L. test

Lemierre syndrome

Lemli-Opitz syndrome

lemniscus, pl. **lemnisci**
> lateral l.

lemon balm

length
> birth l.
> clitoral l.
> crown-heel l.
> cycle l.
> femoral l.
> penile l.
> sinus cycle l.
> stretched penile l.
> stretched phallic l.
> subischial leg l. (SILL)
> supine l.

lengthening
> Achilles tendon l.
> Evans calcaneal l.
> hamstring l.
> l. of hamstring
> heel cord l.
> muscle l.
> l. osteotomy
> tendo Achillis l. (TAL)
> tendon l.

Lennox-Gastaut syndrome

lens
> crystalline l.
> l. dislocation
> Morgan therapeutic l.
> l. opacity
> posterior chamber intraocular l.
>   (PC-IOL)
> Sauflon PW contact l.
> Silsoft extended wear contact l.

Lente
> L. Iletin I, II
> L. L

lenticonus
> anterior l.
> posterior l.

lenticular
> l. cataract
> l. opacity

lentiform nucleus

lentigines (*pl. of* lentigo)

lentiginosis profusa

lentiginous nevus

lentigo, pl. **lentigines**
> agminated l.
> lentigines, atrial myxomas,
>   cutaneous papular myxomas, blue
>   nevi (LAMB)

> lentigines, electrocardiographic
>   abnormalities, ocular hypertelorism,
>   pulmonary stenosis, abnormalities
>   of genitalia, retardation of
>   growth, deafness (LEOPARD)
> lentigines, electrocardiographic
>   abnormalities, ocular hypertelorism,
>   pulmonary stenosis, abnormalities
>   of genitalia, retardation of
>   growth, deafness syndrome

lentis
> ectopia l.
> simple ectopia l.

lentivirus

Lenz microphthalmia syndrome

Leonard catheter

LEOPARD
> lentigines, electrocardiographic
>   abnormalities, ocular hypertelorism,
>   pulmonary stenosis, abnormalities of
>   genitalia, retardation of growth,
>   deafness
>   LEOPARD syndrome

Lepiota

Lepore hemoglobin

lepori
> *Brugia l.*

leprae
> *Mycobacterium l.*

leprechaunism

lepromatous leprosy

leprosum
> erythema nodosum l.

leprosy
> borderline lepromatous l.
> borderline tuberculoid l.
> dimorphous l.
> full lepromatous l.
> full tuberculoid l.
> indeterminate l.
> lepromatous l.
> tuberculoid l.

leptin
> cord plasma l.
> l. receptor

leptomeningeal
> l. angiomatosis
> l. cyst
> l. heterotopia

leptomeningitis
> acute syphilitic l.
> mumps l.

Leptospira
> L. canicola
> L. grippotyphosa
> L. icterohaemorrhagiae
> L. interrogans
> L. pomona

leptospiral
>   l. illness
>   l. meningitis

leptospire

leptospirosis
>   anicteric l.
>   icteric l.

leptotrichosis

LES
>   lower esophageal sphincter
>   LES pressure

Lesch-Nyhan syndrome (LNS)

lesion
>   acquired hypothalamic l.
>   acral skin l.
>   acyanotic l.
>   anesthetic skin l.
>   annular l.
>   arciform l.
>   Bankart l.
>   blanching wheal and flare l.
>   blueberry muffin skin l.
>   brain l.
>   brainstem l.
>   brown skin l.
>   cannonball l.
>   cardiac l.
>   central cord l.
>   cicatricial l.
>   clastic l.
>   clouding of l.
>   coin l.
>   collapse-consolidation l.
>   confetti l.
>   congenital l.
>   coronary artery l. (CAL)
>   correctable l.
>   crescentic l.
>   crusted l.
>   cutaneous l.
>   cyanotic congenital heart l.
>   dermatophyte l.
>   Dieulafoy l.
>   Dieulafoy gastric l.
>   discoid l.
>   discontinuous l.
>   eczematoid l.
>   eczematous skin l.
>   epileptogenic l.
>   erythematous satellite l.
>   exophytic l.
>   extrapyramidal l.

>   flaccid l.
>   gingival l.
>   heart l.
>   hypoesthesic skin l.
>   hypothalamic l.
>   iris l.
>   isodense l.
>   Janeway l.
>   juxtapleural inflammatory l.
>   left-sided l.
>   left-to-right shunt l.
>   linear l.
>   low-grade squamous
>   intraepithelial l. (LSIL)
>   lytic l.
>   macular-papular-vesicular l.
>   maculopapular l.
>   mass l.
>   metaphyseal l.
>   microvascular l.
>   mixing l.
>   morphogenetic l.
>   mucosal l.
>   multifocal white matter
>   inflammatory l.
>   multiple-ring-enhancing mass l.
>   Nelis l.
>   nodulocystic l.
>   oculocutaneous l.
>   osseous BA l.
>   osteochondrotic l.
>   palmar l.
>   papular l.
>   papulonodular l.
>   papulovesicular l.
>   parenchymal brain l.
>   pebbly skin l.
>   photodistributed l.
>   plucked chicken skin l.
>   proliferative l.
>   pseudoencapsulated l.
>   psoriasiform l.
>   punched-out lytic l.
>   pyramidal l.
>   raised l.
>   right-sided l.
>   satellite l.
>   seborrheic-looking skin l.
>   Sinding-Larsen l.
>   single ring-enhancing mass l.
>   skin l.
>   skip l.

L

NOTES

lesion *(continued)*
solitary bone l.
space-occupying l.
target l.
targetoid l.
total mixing l.
tubulointerstitial l.
umbilication of l.
upper GI l.
urticarial raised l.
Van Gehuchten l.
vascular proliferative l.
vasculitic skin l.
vesicobullous skin l.
vesicopustular l.
vesicular palmar l.
vesicular skin l.
vesiculoulcerative l.
violaceous l.
watershed l.
weeping l.
zosteriform l.
lesson
speech l.
Lester-Martin technique
LET
lidocaine, epinephrine, tetracaine
letalis
epidermolysis bullosa l.
Herlitz epidermolysis bullosa l.
let-down
lethal neonatal dwarfism
lethargic
lethargica
encephalitis l.
lethargy
postictal l.
letter chart
Letterer-Siwe disease
leucine
Leuconostoc
leucovorin
calcium l.
leukapheresis
leukemia
acute lymphatic l.
acute lymphoblastic l. (ALL)
acute lymphocytic l. (ALL)
acute megakaryoblastic l.
acute myeloblastic l.
acute myelogenous l.
acute myeloid l. (AML)
acute nonlymphoblastic l. (ANLL)
acute nonlymphocytic l.
aplastic l.
basophilic l.
central nervous system l.
chronic lymphocytic l. (CLL)

chronic myelocytic l.
chronic myelogenous l. (CML)
CNS l.
congenital l.
eosinophilic l.
granulocytic l.
hemoblastic l.
l. infiltrate
juvenile myelomonocytic l. (JMML)
leukopenic l.
lymphatic l.
lymphoblastic l.
lymphocytic l.
lymphosarcoma cell l.
mast cell l.
megakaryoblastic l.
megakaryocytic l.
micromyeloblastic l.
myeloblastic l.
myelocytic l.
myelogenous l.
myeloid l.
myelomonocytic l.
non-Hodgkin l. (NHL)
nonlymphoblastic l.
nonlymphocytic l.
promyelocytic l.
testicular l.
leukemia/lymphoma
adult T-cell l./l. (ATLL)
leukemic
l. blast
l. cell
leukemicus
hiatus l.
leukemogenesis
leukemoid reaction
Leukeran
Leukine
leukoclastic angiitis
leukocoria
leukocyte
l. adherence deficiency
l. adhesion deficiency (LAD)
l. adhesion deficiency-1 (LAD-1)
l. adhesion deficiency-2 (LAD-2)
l. adhesion deficiency 2 syndrome
diapedetic l.
l. esterase dipstick
hexamethyl propylene amine oxime l. (HMPAO)
l. histamine release test
l. infiltration
polymorphonuclear l.
leukocyte-depletion filter
leukocyte hexosaminidase A
leukocyte-removal filter

leukocytoclastic
    l. angiitis
    l. vasculitis
leukocytosis
    extreme l.
    granulocytic l.
    mild l.
    neutrophilic l.
leukocytospermia
leukocyturia
leukodepletion filter
leukoderma acquisitum centrifugum
leukodystrophy
    globoid cell l.
    juvenile metachromatic l.
    Krabbe l.
    metachromatic l. (MLD)
leukoencephalopathy
    focal pontine l.
    multifocal l.
    perinatal telencephalic l.
    progressive multifocal l. (PML)
    l. syndrome
leukoerythroblastic
leukokoria
leukomalacia
    cystic l.
    cystic periventricular l. (cPVL)
    periventricular l. (PVL)
leukopenia
leukopenic leukemia
leukoplakia
    hairy l.
    oral hairy l.
leukorrhea
    physiologic l.
leukostasis
    pulmonary l.
leukotriene
    l. C_4 (LTC$_4$)
    l. D_4 (LTD$_4$)
    l. E_4 (LTE$_4$)
    l. inhibitor
    l. receptor antagonist (LTRA)
leuprolide
leuprorelin acetate
Leustatin
levalbuterol hydrochloride
levamisole
levator palpebrae muscle
Levbid
LeVeen shunt

level
    air-fluid l.
    arousal l.
    bile chenodeoxycholic acid l.
    blood ammonia l.
    blood lead l. (BLL)
    ceruloplasmin l.
    complement C3 l.
    l. of consciousness (LOC)
    cord IgG l.
    cotinine l.
    C-peptide l.
    elevation of blood lead l. (EBLL)
    folate l.
    high gastrin l.
    immunoglobulin E l.
    magnesium l.
    operant l.
    peak l.
    peak and trough l.'s
    phosphatidylglycerol l.
    plasma ornithine l.
    plasminogen l.
    platelet calmodulin l.
    quantitative beta hCG l.
    RBC adenosine deaminase l.
    serum acetaminophen l.
    serum amylase l.
    serum anticonvulsant l.
    serum bile salt l.
    serum carotene l.
    serum copper l.
    serum cortisol l.
    serum digoxin l.
    serum histamine l.
    serum lead l.
    serum leptin l.
    sweat chloride l.
    tacrolimus l.
    therapeutic blood l.
    troponin I l.
    trough tacrolimus l.
    unconjugated estriol l.
    vitamin B_{12} l.
levetiracetam
Levlen contraceptive pill
levoamphetamine
levobunolol
levocardia
levocarnitine
levodopa
Levo-Dromoran

L

NOTES

levofloxacin
levonorgestrel
Levophed
levorphanol
Levo-T
Levothroid
    L. Injection
    L. Oral
levothyroxine test
levre de tapir
Levsin
Levsinex
Levsin/SL
Levy-Hollister syndrome
Lévy-Roussy syndrome
lexical cohesion
lexical-syntactic
    l.-s. deficit
    l.-s. syndrome (LSS)
lexicon
Leyden-Möbius muscular dystrophy
Leydig
    L. cell
    L. cell aplasia
    L. cell atrophy
    L. cell hyperplasia
    L. cell tumor
Leyton Obsessional Inventory
LF
    laparoscopic fundoplication
    low frequency
LFT
    lateral femoral torsion
LGA
    large for gestational age
L-GG
    Lactobacillus rhamnosus strain GG
LGV
    lymphogranuloma venereum
LH
    luteinizing hormone
Lhadi
Lhermitte-Duclos
    L.-D. disease
    L.-D. syndrome
Lhermitte sign
LHON
    Leber hereditary optic neuropathy
    LHON syndrome
LHR
    right lung-to-head circumference ratio
L-5 hydroxytryptophan
liability to pressure palsy
libido
Libman-Sacks
    L.-S. disease
    L.-S. endocarditis

library
    DNA l.
lice (*pl. of* louse)
licensed
    l. practical nurse (LPN)
    l. vocational nurse (LVN)
lichen
    l. nitidus
    l. planus
    l. sclerosus et atrophicus
    l. scrofulosorum
    l. simplex
    l. simplex chronicus
    l. spinulosus
    l. striatus
lichenification
lichenified plaque
lichenoides
    pityriasis l.
lichenoid papule
Lich-Gregoire technique
Liddle syndrome
Lidex
Lidex-E
lid lag
lidocaine
    l., adrenaline, tetracaine (LAT)
    buffered l.
    l. and epinephrine
    l., epinephrine, tetracaine (LET)
    l. and prilocaine
lidocaine-prilocaine cream
lidofilcon B
LidoPen I.M. Injection Auto-Injector
Lieberkuhn
    crypt of L.
lienorenal ligament
LIFE
    longitudinal interval followup evaluation
life
    day of l. (DOL)
    l. events checklist (LEC)
    l. events and difficulties schedule (LEDS)
    L. Events and Difficulty Schedule Interview
    extrauterine l.
LifeScan blood glucose meter
life-support machine
Li-Fraumeni syndrome
lift
    chin l.
    parasternal l.
ligament
    acromioclavicular l.
    anterior cruciate l. (ACL)
    anterior talofibular l. (ATFL)
    calcaneocuboid l.

calcaneofibular l. (CFL)
congenital laxity of l.
coracoclavicular l.
gastrophrenic l.
inguinal l.
lax l.
lienorenal l.
l. of Marshall
medial collateral l. (MCL)
patellar l.
phrenoesophageal l.
posterior talofibular l. (PTFL)
l. of Treitz
ulnar collateral l. (UCL)

ligamentous
l. injury (grade I–III)
l. laxity

ligamentum teres

ligase
DNA l.

ligase-chain
l.-c. reaction (LCR)
l.-c. reaction assay
l.-c. reaction testing

ligation
l. of appendix
endoscopic elastic band l.
endoscopic variceal l. (EVL)
thoracic duct l.

light
ambient l.
bilirubin l.'s
broad-spectrum white l.
l. chain
green l.
l. microscopy
narrow-spectrum blue l.
l. perception (LP)
Questran L.
super blue l.
l. therapy
ultraviolet l.

light-emitting diode

lightning
l. attack
l. pain

Lightwood-Albright syndrome

Lignac syndrome

Likert scale

LIM1 protein

limb
l. abnormality syndrome

l. actigraphy
l. atrophy
l. disproportion
efferent l.
ileal l.
l. lead
l. length inequality
phantom l.
l. salvage
short l.
vertebral, anal, cardiac, tracheal,
    esophageal, renal, l. (VACTERL)

limb-body wall complex (LBWC)

limb-girdle muscular dystrophy

limbi (*pl. of* limbus)

limbic
l. GABAergic system
l. status epilepticus
l. structure

Lim broth

limbus, pl. **limbi**

liminal

limit
l. dextrans
l. dextrinosis

limited
l. neck motion
l. support
l. systemic scleroderma

limp
antalgic l.
l. infant syndrome
psychogenic l.
Trendelenburg l.

limulus lysate test

LINCL
late infantile neural ceroid lipofuscinosis

lindane shampoo

line
arterial l.
Beau l.
Blaschko l.
Burton gum lead l.
central venous l. (CVL)
central venous pressure l.
Chamberlain l.
Dennie l
dentate l.
l. drawing
Harris growth arrest l.
Hilgenreiner l.
indwelling venous l. (IVL)

NOTES

L

line *(continued)*
intravenous l.
Kerley B l.'s
lead l.
midaxillary l.
midclavicular l.
milk l.'s
murine myeloid leukemia cell l.
Pastia l.
pectinate l.
Perkin l.
l. placement
radiolucent l.
railroad track l.
Shenton l.
tympanomastoid suture l.
tympanosquamous suture l.
umbilical venous l. (UVL)
venous l.
lineage
B-cell l.
linear
l. branching pattern
l. gingival erythema
l. growth
l. growth retardation
l. growth velocity
l. hypocalcification
l. hypoplasia
l. IgA dermatosis
l. IgA disease
l. Koebner reaction
l. lesion
l. probe
l. regression analysis
l. scleroderma
l. skull fracture
l. visual analog scale
lineogram
linezolid
lingua, pl. **linguae**
l. nigra
l. plicata
lingual
l. appliance
l. frenulum
l. surface
linguistic
linguistics
lingula
lingular effusion
linoleic acid
linolenic acid
Linton tube
Lioresal
liothyronine
LIP
lipoid interstitial pneumonitis

lymphocytic interstitial pneumonitis
lymphoid interstitial pneumonitis
lip
cleft l.
l. closure
Cupid's bow upper l.
fissured l.'s
l. pit
l. scar revision
vermilion border of l.
lipase
bile salt-stimulated l. (BSSL)
lipoprotein l. (LPL)
l. unit
lipemia
lipid
l. accumulation
l. envelope
l. inclusion
myelin l.
l. myopathy
l. peroxidation
l. storage disease
l. storage disorder
lipid-laden macrophage
lipidosis, pl. **lipidoses**
cerebroside l.
juvenile dystonic l.
lipiduria
lipiodol
Lipisorb
lipoatrophic diabetes
lipoatrophy
insulin l.
localized l.
lipoblastoma
primitive l.
lipochondrodystrophy
lipodystrophy
congenital generalized l.
generalized l.
partial l.
protease inhibitor-induced l.
lipofuscin material
lipofuscinosis
ceroid l.
Haltia-Santavuori neural ceroid l.
hypoadrenalism neural ceroid l.
infantile neural ceroid l.
Jansky-Bielschowsky neural
ceroid l.
juvenile neural ceroid l.
late infantile neural ceroid l.
(LINCL)
neural ceroid l.
neuronal ceroid l. (NCL)
Spielmeyer-Vogt neural ceroid l.
lipogenic dyshepatia

lipoglycan antigen
lipogranulomatosis
    Farber l.
    l. subcutanea
lipoid
    l. interstitial pneumonitis (LIP)
    l. pneumonia
    l. proteinosis
lipoidica
    necrobiosis l.
lipolysis
lipoma
    cord l.
    lumbosacral l.
    macrocephaly l.
lipomatosis
    familial multiple l.
lipomeningocele
Lipomul
lipomyelomeningocele
    skin-covered l.
lipooligosaccharide (LOS)
lipophilic fungus
lipopolysaccharide (LPS)
    l. coat
    Shiga l.
lipoprotein
    high-density l. (HDL)
    l. lipase (LPL)
    l. lipase deficiency
    low-density l. (LDL)
    very low density l. (VLDL)
liposarcoma
    myxoid l.
liposomal amphotericin B
liposome
    amphotericin B l.
Liposyn formula
5-lipoxygenase
lipreading
Liquaemin
liquefaction
liquefactive necrosis
Liquibid
Liqui-Char
liquid
    chylous l.
    Contac Cough Formula L.
    l. feeding
    Gordofilm L.
    l. nitrogen
    Occlusal-HP L.

    perfluorochemical l.
    l. petrolatum
    L. Pred
    Prometh VC Plain L.
    RID l.
    Ryna L.
    l. ventilation (LV)
    X-Prep L.
liquid-assisted high-frequency oscillatory ventilation (LA-HFOV)
liquified powder cocaine
Liquifilm
    HMS L.
    Poly-Pred L.
Liqui-Gel
    Dimetapp 4-Hour L.-G.
Liquiprin
LiquiVent
liquor
    l. carbonis detergens (LCD)
    l. carbonis detergens cream
    l. carbonis detergens ointment
    meconium staining of l.
Lisch nodule
lisinopril
lisp
lispro
    insulin l.
Lissauer tract
lissencephaly
    classical l.
    l. (type I, II)
list
    Amsterdam Depression L. (ADL)
    National Recipient Waiting L.
listening
    dichotic l.
Listeria
    L. monocytogenes
    L. monocytogenes sepsis
listeriosis
Listermint with Fluoride
listless
listlessness
litem
    guardian ad l.
Lithane
lithiasis
    biliary l.
    uric acid l.
lithium
    l. carbonate

L

NOTES

lithium *(continued)*
    l. citrate
    l. resistance
Lithobid
Lithonate
Lithotabs
little
    L. area
    L. disease
    L. League elbow
    L. League shoulder
Livadatis circular myotomy
live
    l. attenuated
    l. poliovirus vaccine
live-attenuated
    l.-a. virus
    l.-a. virus vaccine
livedo reticularis
liver
    acute fatty l.
    l. cirrhosis
    cut-down l.
    enlarged l.
    fatty l.
    fetal l.
    l. flap
    l. infiltrate
    l. parenchyma
    l. phosphorylase deficiency
    shock l.
    l. span
    l. transplant
    l. transplantation
    l. tumor
lividity
    postmortem l.
living
    activities of daily l. (ADL)
Livostin
LJP
    localized juvenile periodontitis
LKS
    Landau-Kleffner syndrome
LLD
    leg length discrepancy
LLDP
    left lateral decubitus position
l-loop
Lloyd-Still index
LLQ
    left lower quadrant
L-M
    Stanford-Binet L-M
LMA
    laryngeal mask airway

LMB
    Laurence-Moon-Biedl
    LMB syndrome
LMP
    last menstrual period
LMW
    low molecular weight
    LMW proteinuria
LMWH
    low molecular weight heparin
LNS
    Lesch-Nyhan syndrome
load
    axial l.
    plasma viral l.
    potential renal solute l. (PRSL)
    pressure l.
    renal solute l. (RSL)
    task l.
    viral l.
    volume l.
loading
    familial l.
lobar
    l. emphysema
    l. panniculitis
    l. pneumonia
    l. sclerosis
lobe
    hepatic l.
    mesial temporal l.
    quadrate hepatic l.
    Riedel l.
    sequestered l.
    temporal l.
lobectomy
    fetal l.
lobster
    l. claw deformity
    l. clawhand
lobular
    l. architecture
    l. capillary hemangioma
lobulation defect
lobule
    sebaceous gland l.
    tense l.
LOC
    level of consciousness
local
    l. anesthesia
    l. education agency (LEA)
    l. inflammatory response
    l. seizure
localization
localization-related epilepsy seizure
localize

localized
- l. albinism
- l. cutaneous leishmaniasis (LCL)
- l. juvenile periodontitis (LJP)
- l. lipoatrophy
- l. pachygyria
- l. peritonitis
- l. scleroderma
- l. vulvar pemphigoid of childhood (LVPC)

localizing sign
loci (*pl. of* locus)
lock
- urokinase-vancomycin l.

locked facet
lockjaw
Locoid Topical
locomotion
locomotor
locoregional node
loculate
locus, pl. **loci**
- l. ceruleus
- quantitative trait loci (QTL)

Locus of Control Scale
locutionary stage
LOD
- logarithm of odds

lodoxamide tromethamine
LoEstrin 1/20
Lofene
Löffler syndrome
Löfgren syndrome
Lofstrand crutches
Log-a-Rhythm Signal Acquisition unit
logarithm of odds (LOD)
Logen
logroll maneuver
lollipop
- fentanyl l.
- Oralet l.

Lomanate
Lomodix
Lomotil
lomustine
Lonalac formula
loneliness
Lone Star tick
long
- l. arm of chromosome
- l. axis
- l. bone

- l. leg cast
- l. leg sitting
- l.- and medium-chain fatty acid coenzyme-A dehydrogenase deficiency (LCAD/MCAD)
- l. Q-T syndrome (LQTS)
- l. thin extremity
- l.- and very-long-chain acyl-CoA dehydrogenase (LCAD/VLCAD)

Long-Acting
- Sinex L.-A.

long-acting thyroid stimulator (LATS)
long-axis view
long-chain
- l.-c. acyl-CoA dehydrogenase (LCAD)
- l.-c. fatty acid
- l.-c. 3-hydroxyacyl-CoA dehydrogenase (LCHAD)
- l.-c. 3-hydroxyacyl-CoA dehydrogenase deficiency
- l.-c. hydroxyacyl-coenzyme A dehydrogenase (LCHAD)
- l.-c. polyunsaturated fatty acid (LCPUFA)
- l.-c. very long-chain acyl-CoA dehydrogenase deficiency

longitudinal
- l. deficiency
- l. dense striation
- l. interval followup evaluation (LIFE)
- l. proton MR spectroscopy
- l. random coefficient model (LRCM)
- l. study

long-segment
- l.-s. aganglionosis
- l.-s. congenital tracheal stenosis (LSCTS)

long-tract sign
longum
- *Bifidobacterium l.*

Loniten Oral
Lonox
look
- anxious l.

loop
- capillary end l.
- dilated intestinal l.
- l. diuretic
- l. diversion

NOTES

loop *(continued)*
    dropout of capillary end l.
    flow-volume l.
    l. of Henle
    ileal l.
    obstructed bowel l.
    rubroolivoccrebellorubral l.
    sentinel l.
looping
    cardiac l.
loose body
Lo/Ovral
    L. contraceptive pill
lop ear
loperamide
    l. hydrochloride
loperamide
Lorabid
loracarbef
loratadine
lorazepam
Lorber criteria
Lorcet
    L. 10/650
    L. Plus
Lorcet-HD
lordosis
    lumbar l.
lordotic deformity
Lorenz night splint
Lorenzo
    L. oil
    L. oil diet
Loroxide
Lortab
    L. 2.5/500
    L. 5/500
    L. 10/500
    L. Elixir
LOS
    lipooligosaccharide
loss
    acute interpersonal l.
    blood l.
    conductive hearing l.
    congenital hearing l.
    l. of consciousness
    l. of correction
    covert l.
    dialysate protein l.
    electrolyte l.
    fetal l.
    gastrointestinal l.
    hearing l.
    high-frequency hearing l.
    high-tone hearing l.
    hysterical visual l.
    insensible water l.

    mixed hearing l.
    nephron l.
    overt l.
    protein l.
    range l.
    renal l.
    sensorineural hearing l. (SNHL)
    sensory l.
    status l.
    stocking-glove sensory l.
    third space l.
    tooth l.
    transepidermal water l. (TEWL)
    visual l.
    water l.
lotion
    BlemErase L.
    calamine l.
    Ovide L.
    Panscol L.
    Sarna l.
    thiosulfate l.
Lotrimin
    L. AF
    L. AF Topical
loudness
Louis-Bar syndrome
louse, pl. **lice**
    body l.
    crab l.
    head l.
    l. infestation
    pubic l.
louse-borne
    l.-b. fever
    l.-b. typhus
Lovaas
    L. method
    L. program
LOVE
    laser office ventilation of ears
LOVE IT
    laser office ventilation of ears with
    insertion of tubes
Lovenox
low
    l. birth weight (LBW)
    l. birth weight infant
    l. blood sugar
    l. cardiac output syndrome
    l. frequency (LF)
    l. imperforate anus
    l. molecular weight (LMW)
    l. molecular weight heparin
    (LMWH)
    l. molecular weight proteinuria
    l. muscle tone
    l. nasal bridge

l. occipital hairline
l. output
l. pressure bladder
l. sensory threshold
l. T3 syndrome
l. vision
low-branched-chain amino acid diet
low-density lipoprotein (LDL)
low-dose
l.-d. dobutamine stress radionuclide ventriculography
l.-d. involved-field irradiation
l.-d. splenic irradiation
Lowe
oculocerebrorenal disease of L.
oculocerebrorenal syndrome of L.
L. syndrome
Löwenstein-Jensen medium
lower
l. airway disease
l. collecting system
l. esophageal sphincter (LES)
l. esophageal transection
l. extremity (LE)
l. lip paralysis
l. motor neuron palsy
l. respiratory illness (LRI)
l. respiratory infection (LRI)
l. respiratory tract
l. respiratory tract infection (LRTI)
low-flow sidestream capnography
low-grade
l.-g. B-cell lymphoma
l.-g. B-cell lymphoma of MALT type
l.-g. diffuse astrocytoma
l.-g. fibrillary astrocytoma
l.-g. squamous intraepithelial lesion (LSIL)
Lowila soap
low-phenylalanine diet
low-pressure breast pump
Low-Quel
low-set ears
low-sodium syndrome
low-vision aid
low-voltage
l.-v. electrocortical activity (LVECoG)
l.-v. fast activity (LVFA)
lozenge
benzocaine l.

Cough-X l.
Suppress l.'s
Lozi-Tab
LP
light perception
lumbar puncture
LPL
lipoprotein lipase
LPL deficiency
LPN
licensed practical nurse
LPS
lipopolysaccharide
LPSS
laryngopharyngeal sensory stimulation
LPSS testing
LQTS
long Q-T syndrome
LR
lateral rotation
LRCM
longitudinal random coefficient model
LRE
least restrictive environment
LRI
lower respiratory illness
lower respiratory infection
LRTI
lower respiratory tract infection
LS
Micro-K LS
L/S
lecithin to sphingomyelin
L/S ratio
LSCTS
long-segment congenital tracheal stenosis
L-shaped cautery
LSIL
low-grade squamous intraepithelial lesion
LSO
lumbosacral orthosis
LSS
lexical-syntactic syndrome
LTC$_4$
leukotriene C$_4$
LTD$_4$
leukotriene D$_4$
LTE$_4$
leukotriene E$_4$
L-thyroxine
LTRA
leukotriene receptor antagonist

NOTES

l-transposition of great arteries
LTS
    laryngotracheal stenosis
LTT
    lateral tibial torsion
lubricant
    ocular l.
Lucarelli risk group
lucency
    white matter l.
lucent band
Lucey-Driscoll syndrome
lucida
    lamina l.
luciferase assay
lucinactant
lucite form
Lückenschadel
Ludorum
Ludwig angina
Luekens trap
Luer lock site
Luft disease
Lugol iodine stain
lumbar
    l. curve
    l. extensor muscle
    l. gibbus
    l. lordosis
    l. meningocele
    l. puncture (LP)
    l. puncture manometry
    l. theca
lumboperitoneal shunt
lumbosacral
    l. agenesis
    l. dimple
    l. junction
    l. lipoma
    l. orthosis (LSO)
    l. sinus
    l. skin pigment change
    l. tuft of hair
lumbricoides
    Ascaris l.
lumen, pl. **lumens, lumina**
    appendiceal l.
Luminal
lumpy jaw
Luna-Parker acid fuscin stain
lunata
    Curvularia l.
Lundh test
lung
    l. aeration
    agenesis of l.
    bubbly l.'s

cystic adenomatoid malformation
    of l.
farmer's l.
l. fluke
l. growth and development
l. hernia
honeycomb l.
hyperlucent l.
hypoplasia of l.
hypoplastic l.
idiopathic diffuse interstitial fibrosis
    of l.
l. infiltrate
Kolobow membrane l.
lymphangiomyomatosis of l.
malt worker's l.
l. morphogenesis
l. overdistention
paraquat l.
premature l.
l. recruitment
sequestered l.
shock l.
SP-A protein of l.'s
SP-B protein of l.'s
SP-C protein of l.'s
surfactant-deficient l.
l. surgery
l. tap
unilateral hyperlucent l.
Lupron
    L. Depot
    L. Depot-3 Month
    L. Depot-4 Month
    L. Depot-Ped
lupus
    ANA-negative l.
    l. angiitis
    l. anticoagulant
    l. anticoagulant syndrome
    l. cerebritis
    discoid l.
    l. erythematosus
    l. erythematosus disseminatus
    l. erythematosus profundus
    l. inhibitor
    l. miliaris disseminatum faciei
    neonatal l.
    l. nephritis
    l. pernio
    l. vulgaris
lupuslike syndrome
LUQ
    left upper quadrant
lurch
    abductor l.
Luride
Luride-SF

Luschka
    foramen of L.
Lusk instrument
luteal phase deficiency
luteinizing hormone (LH)
Lutembacher syndrome
luteotropic hormone
Lutrepulse
Lutz-Splendore-Almeida blastomycosis
Luvox
luxation
    dental extrusion/lateral l.
    extrusion/lateral l.
    extrusive l.
    intrusive l.
    lateral l.
    rotary atlantoaxial l.
luxury perfusion
LV
    left ventricle
    left ventricular
    liquid ventilation
        LV afterload
        LV contractility
        LV dysfunction
        LV preload
LVD
    left ventricular dysfunction
LVECoG
    low-voltage electrocortical activity
LVEF
    left ventricular ejection fraction
LVFA
    low-voltage fast activity
LVN
    licensed vocational nurse
LVOT
    left ventricular outflow tract
LVOTO
    left ventricular outflow tract obstruction
LVPC
    localized vulvar pemphigoid of childhood
LVSWI
    left ventricular stroke work index
lyase
    argininosuccinate l.
Lyell
    L. disease
    L. syndrome
lyer
    side l.

Lyme
    L. arthritis
    L. disease
    L. disease vaccine
    L. enzyme-linked immunosorbent
    assay
    L. meningitis
    L. neuroborreliosis
    L. radiculoneuritis
Lyme-associated peripheral facial nerve palsy
LYMErix
lymph
    l. node
    l. node enlargement
lymphadenectomy
lymphadenitis
    cervical l.
    chronic pyogenic l.
    granulomatous l.
    histocytic necrotizing l.
    inguinal l.
    Kibuchi histocytic necrotizing l.
    mesenteric l.
    necrotizing granulomatous l.
    pyogenic l.
    recurrent pyogenic l.
    regional l.
    submental l.
    suppurative l.
    tuberculous cervical l.
lymphadenopathy
    cervical l.
    diffuse nonmalignant l.
    hilar l.
    mediastinal l.
    shotty cervical l.
    submental l.
    Toxoplasma l.
lymphangiectasia
    congenital pulmonary l.
    pulmonary l.
lymphangiectasis
    congenital pulmonary l.
lymphangiography
    bipedal l.
lymphangioma
    alveolar l.
    l. circumscriptum
    l. cysticum
lymphangiomatosis
lymphangiomyomatosis of lung

L

NOTES

lymphangitis
lymphatic
    l. dysplasia
    l. leukemia
    l. obstruction
lymphedema
    congenital l.
    congenital extremity l.
    extremity l.
    hereditary l.
    intrauterine l.
    l. praecox
    primary l.
    secondary l.
    l. tarda
lymphoblastic
    l. leukemia
    l. lymphoma
lymphoblastoid
lymphocytapheresis
lymphocyte
    B l.
    l. cell
    cytotoxic l. (CTL)
    cytotoxic T l. (CTL)
    l. depleted
    l. immune globulin
    polymorphonuclear l.
    l. predominant
    T l.
lymphocyte-depleted Hodgkin disease
lymphocyte-predominant Hodgkin disease
lymphocytic
    l. choriomeningitis
    l. choriomeningitis virus (LCMV)
    l. gastritis
    l. interstitial pneumonitis (LIP)
    l. leukemia
    l. meningitis
    l. meningoradiculoneuritis
    l. pleocytosis
    l. thyroiditis
    l. vasculitis
lymphocytosis
    infectious l.
lymphogranuloma
    l. inguinale
    l. venereum (LGV)
lymphohematogenous disease
lymphohistiocytic infiltration
lymphohistiocytosis
    familial erythrophagocytic l. (FEL)
    familial hemophagocytic l. (FHLH)
    hemophagocytic l.
lymphoid
    l. hyperplasia
    l. interstitial pneumonitis (LIP)
    l. tissue

lymphokine
lymphoma
    African Burkitt l.
    American Burkitt l.
    anaplastic large cell l.
    B-cell l.
    Burkitt l. (BL)
    central nervous system l.
    colonic B-cell l.
    diffuse small cell cleaved l.
    EBV-related B-cell l.
    endemic Burkitt l.
    extranodal marginal zone B-cell l.
    histiocytic l.
    Hodgkin l.
    immunoblastic l.
    intraocular l.
    large B-cell l.
    large cell anaplastic Ki-1 l.
    large cell immunoblastic l.
    low-grade B-cell l.
    lymphoblastic l.
    Mediterranean l.
    non-Hodgkin l. (NHL)
    primary central nervous system l.
      (PCNSL)
    small cell cleaved l.
    small noncleaved cell l. (SNCCL)
    sporadic Burkitt l.
    T-cell l.
    true histiocytic l.
lymphonodular
    l. hyperplasia
    l. pharyngitis
lymphopenia
lymphopoietic differentiation
lymphoproliferative
    l. disease
    l. disorder
    l. syndrome
lymphoproliferative/myeloproliferative
  disease
lymphoreticular
    l. malignancy
    l. neoplasia
lymphoreticulosis
lymphorrhage
lymphosarcoma cell leukemia
Lynch syndrome
Lyon
Lyon hypothesis
lyonization
lyophilize
lyosomal
Lyphocin Injection
lysate
    endothelial cell l.
lysine 6-oxidase

lysinuric protein intolerance
lysis test
lysome
  hepatocellular l.
lysosomal
  l. metabolite
  l. storage disease
  l. storage disorder
lysosome

lysozyme
lyssa body
lysylbradykinin
lytic
  l. cocktail
  l. infection
  l. lesion
Lytren formula

NOTES

M2 inhibitor
MA
    metatarsus adductus
mA
    milliampere
Maalox
    M. Anti-Gas
    M. Plus Extra Strength
MAb
    monoclonal antibody
MABP
    mean arterial blood pressure
MAC
    midarm circumference
    Mycobacterium avium complex
    Mycobacterium avium-intracellulare
    complex
MacArthur
    M. Longitudinal Twin Study
    M. Story Stem Battery (MSSB)
MacCallum patch
Macewen sign
Machado-Joseph
    M.-J. ataxia
    M.-J. disease
Macherey-Nagel strep test
machine
    BiPAP m.
    CPAP m.
    life-support m.
    Mayo-Gibbon heart-lung m.
machinery murmur
Machupo virus
MacIndoe procedure
Macleod syndrome
macrencephaly
Macrobid
macrocarpon
    Vaccinium m.
macrocephaly
    familial m.
    m. lipoma
macrocirculatory
macrocytic anemia
macrocytosis
macrodactyly
    primary m.
    secondary m.
Macrodantin
Macrodex
macrodontia
macroglobulin
    a-2 m. (a-2M)

macroglossia
    relative m.
    true m.
macrognathia
macrogynecomastia
macrogyria
macrolide therapy
macromineral
macronodular cirrhosis
macronutrient balance
macroorchidism
macrophage
    m. activation syndrome (MAS)
    m. inflammatory protein (MIP)
    m. inflammatory protein-1 alpha
    lipid-laden m.
    m. tropic (M-tropic)
macrophage-targeted glucocerebrosidase
macrophage-tropic strain
macroscopic hematuria
macrosomia
macrosomic
macrostomia
macrothrombocytopenia
macrovascular
MACS
    Multicenter AIDS Cohort Study
macula
    cherry-red m.
macular
    m. atrophy
    m. cherry-red spot
    m. hemangioma
    m. light reflex
    m. pseudocoloboma
    m. rash
    m. stain
    m. star formation
macular-papular-vesicular lesion
macule
    ash-leaf m.
    blanching m.
    bluish-black m.
    crop of m.'s
    erythematous m.
    hypopigmented m.
maculopapular
    m. eruption
    m. exanthem
    m. lesion
    m. nodosa
    m. rash
MadaJet XL needle-free injector
madarosis

M

MADD
Mothers Against Drunk Driving
multiple acyl-coenzyme A dehydrogenase deficiency
Maddacrawler walker
Madelung deformity
madurae
Actinomadura m.
Madura foot
mafenide
Maffucci syndrome
MAG-3
mercaptotriglycine
MAG-3 diuretic renogram
Mag-200
Mag-Carb
Magendie
foramen of M.
magic mouthwash
magna
chorea m.
cisterna m.
coxa m.
dilated cisterna m.
mega cisterna m.
Magnacal formula
magnesia
milk of m. (MOM)
Phillips' Milk of M.
magnesium
m. chloride
m. citrate
m. deficiency
m. hydroxide
intratracheal m. (ITMg)
ionized m.
m. level
m. pemoline
m. sulfate
m. supplement
total m.
magnesium-containing cathartic
magnetic
m. resonance angiography (MRA)
m. resonance cholangiography (MRC)
m. resonance cholangiopancreatography (MRCP)
m. resonance imaging (MRI)
m. resonance spectroscopy (MRS)
m. source imaging (MSI)
magnetoencephalography (MEG)
magnum
asymmetric small foramen m.
foramen m.
Magonate
Mag-Ox 400
Magpi procedure

Mag-Tab SR
Magtrate
MAH
minimal acceptable height
ma huang
MAI
Mycobacterium avium-intracellulare
MAI infection
Maigret-50
main
m. bronchus
m. duct of Wirsung
m. renal vein
Maine
prominent skin discoloration of coast of M.
mainstreaming
Mainz pouch diversion
Maisonneuve fracture
Majewski short rib polydactyly
Majocchi granuloma
major
m. aortopulmonary collateral artery (MAPCA)
m. basic protein (MBP)
m. depressive disorder (MDD)
m. histocompatibility complex (MHC)
Leishmania m.
m. motor seizure
thalassemia m.
majus, pl. **majora**
labium m.
mal
m. de Meleda
grand m.
myoclonic petit m.
petit m.
malabsorption
bile acid m.
carbohydrate m.
fat m.
glucose-galactose m.
isolated congenital folate m. (ICFM)
lactose m.
methionine m.
primary bile acid m.
starch m.
m. syndrome
tryptophan m.
m. workup
malacia
maladaptive coping strategy
maladie
m. de Roger
m. des tics
malaise

malalignment
- patellofemoral m.
- rotational m.
- m. syndrome

malar
- m. distribution
- m. eminence
- m. flush
- m. rash

malaria
- cerebral m.
- chloroquine-resistant m.
- m. endemic
- falciparum m.

malariae
- *Plasmodium m.*

Malassezia
- *M. furfur*
- *M. furfur* pustulosis
- *M.* pachydermatitis

Malatal
malate
- timolol m.

malathion
Malecot tube
male pseudohermaphroditism (MPH)
malformation
- adenomatoid m.
- Arnold-Chiari m.
- arteriovenous m. (AVM)
- arteriovenous fistula m. (AVFM)
- bronchopulmonary m.
- cardiac m.
- cardiovascular m. (CVM)
- cerebral arteriovenous m. (CAVM)
- Chiari m. (type I–IV)
- congenital bronchopulmonary m.
- congenital cardiovascular m. (CCVM)
- congenital cystic adenomatoid m. (CCAM)
- conotruncal cardiac m.
- cystic adenomatoid m. (CAM)
- Dandy-Walker m.
- ductal plate m.
- Ebstein m.
- extracardiac m.
- foregut m.
- GI tract venous m.
- hamartomatous m.
- obstructive m.
- ocular m.

- pulmonary arteriovenous m. (PAVM)
- split cord m. (SCM)
- split spinal cord m. (SSCM)
- submucosal arterial m.
- thyroid gland m.
- vascular m.
- vein of Galen m.
- venous m. (VM)

malformed
- m. ear
- m. pinna
- m. radial head

malfunction
- congenital cystic adenomatoid m.
- shunt m.

Malgaigne fracture
malignancy
- CNS m.
- intraocular m.
- lymphoreticular m.

malignant
- m. arrhythmia
- m. brain edema
- m. brain tumor
- m. epithelial tumor
- m. extrarenal rhabdoid tumor
- m. fibrous histiocytoma (MFH)
- m. germ cell tumor
- m. histiocytosis
- m. hyperphenylalaninemia
- m. hyperpyrexia
- m. hypertension
- m. hyperthermia (MH)
- m. hyperthermic rhabdomyolysis
- m. mesodermal tumor
- m. nerve sheath tumor
- m. neurilemoma
- m. osteoid
- m. otitis externa
- m. phenylalaninemia
- m. pilocytic astrocytoma
- m. schwannoma
- m. teratoma
- m. transformation

malingering
Mallamint
malleable splint
mallei
- *Burkholderia m.*

malleolar ossification center
malleolus, pl. **malleoli**

M

NOTES

malleolus *(continued)*
    lateral m.
    medial m.
Mallergan-VC With Codeine
mallet
    m. finger
    m. toe
malleus
    short process of m.
Mallory-Weiss tear (MWT)
Malmö
    hemoglobin M.
malmoense
    Mycobacterium m.
malnourished
malnutrition
    fetal m.
    protein-calorie m.
    protein-energy m.
malocclusion
malodorous
    m. breath
    m. urine
malondialdehyde (MDA)
Malotuss
malposition
    cardiac m.
malrotation
    m. of bowel
    intestinal m. (IM)
    m. with midgut volvulus
MALT
    mucosa-associated lymphoid tissue
    MALT type
malt
    barley m.
    m. soup extract
    m. worker's lung
maltase
    acid m.
maltophilia
    Stenotrophomonas m.
    Xanthomonas m.
maltreatment
Maltsupex
malunion
MAMC
    mean arm muscle circumference
    midarm muscle circumference
Mamex formula
mammal
mammary
MAMSA, m-AMSA
    amsacrine
man
    elephant m.
management
    airway m.

    anxiety m.
    brace m.
    Family Inventory of Resources
      for M. (FIRM)
    intensive diabetes m. (IDM)
    routine wound m.
manager
    case m.
mandated reporter (of child abuse)
Mandelamine
mandelate
    methenamine m.
mandible
    dislocated m.
    hypoplastic m.
    prominent m.
    underdeveloped m.
mandibular
    m. advancement
    m. dislocation
    m. hypoplasia
    m. prognathism
mandibular-acral dysplasia
mandibulofacial dysostosis
mandrillaris
    Balamuthia m.
maneuver
    Barlow m.
    Credé m.
    doll's eye m.
    doll's head m.
    Frenzel m.
    Gower m.
    Heimlich m.
    jaw thrust-spine stabilization m.
    logroll m.
    Mauriceau-Smellie-Veit m.
    Ortolani m.
    Sellick m.
    vagotonic m.
    Valsalva m.
Manezine
manganese intoxication
mange
    sarcoptic m.
mania
    prepubertal m.
manic
manic-depressive
    m.-d. disorder
    m.-d. illness
manifestation
    extraintestinal m. (EIM)
    extrapyramidal m.
manipulation
    preorthognatic surgery m.
mannitol
mannose-type sugar

mannosidase
mannosidosis
Mann-Whitney U test
manometer
manometric
manometry
  anorectal m.
  esophageal m.
  lumbar puncture m.
  rectal balloon m.
mansoni
  Schistosoma m.
Mantel-Haenszel
  M.-H. procedure
  M.-H. test
mantle
  Acid M.
  m. sclerosis
Mantoux
  M. method
  M. tuberculin skin test
manual
  m. alphabet
  m. differential
  m. English
  m. reduction
  m. splinting of thoracic cage
  m. thrust
  m. ventilation bag (MVB)
manubrium
manuum
  tinea m.
MAOI
  monoamine oxidase inhibitor
Maox
MAP
  mean airway pressure
  mean arterial pressure
Mapap
MAPCA
  major aortopulmonary collateral artery
maple
  m. syrup urine
  m. syrup urine disease (MSUD)
mapping
  brain m.
  brain electrical activity m. (BEAM)
  pressure m.
Maranox
marantic endocarditis
marasmic
marasmus

Marbaxin
marble bone disease
marbled hypopigmented streak
Marburg
  M. disease
  M. virus
Marburg-type MS
Marcaine
marcescens
  Serratia m.
march
  m. hemoglobinuria
  jacksonian m.
Marcillin
Marcus
  M. Gunn jaw-winking ptosis
  M. Gunn pupil
  M. Gunn sign
Marden-Walker syndrome
Marfan
  M. sign
  M. syndrome
Margesic H
margin
  anal m.
  blurring of left psoas m.
  costal m.
  psoas m.
  tentorial m.
marginal
  m. alopecia
  m. insertion
  obtuse m.
  m. sinus
  m. zone
marginatum
  eczema m.
  erythema m.
Marie-Strümpell encephalitis
Marie syndrome
marijuana
Marinesco-Sjögren syndrome
Marinol
marinum
  Mycobacterium m.
Marion disease
mark
  belt m.
  Caitlin m.
  choke m.
  port-wine m.
  strawberry m.

NOTES

M

marked asynchrony
markedly decreased reflex
marker
    neonatal m.
    radiopaque m.
    serological m.
marking
    pulmonary vascular m.
    m. time pattern
Marmine
    M. Injection
    M. Oral
marmorata
    cutis m.
marmoratus
    status m.
marneffei
    Penicillium m.
Maroteaux-Lamy syndrome
marrow
    adult bone m. (ABM)
    bone m.
    fetal bone m. (FBM)
    m. transplantation
marrow-ablative chemotherapy
MARS
    mixed antiinflammatory syndrome
    molecular adsorbent recirculating system
    motion artifact rejection system
    MARS pulse oximetry
Marshall
    ligament of M.
    M. syndrome
    M. and Tanner pubertal stage
    M. and Tanner pubertal staging
Marshall-Smith syndrome
marsupialization
Martin modification
MAS
    macrophage activation syndrome
    meconium aspiration syndrome
masculine
masculinization
Masimo
    M. SET home monitor
    M. SET signal extraction pulse
      oximetry
mask
    m. of atopic dermatitis
    bag and m.
    bag, valve, m. (BVM)
    m. and bag ventilation
    Bili m.
    face m.
    Laerdal m. (0–20
    Neutrogena Acne M.
    nonrebreather face m.
Maslach Burnout Inventory

MASS
    mitral valve, aorta, skeleton, skin
      MASS phenotype
mass
    abdominal m.
    m. accretion
    bilateral flank m.'s
    bone mineral m. (BMM)
    doughnut-shaped m.
    doughy m.
    m. effect
    exophytic m.
    extravesical m.
    extrinsic extravesical m.
    fat m. (FM)
    fat-free m. (FFM)
    flank m.
    hamartomatous m.
    hypoxia, intussusception, brain m.
      (HIB)
    lean body m. (LBM)
    m. lesion
    neonatal abdominal m.
    pyloric m.
    scrotal m.
    m. spectrometer
    m. spectrometry (MS)
    spongy m.
    suprapubic m.
    total fat m. (TFM)
    unilateral flank m.
    vertebral bone m. (VBM)
massage
    cardiac m.
    heart m.
    lacrimal sac m.
    m. therapy
masseter muscle
massive
    m. ascites
    m. atelectasis
    m. intravascular hemolysis
    m. pulmonary embolus
mast
    m. cell
    m. cell disease
    m. cell leukemia
    m. cell stabilizer
MAST blood test
MasterFlex fetal perfusion pump
mastitis neonatorum
mastocytoma
mastocytosis
    bullous m.
    cutaneous m.
    diffuse cutaneous m.
    nasal m.

primary nasal m.
systemic m.

mastoid
m. air cell
m. bone fracture
cloudy m.
m. cortex
m. drainage
m. osteitis
m. process

mastoidectomy

mastoiditis
acute coalescent m.
acute surgical m.
chronic m.
coalescent m.
pneumococcal m.
surgical m.

masturbation

MAT
microscopic agglutination test

mat
mycelial m.

matching
m. familiar figures (MFF)
M. Familiar Figures Test
feature m.
V/Q m.

mater
dura m.
pia m.

material
absorbent gelling m. (AGM)
coffee-ground m.
didactic m.
lipofuscin m.
nonionic contrast m.
other potentially infectious m.
(OPIM)
white pseudomembranous m.

maternal
m. antithyroid antibody
m. cytokinemia
m. diabetes
m. hydramnios
m. hypercalcemia
m. hypertension
m. hypothyroidism
m. IgG antibody
m. serum alpha fetoprotein
(MSAFP)
m. smoking

m. substance abuse
m. tachycardia
m. thyrotropin receptor blocking
antibody-induced congenital
hypothyroidism

maternal-fetal
m.-f. hemorrhage
m.-f. histocompatibility
m.-f. microtransfusion
m.-f. transmission of antibody

maternal-infant
m.-i. attachment
m.-i. bonding

**maternally inherited myopathy and
cardiomyopathy (MIMyCA)**

maternofetal transfusion

Matie-Unna hypotrichosis

matrilineal

matrix, pl. **matrices**
bone m.
calcified m.
germinal m.
m. metalloproteinase (MMP)
nail m.
Raven Progressive Matrices (RPM)
telencephalic subependymal
germinal m.
uncalcified bone m.

matted
m. omentum
m. peritoneum

matter
gray m.
heterotopic gray m.
spongy degeneration of white m.
supratentorial white m.
white m.

mattress
Dräger thermal gel m.

Matulane

maturation
delayed sexual m.
sexual m.
terminal m.

mature
early m.
late m.
m. teratoma

mature-onset diabetes of youth

maturity
Dubowitz Scale for Infant M.

M

NOTES

maturity *(continued)*
    m. onset deafness
    social m.
maturity-onset
    m.-o. diabetes
    m.-o. diabetes of youth (MODY)
Mauriac syndrome
Mauriceau-Smellie-Veit maneuver
Maxafil
Maxidex Ophthalmic
maxilla, pl. **maxillae**
    short m.
maxillary
    m. advancement
    m. bone
    m. hypoplasia
    m. sinus
    m. sinus aspiration
maxima
    protein m.
maximal
    m. cardiac width
    m. chest width
    m. electroshock (MES)
    m. electroshock model
    m. oxygen intake (MOI)
maximum
    M. Strength Nytol
    m. temperature
maximum-intensive phototherapy
Maxipime
Maxitrol Ophthalmic
Maxivate Topical
Maxolon
Maxon suture
Mayaro virus
Mayer-Rokitansky-Küster-Hauser syndrome
Mayer wave
May-Hegglin anomaly
Mayo-Gibbon heart-lung machine
MB
    muscle-brain
      creatine kinase MB
      MB isoenzyme
m-BACOD
    methotrexate, bleomycin, doxorubicin, cyclophosphamide, Oncovin, dexamethasone
MBC
    minimal bacterial concentration
MBD
    minimal brain dysfunction
MBM
    mother's breast milk
MBP
    major basic protein

MBS
    modified barium swallow
MCA
    middle cerebral artery
MCAD
    medium-chain acyl-CoA dehydrogenase
      MCAD deficiency
McAllister grading system
MCAO
    middle cerebral artery occlusion
McArdle disease
McBurney
    M. incision
    M. point
McCarthy
    M. Memory Scale
    M. reflex
    M. Scales of Children's Abilities
McCune-Albright syndrome
MCD
    metastatic Crohn disease
    molybdenum cofactor deficiency
MCDD
    multiple complex developmental disorder
MCFA
    medium-chain fatty acid
McGill forceps
McGoon index
McGrath scale
MCH
    mean corpuscular hemoglobin
MCHC
    mean cell hemoglobin concentration
    mean corpuscular hemoglobin concentration
McKusick-Kaufman syndrome
MCL
    medial collateral ligament
McLeod syndrome
MCLS
    mucocutaneous lymph node syndrome
McMaster Family Assessment Device
McMurray
    M. sign
    M. test
McNemar test
MCNS
    minimal change nephrotic syndrome
MCP
    medical control physician
    metacarpophalangeal
MCT
    medium-chain triglyceride
      MCT oil
      MCT oil formula
MCTD
    mixed connective tissue disease

MCV
    mean corpuscular volume
MD
    medical doctor
MDA
    malondialdehyde
MDAC
    multidose activated charcoal
MDD
    major depressive disorder
MDI
    mental development index
    metered-dose inhaler
MDK
    multicystic dysplastic kidney
MDMA
    methylenedioxy-methamphetamine
MDR
    minimum daily requirement
    multidrug resistance
MDR-TB
    multidrug-resistant tuberculosis
MDS
    myelodysplastic syndrome
MDT
    multidrug therapy
M:E
    myeloid to erythroid
MEA
    mercaptoethylamine
    multiple endocrine abnormalities
    multiple endocrine adenomatosis
Mead Johnson bottle
meal
    ante cibum (before m.'s) (a.c.)
    post cibum (after m.'s) (p.c.)
meal-time skill
mean
    m. age
    m. airway pressure (MAP)
    m. aortic pressure
    m. arm muscle circumference
      (MAMC)
    m. arterial blood pressure (MABP)
    m. arterial pressure (MAP)
    m. birth weight
    m. cell hemoglobin concentration
      (MCHC)
    m. corpuscular hemoglobin (MCH)
    m. corpuscular hemoglobin
      concentration (MCHC)
    m. corpuscular volume (MCV)

    m. developmental quotient
    m. fraction absorption
    m. intercriterion correlation (MIC)
    m. left atrial pressure
    m. length of utterance (MLU)
    m. length of utterance in
      morphemes (MLUm)
    m. platelet volume (MPV)
    m. pulmonary artery pressure
    m. right atrial pressure
means-end problem solving (MEPS)
measles
    atypical m.
    black m.
    m. exanthem
    German m.
    m. inclusion body encephalitis
      (MIBE)
    modified m.
    m., mumps, rubella (MMR)
    m., mumps, rubella immunization
    m., mumps, rubella vaccine
    m. pneumonia
    three-day m.
    typical m.
    uncomplicated m.
    m. virus
    m. virus enzyme-linked
      immunosorbent assay
      (MV(c)ELISA)
measure
    anthropometric m.
    gross motor function m.
    Prematurity Risk Evaluation M.
      (PREM)
    process-oriented m.
measurement
    anthropomorphic m.
    blood pressure m.
    body m.
    bone density m.
    bone mineral m.
    bone strength m.
    noninvasive blood pressure m.
      (NIBPM)
    peak flow m.
    pulse oximetry waveform systolic
      blood pressure m. (POWSBP)
    sequential peak flow m.
    somatic growth m.
Measurin
meatal stenosis

M

NOTES

meatus
>auditory m.
>bilateral atresia of external auditory m.
>external auditory m.
>external urethral m.
>fishmouth m.
>glanular urethral m.
>penile urethral m.
>penopubic urethral m.
>urethral m.

Mebaral
mebendazole
MECA
>Methods for Epidemiology of Child and Adolescent Mental Disorders
>MECA study

mecamylamine
mechanical
>m. birth injury
>m. dead space
>m. obstruction
>m. respirator
>m. suffocation
>m. ventilation

mechanic's hand
mechanism
>cerebroprotective m.
>excitotoxic m.
>Frank-Starling m.
>neural m.
>normal flap-valve m.
>peptide growth factor signaling m.
>Starling m.

mechanobullous
mechlorethamine
>m., Oncovin, procarbazine, prednisone
>m., Oncovin (vincristine), procarbazine, prednisone (MOPP)

Meckel
>M. cave
>M. diverticulum
>M. scan
>M. syndrome

Meckel-Gruber syndrome
meclizine
meconium
>m. aspiration
>m. aspiration syndrome (MAS)
>m. blockage syndrome
>m. ileus (MI)
>m. obstruction
>passage of m.
>m. peritonitis
>m. plug
>m. plug syndrome
>m. stained

>m. staining
>m. staining of liquor

meconium-stained amniotic fluid (MSAF)
MeCP2
>methyl-CpG-binding protein 2

MED
>minimal effective dose

Meda-Cap
Meda Tab
Medela breast pump
Medex
media
>acute otitis m. (AOM)
>acute suppurative otitis m.
>chronic otitis m. (COM)
>chronic suppurative otitis m. (CSOM)
>clostridial otitis m.
>dermatophyte test m. (DTM)
>draining otitis m.
>Dulbecco m.
>Earle m.
>Ham F10 m.
>ionic contrast m.
>mucoid otitis m. (MOM)
>nonionic contrast m.
>otitis m. (OM)
>recurrent otitis m.
>Sabourad dextrose m.
>secretory otitis m.
>serous otitis m.
>suppurative otitis m.
>Whitten m.
>Whittingham m.

medial
>m. collateral ligament (MCL)
>m. collateral ligament syndrome
>m. compartment
>m. condyle
>m. epicondylar fracture
>m. femoral torsion (MFT)
>m. hip rotation
>m. hip rotation in extension
>m. longitudinal arch
>m. longitudinal arch support
>m. malleolus
>m. metaphyseal beak
>m. necrosis
>m. rotation (MR)
>m. rotation clubfoot
>m. snapping hip syndrome
>m. talocalcaneal facet
>m. tibial torsion (MTT)

medialis
>vastus m.

median
>m. alveolar notch

multiples of m. (MOM)
m. plane

mediastinal
m. crunch
m. granuloma
m. lymphadenopathy
m. teratoma
m. tumor
m. widening

mediastinitis
fibrosing m.
pyogenic m.
suppurative m.

mediastinum
narrow m.

MediBottle
Medicaid
medical
m. control physician (MCP)
m. doctor (MD)
m. optical spectroscopy (MOS)
m. optimal imaging (MOI)

Medic-Alert Foundation
medicalization
medically fragile
medicamentosa
rhinitis m.

Medicare
medicated
Zilactin-B M.

medication
anticholinesterase m.
antiemetic m.
antiretroviral m.
antitussive m.
anxiolytic m.
exogenous m.
intrathecal m.
neuroleptic m.
opioid m.
psychostimulant m.
rescue m.

medication-induced stuttering
medicine
Alka-Seltzer Plus Children's
Cold M.
American Institute of Ultrasound
in M. (AIUM)
complementary and alternative m.
(CAM)
doctor of m.
emergency m.

herbal m.
osteopathic m.
pediatric emergency m. (PEM)
pediatric pulmonary m.
pulmonary m.
Reese's Pinworm M.

Medicone
Rectal M.

Medihaler-Epi
Medihaler-ISO Inhalation Aerosol
medinensis
Dracunculus m.

Mediplast Plaster
MediPort catheter
Medipren
Medi-Quick Topical Ointment
meditation
Mediterranean
M. anemia
M. lymphoma
M. myoclonus

Medi-Tuss
medium
Bordet-Gengoi m.
charcoal-blood m.
Löwenstein-Jensen m.
Regan-Lowe m.
selective broth m. (SBM)

medium-chain
m.-c. acyl-CoA dehydrogenase
(MCAD)
m.-c. acyl-CoA dehydrogenase
deficiency
m.-c. fatty acid (MCFA)
m.-c. triglyceride (MCT)
m.-c. triglyceride oil

Med-Neb respirator
Medralone Injection
Medrol Oral
medroxyprogesterone
m. acetate (MPA)
m. injection

medrysone
medulla
adrenal m.
m. oblongata
rostral ventromedial m.

medullaris
tethered conus m.

medullary
m. canal
m. cystic disease

M

NOTES

medullary *(continued)*
   m. dysplasia
   m. necrosis
   m. parenchyma
   m. recycling
   m. sponge kidney
   m. thyroid carcinoma
medulloblastoma
   classic m.
   desmoplastic m.
   melanotic m.
medullomyoblastoma
medusae
   caput m.
MedWatch form
MEE
   middle ear effusion
MEF
   middle ear fluid
mefenamic acid
mefloquine hydrochloride
Mefoxin
MEG
   magnetoencephalography
megacalycosis
mega cisterna magna
megacolon
   aganglionic m.
   congenital aganglionic m.
   toxic m.
megacystis-megaureter syndrome
megacystis, microcolon, intestinal hypoperistalsis (MMIH)
megaesophagus
megahertz (MHz)
megakaryoblastic leukemia
megakaryocyte
megakaryocytic leukemia
megakaryocytopoiesis
megakaryopoiesis
megalencephaly
   primary m.
   unilateral m.
megaloblastic
   m. anemia
   m. crisis
   m. erythropoiesis
megaloblastoid
megaloblastosis
megalocephaly
megalocornea
megalocystis microcolon intestinal hypoperistalsis syndrome
megaloencephaly
megalourethra
meganeurite
megarectum

megaterium
   Bacillus m.
megaureter
   obstructive m.
megavitamin therapy
megestrol acetate
meglumine diatrizoate
meibomian gland
meibomianitis
Meigs syndrome
meiosis
meiotic division
Meissner plexus
mekongi
   Schistosoma m.
melancholia
melancholic depression
melanin-like pigment
melanization
melanocyte
   pigmented m.
melanocytic nevus
melanocytosis
   dermal m.
   meningeal m.
melanoderma
melanoma
   benign juvenile m.
   cutaneous m.
   juvenile m.
melanosarcoma
melanosis
   Becker m.
   cutaneous m.
   neonatal pustular m.
   m. oculi
   pustular m.
   transient neonatal pustular m.
melanotic medulloblastoma
melanura
   Culiseta m.
MELAS
   mitochondrial myopathy, encephalopathy, lactic acidosis, strokelike episodes
   myopathy, encephalopathy, lactic acidosis, strokelike episodes
   MELAS syndrome
melatonin
   urinary excreted m.
Meleda
   mal de M.
melena neonatorum
Meleney synergistic gangrene
melioidosis
melitensis
   Brucella m.
Melkersson-Rosenthal syndrome
Melkersson syndrome

Mellaril
Mellaril-S
mellituria
mellitus
    diabetes m. (type 1, 2) (DM)
    gestational diabetes m.
    insulin-dependent diabetes m.
      (IDDM)
    juvenile-onset diabetes m. (JDM,
      JODM)
    new-onset diabetes m.
    non-insulin-dependent diabetes m.
      (NIDDM)
Melnick-Fraser syndrome
Melnick-Needles
    M.-N. disease
    M.-N. syndrome
melorheostosis
melphalan
membrane
    m. attack complex
    basal m. (BM)
    basement m.
    cloacal m.
    cracked mucous m.
    cricothyroid m.
    cuprophane hemodialyzer m.
    cytoplasmic m.
    Descemet m.
    diphtheritic m.
    dry mucous m.
    extraplacental m.
    glomerular basement m. (GBM)
    milk fat globule m. (MFGM)
    mucous m.
    otitis media with perforated
      tympanic m.
    parched mucous m.
    perforated tympanic m.
    persistent pupillary m.
    plasma m.
    platelet m.
    premature rupture of m.'s (PROM)
    preterm premature rupture of m.'s
      (PPROM)
    preterm spontaneous rupture
      of m.'s (PSROM)
    prolonged premature rupture
      of m.'s (PPROM)
    prolonged rupture of m.'s
    m. protein
    pupillary m.

    red cell m.
    Reissner m.
    subaortic m.
    tympanic m.
membranoproliferative glomerulonephritis
  (MPGN)
membranous
    m. conjunctivitis
    m. croup
    m. glomerulonephritis
    m. laryngotracheobronchitis
    m. lupus nephritis
    m. nephropathy
    m. septum
memory, pl. **memories**
    autobiographical m.
    m. cell
    episodic m.
    recovered m.
    rote m.
    sequential m.
    spatial m.
    visual sequential m.
    visual spatial m.
MEN-2
    multiple endocrine neoplasia type 2
Menadol
menarche
MenCon
    meningococcal conjugate
      MenCon vaccine
mendelian syndrome
Menetrier disease
Menghini technique
Meni-D
Ménière
    M. disease
    M. syndrome
    M. vertigo
meningeal
    m. angiomatosis
    m. carcinomatosis
    m. fibrosis
    m. irritation
    m. melanocytosis
    m. sign
meninges (*pl. of* meninx)
meningioma
    acoustic m.
    optic nerve sheath m.
    perioptic m.
    suprasellar m.

M

NOTES

meningism
meningismus
meningitidis
    Neisseria m.
meningitis, pl. **meningitides**
    aseptic m.
    bacillary m.
    bacterial m.
    basilar m.
    Candida m.
    chronic lymphocytic m.
    chronic syphilitic m.
    coccidioidomycosis m.
    Coxsackie viral m.
    cryptococcal m.
    echoviral m.
    echovirus 9 m.
    m. or encephalitis, metabolic, Reye syndrome (MMR)
    enteroviral m.
    eosinophilic m.
    experimental pneumococcal m.
    exudative m.
    fulminating m.
    fungal m.
    GBS m.
    group B streptococcal m.
    Haemophilus m.
    Haemophilus influenzae m.
    herpes aseptic m.
    herpes zoster m.
    influenzal m.
    leptospiral m.
    Lyme m.
    lymphocytic m.
    meningococcal m.
    Mollaret m.
    neonatal m.
    nosocomial bacterial m.
    pneumococcal m.
    postnatal bacterial m.
    purulent m.
    pyogenic m.
    recurrent bacterial m.
    recurrent fungal m.
    recurrent purulent m.
    Salmonella m.
    septic m.
    serous form of tuberculous m.
    streptococcal m.
    syphilitic m.
    tuberculous m.
    viral m.
meningocele
    cranial m.
    lumbar m.
meningococcal
    m. conjugate (MenCon)
    m. conjugate vaccine
    m. endotoxin
    m. meningitis
    m. multifocal osteomyelitis
    m. polysaccharide
    m. polysaccharide vaccine
    m. septicemia
meningococcemia
    chronic m.
meningococcus, pl. **meningococci**
    serogroup B m.
meningoencephalitic stage
meningoencephalitis
    amebic m.
    aseptic m.
    bacterial m.
    Balamuthia m.
    enteroviral m.
    eosinophilic m.
    granulomatous amebic m.
    mumps m.
    primary amebic m.
    m. syndrome
    viral m.
meningoencephalocele
meningoencephalomyelitis
meningomyelocele
    sacral m.
meningoradiculomyelitis
    chronic m.
meningoradiculoneuritis
    lymphocytic m.
meningovascular syndrome
meningoventriculitis
meninx, pl. **meninges**
meniscal injury
meniscoplasty
meniscus, pl. **menisci**
    discoid m.
    discoid lateral m.
    increased tear m.
    m. tear
Menkes
    M. kinky hair
    M. kinky-hair disease
    M. syndrome
menopause
menorrhagia
menotropin
MenPS vaccine
menses
    absent m.
    irregular m.
menstrual
    m. migraine
    m. pain
    m. pattern
    m. period

menstrual-associated periodic
  hypersomnia
menstruation
     vicarious m.
mentagrophytes
     Trichophyton m.
mental
     m. age
     m. arithmetic test
     m. clouding
     m. deficiency
     m. development
     m. developmental index
     m. development index (MDI)
     m. handicap
     m. health
     m. illness
     m. retardation
     m. retardation syndrome
     m. scale
mentalis habit
MEP
     motor evoked potential
meperidine
     m. hydrochloride
mephenytoin
mephobarbital
Mephyton
mepivacaine
     m. hydrochloride
     m. intoxication
Mepro formula
Mepron
MEPS
     means-end problem solving
mercaptoacetyl triglycine
mercaptoethylamine (MEA)
6-mercaptopurinc
mercaptotriglycine (MAG-3)
Merchant view
Merck respirator
mercurial diuretic
mercuric chloride
mercury-free vaccine
mercury vapor poisoning
Meritene formula
Merkel cell
meroacrania
meroanencephaly
meromelia
meromicrosomia
meropenem

merorachischisis
merosin deficiency
Merrem
MERRF
     myoclonus, epilepsy, ragged red fibers
     myoclonus epilepsy with ragged red
     fibers
      MERRF syndrome
Merrill program
Merthiolate spray
Merzbacher-Pelizaeus disease
MES
     maximal electroshock
MESA
     microsurgical epididymal sperm
     aspiration
mesalamine
mesangial
     m. cell proliferation
     m. hypercellularity
     m. lupus nephritis
     m. proliferative glomerulonephritis
     m. sclerosis
mesangiocapillary glomerulonephritis
  (type I, II) (MPGN)
mesangium
Mesantoin
mesencephalic-diencephalic junction
mesencephalic tectum
mesencephalon
mesenchymal
     m. cell
     m. hamartoma
mesenchyme
mesenrhomboencephalitis
mesenteric
     m. adenitis
     m. lymphadenitis
     m. root
     m. stalk
     m. vein
mesenteroaxial volvulus
mesentery
     ventral m.
mesial
     m. temporal lobe
     m. temporal sclerosis (MTS)
Mesigyna
mesna
Mesnex
mesoblastic nephroma
mesocardia

M

NOTES

mesocaval shunt
mesocephalic
mesoderm
mesodermal
    m. heterotopia
    m. tumor
mesolimbic dopamine tract
mesomelic
    m. dysplasia
    m. shortening
mesonephric cyst
mesonephros
mesoporphyrin
    tin m. (SnMP)
mesoridazine
mesothelioma
messenger ribonucleic acid (mRNA)
Mestinon
    M. Injection
    M. Oral
mesylate
    benztropine m.
    Desferal M.
metaanalysis
metabolic
    m. acidosis
    m. bone disease
    m. disease in newborn
    m. disorder
    m. disorder with hepatic
      dysfunction
    m. disorder with neurologic
      dysfunction
    m. myopathy
    m. response
    m. syndrome X
    m. test
metabolism
    aberrant vitamin D m.
    amino acid m.
    bone mineral m.
    cerebral glucose m.
    copper m.
    defective purine m.
    energy m.
    glycolipid m.
    inborn error of m. (IEM)
    methionine m.
    partition of energy m.
    purine m.
metabolite
    lysosomal m.
metacarpal
    m. fracture
    m. shortening
metacarpophalangeal (MCP)
    m. dislocation
    m. joint

metacercaria excyst
metachromatic leukodystrophy (MLD)
metacognition
metacognitive
Metadate ER tablets
metaiodobenzylguanidine (MIBG, MIGB)
metal
    m. intoxication
    m. poisoning
    trace m.
metalloenzyme
metalloproteinase
    matrix m. (MMP)
metalloprotein dimer
metamorphopsia
Metamucil Instant Mix
metamyelocyte
    m. cell
    giant m.
metanephros
metaphase
metaphyseal
    m. aspiration
    m. cortex
    m. dysostosis
    m. dysplasia
    m. dystosis
    m. fibrous defect
    m. flaring
    m. fracture
    m. lesion
    m. lesion of distal femur
metaphyseal-diaphyseal angle
metaphysical sclerosis
metaphysis, pl. metaphyses
    m. angulation
    cupped m.
    popcorn m.
    rachitic m.
    tibial m.
    widened m.
metaplasia
    agnogenic myeloid m. (AMM)
    intestinal m.
    squamous m.
Metaprel
metaproterenol
    Arm-a-Med M.
    Dey-Dose M.
metastasis, pl. metastases
    hematogenous m.
    tumor, node, metastases (TNM)
metastatic
    m. Crohn disease (MCD)
    m. tuberculous abscess
    m. tumor

metatarsal
- m. head osteochondritis
- m. shortening

metatarsophalangeal joint

metatarsus
- m. adductus (MA)
- m. primus varus

metatropic
- m. dwarfism
- m. dysplasia

metencephalon

meter
- Airshields jaundice m.
- Astech Peak Flow M.
- Health Scan Assess Plus peak flow m.
- LifeScan blood glucose m.
- Mini-Wright Peak Flow M.
- Parkinson-Cowan dry gas m.
- peak flow m. (PFM)
- Pocketpeak peak flow m.
- transcutaneous jaundice m.

metered-dose inhaler (MDI)

metformin

methacholine
- m. challenge
- m. provacative testing

methadone

methamphetamine

methapyrilene

methemoglobinemia
- hereditary m.

methemoglobin reduction test

methenamine
- m. hippurate
- m. mandelate
- m. silver stain

methicillin-resistant *Staphylococcus aureus* **(MRSA)**

methicillin sodium

methimazole

methionine
- m. malabsorption
- m. metabolism
- m. synthase deficiency

methioninemia

methocarbamol

method
- arithmetic m.
- barrier m.
- Bayley and Pinneau height-predicting m.
- bone-age determination m.
- cluster-stratified sampling m.
- Cobb m.
- cotton swab m.
- end-point dilution m.
- M.'s for the Epidemiology of Child and Adolescent Disorders T score
- M.'s for Epidemiology of Child and Adolescent Mental Disorders (MECA)
- Ferber m.
- flush m.
- Gibson-Coke m.
- growth-remaining m.
- hemoglobin subtype m.
- Kaplan-Meier m.
- Kibrick m.
- Kirby-Bauer m.
- Lovaas m.
- Mantoux m.
- Narula m.
- oscillometric m.
- pilocarpine iontophoresis m.
- m. of Politzer
- simplistic m.
- straight-line graph m.
- Strauss m.
- Tanner and Whitehouse II bone-age determination m.
- thermodilution m.
- Volpe m.
- Yuzpe m.

methodology study

methohexital

methotrexate (MTX)
- m., bleomycin, doxorubicin, cyclophosphamide, Oncovin, dexamethasone (m-BACOD)
- intrathecal m.

methoxamine

methoxyflurane

methsuximide

methylation

methylbutyrate
- hydroxy beta m. (HMB)

methylcellulose drops

methylcobalamin

methyl-CpG-binding protein 2 (MeCP2)

methyldopa

M

NOTES

methylene
    m. blue
    m. tetrahydrofolate reductase
methylenedioxy-methamphetamine (MDMA)
3-methylglutaconic aciduria
Methylin
    M. C, ER
methylmalonic
    m. acid
    m. acidemia
    m. aciduria (MMA)
methylmercury intoxication
methylphenidate (MPH)
    extended-release m.
    m. hydrochloride
methylprednisolone
    m. acetate
    m. base
    pulse m.
methylsuccinic acid
methyltransferase
    thiopurine m. (TPMT)
methylxanthine
Meticorten
metoclopramide
metolazone
metopic craniosynostosis
metoprolol
Metreton Ophthalmic
metrizamide
Metrodin
MetroGel Topical
MetroGel-Vaginal
Metro I.V. Injection
metromenorrhagia
metronidazole
metroplasty
    abdominal m.
    Jones wedge m.
    Strassman m.
    Tompkins m.
metyrapone
mevalonic
    m. acidemia
    m. aciduria
mexicana
    Leishmania m.
mexiletine
Mexitil
meyeri
    Actinomyces m.
Meyerson nevus
Mezlin
mezlocillin sodium
M.F.
    K-Phos M.F.

MFF
    matching familiar figures
MFG
    milk fat globule
MFGM
    milk fat globule membrane
MFH
    malignant fibrous histiocytoma
M-FISH
    multispectral fluorescent in situ hybridization
MFNS
    mometasone furoate aqueous nasal spray
MFPR
    multifetal pregnancy reduction
MFT
    medial femoral torsion
MGD
    mixed gonadal dysgenesis
MH
    malignant hyperthermia
MHA-TP
    microhemagglutination assay for antibodies to *Treponema pallidum*
MHC
    major histocompatibility complex
        MHC class I antigen deficiency
MHP
    hyperphenylalaninemia
MHz
    megahertz
MI
    meconium ileus
    migration index
    myocardial infarction
Miacalcin Nasal Spray
Miami Moss instrumentation
MIBE
    measles inclusion body encephalitis
Mibelli
    angiokeratoma of M.
    M. angiokeratoma
    porokeratosis of M.
MIBG
    metaiodobenzylguanidine
        MIBG scan
MIC
    mean intercriterion correlation
    minimal inhibitory concentration
Micatin Topical
micdadei
    Legionella m.
micelle
Michaelis-Menten dissociation constant
Michel
    M. anomaly
    M. aplasia
miconazole gel

MICRhoGAM
microabscess
      Munro m.
microaerophilic
microalbuminuria
microangiopathic
      m. hemolytic anemia
      m. hemolytic uremic syndrome
      m. process
microangiopathy
      HIV m.
      mineralizing m.
      thrombotic m. (TMA)
microarousal
microaspiration
microassisted fertilization
microatelectasis
microbe
microbial
microbrachycephaly
microbubble
      gelatin-encapsulated m.
microcephalic idiocy
microcephalus
microcephaly
      primary m.
      secondary m.
microcirculation
microcirculatory
      m. compromise
      m. dysfunction
microcolon
microcomedone
microcoria
microcornea
microcrystalline
      griseofulvin m.
microcytic anemia
microcytosis
microdactyly
microdeletion
      chromosome m.
      m. of chromosome 22q11
      m. syndrome
microdialysis
microdontia
microdysgenesis
microencephaly
microfilament
microflora
      fecal m.

microfracture
      vertebral m.
microgastria
microglia
microglossia
micrognathia
      severe m.
microgyria
microhamartoma
      biliary m.
microhemagglutination
      m. assay for antibodies to
            Treponema pallidum (MHA-TP)
      m. test
microhyphema
microimmunofluorescence (MIF)
      m. test
microinfarct
Micro-K
      M.-K 10 Extencaps
      M.-K LS
microlipid
      M. formula
microlithiasis
      biliary m.
      pulmonary alveolar m.
Micro-Mist disposable nebulizer
micromyeloblastic leukemia
microneedle
microNefrin
micronodular
      m. gastritis
      m. liver cirrhosis
Micronor
micronutrient deficiency
microorganism
micropenis
microphallus
microphthalmia
microphthalmia
      anterior m.
microphthalmos
micropinocytosis
micropolygyria
micropreemie
microscope
      H-7000 electron m.
microscopic
      m. agglutination test (MAT)
      m. fat
      m. polyarteritis

M

NOTES

microscopy
    darkfield m.
    electron m.
    light m.
    phase-contrast m.
    transmission electron m. (TEM)
microsomia
    hemifacial m.
microspherocyte
microsractphakia
microsporidial keratoconjunctivitis
Microsporum
    M. audouinii
    M. canis
microstomia
Microstream capnograph
microsurgical epididymal sperm aspiration (MESA)
microthrombocytopenia
microthromboembolism
microti
    Babesia m.
microtia
    aural m.
microtransfusion
    maternal-fetal m.
microtrauma
microvascular lesion
microvasculopathy
microvesicular steatosis
microvessel
microvillus, pl. **microvilli**
    m. atrophy (MVA)
    m. inclusion disease (MID)
Microzide
micturition syncope
MID
    microvillus inclusion disease
Midamor
midarm
    m. circumference (MAC)
    m. muscle circumference (MAMC)
midaxillary line
midazolam
    m. nasal spray
    transmucosal m.
midbrain
midclavicular line
middiastolic
    m. murmur
    m. rumble
middle
    m. cerebellar peduncle
    m. cerebral artery (MCA)
    m. cerebral artery occlusion (MCAO)
    m. ear

    m. ear effusion (MEE)
    m. ear fluid (MEF)
    m. ear infection
    m. finger
    m. meatus nasal antral window
    m. one-third of face underdevelopment
midface hypoplasia
midfacial hypoplasia
midfoot breech
midforceps
midgestational
midgut volvulus
midline
    m. cleft palate
    m. craniofacial tumor
    m. facial defect
    m. shift
Midol IB
midstream urine sample
midsupination
midsystolic click
midtemporal epilepsy
midureteral stricture
midvaginal transverse septum
Miege disease
MIF
    microimmunofluorescence
    migration inhibitory factor
    müllerian inhibiting factor
    MIF test
mifepristone
MIGB
    metaiodobenzylguanidine
    MIGB imaging
migraine
    abdominal m.
    acute confusional m.
    basilar artery m.
    classic m.
    classical m.
    common m.
    complicated m.
    confusional m.
    familial hemiplegic m. (FHM)
    footballer m.
    m. headache
    hemiplegic m.
    menstrual m.
    ophthalmoplegic m.
    m. sine hemicrania
    m. syndrome
    m. variant
    m. with aphasia
    m. with aura
    m. without aura
migraine-type headache

migrainous
    m. attack
    m. headache
migrans
    cutaneous larva m.
    erythema m.
    erythema chronicum m. (ECM)
    ocular larva m.
    visceral larva m.
migration
    m. index (MI)
    m. inhibitory factor (MIF)
migratory
    m. path
    m. peripheral arthritis
    m. polyarthritis
Mikity-Wilson syndrome
Mikulicz
    M. disease
    M. procedure
    M. syndrome
mild
    m. acetabular dysplasia
    m. anemia
    m. anorexia nervosa
    m. dehydration
    m. downslant to palpebral fissure
    m. leukocytosis
    m. mental retardation
    m. pulmonic stenosis
    m. scoliosis
    m. spastic diplegic cerebral palsy
    m. ulcerative colitis
mild-to-moderate obesity
Miles Nervine Caplets
milestone
    cognitive developmental m.
    developmental m.
    early language m. (ELM)
milia (*pl. of* milium)
miliaria
    M. crystallina
    m. crystalloid
    m. rubra
    sebaceous m.
    sudoral m.
miliary
    m. infiltrate
    m. sudamina
    m. tuberculosis
milieu therapy
milium, pl. **milia**

milk
    m. allergy
    banked m.
    m. bolus obstruction
    breast m.
    m. ejection reflex
    m. fat globule (MFG)
    m. fat globule membrane (MFGM)
    human m.
    icterogenic breast m.
    m. lines
    m. lines of abdomen
    m. lines of thorax
    m. of magnesia (MOM)
    mother's breast m. (MBM)
    nonfat m.
    m. precipitin disease
    m. protein hydrolysate (MPH)
    m. protein intolerance
    m. scan
    soy m.
    m. stool
    m. triglyceride
    volume percent of cream in m. (CRCT)
    witch's m.
milk-alkali syndrome
milk-based formula
milk-fed
    human m.-f.
milking of umbilical cord
Milkinol
milkmaid's
    m. grip
    m. hand
    m. sign
milk-protein allergy
milk/soy-protein allergy
milky fluid
Millar catheter
Miller
    M. Assessment for Preschoolers
    M. blade (#0, #1)
Miller-Dieker syndrome
Miller-Fisher
    M.-F. syndrome
    M.-F. variant
milleri
    Streptococcus m.
milliampere (mA)
milliliter (mL)

M

NOTES

million
    parts per m. (ppm)
Millipore filter
milrinone
Milroy disease
MILTA
    mucosal intact laser tonsillar ablation
Milupa formula
Milwaukee brace
Mima polymorpha
mimicry
    antigenic m.
    molecular m.
MIMyCA
    maternally inherited myopathy and
      cardiomyopathy
    MIMyCA syndrome
Minamata disease
mind
    theory of m.
mineral
    m. balance study
    m. oil
mineralization
    skeletal m.
mineralizing microangiopathy
mineralocortical deficiency
mineralocorticoid-deficiency RTA
minicore myopathy
Mini-Dose
    HypRho-D M.-D.
minifluoroscopy
Mini-Gamulin Rh
minima
    protein m.
minimal
    m. acceptable height (MAH)
    m. bacterial concentration (MBC)
    m. brain damage
    m. brain dysfunction (MBD)
    m. cerebral dysfunction
    m. change disease
    m. change nephrotic syndrome
      (MCNS)
    m. effective dose (MED)
    m. inhibitory concentration (MIC)
    m. lesion nephrotic syndrome
      (MLNS)
Mini-Med tubing
minimum
    m. daily requirement (MDR)
    m. inhibitory concentration
mini-Pena procedure
mini-pill
Minipress
Minitran Patch
Mini-Wright Peak Flow Meter

Minnesota
    M. Multiphasic Personality
      Inventory (MMPI)
    M. Multiphasic Personality
      Inventory-Adolescent (MMPI-A)
minocycline
minor
    m. cerebral dysfunction
    chorea m.
    emancipated m.
    m. group antigen incompatibility
    m. motor seizure
    thalassemia m.
minora (*pl. of* minus)
minoxidil
Mintezol
minus, pl. **minora**
    labium m., pl. labia minora
    Spirillum m.
Minute-Gel
minutissimum
    Corynebacterium m.
Miochol-E
miosis
    congenital m.
    ipsilateral m.
MIP
    macrophage inflammatory protein
MIP-1 alpha
    recombinant human MIP-1 alpha
mirabilis
    Proteus m.
MiraLax
mirror
    m. laryngoscopy
    pharyngeal m.
    m. syndrome
mirror-image dextrocardia
misarticulation
misbehavior
mismatch
    ventilation-perfusion m.
    V/Q m.
misoprostol
MISS
    Modified Injury Severity Score
missense mutation
missing teeth
mist
    Afrin Saline M.
    AsthmaHaler M.
    Ayr saline nasal m.
    Bronitin M.
    Bronkaid M.
    HuMist Nasal M.
    Ocean Nasal M.
    Primatene M.

m. tent
m. therapy
mite
dust m.
house dust m.
scabies m.
Mithracin
mitis Ehlers-Danlos syndrome
mitochondrial
m. cytopathy
m. deoxyribonucleic acid (mtDNA)
m. disease
m. DNA (mtDNA)
m. encephalomyelopathy, lactic acidosis, strokelike symptoms
m. encephalomyopathy
m. encephalopathy, lactic acidosis, stroke
m. glycine cleavage system
m. inheritance
m. injury
m. myopathy
m. myopathy, encephalopathy, lactic acidosis, strokelike episodes (MELAS)
m. oxidative phosphorylation
m. respiratory chain defect
mitochondrion, pl. **mitochondria**
abnormal m.
mitogen
poke weed m. (PWM)
mitogenic
m. effect
m. peptide
mitomycin
m. C
mitosis
crypt cell m.
mitoxantrone
mitral
m. insufficiency
m. stenosis
m. valve
m. valve, aorta, skeleton, skin (MASS)
m. valve prolapse (MVP)
Mitrofanoff technique
Mitsuda reaction
mittelschmerz
Mittendorf dot
mitten-hand deformity
Mivacron

mivacurium
mix
Metamucil Instant M.
mixed
m. antiinflammatory syndrome (MARS)
m. cellularity Hodgkin disease
m. cerebral palsy
m. connective tissue disease (MCTD)
m. cystic/solid architecture
m. flexor/extensor fit
m. gonadal dysgenesis (MGD)
m. hearing impairment
m. hearing loss
m. hyperlipidemia
m. hypothyroidism
m. infantile spasm
m. obstructive apnea/hypopnea index (MOAHI)
m. porphyria
m. receptive-expressive language disorder (MRELD)
m. sensory polyneuritis
m. sleep apnea
m. venous oxygen content
mixed-type cerebral palsy
mixing lesion
mizoribine (MZB)
ML
mucolipidosis
mL
milliliter
MLD
metachromatic leukodystrophy
juvenile MLD
late infantile MLD
ML-II
mucolipidosis II
ML-III
mucolipidosis III
MLNS
minimal lesion nephrotic syndrome
mucocutaneous lymph node syndrome
MLU
mean length of utterance
MLUm
mean length of utterance in morphemes
MMA
methylmalonic aciduria
MMF
mycophenolate mofetil

NOTES

MMIH
megacystis, microcolon, intestinal hypoperistalsis
MMIH syndrome
M-mode echocardiography
MMP
matrix metalloproteinase
MMPI
Minnesota Multiphasic Personality Inventory
MMPI-A
Minnesota Multiphasic Personality Inventory-Adolescent
MMR
measles, mumps, rubella
meningitis or encephalitis, metabolic, Reye syndrome
MMR vaccine
M-M-R II vaccine
M-O
Haley's M-O
MOA
monoamine oxidase inhibitor
MOAHI
mixed obstructive apnea/hypopnea index
mobility
m. aid
m. specialist
mobilization
gastric m.
tarsometatarsal m.
Mobitz I, II block
Möbius, Moebius
M. syndrome
modafinil acetamide
modality
Modane
M. Bulk
M. Soft
mode
polygenic m.
pressure support m.
model
APLS m.
cognitive-diathesis m.
Cox proportional hazard m.
Gesell Developmental M.
longitudinal random coefficient m. (LRCM)
maximal electroshock m.
murine m.
random regression m.
moderate
m. dehydration
m. hirsutism
m. mental retardation
m. ulcerative colitis

modification
behavior m.
Martin m.
posttranslational m.
modified
m. barium swallow (MBS)
m. barium swallow with videofluoroscopy
m. Blalock-Taussig shunt
m. bovine surfactant extract
m. Dieterle stain
m. Fontan operation
m. Fontan procedure
m. Gomori trichrome reaction
M. Injury Severity Score (MISS)
m. Kinyoun acid-fast stain
m. measles
m. trichrome stain
MODS
multiorgan dysfunction syndrome
multiple organ dysfunction syndrome
Modical formula
modulator
cytokine m.
MODY
maturity-onset diabetes of youth
Moebius (*var. of* Möbius)
Moeller-Barlow disease
mofetil
mycophenolate m. (MMF, MPM, RS-61443)
Mogen clamp
Mohr syndrome
MOI
maximal oxygen intake
medical optimal imaging
multiplicity of infection
moist
Nasal M.
Moisturel
moisturizer
Betadine First Aid Antibiotics + M.
molar
first permanent m.
first primary m.
hutchinsonian m.
mulberry m.
permanent m.
primary m.
second permanent m.
second primary m.
third permanent m.
mold spore
molecular
m. adsorbent recirculating system (MARS)
m. genetic study

m. mimicry
m. regulation

molecule

cell adhesion m. (CAM)
intercellular adhesion m. 1 (ICAM-1)
vascular cell adhesion m. (VCAM)

molestation

Mol-Iron

Moll

apocrine gland of M.
M. gland

Mollaret meningitis

Mollifene Ear Wax Removing Formula

molluscum

m. contagiosum
m. fibrosum pendulum
Staphylococcus aureus m.

molybdenum

m. cofactor
m. cofactor deficiency (MCD)

Molypen

MOM

milk of magnesia
mucoid otitis media
multiples of median

mometasone

m. furoate
m. furoate aqueous nasal spray (MFNS)

Monafed

Monaghan respirator

monarticular arthritis

Monday morning colic

Mondini

M. anomaly
M. aplasia

Mongolian spot

mongolism

mongoloid slant

monilethrix

monilia

monilial

m. diaper dermatitis
m. diaper rash
m. esophagitis

moniliasis

oral m.

moniliformis

Streptobacillus m.

Monistat

M. I.V. Injection
M. Vaginal

Monistat-Derm Topical

monitor

apnea m.
Baby Sense m.
BASC m.
Behavior Assessment System for Children m.
blood pressure m.
CA m.
Camino m.
cardiac-apnea m.
cardiac event m.
cardiorespiratory m.
cerebral function m. (CFM)
Cue Fertility M.
event m.
fetal m.
Finapres blood pressure m.
Holter m.
home cardiorespiratory m. (HCRM)
Ladd m.
Masimo SET home m.
Nellcor N-200 home m.
Nellcor N-3000 home m.
Nellcor Puritan Bennett home m.
peak flow meter m.
Propaq Encore vital signs m.
VitaGuard m.

monitoring

ambulatory blood pressure m. (ABPM)
beat-to-beat continuous blood pressure m.
continuous blood gas m.
continuous long-term m. (CLTM)
distal esophageal pH m.
EEG/polygraphic/video m.
fetal scalp m.
home blood glucose m.
home uterine activity m. (HUAM)
ICP m.
jugular bulb m.
prolonged EEG m.
pulmonary artery pressure m.
transtelephonic m. (TTM)
video m.

monkeybars

monkey polyoma virus

NOTES

M

mono
    mononucleosis
monoamine oxidase inhibitor (MAOI, MOA)
monoaminergic
monoarticular synovitis
monochorionic twin
Monoclate-P
monoclonal
    m. antibody (MAb)
    m. antiendotoxin antibody
    m. anti-IgE antibody
monoclonic seizure
monocular
    m. diplopia
    m. nystagmus
monocyte cell
monocytogenes
    Listeria m.
monocytopenia
monocytosis
Monodox
monogenic disorder
monoglutamate
monohydrate
    cefadroxil m.
    lactose m.
monolaurin
monomorphous papular eruption
mononeuritis, pl. **mononeuritides**
    m. multiplex
    m. with paralysis
mononeuropathy
    multiple m.'s
mononuclear
    m. phagocyte
    m. pleocytosis
mononucleosis (mono)
    infectious m. (IM)
mononucleosis-type syndrome
monophasic R wave
monophonic
    m. wheeze
    m. wheezing
monophosphate
    cyclic adenosine m. (cAMP)
monoplegia
    spastic m.
monoploid
monosialoganglioside
monosodium glutamate poisoning
monosomy 7 syndrome
Monospot
    M. screen
    M. test
Monosticon Dri-Dot
monostotic
monosymptomatic

monotherapy
    digoxin m.
monovular twin
monoxide
    carbon m. (CO)
    end-tidal breath carbon m.
monozygotic twin
Monro
    foramen of M.
monsplasty
mons pubis
monster cell
Monteggia
    M. fracture
    M. fracture dislocation
montelukast
Montenegro skin test
Montgomery County virus
month
    Lupron Depot-3 M.
    Lupron Depot-4 M.
mood
    m. disorder
    dysphoric m.
    m. lability
mood-congruent psychotic feature
moodiness
moon facies
moon-shaped facies
MOPP
    mechlorethamine, Oncovin (vincristine), procarbazine, prednisone
    MOPP chemotherapy protocol
Moraxella catarrhalis
morbidity
    asthma m.
morbilliform skin rash
Morbillivirus
morbillorum
    Gemella m.
Morch respirator
More-Dophilus
Morgagni
    foramen of M.
    M. hernia
Morgagni-Adams-Stokes syndrome
Morgan therapeutic lens
moribund
moricizine
Morison pouch
morning
    m. glory disk anomaly
    m. osmolality
Moro
    M. reflex
    M. response
morphea scleroderma

morpheme
  mean length of utterance in m.'s
    (MLUm)
morphine sulfate
morphogenesis
  branching m.
  lung m.
  parenchymal lung m.
morphogenetic lesion
morphological
morphology
  QRS m.
morphometric
Morquio
  M. disease
  M. syndrome
Morquio-Ullrich syndrome
Morsch-Retec respirator
mortality
  Pediatric Risk of M.
  postneonatal m.
mortise view
morula
MOS
  medical optical spectroscopy
mosaic
  m. perfusion
  Turner m.
  m. verruca
mosaicism
  erythrocyte m.
  germ cell m.
  gonadal m.
  placental m.
  somatic m.
  Turner m.
  m. for XXX
  45,X/46,XY m.
MOSF
  multiple organ system failure
mossy fiber sprouting
mothball
  naphthalene m.
mother
  M. Against Drunk Driving
    (MADD)
  m. breast milk (MBM)
  m. burnout
  infant of diabetic m. (IDM)
  infant of substance-abusing m.
    (ISAM)
  Rh-negative m.

mother-child interaction
motherease speech
mother-infant transmission
motilin receptor agonist
motility
  altered gastric m.
  decreased gastrointestinal m.
  m. disorder
  gut m.
  intestinal m.
  receptor for hyaluronan-mediated m.
    (RHAMM)
motility-related dysphagia
motion
  m. artifact rejection system
    (MARS)
  chest wall m.
  limited neck m.
  paradoxical chest wall m.
  passive range of m.
  range of m. (ROM)
  scapulothoracic m.
  m. sickness
motion-resistant pulse oximetry
motoneuron
motor
  m. automatism
  m. control
  m. cortex
  m. disability
  m. evoked potential (MEP)
  fine m.
  gross m.
  m. hyperactivity
  m. nerve
  m. neuron
  m. neuron disease
  m. neuron palsy
  m. neuron sign
  oral m.
  m. pattern
  m. perception
  m. perception dysfunction
  m. planning
  m. restlessness
  m. scale
  m. seizure
  m. skill
  m. tic
motor-axonal neuropathy
motor-sensory axonal neuropathy

M

NOTES

Motrin
  Children's M.
  M. IB
  Ibu-Tab Junior Strength M.
MOTT
  mycobacteria other than tuberculosis
mottled
  m. enamel
  m. retina
mottling
mount
  chest m.
  direct wet m.
  wet m.
mountain sickness
mousse
  RID M.
mouth
  m. breathing
  downturned m.
  fish-shaped m.
  m. guard
  inverted-V m.
  nothing by m. (non per os)
    (n.p.o.)
  open m.
  by m. (per os) (p.o.)
  purse-string m.
  tapir m.
  trench m.
Mouth-Aid
  Orajel M.-A.
mouthing
mouthpiece
mouth-to-mask breathing
mouth-to-mouth resuscitation
mouth-to-nose/mouth resuscitation
mouthwash
  magic m.
movement
  adventitious choreiform m.
  angular m.
  athetoid m.
  bicycling m.
  chaotic eye m.
  choreic m.
  choreiform m.
  choreoathetoid m.
  choreoathetotic m.
  circumduction m.
  clonic m.
  compensatory m.
  dancing eye m.
  deviant volitional m.
  dissociated m.
  equal ocular m. (EOM)
  extraocular m. (EOM)
  extrapyramidal m.
  eye m.
  gliding m.
  hand-to-mouth m.
  hand-wringing m.
  involuntary m.
  irregular stereotyped m.
  multifocal clonic m.
  nonrapid eye m. (NREM)
  opposition m.
  pedaling m.
  rapid alternating m.
  rapid eye m. (REM)
  rapid succession m.
  reciprocal m.
  respiratory m.
  rotation m.
  sleep with rapid eye m.
  stereotypical m.
  swimming m.
  symmetrical m.
  unifocal clonic m.
  volitional m.
moxa herb
moxalactam
moxibustion
moyamoya
  m. disease
  m. syndrome
Moynihan
  M. respirator
  M. syndrome
MPA
  medroxyprogesterone acetate
MPGN
  membranoproliferative
    glomerulonephritis
  mesangiocapillary glomerulonephritis
    (type I, II)
MPH
  male pseudohermaphroditism
  methylphenidate
  milk protein hydrolysate
MPHD
  multiple pituitary hormone deficiency
MPIAS
  multiparameter intraarterial sensor
MPM
  mycophenolate mofetil
MPO
  myeloperoxidase
    MPO deficiency
MPQ
  Multidimensional Personality
    Questionnaire
M-Prednisol Injection
M protein factor
MPS
  mucopolysaccharide

MPT
  multipuncture test
MPV
  mean platelet volume
MR
  medial rotation
MRA
  magnetic resonance angiography
MRC
  magnetic resonance cholangiography
MRCP
  magnetic resonance
    cholangiopancreatography
    MRCP using HASTE with a
      phased array coil
MRELD
  mixed receptive-expressive language
    disorder
MRI
  magnetic resonance imaging
    diffuse tensor brain MRI
    functional MRI (fMRI)
    ^{31}P MRI
mRNA
  messenger ribonucleic acid
    posttranslational modification of
      mRNA
MRS
  magnetic resonance spectroscopy
    phosphorus MRS
    proton MRS
MRSA
  methicillin-resistant *Staphylococcus*
    aureus
MS
  mass spectrometry
  multiple sclerosis
    acute MS
    MS Contin Oral
    Marburg-type MS
MSAF
  meconium-stained amniotic fluid
MSAFP
  maternal serum alpha fetoprotein
MSBP
  Münchausen syndrome by proxy
MSD Enteric Coated ASA
MSEL
  Mullen Scales of Early Learning
MSI
  magnetic source imaging
MSIR Oral

MSK
  musculoskeletal
MSLSS
  Multidimensional Student Life
    Satisfaction Scale
MSLT
  Multiple Sleep Latency Test
MSP
  Münchausen syndrome by proxy
MSPS
  musculoskeletal pain syndrome
MSPSS
  Multidimensional Scale of Perceived
    Social Support
MSSB
  MacArthur Story Stem Battery
MST
  multiple subpial transection
  multisystemic therapy
MSUD
  maple syrup urine disease
MT
    Pancrease MT
    Ultrase MT
MTC
  multilocular thymic cyst
mtDNA
  mitochondrial deoxyribonucleic acid
  mitochondrial DNA
M.T.E.-4, -5, -6
M-tropic
  macrophage tropic
    M-tropic strain
MTS
  mesial temporal sclerosis
MTT
  medial tibial torsion
MTX
  methotrexate
Mucha-Habermann disease
mucin clot test
mucociliary
    m. clearance
    m. function
mucocolpos
mucocutaneous
    m. candidiasis
    m. junction
    m. lymph node
    m. lymph node syndrome (MCLS,
      MLNS)
    m. pigmentation

M

NOTES

mucoepidermoid carcinoma
Muco-Fen-LA
mucoid
    m. otitis media (MOM)
    m. sputum
mucolipidosis (ML)
    m. II (ML-II)
    m. III (ML-III)
mucolytic
mucomycosis
Mucomyst solution
mucopeptide
mucoperichondrium
mucopolysaccharide (MPS)
    aggregated m.
    m. pattern
    m. protein
    urine m.
mucopolysaccharidosis,
  pl. mucopolysaccharidoses
    m. IH
    m. II
    m. IIIA
    m. IS
mucoprotein
mucopurulent cervicitis
Mucor
mucormycosis
    cutaneous m.
    pulmonary m.
    rhinocerebral m.
mucosa
    atrophic vaginal m.
    buccal m.
    ectopic gastric m.
    gastric m.
    genital m.
    intestinal m.
    necrotic m.
    palatal m.
    rugated vaginal m.
    thin vaginal m.
    vaginal m.
mucosa-associated lymphoid tissue
  (MALT)
mucosae
    hyalinosis cutis et m.
mucosal
    m. biopsy
    m. bleeding
    m. intact laser tonsillar ablation
      (MILTA)
    m. leishmaniasis
    m. lesion
    m. neuroma syndrome
    m. rosette
    m. sloughing

mucosalis
    Campylobacter m.
Mucosil
mucositis
mucosulfatidosis
mucous
    m. inspissation
    m. membrane
    m. membrane provocation
    m. membrane wart
    m. retention cyst
mucoviscidosis
mucus
    m. aspirator
    cervical m.
    m. plug
muffled heart sound
MUGA
    multiple gated acquisition
    MUGA scan
mulberry
    m. molar
    m. tumor
Mulibrey
    muscle, liver, brain, eye
    Mulibrey nanism
Mullen Scales of Early Learning
  (MSEL)
müllerian
    m. duct
    m. inhibiting factor (MIF)
Mullins long transseptal sheath
Multe-Pak-4
Multicenter AIDS Cohort Study
  (MACS)
multicentric Castleman disease
multicore myopathy
multicystic
    m. dysplastic kidney (MDK)
    m. encephalomalacia
    m. kidney
    m. kidney disease
    m. renal dysplasia
multidimensional
    M. Personality Questionnaire
      (MPQ)
    M. Scale of Perceived Social
      Support (MSPSS)
    M. Student Life Satisfaction Scale
      (MSLSS)
multidisciplinary team
multidose activated charcoal (MDAC)
multidrug
    m. chemotherapy
    m. resistance (MDR)
    m. therapy (MDT)
multidrug-resistant tuberculosis (MDR-
  TB)

multielectrode
ESA Coulochem m.
multifactorial disorder
multifetal pregnancy reduction (MFPR)
multifocal
m. atrial tachycardia
m. clonic convulsion
m. clonic movement
m. clonic seizure
m. leukoencephalopathy
m. osteomyelitis
m. spike
m. white matter inflammatory
lesion
multiforme
bullous erythema m.
erythema m. (EM)
glioblastoma m.
multigenerational
multihandicapped
multilocularis
Echinococcus m.
multilocular thymic cyst (MTC)
multimodal treatment plan
multinuclearity
hereditary erythroblastic m.
multinucleated
m. cell encephalitis
m. giant cell
multiorgan
m. dysfunction syndrome (MODS)
m. system failure
multipara
multiparameter intraarterial sensor (MPIAS)
multiple
m. acyl-coenzyme A dehydrogenase
deficiency (MADD)
m. basal cell nevoid syndrome
m. birth
m. bone enchondromata
m. carboxylase deficiency
m. cartilaginous exostosis
m. complex developmental disorder
(MCDD)
m. dislocations
m. endocrine abnormalities (MEA)
m. endocrine adenomatosis (MEA)
m. endocrine neoplasia
m. endocrine neoplasia type 2
(MEN-2)
m. epiphyseal dysplasia

m. gastrointestinal polyps
m. gated acquisition (MUGA)
m. gestation
m. hamartoma syndrome
m. lentigines syndrome
m.'s of median (MOM)
m. mononeuropathies
m. myofibromatosis
m. neuroma syndrome
m. opportunistic pathogen infection
m. oral frenula
m. organ dysfunction syndrome
(MODS)
m. organ system failure (MOSF)
m. osteomas
m. pituitary hormone deficiency
(MPHD)
m. pterygium syndrome
m. sclerosis (MS)
M. Sleep Latency Test (MSLT)
m. subpial transection (MST)
m. sulfatase deficiency
m. tics
m. villous infarcts
m. X syndrome
multiple-ring-enhancing mass lesion
multiplex
arthrogryposis m.
dysostosis m.
mononeuritis m.
paramyoclonus m.
steatocystoma m.
multiplicity of infection (MOI)
multipuncture
m. technique
m. test (MPT)
multispectral fluorescent in situ hybridization (M-FISH)
multisymptomatic
multisystemic therapy (MST)
multivalent
multivorans
Burkholderia m.
multocida
Pasteurella m.
Prevotella m.
mummy wrap
mumps
m. arthritis
m. encephalitis
m. leptomeningitis
m. meningoencephalitis

NOTES

M

Münchausen
> M. disease
> M. disease by proxy
> M. syndrome
> M. syndrome by proxy (MSBP, MSP)

munching pattern
munity
Munro microabscess
Munson sign
mupirocin
mural
> m. endocardium
> m. thrombosis

murine
> M. Ear Drops
> m. leukemia virus
> m. model
> m. myeloid leukemia cell line
> m. typhus

murmur
> apical presystolic m.
> Austin Flint m.
> blowing decrescendo diastolic m.
> cardiac m.
> continuous shunt m.
> crescendo m.
> decrescendo diastolic m.
> diamond-shaped m.
> diastolic m.
> flow m.
> functional m.
> Gibson m.
> Graham Steell m.
> harsh pansystolic m.
> heart m.
> holosystolic m.
> innocent m.
> machinery m.
> middiastolic m.
> musical m.
> pansystolic m.
> presystolic m.
> pulmonary m.
> pulmonic m.
> rumbling m.
> Still m.
> systolic continuous m.
> systolic ejection m. (SEM)
> to-and-fro m.
> m. of valvulitis
> vibratory m.

muromonab-CD3
Muro 128 Ophthalmic
Muroptic-5
Murphy sign

muscarinic
> m. action
> m. effect

muscle
> absence of rectal m.'s
> accessory m.
> m. actin
> m. adenosine monophosphate deaminase deficiency
> airway smooth m.
> antagonistic m.
> m. atrophy
> biceps femoris m.
> m. biopsy
> m. bulk
> m. carnitine palmityltransferase deficiency
> ciliary m.
> conal m.
> concave temporalis m.
> m. cylinder
> deltoid m.
> depressor anguli oris m.
> diarthrodial m.
> divergent rectus m.
> m. enlargement
> m. enzyme test
> external sphincter m.
> extraocular m.
> eyelid m.
> m. fasciculation
> gastrocnemius m.
> genioglossus m.
> gluteal m.
> gluteus maximus m.
> gluteus medius m.
> gluteus minimus m.
> gracilis m.
> m. herniation
> ipsilateral lateral rectus m.
> lateral rectus m.
> m. lengthening
> levator palpebrae m.
> m., liver, brain, eye (Mulibrey)
> m., liver, brain, eye nanism
> lumbar extensor m.
> masseter m.
> m. necrosis
> obturator internus m.
> papillary m.
> m. paralysis
> pharyngeal m.
> m. phosphofructokinase deficiency
> m. proprioceptor
> quadratus labiae superioris m.
> rectus femoris m.
> m. relaxant
> m. rigidity

scalene m.
scalloped temporalis m.
SCM m.
semimembranosus m.
semitendinosus m.
sphincter m.
superior oblique m.
m. surgery
temporalis m.
m. testing
m. tone
unilateral hypoplastic pectoral m.
vastus lateralis m.
zygomatic head of quadratus labiae
  superioris m.

muscle-brain (MB)
muscle-brain isoenzyme

muscle-eye-brain
m.-e.-b. disease
m.-e.-b. disease of Santavuori

muscular
m. atrophy
m. cuff
m. dystrophy
m. hypotonia
m. torticollis
m. ventricular septum

muscularis
musculocutaneous nerve
musculoskeletal (MSK)
m. pain syndrome (MSPS)

Muse pellet
mushroom
Amanita m.
m. gyrus

musical murmur
mustard
M. atrial switch procedure
nitrogen m.
M. operation
M. technique

Mustardé procedure
Mustargen Hydrochloride
mutagenesis
mutagenic treatment
Mutamycin
mutans
Streptococcus m.

mutant
m. homoplasmy
Hoxa-5 null m.

mutation
autosomal recessive m.
chromosome 17 m.
Drosophila m.
dynamic m.
factor V Leiden m.
full m.
gene m.
121ins2 m.
interleukin-2 receptor alpha
  chain m.
missense m.
prothrombin gene m.
m. testing

mute
mutilans
keratoma hereditarium m.

mutilating keratoderma
mutilation
female genital m.

mutism
akinetic m.
cerebellar m.
selective m.
transient m.

MVA
microvillus atrophy

MVB
manual ventilation bag

MV(c)ELISA
measles virus enzyme-linked
  immunosorbent assay

MVP
mitral valve prolapse

MWT
Mallory-Weiss tear

myalgia cruris epidemica
Myambutol
Myapap
myasthenia
congenital m.
m. gravis
juvenile m.
transient neonatal m.

myasthenia-like syndrome
myasthenic syndrome
Mycelex-G
M.-G Topical
M.-G Vaginal

Mycelex Troche
mycelial mat

M

NOTES

mycetoma
    renal m.
Mycifradin Sulfate
Mycinettes
Mycitracin Topical
mycobacteria (*pl. of* mycobacterium)
mycobacterial
    m. organism
Mycobacterium
    M. abscessus
    M. africanum
    M. avium
    M. avium complex (MAC)
    M. avium-intracellulare (MAI)
    M. avium-intracellulare complex
      (MAC)
    M. bovis
    M. chelonae
    M. fortuitum
    M. fortuitum complex
    M. kansasii
    M. leprae
    M. malmoense
    M. marinum
    M. scrofulaceum
    M. tuberculosis
    M. ulcerans
    M. xenopi
mycobacterium, pl. **mycobacteria**
    atypical mycobacteria
    nontuberculous m. (NTM)
    nontuberculous mycobacteria (NTM)
    mycobacteria other than tuberculosis
      (MOTT)
Mycobutin
mycophenolate mofetil (MMF, MPM,
    RS-61443)
mycophenolic acid
Mycoplasma
    M. fermentans
    M. genitalium
    M. hominis
    M. penetrans
    M. pneumonia
    M. pneumoniae
mycoplasmal antibody
mycosis
    m. fungoides
    hypopigmented m.
Mycostatin
mycotic aneurysm
Mydfrin
    M. Ophthalmic
    M. Ophthalmic Solution
Mydriacyl
mydriasis
    congenital m.
    unilateral m.

mydriatic
myelin
    m. lipid
    m. sheath
myelination
myelinization
myelinoclastic diffuse cerebral sclerosis
myelinolysis
    central pontine m.
myelitis
    acute transverse m.
    transverse m.
    zoster m.
myeloblast cell
myeloblastic leukemia
myelocele
myelocyte cell
myelocytic leukemia
myelodysplasia
    pediatric m.
myelodysplastic syndrome (MDS)
myelofibrosis
myelogenous leukemia
myelogram
myelograph
myelography
myeloid
    m. to erythroid (M:E)
    m. to erythroid ratio
    m. leukemia
myelokathexis
myelomalacia
myelomeningocele
myelomonocytic leukemia
myeloneuropathy
    human T-cell lymphotropic virus 1
      tropic m.
myeloopticoneuropathy
    subacute m.
myelopathy
    compression m.
    craniocervical m.
    delayed m.
    HTLV-I associated m. (HAM)
    human T-cell lymphotrophic virus
      type I associated m. (HAM)
    postirradiation m.
    schistosomal m.
    tropical spastic paraparesis/HTLV-I
      associated m. (TSP/HAM)
    vacuolar m.
    vascular m.
myeloperoxidase (MPO)
    m. deficiency
myelophthisis
myelopoiesis
    ineffective m.
myeloproliferative syndrome

myeloradiculitis
    acute m.
myeloschisis
    dorsal m.
myelosuppression
myelotoxicity
myenteric
    m. plexus
    m. plexus neuropathy
myiasis
Mykrox
Mylanta Gas
Mylanta-II
Mylar glove
Myleran
Mylicon
myoblast transfer therapy
myocardial
    m. abscess
    m. contusion
    m. fiber degeneration
    m. infarction (MI)
    m. ischemia
    m. muscle creatine kinase
      isoenzyme (CK-MB)
    m. siderosis
    m. steal syndrome
    m. stunning
myocarditis
    acute interstitial m.
    diphtheritic toxic m.
    enteroviral m.
    Fiedler m.
    giant cell m.
    infectious m.
    interstitial m.
    silent m.
    toxic m.
    viral m.
myocardium
    stunned m.
Myochrysine
myoclonic
    m. absence
    m. ataxia
    m. convulsion
    m. dystonia
    m. encephalopathy
    m. epilepsy
    m. jerk
    m. petit mal

    m. seizure
    m. spasm
myoclonic-astatic seizure
myoclonus
    Baltic m.
    cortical reflex m.
    m. epilepsy
    m., epilepsy, ragged red fibers
      (MERRF)
    m. epilepsy with ragged red fibers
      (MERRF)
    epileptic m.
    essential m.
    intention m.
    jaw m.
    Mediterranean m.
    nocturnal m.
    nonepileptic m.
    ocular m.
    reflex m.
    reticular reflex m.
    sleep m.
    m. syndrome
myocytic hypertrophy
myocytolysis
    coagulative m.
myoepithelial
myofascial release
myofiber disarray
myofibril
myofibromatosis
    congenital multiple m.
    infantile m.
    multiple m.
    periorbital infantile m
    renal m.
    solitary renal m.
myofilament
myogenic
myoglobin
myoglobinuria
    recurrent m.
    sporadic m.
myoinositol
myokymia
    interictal m.
myometrium
myonecrosis
    clostridial m.
myopathy
    cardioskeletal m.
    centronuclear m.

M

NOTES

myopathy *(continued)*
    congenital m.
    dysmaturative m.
    m., encephalopathy, lactic acidosis,
      strokelike episodes (MELAS)
    familial visceral m.
    fatal infantile m.
    holovisceral m.
    hypothyroid m.
    infantile myofibrillar m.
    lipid m.
    metabolic m.
    minicore m.
    mitochondrial m.
    multicore m.
    myotubular m.
    nemaline rod m.
    nonfamilial visceral m.
    ocular m.
    Proteus syndrome m.
    ragged red m.
    Sengers mitochondrial m.
    steroid-induced m.
    visceral m.
    X-linked cardioskeletal m.
    X-linked myotubular m.
myopericarditis
myophosphorylase deficiency
myopia
    high m.
    severe m.
myosin
myosis
myositis
    eosinophilic m.
    inflammatory m.
    intrauterine viral m.
    m. ossificans
    m. ossificans circumscripta
    m. ossificans progressiva

myotomy
    Heller m.
    Livadatis circular m.
Myotonachol
myotonia
    chondrodystrophic m.
    cold-induced m.
    m. congenita
    grip m.
    m. neonatorum
    percussion m.
myotonic
    m. chondrodystrophy
    m. muscular dystrophy
myotubular myopathy
Myphetapp
myringitis
    bullous m.
myringotomy
    laser m.
    laser-assisted m. (LAM)
    Otoscan laser-assisted m. (OtoLAM)
    m. tube
    wide-field m.
Mysoline
Mytussin DM
myxedema
    m. coma
    infantile m.
myxoid
    m. dysplasia
    m. histopathologic subtype
    m. liposarcoma
myxoma
    familial cardiac m.
MZB
    mizoribine

NA
nosocomially acquired
Na
sodium
NAA
nucleic acid amplification
NAA test
Nabi-HB
N-acetylaspartate
N-acetylaspartic acid
N-acetylglutamate
N-a. deficiency
N-a. synthetase
nadir
Nadolol
NADPH
nicotinamide adenine dinucleotide
phosphate
NADPH oxidase
Naegleria fowleri
naeslundii
Actinomyces n.
Nafazair Ophthalmic
Nafcil Injection
nafcillin sodium
naftifine
Naftin
Nager
N. acrofacial dysostosis
N. syndrome
NaHCO₃
sodium bicarbonate
nail
n. bed cyanosis
n. bed telangiectasia
brittle n.
clubbing of n.'s
n. defect
dystrophic n.
n. dystrophy
n. fold telangiectasia
hippocratic n.
hypertrophic n.
hypoplastic n.
n. matrix
pachyonychia congenita syndrome
of n.
n. pitting
n. ringworm
shedding of n.'s
spoon-shaped n.
titanium elastic n.
n. trephination
yellow n.

nail-fold
n.-f. capillary
n.-f. infection
nailing
titanium elastic n. (TEN)
nail-patella syndrome
naive
nalbuphine
Naldecon
N. DX Children's
N. DX Pediatric Drops
N. EX Children's Syrup
N. EX Pediatric Drops
N. Senior DX
N. Senior EX
nalidixic
n. acid
n. acid agar
Nallpen Injection
nalorphine
naloxone hydrochloride
NALT
nasopharyngeal-associated lymphoid
tissue
naltrexone
NAMCS
National Ambulatory Medical Care
Survey
NAME
nevi, atrial myxomas, myxoid
neurofibromas, ephelides
NAME syndrome
naming speed deficit
Nan
N. 2 formula
N. 1 LP formula
NANBH
non-A, non-B hepatitis
nanism
Mulibrey n.
muscle, liver, brain, eye n.
nanogram
naphazoline
Naphcon Forte Ophthalmic
naphthalene mothball
naphthoquinone
NAPI
Neurodevelopmental Assessment of
Preterm Infants
NAPNAP
National Association of Pediatric Nurse
Associates and Practitioners
naproxen
Na⁺ pump
Narcan

N

narcissus
narcolepsy
narcoleptic
    n. attack
    n. sleep
narcosis
narcotic drug
naris, pl. nares
    anteverted n.
NARP
    neuropathy, ataxia, retinitis pigmentosa
    NARP syndrome
narrow
    n. band spectrophotometer
    n. bifrontal diameter
    n. complex supraventricular
    tachycardia
    n. foot
    n. hand
    n. mediastinal waist
    n. mediastinum
    n. mesenteric stalk
    n. palate
    n. pulmonary outflow tract (NPOT)
narrowness
    intermaxillary n.
narrow-spectrum blue light
Narula method
NAS
    Neonatal Abstinence Score
    neonatal abstinence syndrome
Nasacort AQ
Nasahist B
NaSal
nasal
    n. air emission
    n. ala
    n. alar cartilage cleft
    n. antral window
    n. antrum
    Ayr N.
    n. bone
    n. bridge
    n. cannula
    n. cauterization
    n. consonant
    n. continuous positive airway
    pressure (n-CPAP)
    n. CPAP
    n. decongestant
    n. diphtheria
    n. encephalocele
    n. flaring
    n. lavage
    n. mastocytosis
    N. Moist
    n. obstruction
    n. packing

    n. polyp
    n. polyposis
    Privine N.
    n. prong continuous positive airway
    pressure (NP-CPAP)
    n. pyriform aperture stenosis
    n. regurgitation
    n. retractor
    n. root
    n. septum
    n. smear
    n. speculum
    n. swab
    n. swab culture
    n. tampon
    n. tip thermistor
    n. turbinate
    n. ulceration
    n. voice
    n. wash
Nasalcrom
Nasalide Nasal Inhaler
Nasarel Nasal Spray
NASBA
    nucleic acid sequence-based amplification
nascentium
    trismus n.
NASH
    nonalcoholic steatohepatitis
nasi
    alae n.
    flaring of alae n.
nasion
nasoendoscopy
nasofrontal suture
nasogastric (NG)
    n. aspirate
    n. drainage
    n. drip feeding
    n. tube (NGT)
    n. tube feeding
nasojejunal (NJ)
    n. tube
nasolacrimal
    n. duct
    n. duct obstruction
    n. sac
Nasonex
nasoorbitoethmoid (NOE)
nasopharyngeal
    n. aspirate (NPA)
    n. carcinoma
    n. fibroma
    n. reflux (NPR)
    n. suction
    n. suctioning
    n. swab
    n. wash

nasopharyngeal-associated lymphoid tissue (NALT)
nasopharyngitis
nasopharyngolaryngoscopy (NPL)
nasopharynx
nasotracheal intubation
NASPGN
North American Society for Pediatric Gastroenterology and Nutrition
nata
pro re n. (as the occasion arises) (p.r.n.)
natal teeth
National
N. Acute Spinal Cord Injury Study
N. Ambulatory Medical Care Survey (NAMCS)
N. Association of Pediatric Nurse Associates and Practitioners (NAPNAP)
N. Center for Child Abuse and Neglect (NCCAN)
N. Clearing House on Child Abuse and Neglect
N. Educational Longitudinal Survey (NELS)
N. Health and Nutrition Examination Survey (NHANES)
N. Institute of Child Health and Human Development (NICHD)
N. Institute of Child Health and Human Development Neonatal
N. Institute of Mental Health (NIMH)
N. Institutes of Health (NIH)
N. Joint Committee on Learning Disabilities (NJCLD)
N. Organization for Rare Disorders (NORD)
N. Pediatric Trauma Registry (NPTR)
N. Recipient Waiting List
N. Vaccine Advisory Committee (NVAC)
N. Wilms Tumor Study Group (NWTS)
Nativa formula
native ileum
NATP
neonatal alloimmune thrombocytopenic purpura
natriuresis

natriuretic peptide
natural
n. environment
n. killer (NK)
n. killer cell (NKC)
n. killer T cell
nausea
Navane
navel
navicular
accessory n.
n. bone
carpal n.
navicularis
fossa n.
naviculocuneiform joint
NB
neuroblastoma
NBAS
Neonatal Behavioral Assessment Scale
Newborn Behavior Assessment Scale
NBI
nosocomial bacterial infection
NBIC
newborn intensive care
NBICU
newborn intensive care unit
NBRS
Nursery Neurobiological Risk Score
NBS
neonatal Bartter syndrome
New Ballard Score
Nijmegen breakage syndrome
NBSCU
newborn special care unit
NBT
nitroblue tetrazolium
NBT dye test
NBTV
nonbacterial thrombotic vegetation
NCAH
nonclassical adrenal hyperplasia
NCCAN
National Center for Child Abuse and Neglect
NCCDS
North American Collaborative Crohn Disease Study
NCL
neuronal ceroid lipofuscinosis
adult NCL
infantile NCL

N

NOTES

NCL *(continued)*
    juvenile NCL
    late infantile NCL
n-CPAP
    nasal continuous positive airway pressure
      n-CPAP prongs
NCSE
    nonconvulsive status epilepticus
NCV
    nerve conduction velocity
NDH
    neurogenic dysplasia of hip
ND-Stat
NDT
    neurodevelopment therapy
NDW
    number of different words
NE
    neonatal encephalopathy
NE-8000 analyzer
near
    n. drowning
    n. gaze reflex
    n. infrared photoplethysmography
      (NIRP)
    n. vision
near-infrared spectroscopy
near-miss
    n.-m. phenomenon
    n.-m. SIDS
near-myeloablative chemotherapy
nearsightedness
neat pincer grasp
Nebcin Injection
Nebules
    Ventolin N.
nebulization
    ipratropium n.
nebulized prostacyclin
nebulizer
    compressed air-driven n.
    Hudson T Up-Draft II
     disposable n.
    jet n.
    Micro-Mist disposable n.
    Pari LC Plusjet n.
    Pulmo-Aide n.
    PulmoMate n.
    Respirgard II n.
    Schuco n.
NebuPent Inhalation
NEC
    necrotizing enterocolitis
    Neurological Examination for Children
Necator americanus
necessitatis
    empyema n.

neck
    femoral n.
    n. reflex
    n. response
    n. of Scotty dog
    short n.
    stiff n.
    thick n.
    twisted n.
    webbed n.
    wry n., wryneck
necklace
    Casal n.
neck-righting reflex
neck-shaft angle (NSA)
necrobiosis
    n. lipoidica
    n. lipoidica diabeticorum (NLD)
necrolysis
    erythema multiforme/toxic
     epidermal n. (EM/TEN)
    toxic epidermal n. (TEN)
necrophorum
    Fusobacterium n.
necropsy
necrosis
    acute tubular n. (ATN)
    aseptic n.
    avascular n. (AVN)
    basal ganglia n.
    bone avascular n.
    caseating n.
    centrilobular n.
    cerebral cortical n.
    cortical n.
    cystic medial n.
    excitotoxic n.
    fat n.
    fibrinoid n.
    hepatic n.
    idiopathic juvenile avascular n.
    ischemic n.
    juvenile avascular n.
    liquefactive n.
    medial n.
    medullary n.
    muscle n.
    neuronal n.
    papillary n.
    pituitary n.
    pontosubicular neuron n. (PSN)
    progressive outer retinal n. (PORN)
    pulp n.
    radiation n.
    renal cortical n.
    selective neuronal n.
    spotty n.
    subcutaneous fat n.

tissue n.
tubular n.
tumor n.

necrotic
    n. arachnidism
    n. coagulum
    n. mucosa

necrotizing
    n. adrenalitis
    n. arteriolitis
    n. arteritis
    n. colitis
    n. encephalopathy
    n. enterocolitis (NEC)
    n. erysipelas
    n. factor
    n. gingivitis
    n. glomerulonephritis
    n. granulomatous lymphadenitis
    n. granulomatous vasculitis
    n. jejunitis
    n. myositis fasciitis
    n. pneumonia
    n. ulcerating gingivitis (NUG)

nedocromil
    n. sodium
    n. sodium ophthalmic solution

need
    Carolina Curriculum for Infants and Toddlers with Special N.'s
    Children with Special Health Care N.'s (CWSN)
    special n.

needle
    butterfly scalp vein n.
    n. cricothyroidotomy
    n. cricothyrotomy
    Dieckmann intraosseous n.
    disposable 23-gauge butterfly n.
    21-gauge hypodermic n.
    n. holder
    intraosseous n.
    screw-tipped intraosseous n.
    short-bevel 21-gauge n.
    spinal n.
    splittable n.
    Sur-Fast n.
    n. thoracentesis

Neer view
nefazodone
negative
    n. affectivity

n. balance
n. balance of body fluid
false n.
n. inspiratory pressure
polyarthritis, RF n.
n. reinforcement

negative-pressure respirator
negativism
negevensis
    Simkania n.
NegGram
neglect
    child abuse and n.
    National Center for Child Abuse and N. (NCCAN)
    National Clearing House on Child Abuse and N.
    suspected child abuse or n. (SCAN)
Negri body
Neisseria
    N. gonorrhoeae
    N. meningitidis
neisserial infection
nelfinivir (NFV)
Nelis lesion
Nellcor
    N. N-200 home monitor
    N. N-3000 home monitor
    N. N20, N200 pulse oximeter
    N. Puritan Bennett home monitor
NELS
    National Educational Longitudinal Survey
nemaline
    n. rod
    n. rod disease
    n. rod myopathy
nematode endophthalmitis
Nembutal
NEMD
    nonspecific esophageal motility disorder
neoadjuvant
neoaneurysm
neoantigen
neoaorta formation
neoaortic valve
neobladder diversion procedure
Neo-Calglucon syrup
NeoCare formula
Neocate One+ formula
Neofed

N

NOTES

neoformans
  Cryptococcus neoformans var. *n.*
Neo-fradin
neologism
Neoloid
Neomixin Topical
neomucosa
neomycin
  n., (bacitracin) polymyxin B, hydrocortisone
  n. and polymyxin B
  n., polymyxin B, bacitracin
  n., polymyxin B, prednisolone
  n. sulfate
neomycin-polymycin combination otic solution
neonatal
  n. abdominal mass
  N. Abstinence Score (NAS)
  n. abstinence sign
  n. abstinence syndrome (NAS)
  n. acne
  n. adjuvant life support
  n. adrenoleukodystrophy
  n. alloimmune thrombocytopenia
  n. alloimmune thrombocytopenic purpura (NATP)
  n. amblyogenic stimulus
  n. apnea
  n. asphyxia
  n. autoimmune neutropenia
  n. Bartter syndrome (NBS)
  N. Behavioral Assessment Scale (NBAS)
  n. blood volume
  n. brain injury
  n. breast hyperplasia
  n. bullous dermatitis
  n. candidiasis
  n. chest disease
  n. cholestasis
  n. cholestatic jaundice
  n. chronic idiopathic neutropenia
  n. cold injury
  n. conjunctivitis
  n. cyanotic congenital heart disease
  n. dermatology
  n. elastin deposition
  n. encephalopathy (NE)
  Exosurf N.
  n. facial coding system (NFCS)
  n. gonococcal disease
  n. Guillain-Barré syndrome
  n. Guthrie card
  n. gynecomastia
  n. hemochromatosis (NH)
  n. hepatitis
  n. hepatitis syndrome
  n. herpes simplex
  n. herpes simplex virus
  n. herpes simplex virus infection
  n. hyperbilirubinemia
  n. hyperthermia
  n. hypocalcemia
  n. hypoglycemia
  n. hypoxic-ischemic encephalopathy
  N. Infant Pain Scale (NIPS)
  n. intensive care unit (NICU)
  n. iron-storage disease (NISD)
  n. isoimmune thrombocytopenia
  n. leukemoid reaction
  n. lupus
  n. lupus erythematosus (NLE)
  n. Marfan syndrome
  n. marker
  n. maturity classification of Dubowitz
  n. meningitis
  n. mortality risk (NMR)
  n. myasthenia gravis
  n. myasthenic syndrome
  n. narcotic pack
  National Institute of Child Health and Human Development N.
  n. neuroblastoma
  n. nongoitrous hypothyroidism
  n. ophthalmia
  n. pemphigus vulgaris
  N. Perception Inventory (NPI)
  n. period
  n. pneumonia
  n. polycythemia
  n. purpura fulminans
  n. pustular melanosis
  n. RDS
  n. respiratory distress syndrome
  n. resuscitation
  n. scabies
  n. scalp abscess
  n. seizure
  n. sepsis
  n. septic arthritis
  N. Skin Assessment Score
  n. small left colon syndrome
  n. stadiometer
  n. stress
  n. tetanus
  n. tetany
  n. thyrotoxicosis
  n. torticollis
  n. transport
  n. varicella
  n. vascular accident
  n. volvulus
  N. Withdrawal Inventory (NWI)

neonate
> athyrotic n.
> N. One Plus
> seronegative n.
> stress n.
> surgical n.

neonatologist

neonatology

neonatorum
> acne n.
> adiponecrosis subcutanea n.
> anemia n.
> apnea n.
> asphyxia n.
> eczema n.
> edema n.
> erythema toxicum n.
> erythroblastosis n.
> gonococcal ophthalmia n.
> icterus gravis n.
> impetigo n.
> keratolysis n.
> mastitis n.
> melena n.
> myotonia n.
> noma n.
> ophthalmia n. (type 1, 2)
> pemphigus n.
> scleredema n.
> sclerema n.
> tetanus n.
> trismus n.
> volvulus n.

neoplasia
> lymphoreticular n.
> multiple endocrine n.
> multiple endocrine n. type 2 (MEN-2)
> syndrome of multiple endocrine n.

neoplasm
> benign vascular n.
> cerebellar n.
> cystic cerebellar n.
> germ cell n.
> gonadal germ cell n.
> vascular n.

neoplastic fibrosis

neopterin

Neoral

Neosar

Neo-Sert umbilical vessel catheter insertion set

Neosporin
> N. Cream
> N. G.U. Irrigant
> N. Ophthalmic Ointment
> N. Topical Ointment

neostigmine

NeoSure nutritional supplement

Neo-Synephrine
> N.-S. 12 Hour Nasal Solution
> N.-S. Ophthalmic Solution

Neo-Tabs

Neotrace-4

Neotrend system

neovascularization of disk (NVD)

nephrectomy

nephritis
> acute postinfectious n.
> autoimmune interstitial n.
> diffuse proliferative lupus n.
> focal lupus n.
> hereditary n.
> interstitial n.
> lupus n.
> membranous lupus n.
> mesangial lupus n.
> postinfectious n.
> proliferative lupus n.
> pyoderma-associated n.
> shunt n.
> tubulointerstitial n. (TINU)

nephritogenic

nephroblastoma

nephroblastomatosis

Nephro-Calci

nephrocalcinosis

Nephrocaps

Nephro-Fer

nephrogenesis

nephrogenic
> n. diabetes insipidus
> n. rest

nephrolithiasis
> uric acid n.
> X-linked hypercalciuric n. (XLHN)
> X-linked recessive n.

nephrologist

nephroma
> congenital mesoblastic n.
> cystic n.
> mesoblastic n.

N

NOTES

nephron
    cortical n.
    n. loss
nephronophthisis (NPH)
nephronophthisis type 1 (NPH1)
nephropathy
    familial juvenile hyperuricemic n.
    HIV-associated n.
    immunoglobulin A n.
    membranous n.
    pediatric lupus n.
    reflux n.
    renal cortical n.
    sickle cell n.
    thin basement membrane n.
    urate n.
nephrophthisis
    familial juvenile n.
nephrosis
nephrostomy
    percutaneous n.
nephrotic syndrome
nephrotoxicity
    aminoglycoside n.
NERICP
    New England Regional Infant Cardiac
    Program
neridronate
nerve
    abducens n.
    acoustic n.
    auditory n.
    n. block
    ciliary n.
    n. conduction study
    n. conduction velocity (NCV)
    cranial n. (II–XII)
    n. dysplasia
    genitofemoral n.
    glioma of optic n.
    infraorbital n.
    n. injury
    laryngeal n.
    motor n.
    musculocutaneous n.
    nociceptive sensory n.
    oculomotor n.
    optic n.
    n. palsy
    n. paralysis
    paralysis of superior laryngeal n.
    phrenic n.
    postauricular n.
    preauricular n.
    sciatic n.
    sensory n.
    n. sheath tumor
    superior laryngeal n.

    n. thickening
    n. tract
    trigeminal n.
    trochlear n.
    vagus n.
    vestibular n.
    vestibulocochlear n.
Nervocaine Injection
nervorum
    vasa n.
nervosa
    anorexia n. (AN)
    bulimia n. (BN)
    eructio n.
    mild anorexia n.
nervous
    n. colon
    n. system
    n. system sarcoidosis
    n. tissue nevus
nesidioblastosis
Nestac formula
Nestrex
net
    Chiari n.
    n. ultrafiltration pressure
Netherton syndrome
netilmicin
netting
    Baby Air mesh n.
Nettleship-Falls ocular albinism
Nettleship syndrome
network
    Cooperative Human Tissue N.
        (CHTN)
    Research N.
    trans-Golgi n.
Neucalm-50
neuii
    Actinomyces n.
Neu-Laxova syndrome
Neupogen
neural
    n. arch joint
    n. axis
    n. ceroid lipofuscinosis
    n. crest cell
    n. discharge
    n. index
    n. mechanism
    n. plate
    n. reflex pathway
    n. retina
    n. tissue accretion
    n. tube
    n. tube closure
    n. tube defect (NTD)

n. tube disorder
n. tube rupture
neuralgia
postherpetic n.
neurally
n. mediated hypotension
n. mediated syncope (NMS)
neuraminic acid
neuraminidase
n. deficiency
n. inhibitor
neuraxial anesthesia
neuraxis tumor imaging
neurectomy
neurenteric cyst
neurilemoma
malignant n.
neurinoma
neuritic cytoplasmic process
neuritis
acute n.
bilateral optic n.
cranial n.
intraocular optic n.
optic n.
peripheral n.
retrobulbar n.
subacute n.
unilateral optic n.
neuroacanthocytosis
neuroanatomical
neuroaxonal dystrophy
neurobiological
neuroblastoma (NB)
n. cell
central n.
familial n.
neonatal n.
occult n.
peripheral n.
neuroborreliosis
Lyme n.
neurocardiogenic syncope
neurochemical
neurocognitive impairment
neurocristopathy
neurocutaneous
n. disorder
n. melanosis syndrome
NeuroCybernetic prosthesis
neurocysticercosis
intraventricular n.

neurodermatitis
circumscribed n.
neurodevelopmental
n. assessment
N. Assessment of Preterm Infants (NAPI)
N. Assessment Procedure for Preterm Infants
n. deficit
n. delay
n. sequela
n. treatment
neurodevelopment therapy (NDT)
neuroectoderm
neuroectodermal tumor
neuroendocrine response
neuroepithelioma
peripheral n.
neuroepithelium
telencephalic n.
neurofibrillary tangle
neurofibroma
plexiform n.
subcutaneous n.
neurofibromatosis
central n.
familial spinal n.
peripheral n.
segmental n.
spinal n.
n. syndrome
n. type 1 (NF1)
n. type 2 (NF2)
neurofibrosarcoma
neurofunctional
neurogenic
n. atrophy
n. bladder
n. bowel
n. clubfoot
n. dysplasia of hip (NDH)
n. equinus deformity
n. hip disease
n. hip dysplasia
n. polydipsia
n. pulmonary edema
n. respiratory failure
n. sarcoma
n. stuttering
n. talipes equinovarus
neuroglial heterotopia

NOTES

N

neurogram
    pudendal n.
neurohormonal
neurohypophysis
neuroid nevus
neuroimaging study
neuroleptic
    n. drug
    n. malignant syndrome (NMS)
    n. medication
neurologic
    n. demyelinating disease
    n. shellfish poisoning
neurological
    n. disorder
    N. Examination for Children
      (NEC)
neurologist
    pediatric n.
neurology
    American Board of Psychiatry
      and N. (ABPN)
neuroma
    acoustic n.
    bilateral acoustic n.'s
    incisional n.
neuromelanin
neuromelanogenesis
neuromotor dysfunction
neuromuscular
    n. blockade
    n. blocking agent
    n. disorder
    n. imbalance
    n. junction (NMJ)
    n. maturity assessment
    n. scoliosis
    n. scoliosis syndrome
neuromyelitis optica
neuron
    Cajal-Retzius n.
    hippocampal n.
    motor n.
    oxytocin-secreting n.
    n. palsy
    parasympathetic n.
neuronal
    n. ceroid lipofuscinosis (NCL)
    n. damage
    n. dysplasia
    n. migration disorder
    n. necrosis
neuronitis
    vestibular n.
neuronophagia
neuronophagy
neuron-specific enolase
Neurontin

neuropathic
    n. anhidrosis
    n. bladder
    n. cystinosis
neuropathy
    acute motor-axonal n. (AMAN)
    acute motor-sensory axonal n.
      (AMSAN)
    n., ataxia, retinitis pigmentosa
      (NARP)
    autonomic n.
    bulbar hereditary motor n. (type I,
      II)
    chronic peripheral n.
    congenital hypomyelinating n.
      (CHN)
    congenital sensory n.
    distal symmetric sensorimotor n.
    familial visceral n.
    giant axonal n.
    glue-sniffing n.
    hereditary autonomic n.
    hereditary motor-sensory n.
    hereditary motor-sensory n. (type
      IA, III–VII) (HMSN)
    hereditary sensory and
      autonomic n.
    hereditary sensory radicular n.
    Leber hereditary optic n. (LHON)
    Leber optic n.
    motor-axonal n.
    motor-sensory axonal n.
    myenteric plexus n.
    optic n.
    postdiphtheritic n.
    radicular n.
    reflux n.
    sensory n.
    tomaculous n.
    toxic n.
    tropical ataxic n.
    ulnar n.
neuropeptide
    enteric n.
neurophysiology
neuroprotection
neuropsychiatric disorder
neuropsychiatry
neuropsychologic
neuropsychological profile
neuropsychology
    clinical assessment in n.
neuroretinitis
    optic n.
neurosarcoidosis
neuroschisis
neurosecretory

neurosensory
   n. deafness
   n. impairment (NSI)
neurosis, pl. **neuroses**
   battle n.
neurosonographic
neurosurgeon
neurosurgical
   n. closure
   n. shunt
neurosyphilis
   congenital paretic n.
   congenital tertiary n.
neurotic
neurotoxicity
neurotoxic shellfish poisoning
neurotoxin
   botulinus n.
   tetanus n.
neurotransmitter precursor
neurotrauma
neurotrophic keratitis
neurovascular
   n. compromise
   n. dystrophy
neurovegetative
   n. functioning or symptom
   n. symptom
neurulation
Neut Injection
neutral
   FluoroCare N.
   K-Phos N.
   n. lipid storage disease
   n. pH
   n. pH of vagina
   n. position
   n. rotation
neutralize
Neutra-Phos
Neutra-Phos-K
Neutrogena
   N. Acne Mask
   N. T/Derm
neutropenia
   alloimmune neonatal n. (ANN)
   autoimmune n. (AIN)
   benign n.
   cardioskeletal n.
   chemotherapy-related n.
   chronic benign n.
   chronic idiopathic n.

congenital n.
cyclic n.
idiopathic n.
immune n.
immune-mediated n.
Kostmann n.
neonatal autoimmune n.
neonatal chronic idiopathic n.
peripheral n.
persistent n.
severe chronic n. (SCN)
severe congenital n.
transient n.
X-linked cardioskeletal myopathy
   and n.
neutropenic
neutrophil
   n. actin deficiency
   n. actin dysfunction
   band form n.
   n. chemotactic deficiency
   circulating n.'s
   n. egress
   n. G6PD deficiency
   n. granulopoiesis
   hypersegmented n.
   n. protease-3
   segmented n.
   n. transfusion
neutrophilia
   acute acquired n.
neutrophilic
   n. leukocytosis
   n. pleocytosis
   n. rhinitis
NEV
   noninvasive extrathoracic ventilator
nevi (*pl. of* nevus)
nevirapine (NVP)
nevocellular nevus
nevoid basal cell carcinoma syndrome
nevomelanocyte
nevoxanthoendothelioma
nevus, pl. **nevi**
   achromic n.
   acquired melanocytic n. (AMN)
   n. anemicus
   angiomatous involuting n.
   n. araneus
   nevi, atrial myxomas, myxoid
      neurofibromas, ephelides (NAME)
   atypical melanocytic n.

N

NOTES

nevus *(continued)*
  Becker n.
  blue rubber bleb n.
  cellular blue n.
  combined n.
  n. comedonicus
  common blue n.
  compound n.
  congenital melanocytic n.
  congenital pigmental n.
  conjunctival n.
  connective tissue n.
  cutaneous n.
  depigmented n.
  n. depigmentosus
  dermal n.
  dysplastic n.
  eczematous halo n.
  epidermal n.
  epithelioid cell n.
  eruptive n.
  n. flammeus
  giant congenital pigmented n.
  halo n.
  intradermal n.
  involuting n.
  Ito n.
  n. of Ito
  n. of Jadassohn
  junctional n.
  lentigines, atrial myxomas,
    cutaneous papular myxomas, blue
    nevi (LAMB)
  lentiginous n.
  melanocytic n.
  Meyerson n.
  nervous tissue n.
  neuroid n.
  nevocellular n.
  organoid n.
  n. of Ota
  pigmented n.
  port-wine n.
  rubber bleb n.
  satellite melanocytic n.
  sebaceous n.
  n. simplex
  speckled lentiginous n.
  spider n.
  n. spilus
  spindle cell epithelioid n.
  Spitz n.
  strawberry n.
  telangiectatic n.
  vascular n.
  verrucous streaky epidermal n.
  woolly hair n.
  zosteriform lentiginous n.

new
  N. Ballard Score (NBS)
  N. England Regional Infant
    Cardiac Program (NERICP)
  n. MacArthur emotion story-stems
  n. variant CJD
  n. variant Creutzfeldt-Jakob disease
    (nvCJD)
newborn
  N. Behavior Assessment Scale
    (NBAS)
  congenital anemia of n.
  cyanotic n.
  full-term n.
  gingival cyst of n.
  gonococcal arthritis of n.
  hemolytic disease of n.
  hemorrhagic disease of n. (HDN)
  horizontal suspension in n.
  hyperthermia in n.
  n. intensive care (NBIC)
  n. intensive care unit (NBICU)
  metabolic disease in n.
  nonfollicular pustulosis of n.
  Parrot atrophy of n.
  n. period
  persistent pulmonary hypertension
    of n. (PPHN)
  n. platelet antigen typing
  pulmonary hypertension of n.
  n. respiratory distress syndrome
  respiratory distress syndrome of n.
  retinopathy of n.
  Rh disease of n.
  n. special care unit (NBSCU)
  transient tachypnea of n. (TTN)
  transient tyrosinemia of n.
  transitory fever of n.
Newman-Keuls analysis
new-onset
  n.-o. diabetes mellitus
  n.-o. hydrocephalus
  n.-o. JDM
newport
  Salmonella n.
Newport Wave ventilator
newtonian aberration
Newtrition
  N. Isofiber formula
  N. Isotonic formula
NextStep Soy Toddler formula
Nezelof syndrome
NF1
  neurofibromatosis type 1
NF2
  neurofibromatosis type 2
NFAT
  nuclear factor of activated T cell

NFCS
　neonatal facial coding system
NFV
　nelfinivir
NG
　nasogastric
　　NG tube
NGHD-SS
　non-growth hormone-deficient short
　　stature
NGT
　nasogastric tube
NH
　neonatal hemochromatosis
NHANES
　National Health and Nutrition
　　Examination Survey
NHL
　non-Hodgkin leukemia
　non-Hodgkin lymphoma
Niacels
niacin poisoning
NIBPM
　noninvasive blood pressure measurement
nicardipine
N'ice
NICHD
　National Institute of Child Health and
　　Human Development
niche
　　ontogenetic n.
nickel dermatitis
Niclocide
niclosamide
Nicobid
Nicolar
nicotinamide
　　n. adenine dinucleotide phosphate
　　　(NADPH)
nicotine
Nicotinex
nicotinic acid
Nico-Vert
NICU
　neonatal intensive care unit
NIDDM
　non-insulin-dependent diabetes mellitus
nidulans
　　Aspergillus n.
nidus
Niemann-Pick
　　N.-P. C disease

N.-P. cell
N.-P. disease (NPD)
N.-P. disease type A (NPA)
N.-P. disease type B (NPB)
N.-P. disease type C (NPC)
N.-P. disease type D (NPD)
N.-P. disease (type I, II)
nifedipine
nifurtimox
niger
　　Aspergillus n.
night
　　n. blindness
　　n. pain
　　n. splint
　　n. splinting
　　n. sweat
　　n. terror
nightmare
nigra
　　lingua n.
　　substantia n.
nigricans
　　acanthosis n.
　　hirsutism, androgen excess, insulin
　　　resistance, acanthosis n. (HAIR-
　　　AN)
　　pseudoacanthosis n.
nigripalpus
　　Culex n.
nigrostriatal tract
NIH
　National Institutes of Health
NIHF
　nonimmune hydrops fetalis
Nijmegen breakage syndrome (NBS)
Nikolsky sign
Nilstat
Nimbex
NIMH
　National Institute of Mental Health
　　NIMH global scale
NIMV
　noninvasive motion ventilation
nine
　　rule of n.'s
nipple
　　accessory n.
　　n. eczema
　　n. feeding
　　n. flow rate
　　O_2 flowmeter n.

N

NOTES

nipple *(continued)*
    preemie n.
    supernumerary n.
nippling
Nipride
NIPS
    Neonatal Infant Pain Scale
NIRP
    near infrared photoplethysmography
NIS-2
    Second National Incidence Study
NISD
    neonatal iron-storage disease
Nissen fundoplication
Nissl granule
nit
2-nite
    Sleepwell 2-n.
nitidus
    lichen n.
nitrate
    silver n.
nitric
    n. oxide (NO)
    n. oxide oxidation
nitrite
    amyl n.
    plasma n.
Nitro-Bid
    N.-B. I.V. Injection
    N.-B. Ointment
nitroblue
    n. tetrazolium (NBT)
    n. tetrazolium dye reduction test
nitrocellulose
Nitrodisc Patch
Nitro-Dur Patch
nitrofurantoin
Nitrogard Buccal
nitrogen
    blood urea n. (BUN)
    n. dioxide inhalation
    liquid n.
    n. mustard
    serum urea n. (SUN)
    urea n.
    n. washout test
nitroglycerin
    n. paste
    topical n.
Nitroglyn Oral
Nitrolingual Translingual Spray
Nitrol Ointment
Nitrong Oral Tablet
Nitropress
nitroprusside
    sodium n. (SNP)
    n. sodium

Nitrostat Sublingual
nitrotyrosine
nitrous oxide
Nivea cream
Nix Creme Rinse
nizatidine
Nizoral
NJ
    nasojejunal
    NJ tube
NJCLD
    National Joint Committee on Learning
    Disabilities
NK
    natural killer
    NK cell
NKC
    natural killer cell
NKH
    nonketotic hyperglycinemia
NLD
    necrobiosis lipoidica diabeticorum
NLE
    neonatal lupus erythematosus
NLP
    no light perception
NMJ
    neuromuscular junction
NMN
    Novy-McNeal-Nicolle
    NMN biphasic blood agar
NMR
    neonatal mortality risk
NMS
    neurally mediated syncope
    neuroleptic malignant syndrome
n,n-diethyl-m-toluamide (DEET)
NNRTI
    nonnucleoside reverse transcriptase
    inhibitor
NO
    nitric oxide
no
    n. light perception (NLP)
    N. Pain-HP
    n. tears
Noack syndrome
Nocardia
    N. asteroides
    N. brasiliensis
    N. caviae
    N. farcinica
    N. nova
    N. otidiscaviarum
    N. transvalensis
nocardiosis
nociception

nociceptive
    n. sensory nerve
    n. stimulus
nociferous cortex
Noctec
nocturnal
    n. angina
    n. asthma
    n. enuresis
    n. epilepsy
    n. leg cramp
    n. myoclonus
    n. pulse oximetry
    n. retrosternal chest pain
    n. sweating
nocturnus
    pavor n.
nodal tachycardia
node
    atrioventricular n.
    caseous n.
    Hensen n.
    locoregional n.
    lymph n.
    mucocutaneous lymph n.
    Osler n.
    parapharyngeal lymph n.
    retropharyngeal lymph n.
    Schmorl n.
    sinoatrial n. (SA)
nodosa
    distal trichorrhexis n.
    infantile periarteritis n.
    infantile polyarteritis n. (IPN)
    maculopapular n.
    periarteritis n.
    polyarteritis n. (PAN)
    trichorrhexis n.
nodosum
    amnion n.
    erythema n.
nodular
    n. adrenal hyperplasia
    n. cortical sclerosis
    n. fasciitis
    n. gastritis
    n. infiltration
    n. lymphoid hyperplasia
    n. nerve thickening
    n. nonsuppurative panniculitis
    n. sclerosing Hodgkin disease

nodule
    Aschoff n.
    blueberry muffin n.
    Bohn n.
    Brown n.
    cold n.
    cutaneous n.
    hot n.
    iris Lisch n.
    Lisch n.
    palpable n.
    parenchymal n.
    rheumatoid n.
    subcutaneous n.
    thyroid n.
    vocal n.
nodulocystic lesion
NOE
    nasoorbitoethmoid
    NOE fracture
NOFT, NOFTT
    nonorganic failure to thrive
noir
    tache n.
noise
    upper airway n.
noma neonatorum
nomogram
    Done n.
    Rumack-Matthew n.
non-A
    n.-A hepatitis
    n.-A, non-B hepatitis (NANBH)
    n.-A, non-B hepatotropic virus
non-ABCDE hepatitis
nonaccidental spiral tibial fracture
nonalcoholic steatohepatitis (NASH)
nonallergenic
    n. perineal rhinitis
    n. rhinitis with eosinophilia
nonallergic rhinitis
non-alpha cell tumor
nonambulatory
nonangiitic vasculopathic condition
nonanion gap metabolic acidosis
nonatopic
nonautonomous attachment
nonbacterial
    n. thrombotic endocarditis
    n. thrombotic vegetation (NBTV)
non-B hepatitis
nonbilious vomiting

N

NOTES

nonbranching pseudohypha
non-breathhold MR cholangiography
nonbronchoscopic bronchoalveolar lavage
nonbullous
    n. congenital ichthyosiform
      erythroderma
    n. impetigo
noncalcific vasculopathy
noncardiac pulmonary edema
noncarrier
noncaseating sarcoidlike granuloma
noncategorical placement
noncirrhotic ascitic disease
nonclassical
    n. adrenal hyperplasia (NCAH)
    21-OH n. adrenal hyperplasia
noncleft median face syndrome
noncoiled cord
noncommunicating
    n. cyst
    n. hydrocephalus
noncompliance
noncontact ultrasound
nonconvulsive
    n. seizure
    n. status epilepticus (NCSE)
noncyanotic congenital heart disease
nondepolarizing paralyzing agent
nondirective supportive psychotherapy
nondisjunction
    chromosomal n.
    n. trisomy 21
Non-Drowsy
    Drixoral N.-D.
nonencephalitogenic cell
nonepileptic
    n. myoclonus
    n. seizure
nonessential amino acid
nonexudative conjunctival injection
nonfamilial
    n. aniridia
    n. hyperinsulinemic hypoglycemia
    n. hyperinsulinism of infancy
    n. visceral myopathy
nonfat milk
nonfixing eye
nonfollicular
    n. pustulosis
    n. pustulosis of newborn
nongamma Coombs test
nongenotoxic
nongonococcal urethritis
non-growth hormone-deficient short
stature (NGHD-SS)
nonhaem iron
nonhematogenous tumor
nonhemolytic reaction

non-Hodgkin
    n.-H. leukemia (NHL)
    n.-H. lymphoma (NHL)
nonhydropic fetus
nonhyperinsulinemic hypoglycemia
non-IgE-mediated food allergy
nonimmune
    n. hemolysis
    n. hydrops
    n. hydrops fetalis (NIHF)
non-insulin-dependent
    n.-i.-d. diabetes
    n.-i.-d. diabetes mellitus (NIDDM)
noninvasive
    n. blood pressure measurement
      (NIBPM)
    n. extrathoracic ventilator (NEV)
    n. motion ventilation (NIMV)
    n. test
nonionic
    n. contrast material
    n. contrast media
nonirritating
nonisomorphic presentation
nonketotic
    n. hyperglycinemia (NKH)
    n. hyperosmolar coma
    n. hypoglycemia
nonkinesigenic
nonlymphoblastic leukemia
nonlymphocytic leukemia
nonmaleficence
nonmigrainous headache
nonmusical
    n. wheeze
    n. wheezing
nonmutogenic
nonnarcotic abstinence syndrome
nonneural congenital defect
nonneurogenic
    n. dysphagia
    n. neurogenic bladder
nonnucleoside reverse transcriptase
inhibitor (NNRTI)
nonnutritional rickets
nonnutritive sucking opportunity (NSO)
nonobstruction
    large-volume n.
nonobstructive pyelonephritis
nonoliguric ARF
nonorganic failure to thrive (NOFT,
NOFTT)
nonossifying fibroma
nonoxynol-9
nonpalpable testis
nonparalytic
    n. hypotonia

n. poliomyelitis
n. strabismus
nonpathologic fracture
nonphotogenic seizure
nonpitting induration
non-PKU phenylalaninemia
nonpolio enterovirus
nonprogressive
n. hypoplastic syndrome
n. motor impairment syndrome
n. ventriculomegaly
nonproliferative diabetic retinopathy
nonpsychotic
non-Q-wave AMI
nonrapid eye movement (NREM)
nonrebreather
n. face mask
high-flow n.
nonreciprocal gait
non-REM
nonrhabdomyogenic soft tissue sarcoma
nonrhabdomyomatous sarcoma
nonrhabdomyosarcoma soft tissue sarcoma (NRSTS)
nonseptated
nonspastic paraparesis
nonspecific
n. arrhythmia (NSA)
n. encephalopathy
n. esophageal motility disorder (NEMD)
n. ileitis
n. mental retardation
n. vaginitis
n. vulvovaginitis
nonspherical congruent hips
nonspherocytic anemia
nonsteroidal antiinflammatory drug (NSAID)
nonstreptococcal pharyngitis
nonstress test (NST)
nonsuppurative panniculitis
nonsusceptible
nonsustained ventricular tachycardia
non-syncytium-inducing (NSI)
n.-s.-i. strain
nonsyndromic
n. bile duct paucity
nontension pneumothorax
nonthyroidal illness (NTI)
nontoxic
nontreponemal test

nontuberculous
n. mycobacteria (NTM)
n. mycobacterial infection
n. mycobacterium (NTM)
nontypeable organism
non-typhi *Salmonella* (NTS)
nontyphoidal *Salmonella*
nonunion
nonvalent pneumococcal conjugate vaccine (PnCV)
nonvascular
nonverbal
n. communication
n. developmental index
n. learning disability (NVLD)
n. perceptual-organization-output disorder
nonvertiginous condition
nonvesicular rash
non-Wessel colic
Noonan-Ehmke syndrome
Noonan syndrome
noradrenaline
plasma n.
noradrenergic
n. locus ceruleus
n. system
Norcet
Norcuron
NORD
National Organization for Rare Disorders
Nordette contraceptive pill
Nordiate
Norditropin Injection
Nordryl
N. Injection
N. Oral
no-reflow phenomenon
norepinephrine
norethindrone
norimbergensis
Burkholderia n.
Norisodrine
normal
n. blood pressure
n. female sex chromosome type (XX)
n. fetal development
n. flap-valve mechanism
n. gastroesophageal reflux of infancy
n. intelligence

N

NOTES

normal *(continued)*
  n. male sex chromosome type (XY)
  n. saline
  n. saline solution (NSS)
  n. spontaneous vaginal delivery (NSVD)
  n. temperature
  n. vaginal delivery
normal-pressure hydrocephalus
Norman-Wood syndrome
normobaric oxygen
normoblast cell
normoblastemia
normocalcemic
normocapnia
normocephalic
normochromic anemia
normocytic anemia
Normodyne
normoglycemia
normophosphatemic
normotensive
Normotest
normothermia
normothrombocytopenia
norm-referenced test
Norpace CR
Norplant II
Norpramin
NOR-QD
Norrbottnian Gaucher disease
Norrie
  N. disease
  N. syndrome
Norris-Carrol criteria
Nor-tet Oral
North
  N. American Collaborative Crohn Disease Study (NCCDS)
  N. American Society for Pediatric Gastroenterology and Nutrition (NASPGN)
  N. Asian tick typhus
Northern blot
Northway (stage I–IV)
nortriptyline hydrochloride
Norvir
  N. capsule
  N. oral solution
Norwalk
  N. agent
  N. virus
Norwegian scabies
Norwood
  N. operation
  N. palliation

  N. procedure
  N. stage
Norzine
nose
  beaked n.
  broad flat n.
  flat n.
  prominent n.
  rabbit n.
  saddle n.
  short beaked n.
nosebleed
nosocomial
  n. bacterial infection (NBI)
  n. bacterial meningitis
  n. diarrhea
  n. infection
  n. pneumonia
  n. sepsis
nosocomially acquired (NA)
nosology
Nostrilla
Nostril Nasal Solution
notch
  alveolar n.
  interarytenoid n.
  intercondylar n.
  median alveolar n.
  N. receptor
  suprasternal n.
notched P wave
notching
  rib n.
note
  hyperresonant calvarial percussion n.
nothing by mouth (non per os) (n.p.o.)
notochord
nova
  Nocardia n.
Novahistine
Novantrone
novo
  de n.
novobiocin
Novolin
  N. 70/30
  N. L, N, R
  N. N, R PenFil
  N. 70/30 PenFil
Novy-McNeal-Nicolle (NMN)
  N.-M.-N. biphasic blood agar
noxae
  embryonic n.
NP-27
NPA
  nasopharyngeal aspirate
  Niemann-Pick disease type A

NPB
  Niemann-Pick disease type B
NPC
  Niemann-Pick disease type C
NP-CPAP
  nasal prong continuous positive airway
  pressure
NPD
  Niemann-Pick disease
  Niemann-Pick disease type D
NPH
  nephronophthisis
    NPH Iletin I, II
    NPH Insulin
    Pork NPH
NPH1
  nephronophthisis type 1
NPH-N
NPI
  Neonatal Perception Inventory
NPL
  nasopharyngolaryngoscopy
n.p.o.
  nothing by mouth (non per os)
NPOT
  narrow pulmonary outflow tract
NPR
  nasopharyngeal reflux
NPTR
  National Pediatric Trauma Registry
NR
    Organidin NR
    Tussi-Organidin DM NR
NREM
  nonrapid eye movement
    NREM arousal parasomnia
NRSTS
  nonrhabdomyosarcoma soft tissue
  sarcoma
NRTI
  nucleoside reverse transcriptase inhibitor
    thymidine analog NRTI
NSA
  neck-shaft angle
  nonspecific arrhythmia
    NSA of femur
NSAID
  nonsteroidal antiinflammatory drug
NSI
  neurosensory impairment
  non-syncytium-inducing
    NSI strain

NSO
  nonnutritive sucking opportunity
NSS
  normal saline solution
NST
  nonstress test
NSVD
  normal spontaneous vaginal delivery
NTD
  neural tube defect
N-telopeptide
NTI
  nonthyroidal illness
NTM
  nontuberculous mycobacteria
  nontuberculous mycobacterium
NTS
  non-typhi *Salmonella*
NTZ Long Acting Nasal Solution
Nubain
nuchal
    n. pad thickening
    n. rigidity
    n. translucency
nuchal-spinal sign
Nuck
    canal of N.
nuclear
    n. atypia
    n. debris
    n. degeneration
    n. dust
    n. factor of activated T cell
    (NFAT)
    n. magnetic resonance spectroscopy
nucleated red blood cell
nuclei (*pl. of* nucleus)
nucleic
    n. acid amplification (NAA)
    n. acid amplification test
    n. acid hybridization
    n. acid probe
    n. acid sequence-based amplification
    (NASBA)
nucleoside
    n. analog
    n. phosphorylase
    n. reverse transcriptase inhibitor
    (NRTI)
nucleotide
    adenine n.
    antisense n.

NOTES

N

nucleotide *(continued)*
    cytosine n.
    guanine n.
    thymine n.
nucleotide-fortified formula
nucleotidylexotransferase
    DNA n.
nucleotidyltransferase
    DNA n.
nucleus, pl. **nuclei**
    n. accumbens
    n. accumbens septi
    caudate n.
    cerebellar n.
    cranial nerve n.
    dentate n.
    disorganized brainstem nuclei
    Edinger-Westphal n.
    inferior olivary n.
    lentiform n.
    olivary nuclei
    owl's eye n.
    red n.
    n. reticularis gigantocellularis
    n. retroambiguus
    superior olivary n.
    n. tractus solitarius
NucliSens assay
NUG
    necrotizing ulcerating gingivitis
NuLYTELY
number
    n. of different words (NDW)
    Reynolds n.
numbing
Numby Stuff
nummular
    n. dermatitis
    n. eczema
Numzitdent
Numzit Teething
Nupercainal
Nuprin
Nuromax Injection
nurse
    licensed practical n. (LPN)
    licensed vocational n. (LVN)
    public health n. (PHN)
    registered n. (RN)
nursemaid's elbow
nursery
    intensive care n. (ICN)
    intensive special care n. (ISCN)
    N. Neurobiological Risk Score (NBRS)
    well baby n. (WBN)
Nursette prefilled disposable bottle

nursing
    Association of Women's Health, Obstetrics, and Neonatal N. (AWHONN)
Nursoy formula
nurturant
nurture
Nuss technique
nutans
    spasmus n.
nutcracker esophagus
Nutracort Topical
Nutraderm cream
Nutramigen formula
Nutrapak formula
Nutren
    N. 1.0, 1.5, 2.0 formula
    N. Jr.
    N. Junior formula
    N. Junior with Fiber formula
Nutricia formula
nutrient
    intraluminal n.
Nutrilipid
Nutriset supplement
nutrition
    central venous n. (CVN)
    European Society of Paediatric Gastroenterology, Hepatology, and N. (ESPGHAN)
    home parenteral n. (HPN)
    North American Society for Pediatric Gastroenterology and N. (NASPGN)
    parenteral n. (PN)
    total parenteral n. (TPN)
    total peripheral parenteral n. (TPPN)
nutritional
    n. deprivation syndrome
    n. hepatotoxicity
    n. immunology
    n. rickets
    n. supplement
nutritionist
Nutropin AQ Injection
NVAC
    National Vaccine Advisory Committee
nvCJD
    new variant Creutzfeldt-Jakob disease
NVD
    neovascularization of disk
NVLD
    nonverbal learning disability
NVP
    nevirapine
NWI
    Neonatal Withdrawal Inventory

NWTS
National Wilms Tumor Study Group
NX
Talwin NX
nyctalopia
Nydrazid Injection
nystagmus
acquired n.
asymmetric n.
congenital jerky n.
congenital pendular n.
convergent n.
downbeat n.
fixation n.
gaze-evoked n.
gaze-paretic n.
horizontal n.
jerk n.
latent n.
monocular n.

optokinetic n.
pendular n.
positional n.
railroad n.
retractive n.
n. retractorius
seesaw n.
spontaneous n.
unilateral optokinetic n.
upbeat n.
vertical n.
vestibular n.
Nystatin
Nystat-Rx
Nystex
Nytol
Maximum Strength N.
Nytone enuretic control unit
Nyton Oral

NOTES

N

O₂
oxygen
O_2 flowmeter nipple
hood O_2
pressure of O_2
O_2 saturation
OA
ocular albinism
osteoarthritis
OAAS
Observer Assessment of Alertness and Sedation
OAD
overanxious disorder
OADP-CDS
Oregon Adolescent Depression Project-Conduct Disorder Screener
OAE
otoacoustic emission
OAE testing
O antigen
OAR
Ottawa Ankle Rules
Oasthouse urine disease
OB
osteoblast
osteoblastoma
obese
obesity
adolescent o.
exogenous o.
o. hypoventilation syndrome
mild to moderate o.
progressive o.
truncal o.
obesity-related hyposomatotropism
Obetrol
obidoxime chloride
object
o. assembly test
o. constancy
o. permanence
unidentified bright o.
objective
obligatory
o. heel valgus
o. primitive reflex
o. tonic neck reflex
oblique
left anterior o. (LAO)
o. radiograph
right anterior o. (RAO)
o. view
obliterans
bronchiolitis o.

obliterated
o. processus vaginalis
o. vein
obliteration
o. of apophyseal space
vessel o.
obliterative
o. bronchitis
o. coronary artery disease
o. endarteritis
o. fibroproliferative bronchiolitis
oblongata
medulla o.
observation
o. hip
prelinguistic autism diagnostic o. (PL-ADOS)
Observer Assessment of Alertness and Sedation (OAAS)
obsession
obsessionality
obsessive-compulsive
o.-c. behavior (OCB)
o.-c. disorder (OCD)
o.-c. personality disorder (OCPD)
obstetric
obstetrical
o. palsy
o. paralysis
obstetrician
obstetrics
obstipation
obstructed bowel loop
obstruction
airway o.
o. of appendix
arterial o.
bowel o.
check valve o.
closed-loop o.
congenital lacrimal duct o.
congenital nasolacrimal duct o. (CNLDO)
distal intestinal o. (DIOS)
duodenal o.
extrahepatic portal vein o.
extrahepatic presinusoidal o.
functional outlet o.
glottal o.
hypopharyngeal-glottal o.
incomplete bowel o.
infravesical o.
intestinal o.
intrabronchial o.
intrabronchiolar o.

O

obstruction *(continued)*
    intraluminal o.
    intrauterine ureteral o.
    lacrimal duct o.
    left ventricular outflow tract o. (LVOTO)
    left ventricular outlet o.
    lymphatic o.
    mechanical o.
    meconium o.
    milk bolus o.
    nasal o.
    nasolacrimal duct o.
    outflow o.
    portal vein o. (PVO)
    positional airways o.
    presinusoidal o.
    pseudointestinal o.
    pulmonary venous o.
    renal o.
    right ventricular outflow tract o.
    strangulating o.
    o. syndrome
    systemic outflow o.
    tracheobronchial o.
    unilateral ureteral o. (UUO)
    UPJ o.
    ureteral o.
    ureteropelvic junction o.
    ureterovesical junction o.
    urinary o.
    uterine outflow o.
    valve o.
    vein o.
    venous o.
    ventricular outflow o.
obstructive
    o. apnea
    o. atelectasis
    o. hydrocephalus
    o. malformation
    o. megaureter
    o. overinflation
    o. respiratory disease
    o. sleep apnea (OSA)
    o. sleep apnea/hypoventilation (OSA/H)
    o. sleep apnea syndrome (OSAS)
    o. symptom
    o. uropathy
obtundation
obtunded
obturator
    o. internus
    o. internus muscle
    plastic o.
    o. sign
obtuse marginal

OCA
    oculocutaneous albinism
    yellow OCA
OCB
    obsessive-compulsive behavior
occipital
    o. bossing
    o. horn syndrome
    o. osteodiastasis
    o. plagiocephaly
occipitoatlantal instability
occipitofrontal
    o. circumference (OFC)
    o. diameter
occipitomental view
occiput
    flattened o.
occluder
    Amplatzer septal o.
occlusal
    o. problem
    o. radiograph
Occlusal-HP Liquid
occlusion
    airway o.
    o. amblyopia
    Angle classification of o.
    arteriolar o.
    basal arterial o.
    cerebral artery o.
    coil o.
    constant flow end-inspiratory airway o.
    o. dermatitis
    end-inspiratory airway o.
    fetal tracheal o.
    middle cerebral artery o. (MCAO)
    surgical tape o.
    tracheal o.
occlusive
    o. dressing
    o. vascular disease
    o. vasculitis
occult
    o. bacteremia
    o. blood
    o. dysraphism
    o. neuroblastoma
    o. neurogenic bladder
    o. spinal dysraphism
    o. trauma, postanoxia, ventriculoperitoneal (OPV)
    o. trauma, postictal ventriculoperitoneal
occulta
    spina bifida o.
occultum
    cranium bifidum o.

occupational
    o. acne
    o. therapy (OT)
occurrence
    inconsequential o.
OCD
    obsessive-compulsive disorder
    osteochondritis dissecans
Ocean Nasal Mist
Ochrobactrum anthropi
ochronosis
Ockelbo virus
OCL
    oral colonic lavage
OCP
    oral contraceptive pill
OCPD
    obsessive-compulsive personality
      disorder
OCRL
    oculocerebrorenal
      OCRL syndrome
OCT
    oral contraceptive therapy
Octamide
Octicair Otic
Octocaine Injection
octreotide
    o. acetate
    o. therapy
Ocu-Carpine Ophthalmic
OcuClear Ophthalmic
Ocufen Ophthalmic
Ocuflox ophthalmic solution
ocular
    o. albinism (OA)
    o. alignment
    o. aspergillosis
    o. bobbing
    o. coloboma
    o. flutter
    o. hypertelorism
    o. hypotony
    o. larva migrans
    o. lubricant
    o. malformation
    o. motor dysmetria
    o. muscular dystrophy
    o. myoclonus
    o. myopathy
    o. nonnephropathic cystinosis
    o. oscillation

    o. pain
    o. paresis
    o. prosthesis
    o. sarcoidosis
    o. toxoplasmosis
oculi
    melanosis o.
oculoauriculovertebral
    o. dysplasia
    o. syndrome
oculocephalic reflex
oculocerebral
    o. dystrophy
    o. syndrome
oculocerebrorenal (OCRL)
    o. disease of Lowe
    o. dystrophy
    o. syndrome
    o. syndrome of Lowe
oculocutaneous
    o. albinism (OCA)
    o. lesion
    o. telangiectasia
    o. tyrosinemia
oculodentodigital
    o. dysplasia
    o. syndrome
oculofacial paralysis
oculoglandular tularemia
oculogyric crisis
oculomandibulofacial (OMF)
    o. syndrome
oculomotor
    o. apraxia
    o. dysfunction
    o. nerve
oculopharyngeal muscular dystrophy
oculoplethysmography
oculosympathetic paresis
oculus
    o. dexter (right eye) (o.d., OD)
    o. sinister (left eye) (o.s., OS)
    o. unitas (both eyes) (o.u., OU)
    o. uterque (each eye) (o.u., OU)
Ocu-Pentolate
Ocusert
    O. Pilo-20 Ophthalmic
    O. Pilo-40 Ophthalmic
Ocutricin
    O. HC Otic
    O. Topical Ointment
Ocu-Trol Ophthalmic

O

NOTES

Ocu-Tropine Ophthalmic
o.d., OD
  oculus dexter (right eye)
ODD
  oppositional defiant disorder
odd
    logarithm of o.'s (LOD)
    o.'s ratio (OR)
odontogenesis
odontogenic keratocyst
odontoid
    o. process
    o. process hypoplasia
odontoideum
    os o.
odontolyticus
    Actinomyces o.
odor
    acrid o.
    amine o.
    fruity breath o.
odorant
odorous
ODT
    Zofran ODT
odynophagia
OE
    otitis externa
OFC
    occipitofrontal circumference
OFD
    orofaciodigital
    OFD syndrome, type I–III
offender
    extrafamily o.
    intrafamily o.
officer
    guidance o.
Office of Special Education Programs (OSEP)
offspring psychopathology
ofloxacin
OG
    oral gastric
    OG tube
OH
    hydroxyl radical
Ohio
    O. bed
    O. warmer
Ohmeda
    O. Minx pulse oximeter
    O. 3800 pulse oximeter
    O. SoftProbe probe
OI
    osteogenesis imperfecta
    oxygenation index

OIA
    optical immunoassay
    Biostar Flu OIA
oil
    algal o.
    BAL in O.
    castor o.
    evening primrose o. (EPO)
    fish o.
    Fleet Flavored Castor O.
    fungal o.
    immersion o.
    Lorenzo o.
    MCT o.
    medium-chain triglyceride o.
    mineral o.
    T-Derm body o.
Oilatum soap
ointment
    AK-Spore Ophthalmic O.
    hydrophilic o.
    LCD o.
    liquor carbonis detergens o.
    Medi-Quick Topical O.
    Neosporin Ophthalmic O.
    Neosporin Topical O.
    Nitro-Bid O.
    Nitrol O.
    Ocutricin Topical O.
    oxytetracycline/polymyxin o.
    Panscol O.
    Polysporin o.
    Posterisan o.
    Salacid O.
    salicylic acid o.
    Septa Topical O.
    Sutilains O.
    tioconazole 6.5% o.
    triamcinolone acetonide o.
    Triple Paste o.
    undecylenic acid o.
    Whitfield o.
    Xylocaine Topical O.
    zinc oxide o.
OIS
    Organ Injury Scaling
Oka
    O. strain
    O. strain varicella vaccine
Oklahoma ankle joint
OKT3
    Orthoclone O.
olanzapine
OLB
    open lung biopsy
Olean
oleate-condensate
    triethanolamine polypeptide o.-c.

olecranon
  o. apophysitis
  o. fossa
  o. fracture
olestra
olfaction
olfactory hallucination
oligemia
oligoamnion
oligoanuria
oligoarthritis
oligoarticular
  o. arthritis
  o. disease
oligoasthenospermia
oligoclonality
oligodactyly
oligodendrocyte
oligodendroglia
oligodendroglial degeneration
oligodendroglioma
  anaplastic o.
oligodeoxynucleotide
  antisense o.
oligohydramnios
oligomeganephronia
oligomenorrhea
oligonucleotide probe analysis
oligophrenia
oligosaccharide
oligospermia
  eugonadotropic o.
oliguria
  transient o.
oliguric ARF
olivary nuclei
olive
  pyloric o.
  superior o.
olivopontocerebellar
  o. atrophy (OPCA)
  o. degeneration
Ollier
  O. disease
  O. syndrome
olopatadine hydrochloride
olpadronate
olsalazine sodium
OLTx
  orthotopic liver transplantation
olympian brow

Olympus GIF-XP10 video endoscope
OM
  otitis media
OME
  otitis media with effusion
omega-3 fatty acid
omega fatty acid
omega-shaped epiglottis
Omenn syndrome
omenta (*pl. of* omentum)
omental cyst
omentectomy
omentum, pl. omenta
  matted o.
omeprazole
OMF
  oculomandibulofacial
Ommaya reservoir
Omnicef
OmniHIB vaccine
Omnipaque
Omnipen
Omnipen-N
omovertebral bone
omphalitis
omphalocele
omphalomesenteric
  o. duct
  o. duct remnant
Omsk
  O. hemorrhagic fever
  O. virus
OMS Oral
Oncaspar
Onchocerca volvulus
onchocerciasis
oncogenous rickets
oncotic
  o. force
  o. pressure
Oncovin
ondansetron
Ondine
  curse of O.
  O. curse
Ondine-Hirschsprung syndrome
one-way valve
onion bulb formation
onion-skin appearance
onionskinning
onlay island flap

O

NOTES

onset
    infantile o.
    juvenile o.
ontogenesis
ontogenetic
    o. niche
    o. shift
OnTrak
onychatrophia
onychia
onycholysis
    distal o.
onychomycosis
    candidal o.
    proximal white subungual o.
    sublingual o.
    superficial o.
    white superficial o.
onychophagia
o'nyong-nyong virus
oocyte atresia
oolemma
oophoritis
O&P
    ova and parasites
Op
    osmotic pressure
opacification
    corneal o.
opacity
    corneal o.
    fine lens o.
    lens o.
    lenticular o.
    punctate lenticular o.
Opalski cell
opaque white exudate
OPC
    oropharyngeal candidiasis
OPCA
    olivopontocerebellar atrophy
Opcon Ophthalmic
open
    o. biopsy
    o. bite
    o. comedo
    o. dermal sinus
    o. endotracheal suction
    o. endotracheal suctioning
    o. flap drainage
    o. fracture
    o. gastrostomy tube placement
    o. heart surgery
    o. lung biopsy (OLB)
    o. mouth
    o. pericardial drainage
opening
    glottic o.

    tentorial o.
    o. wedge osteotomy
open-mouth view
open-tube bronchoscopy
operant level
operation (*See also* procedure)
    Alexander o.
    arterial switch o.
    atrial switch o.
    Blalock-Hanlon o.
    Blalock-Taussig o.
    Damus-Kaye-Stansel o.
    Fontan o.
    Glenn o.
    Heller-Nissen o.
    Jatene o.
    Kasai o.
    King o.
    Ladd o.
    modified Fontan o.
    Mustard o.
    Norwood o.
    Ramstedt o.
    Rastelli o.
    Ross o.
    Ross-Konno o.
    Senning o.
    Sistrunk o.
    Thiersch o.
    two-stage arterial switch o.
    vaginal switch o.
    window o.
opercular syndrome
operculum, pl. **opercula**
OPG
    osteoprotegerin
ophiasis
Ophthacet
Ophthaine
Ophthalgan Ophthalmic
ophthalmia
    neonatal o.
    o. neonatorum (type 1, 2)
ophthalmic
    Achromycin O.
    Acular O.
    Adsorbocarpine O.
    Adsorbonac O.
    Akarpine O.
    AK-Beta O.
    AK-Chlor O.
    AK-Con O.
    AK-Dex O.
    AK-Poly-Bac O.
    AK-Pred O.
    AKTob O.
    AK-Tracin O.

AK-Trol O.
Albalon Liquifilm O.
Atropair O.
Atropine-Care O.
Atropisol O.
Betagan Liquifilm O.
Chloroptic O.
Ciloxan O.
Comfort O.
Decadron Phosphate O.
Degest 2 O.
Dexacidin O.
Dexasporin O.
Econopred Plus O.
Estivin II O.
o. herpes
I-Naphline O.
Infectrol O.
Inflamase Forte O.
Inflamase Mild O.
Isopto Atropine O.
Isopto Carpine O.
I-Tropine O.
Maxidex O.
Maxitrol O.
Metreton O.
Muro 128 O.
Mydfrin O.
Nafazair O.
Naphcon Forte O.
Ocu-Carpine O.
OcuClear O.
Ocufen O.
Ocusert Pilo-20 O.
Ocusert Pilo-40 O.
Ocu-Trol O.
Ocu-Tropine O.
Opcon O.
Ophthalgan O.
Ophthochlor O.
Osmoglyn O.
Pilagan O.
Pilocar O.
Pilopine HS O.
Piloptic O.
Pilostat O.
Polysporin O.
Pred Forte O.
Pred Mild O.
Timoptic O.
Timoptic-XE O.
Tobrex O.

VasoClear O.
Vasocon Regular O.
Viroptic O.
Visine L.R. O.
Voltaren O.
ophthalmicus
herpes zoster o. (HZO)
ophthalmitis
ophthalmologist
ophthalmopathy
thyroid o.
thyroid-related o. (TRO)
ophthalmoplegia
chronic progressive external o. (CPEO)
external o.
internal o.
internuclear o.
o. plus
progressive external o. (PEO)
ophthalmoplegic migraine
ophthalmoscope
direct o.
indirect o.
indirect laser o.
ophthalmoscopy
indirect o.
Ophthetic
Ophthochlor Ophthalmic
opiate
OPIM
other potentially infectious material
opioid
endogenous o.
o. medication
opisthorchiasis
Opisthorchis
opisthotonic posturing
opisthotonos, opisthotonus
Opitz-Frias syndrome
Opitz-Kaveggia syndrome
Opitz syndrome
opium
alcoholic tincture of o.
o. tincture
Oppenheim
O. congenital hypotonia
O. disease
O. reflex
opponens splint
opportunistic infection

NOTES

opportunity
nonnutritive sucking o. (NSO)
opposition
finger o.
o. movement
precise finger o.
oppositional
o. defiant disorder (ODD)
o. disorder
oppositionalism
OPS
orthogonal polarization spectral
OPS imaging
opsoclonus
transient o.
opsoclonus-myoclonus
o.-m. etiology
syndrome of o.-m.
opsomyoclonus
opsonin defect
opsonization
poor o.
opsonophagocytosis
optic
o. chiasma
o. disk
o. disk hyperemia
o. nerve
o. nerve aplasia
o. nerve atrophy
o. nerve cupping
o. nerve disease
o. nerve dysplasia
o. nerve edema
o. nerve glioma
o. nerve hypoplasia
o. nerve sheath
o. nerve sheath meningioma
o. nerve tumor
o. neuritis
o. neuropathy
o. neuroretinitis
o. pathway glioma
o. pathway tumor
optica
neuromyelitis o.
optical
o. immunoassay (OIA)
o. prism
o. spectroscopy
o. tomography
optician
Opticrom
optimality score
Optochin-resistant *Streptococcus*
pneumoniae **(ORSP)**
Optochin test

optode
indwelling o.
optokinetic nystagmus
optometrist
optosis
spinal o.
OPV
occult trauma, postanoxia,
ventriculoperitoneal
oral polio vaccine
oral poliovirus vaccine
Sabin OPV
OPV shunt
OPV vaccine
OR
odds ratio
Orabase
O. gel
O. HCA Topical
Kenalog in O.
Orabase-B, -O
Oracit
Orajel
O. Brace-Aid Oral Anesthetic
O. Maximum Strength
O. Mouth-Aid
O. Perioseptic
oral
Achromycin V O.
Adapin O.
Aller-Chlor O.
o. allergy syndrome
AllerMax O.
AL-Rr O.
Amen O.
Ansaid O.
Anxanil O.
Apresoline O.
Aquasol E O.
Aristocort O.
Asacol O.
Atarax O.
Atolone O.
o. attenuated *Salmonella typhi*
vaccine
Banophen O.
Belix O.
Benadryl O.
Bentyl Hydrochloride O.
Blocadren O.
o. bronchodilator
Calm-X O.
o. candidiasis
o. candidosis
Cataflam O.
Catapres O.
o. cavity
Ceftin O.

Celestone O.
Chlo-Amine O.
Chlorate O.
Chlor-Trimeton O.
Cipro O.
o. colonic lavage (OCL)
o. contraceptive pill (OCP)
o. contraceptive therapy (OCT)
Cortef O.
o. Crohn disease
Curretab O.
Cycrin O.
Cytomel O.
Decadron O.
Delta-Cortef O.
Demadex O.
Dexameth O.
Diamine T.D. O.
Dilaudid O.
Dimetabs O.
Di-Spaz O.
Dormarex 2 O.
Dormin O.
Durrax O.
Edecrin O.
o. enanthem
o. epithelium
o. exploration
Flagyl O.
Flumadine O.
o. gastric (OG)
o. gastric tube
Genahist O.
o. glucose tolerance test
Gly-Oxide O.
o. hairy leukoplakia
Hydrocortone O.
Hy-Pam O.
Indocin SR O.
o. intake
Kenacort O.
Kloromint O.
Laniazid O.
Lasix O.
Levothroid O.
Loniten O.
Marmine O.
Medrol O.
Mestinon O.
o. moniliasis
o. motor
MS Contin O.

MSIR O.
o. mucosa cyanosis
o. mucous membrane graft
Nitroglyn O.
Nordryl O.
Nor-tet O.
Nyton O.
OMS O.
Oramorph SR O.
o. osmotic (OROS)
Panmycin O.
PediaCare O.
Pediapred O.
Pentasa O.
Phendry O.
Phenergan O.
Phenetron O.
o. play
o. poliomyelitis vaccine
o. polio vaccine (OPV)
o. poliovirus vaccine (OPV)
Prelone O.
Proglycem O.
Provera O.
Proxigel O.
o. reflex
o. rehydration solution (ORS)
o. rehydration therapy (ORT)
Rheumatrex O.
Robitet O.
Roxanol SR O.
Salagen O.
Siladryl O.
Sinequan O.
Sleep-eze 3 O.
Sominex O.
o. stimulation
Sumycin O.
Synthroid O.
o. tactile defensiveness
Tega-Vert O.
Telachlor O.
Teldrin O.
Teline O.
o. temperature
Tetracap O.
Tetralan O.
o. thrush
Toradol O.
o. transmucosal fentanyl citrate (OTFC)
Trimazide O.

NOTES

oral *(continued)*
    Twilite O.
    Ucephan O.
    o. ulcer
    o. ulceration
    Unipen O.
    Urolene Blue O.
    Valium O.
    Vamate O.
    Vancocin O.
    Vasotec O.
    Videx O.
    Vistaril O.
    Voltaren O.
    Voltaren-XR O.
    Xylocaine O.
Oralet
    Fentanyl O.
    O. lollipop
oral-motor dysfunction
Oraminic II
Oramorph SR Oral
oranienburg
    Salmonella o.
Orap
Orapred
Orasept
Orasol
Orasone
Oratect
Orazinc
orbiculare
    Pityrosporum o.
orbit
orbital
    o. blowout
    o. blowout fracture
    o. bone hypoplasia
    o. cellulitis
    o. floor
    o. hemorrhage
    o. hypotelorism
    o. inflammation
    o. septum
    o. subperiosteal abscess
    o. tumor
    o. wall fracture
orbitofrontal gyri
orchidectomy
orchiditis
orchidoblastoma
orchidoepididymitis
orchidometer
    Prader o.
orchiopexy, orchidopexy
    Fowler-Stephens o.
    scrotal o.

orchitis
orciprenaline oral suspension
Ordinal Scales of Intellectual Development
Oregon Adolescent Depression Project-Conduct Disorder Screener (OADP-CDS)
Oretic
organ
    O. Injury Scaling (OIS)
    pelvic o.
    o. situs
    Zuckerkandl o.
organelle
organic
    o. acidemia
    o. acidosis
    o. aciduria
    o. arsenical
    o. brain disease
    o. heart disease
    o. hyperkinetic syndrome
    o. lead
    o. mental syndrome
    o. mercury poisoning
    o. tricuspid incompetence
Organidin NR
organism
    antibiotic-resistant gram-negative o. (ARGNO)
    coliform o.
    comma-shaped o.
    mycobacterial o.
    nontypeable o.
    parasitic o.
organization
    World Health O. (WHO)
organoaxial volvulus
organochlorine pesticide
organogenesis
    fetal o.
organoid nevus
organomegaly
organophosphate
    o. ingestion
    o. insecticide
oriental
    o. sore
    O. spotted fever
orientation
    child-centered literary o. (CCLO)
    spatial o.
Orientia tsutsugamushi
orienting
orifice
    eccentric o.
orificial tuberculosis

origin
    fever of undetermined o. (FUO)
    fever of unknown o. (FUO)
    somatropin of rDNA o.
original
    K-Phos O.
Orimune poliovirus vaccine
oris
    depressor anguli o.
    fetor o.
ORLAU
    Orthotic Research and Locomotor
        Assessment Unit
    ORLAU swivel walker
Ormazine
ornidazole
ornipressin
ornithine
    o. decarboxylase
    difluoromethyl o. (DFMO)
    o. transcarbamylase (OTC)
    o. transcarbamylase deficiency
ornithine-ketoacid aminotransferase
    deficiency
ornithosis
orodigitofacial dysostosis
orofacial
    o. cleft
    o. dyskinesia
orofaciodigital (OFD)
    o. syndrome
orogastric
orolabial herpes
oroleukokeratosis
oromandibular dystonia
oromotor sign
oronasal
oropharyngeal
    o. candidiasis (OPC)
    o. tularemia
oropharynx
OROS
    oral osmotic
    OROS methylphenidate
        hydrochloride
orotic
    o. acid
    o. acidemia
    o. aciduria
oroticaciduria
orotracheal intubation
Oroya fever

orphan
    o. drug
    enteric cytopathogenic human o.
        (ECHO)
orphanage
orphenadrine
ORS
    oral rehydration solution
ORSP
    Optochin-resistant *Streptococcus*
        pneumoniae
ORT
    oral rehydration therapy
Ortho-Cept
Orthoclone OKT3
orthodeoxia
orthodiagram
orthodontic appliance
orthodontist
orthodromic conduction
Orthoglass splint
orthognathic surgery
orthogonal
    o. polarization spectral (OPS)
    o. polarization spectral imaging
orthographic
orthomolecular therapy
orthomyxovirus
orthopedically disabled
orthopedic appliance
orthopedics
orthopedist
orthophoria
Orthoplast jacket
orthoplasty
orthopnea
orthopoxvirus
orthoroentgenogram
orthosis, pl. **orthoses**
    ankle-foot o. (AFO)
    Atlanta Scottish Rite Hospital o.
    Boston o.
    cranial o.
    CranioCap cranial o.
    foot o. (FO)
    hip-knee-ankle-foot o. (HKAFO)
    knee-ankle-foot o.
    lumbosacral o. (LSO)
    reciprocating gait o. (RGO)
    soft Boston o.
    supramalleolar o. (SMO)
    thoracolumbosacral o. (TLSO)

NOTES

orthostasis
orthostatic
    o. dizziness
    o. hypotension
    o. intolerance
    o. proteinuria
    o. tachycardia syndrome
    o. test
orthosympathetic
Orthotic Research and Locomotor Assessment Unit (ORLAU)
orthotonos, orthotonus
orthotopic
    o. heart transplantation
    o. liver transplantation (OLTx)
Ortolani
    O. maneuver
    O. sign
    O. technique
    O. test
Or-Tyl Injection
o.s., OS
    oculus sinister (left eye)
os
    o. odontoideum
    o. subfibulare
    o. trigonum
OSA
    obstructive sleep apnea
OSA/H
    obstructive sleep apnea/hypoventilation
OSAS
    obstructive sleep apnea syndrome
Osborne wave
Os-Cal
    O.-C. 500
oscillation
    flutterlike o.
    high-frequency o. (HFO)
    ocular o.
oscillator
    Babylog 8000 o.
    high-frequency o.
    Infant Star 8000 o.
    Sensormedic 3100A 8000 o.
    Stephanie 8000 o.
oscillatory
    high-frequency o.
    o. ventilation
oscillometric
    o. method
    o. technique
oscilloscope
    cathode ray o. (CRO)
OSD
    Osgood-Schlatter disease
oseltamivir

OSEP
    Office of Special Education Programs
Osgood-Schlatter
    O.-S. disease (OSD)
    O.-S. syndrome
Osler node
Osler-Weber-Rendu
    O.-W.-R. disease
    O.-W.-R. syndrome (OWRS)
Osler-Weber syndrome
osmiophilic body
Osmitrol Injection
Osmoglyn Ophthalmic
osmolality
    morning o.
    serum o.
Osmolite HN Plus formula
osmotic
    o. diarrhea
    o. diuresis
    o. gap
    oral o. (OROS)
    o. pressure (Op)
Osp
    outer surface protein
OspA
    outer surface protein A
    recombinant OspA
osseous
    o. BA lesion
    o. coalition
ossicle
    auditory o.'s
ossicular
    o. discontinuity
    o. disruption
ossiculum terminale
ossificans
    myositis o.
ossification
    appositional o.
    enchondral o.
    endochondral o.
    extra o.
ossifying fibroma
ossium
    fragilitas o.
ostectomy
osteitis
    acute mastoid o.
    alveolar o.
    o. fibrosa
    o. fibrosis cystica
    mastoid o.
    o. pubis
    rarefying o.
osteoarthritis (OA)
    degenerative o.

osteoarthropathy
    hypertrophic o. (HOA)
osteoarthrophthalmopathy
    hereditary o.
osteoblast (OB)
osteoblastic osteosarcoma
osteoblastoma (OB)
Osteocalcin
osteocalcin
    serum o.
osteochondral fracture
osteochondritis
    capitellar o.
    o. of capitellum
    o. deformans juvenilis
    o. dissecans (OCD)
    metatarsal head o.
    radial head o.
    tarsal navicular o.
osteochondrodysplasia
osteochondrodystrophy
    familial o.
osteochondroma
osteochondrosis, pl. **osteochondroses**
    o. deformans tibiae
osteochondrotic lesion
osteoclast
osteoclastic
osteoclastogenesis
osteodiastasis
    occipital o.
osteodystrophia juvenilis
osteodystrophy
    Albright hereditary o.
    azotemic o.
    renal o.
osteofibrous dysplasia
osteogenesis
    o. imperfecta (OI)
    o. imperfecta congenita syndrome
    o. imperfecta cystica
osteogenic sarcoma
osteoid
    malignant o.
    o. osteoma
    o. seam
osteoma
    multiple o.'s
    osteoid o.
osteomalacia
    juvenile o.

osteomyelitis
    acute o.
    calvarial o.
    chronic o.
    chronic recurrent multifocal o. (CRMO)
    diaphyseal o.
    hematogenous o.
    meningococcal multifocal o.
    multifocal o.
    Pasteurella multocida o.
    pyogenic o.
    Salmonella o.
    sclerosing o.
    spinal o.
    subacute o.
    tuberculous o.
    vertebral o.
osteonecrosis
osteoonchodysostosis
osteopathia striata
osteopathic medicine
osteopenia
    ground-glass o.
    juxtaarticular o.
osteopetrosis
    congenital o.
    o. tarda
osteopoikilosis
osteoporosis
    juvenile o.
    o. pseudoglioma syndrome
osteoprotegerin (OPG)
osteoradionecrosis
osteosarcoma
    chondroblastic o.
    femoral o.
    fibroblastic o.
    osteoblastic o.
    secondary o.
    small cell o.
    telangiectatic o.
osteotomy
    derotation o.
    derotation femoral o.
    diaphyseal fibular o.
    femoral o.
    fibular o.
    innominate o.
    lengthening o.
    opening wedge o.
    pelvic lengthening o.

O

NOTES

osteotomy *(continued)*
    plantarflexion o.
    proximal humeral derotation o.
    rotational o.
    shortening dorsal wedge radial o.
    tibial valgus o.
    transiliac lengthening o.
    valgus o.
    varus o.
    wedge o.
ostiomeatal complex
ostium, pl. **ostia**
    follicular o.
    o. primum
    o. primum ASD
    o. primum defect
    o. secundum
    o. secundum defect
    o. venosus defect
    vessel o.
ostomy
    intestinal o.
OT
    occupational therapy
Ota
    nevus of O.
otalgia
OTC
    ornithine transcarbamylase
    over the counter
OTFC
    oral transmucosal fentanyl citrate
other
    o. cerebral palsy
    o. potentially infectious material
    (OPIM)
otic
    AK-Spore H.C. O.
    AntibiOtic O.
    Bacticort O.
    Cerumenex O.
    Cipro HC O.
    Cortatrigen O.
    Cortisporin O.
    Debrox O.
    Drotic O.
    Floxin O.
    LazerSporin-C O.
    Octicair O.
    Ocutricin HC O.
    Otocort O.
    Otomycin-HPN O.
    Otosporin O.
    PediOtic O.
oticus
    herpes zoster o.
otidiscaviarum
    Nocardia o.

Otis-Lennon Intelligence Test
otitic hydrocephalus
otitidis
    Alloiococcus o.
otitis
    adhesive o.
    o. externa (OE)
    external o.
    o. media (OM)
    o. media with effusion (OME)
    o. media without effusion
    o. media with perforated tympanic
    membrane
otitis-conjunctivitis syndrome
otoacoustic
    o. emission (OAE)
    o. emission testing
Otobiotic
Otocalm Ear
Otocort Otic
otogenic brain abscess
OtoLAM
    Otoscan laser-assisted myringotomy
otolaryngologist
otolaryngology
otologist
Otomycin-HPN Otic
otomycosis
otopalatodigital syndrome
otorhinolaryngologist
otorrhea
    CSF o.
Otoscan laser-assisted myringotomy (OtoLAM)
otosclerosis syndrome
otoscope
    Siegel o.
otoscopy
    pneumatic o.
otospongiosis syndrome
Otosporin Otic
ototoxic drug
ototoxicity
Otovent negative pressure treatment
Oto-wick
    Pope O.-w.
Ottawa Ankle Rules (OAR)
o.u., OU
    oculus unitas (both eyes)
    oculus uterque (each eye)
Oucher scale
out
    toeing o.
outcome
    Bayley cognitive o.
outer
    o. canthus
    o. ear

o. surface protein (Osp)
o. surface protein A (OspA)

outflow
o. obstruction
o. tract

outlet
o. foramina
o. septum

outpatient

output
cardiac o.
decreased urine o.
high o.
hyperdynamic ventricle with
  high o.
low o.
urine o.
urine acid o. (UAO)

outtoe gait

outtoeing

ova (*pl. of* ovum)

oval
o. scaling
o. window

ovale
foramen o.
patent foramen o.
Pityrosporum o.
Plasmodium o.

ovalis
fossa o.

ovalocytosis
Southeast Asian o. (SAO)

ovarian
o. cyst
o. dysgenesis
o. dysgerminoma
o. hyperandrogenism
o. rupture
o. teratoma
o. torsion
o. tumor
o. vasculitis

ovariectomy

ovary
autoamputation of o.
o. in inguinal hernia
juvenile granulosa cell tumor of o.
polycystic o. (PCO)
torsion of o.

overactivity

overaeration

overanxious
o. disorder (OAD)
o. disorder of childhood

overcirculation
pulmonary o.

overcorrection

over the counter (OTC)

overcrowding

overdistention
lung o.

overdose syndrome

overfeeding

overflow
o. proteinuria
tear o.

overgrowth
cyclosporine-induced gingival o.
gingival o.
phenytoin-induced gingival o.
small bowel o.

overheating

overhydration

overinflation
congenital lobar o. (CLO)
generalized obstructive o.
obstructive o.

overlap
criterion o.

overlapping toe

overload
diastolic o.
iron o.
o. pattern
sensory o.
systolic o.

overloading
carbohydrate o.

overmature gamete

overpressuring

overprotection

overriding
o. aorta
o. finger
o. toe

overshadowing
diagnostic o.

overstimulated

overt
o. bilirubin encephalopathy
o. loss

over-the-needle catheter

overtraining syndrome

NOTES

413

overuse syndrome
overwhelming infection
Ovide lotion
ovotestis
    dysgenetic o.
Ovral contraceptive pill
Ovrette contraceptive pill
O-V Staticin
Ovudate fertility test kit
ovum, pl. ova
    ova and parasites (O&P)
ovumeter
Ovustick
owl's
    o. eye nucleus
    o. eyes view of hydrocele
Owren disease
OWRS
    Osler-Weber-Rendu syndrome
oxacillin sodium
oxalate
oxalosis
    primary o.
oxandrolone
Oxepa formula
Oxford diagnostic criteria
oxidase
    catechol o.
    cytochrome *c* o.
    NADPH o.
6-oxidase
    lysine 6-o.
oxidation
    o. disorder
    fatty acid o. (FAO)
    nitric oxide o.
oxidative
    o. brain injury
    o. phosphorylation (OXPHOS)
    o. phosphorylation disease
oxidative-reductase activity
oxide
    inhaled nitric o. (iNO, I-NO)
    nitric o. (NO)
    nitrous o.
    zinc o.
oxime
    technetium hexamethylpropyleneamine o.
oximeter
    INVOS 3100 cerebral o.
    Nellcor N20, N200 pulse o.
    Ohmeda Minx pulse o.
    Ohmeda 3800 pulse o.
    Oxytrak pulse o.
    pulse o.
    RPO o.
oximetric data

oximetry
    cerebral o.
    MARS pulse o.
    Masimo SET signal extraction pulse o.
    motion-resistant pulse o.
    nocturnal pulse o.
    pulse o.
    reflectance pulse o. (RPO)
    signal extraction pulse o.
    stress o.
    transcutaneous o.
5-oxoprolinase deficiency
OXPHOS
    oxidative phosphorylation
ox's eye
oxtriphylline
Oxy-5
    O.-5 Advanced Formula for Sensitive Skin
    O.-5 Tinted
Oxy-10 Advanced Formula for Sensitive Skin
oxybutynin
Oxycel gauze
oxycephaly
oxycodone
    o. and acetaminophen
    o. and aspirin
oxygen (O_2)
    alveolar-arterial difference in partial pressure of o. (AADPPO)
    blow-by o.
    cerebral arteriovenous difference for o. (Ca-vDO_2)
    o. consumption per minute (Vo_2)
    o. deprivation
    fraction of inspired o. (FIO_2, FiO_2)
    free-flow o.
    helium and o. (heliox)
    o. hood
    hyperbaric o.
    inspired o.
    normobaric o.
    partial pressure alveolar o. (PaO_2)
    partial pressure arterial o. (PaO_2)
    pressure of o. (PO_2)
    o. saturation
    o. tent
    o. therapy
    o. toxicity
oxygenase
    heme o. (HO)
oxygenated blood
oxygenation
    extracorporeal membrane o. (ECMO)

fetal cerebral o.
   o. index (OI)
oxygen-free radical
oxyhemoglobin saturation
oxymetazoline
oxymetholone
oxytetracycline/polymyxin ointment

oxytocin
oxytocin-secreting neuron
Oxytrak pulse oximeter
Oxy 10 Wash
Oyst-Cal 500
Oystercal 500

NOTES

O

P
> P protein
> P wave

P2

P$_{ao}$
> airway opening pressure

4p
> 4p syndrome

PA
> posteroanterior
> pulmonary artery
> > PA pressure

P & A
> protection and advocacy

PAAS
> Pediatric Acute Admission Severity
> > PAAS classification

Paas disease

Pabafilm

Pabanol

PAC
> papular acrodermatitis of childhood
> premature atrial contraction

pacchionian granulation

paced auditory serial addition test

pacemaker
> wandering atrial p.

pachydermatitis
> *Malassezia* p.

pachygyria
> localized p.

pachyonychia
> p. congenita
> p. congenita syndrome
> p. congenita syndrome of nail

Pacific Islander

pacificus
> *Ixodes* p.

pacifier
> sucrose p.
> sugar-dipped p.
> sweetened p.
> water p.

pacing
> epicardial p.
> phrenic nerve p.
> transvenous p.

pack
> E-Z Heat hot p.
> neonatal narcotic p.
> respiratory therapy p.

packed
> p. red blood cell (PRBC)
> p. red blood cell transfusion

packing
> anterior nasal p.
> nasal p.
> posterior nasal p.

paclitaxel

PACNS
> primary angiitis of CNS

PaCO$_2$
> partial pressure of carbon dioxide in
> arterial gas

pad
> arch insole p.
> Breathe Easy foam p.
> Bumpa Bed crib bumper p.
> scaphoid p.
> Sleep Guardian foam p.
> sucking p.
> suprapubic fat p.

Paecilomyces

paediatric (*var. of* pediatric)

Paediatric Crohn Disease Activity Index (PCDAI)

paediatrics (*var. of* pediatrics)

PAG
> pictorial anticipatory guidance

Paget disease

PAH
> phenylalanine hydroxylase

PAI
> partial (incomplete) androgen
> insensitivity
> plasminogen activator inhibitor
> > PAI deficiency

pain
> abdominal p.
> asymbolia to p.
> bone p.
> chest p.
> colicky abdominal p.
> congenital insensitivity to p.
> p. disorder
> facial p.
> flank p.
> functional abdominal p.
> heel p.
> lightning p.
> menstrual p.
> night p.
> nocturnal retrosternal chest p.
> ocular p.
> patellofemoral malalignment p.
> psychogenic p.
> recurrent abdominal p. (RAP)
> retrosternal chest p.

P

pain *(continued)*
 p. threshold
 visceral p.
painful joint
Pain-HP
 No P.-HP
painless hematuria
paint
PAIR
 percutaneous aspiration, instillation of
 hypertonic saline, respiration
Paired Associate Learning Task (PALT)
PAIVS
 pulmonary atresia with intact ventricular
 septum
palaeartica
palatal
 p. expansion
 p. fistula
 p. fistula closure
 p. mucosa
 p. paresis
 p. petechia
palate
 abnormal p.
 cleft p. (CP)
 cleft lip and p. (CLP)
 conotruncal cardiac defect,
  abnormal face, thymic hypoplasia,
  cleft p. (CATCH 22)
 high-arched p.
 isolated cleft p.
 midline cleft p.
 narrow p.
 p. repair
 soft p.
 submucous cleft p.
palatine
palatorespiratory dysfunction
pale stool
palilalia
palisading granuloma
palivizumab
palliation
 p. of great vessels
 Norwood p.
palliative
 p. procedure
 p. shunt
 p. surgery
pallid
 p. breathholding spell
pallidal degeneration
pallidin
pallidotomy

pallidum
 microhemagglutination assay for
  antibodies to *Treponema p.*
  (MHA-TP)
 Treponema p.
pallidus
 globus p.
Pallister-Hall syndrome
Pallister-Killian syndrome
pallor
 blanching p.
 circumoral p.
 placental p.
 white matter p.
 yellow-green p.
palmar
 p. crease
 p. erythema
 p. grasp
 p. grasp reflex
 p. hyperlinearity
 p. lesion
 p. and plantar punctate
  hyperkeratosis
 p. pustulosis
 p. xanthoma
palmaris
 keratosis p.
 pustulosis p.
 tinea nigra p.
 xanthoma striata p.
palmar-plantar sign
Palmaz stent
palmitate
 colfosceril p.
Palmitate-A 5000
palmitic acid
palmitoyltransferase
 carnitine p. (CPT)
 carnitine p. I (CPT I)
 carnitine p. II (CPT II)
palmoplantar
 p. keratoderma
 p. pustulosis
palpable
 p. bony abnormality
 p. gonad
 p. kidney
 p. nodule
 p. purpura
 p. spongy mass sign
palpably enlarged kidney
palpate
palpebral
 p. conjunctiva
 p. conjunctivitis
 p. fissure

p. reflex
p. slant

palpebrum
pediculosis p.

palpitation

PALS
pediatric advanced life support

palsy
abducens p.
acquired abducens p.
acquired 6th nerve p.
ataxic cerebral p.
athetoid cerebral p.
atonic cerebral p.
Bell p.
brachial plexus p.
bulbar p.
cerebellar cerebral p.
cerebral p. (CP)
choreoathetoid cerebral p.
congenital 6th nerve p.
cranial nerve p.
diaphragm p.
double elevator p.
dyskinetic cerebral p.
dystonic cerebral p.
Erb p.
Erb-Duchenne p.
Erb-Klumpke p.
extrapyramidal cerebral p.
facial nerve p.
gaze p.
hemiparetic cerebral p.
hemiplegic cerebral p.
hereditary neuropathy with liability
  to pressure p. (HNPP)
horizontal supranuclear gaze p.
hypotonic cerebral p.
Klumpke brachial p.
lateral rectus p.
liability to pressure p.
lower motor neuron p.
Lyme-associated peripheral facial
  nerve p.
mild spastic diplegic cerebral p.
mixed cerebral p.
mixed-type cerebral p.
motor neuron p.
nerve p.
neuron p.
obstetrical p.
other cerebral p.

peripheral facial nerve p. (PFNP)
phrenic nerve p.
postinfectious abducens p.
pressure p.
progressive bulbar p.
pseudobulbar p.
pyramidal cerebral p.
rectus p.
rigid cerebral p.
spastic cerebral p.
supranuclear p.
trochlear nerve p.
vertical gaze p.

PALT
Paired Associate Learning Task

Paludrine

Pamelor

pamidronate

pamoate
pyrantel p.

pampiniform plexus

Pamprin IB

PAN
polyarteritis nodosa

panagglutinin

panamensis
Leishmania p.

p-ANCA
perinuclear antineutrophil cytoplasmic
  antibody

pancarditis
acute p.

pancreas
annular p.
direct stimulation of p.
p. divisum
p. sufficient (PS)

Pancrease MT

pancreatic
p. agenesis
p. duct stent
p. dysfunction
p. exocrine deficiency
p. exocrine insufficiency
p. head resection
p. islet cell
p. panniculitis
p. pseudocyst
p. ring
p. sequestrum
p. tumor
p. ultrasound

NOTES

P

pancreaticobiliary anomaly
pancreaticojejunostomy
pancreatin
pancreatitis
    acute hemorrhagic p.
    choledochal cyst-induced p.
    chronic p.
    cyst-induced p.
    drug-induced p.
    gallstone p.
    hereditary p.
    infectious p.
Pancrecarb
pancrelipase
pancuronium
    p. bromide
pancytopenia
    aplastic p.
    Fanconi p.
    p. syndrome
PANDAS
    pediatric autoimmune neuropsychiatric
        disorders associated with streptococcus
pandemic
Pandoraea
    P. apista
    P. pnomenusa
    P. pulmonicola
    P. sputorum
panel
    streptococcal antigen p.
    von Willebrand p.
panencephalitis
    progressive rubella p.
    rubella p.
    sclerosing p.
    subacute sclerosing p. (SSPE)
Paneth cell inclusion
panhypogammaglobulinemia
panhypopituitarism
    familial p.
panic
    p. attack
    p. disorder
panlobar disarray
Panmycin Oral
Panner disease
panniculitis
    cold p.
    factitial p.
    lobar p.
    nodular nonsuppurative p.
    nonsuppurative p.
    pancreatic p.
    popsicle p.
    poststeroid p.
    relapsing nodular nonsuppurative p.
    septal p.

pannus
panopacification
panophthalmitis
panoramic radiograph
Panorex view
PanOxyl-AQ
PanOxyl Bar
Panscol
    P. Lotion
    P. Ointment
pansystolic murmur
pantothenic acid
panty spica
panuveitis
PaO$_2$
    partial pressure alveolar oxygen
    partial pressure arterial oxygen
PAOP
    pulmonary artery occluded pressure
PAP
    pulmonary alveolar proteinosis
        acquired PAP
        primary PAP
        secondary PAP
Pap
    Papanicolaou
    Pap smear
PAPA
    preschool-age psychiatric assessment
Papanicolaou (Pap)
    P. smear
papaverine
paper
    filter p. (FP)
papG allele
Papile grading
papilla, pl. **papillae**
    Bergmeister p.
    edematous p.
    fungiform p.
    p. of Vater
papillary
    p. muscle
    p. muscle dysfunction
    p. necrosis
    p. variant
papilledema
    chronic p.
papilliferum
    syringocystadenoma p.
papillitis
papillocarcinoma
    choroid plexus p.
papilloma
    choroid plexus p. (CPP)
    laryngeal p.
    raided raspberry-like p.
    raspberry-like p.

respiratory p.
tan p.

papillomacular bundle

papillomatosis
benign p.
laryngeal p.
recurrent respiratory p. (RRP)
respiratory p.

papillomavirus
human p. (HPV)

Papillon-Léage-Psaume syndrome

Papillon-Lefèvre syndrome

papoose

papovavirus BK

PAPP-A
pregnancy-associated plasma protein A

papular
p. acrodermatitis
p. acrodermatitis of childhood (PAC)
p. eruption
p. exanthem
p. lesion
p. rash
p. urticaria

papule
acral keratotic p.
acuminate p.
blue p.
crop of p.'s
erythematous p.
filiform p.
flesh-colored p.
genital p.
Gottron p.
keratotic p.
lichenoid p.
polygonal p.
satellite p.
verrucous p.
violaceous polygonal p.
white p.

papulonecrotica
tuberculosis p.

papulonecrotic tuberculid

papulonodular lesion

papulosis
bowenoid p.

papulosquamous
p. eruption
p. skin change

papulovesicle

papulovesicular
p. acrodermatitis
p. lesion

PAQLQ
Pediatric Asthma Quality of Life Questionnaire

para

paraaminosalicylic acid

paraben

paracentesis

paracetamol (*var. of* parecetamol)

parachute
p. mitral valve
p. reflex
p. response

Paracoccidioides brasiliensis

paracoccidioidin skin testing

paracoccidioidomycosis

paracrine

paracrine-acting growth factor

paracrystalline inclusion

paradoxical
p. aciduria
p. breathing
p. chest wall motion
p. pulse
p. pupil reaction

paradoxic respiration

paradoxus
pulsus p.

paraductal acanthosis

paraduodenal hernia

paraesophageal hiatal hernia

Paraflex

Parafon Forte DSC

paraganglioma

paragonimiasis
cerebral p.

Paragonimus westermani

parahaemolyticus
Vibrio p.

parahemophilia

parainfluenza
p. virus (PIV)
p. virus type 1 (PF1)
p. virus type 2 (PF2)
p. virus type 3 (PF3)
p. virus type 4 (PF4)

parakeratosis

Paral

paraldehyde

NOTES

P

parallel
    p. circulation
    p. play
    p. speech
    p. study arm
paralysis, pl. **paralyses**
    abducens facial p.
    acute flaccid p.
    anal sphincter p.
    bladder sphincter p.
    bulbar p.
    ciliary p.
    congenital abducens facial p.
    congenital oculofacial p.
    congenital unilateral lower lip p.
    p. of conjugate upward gaze
    deltoid p.
    diaphragm p.
    Erb-Duchenne p.
    facial p.
    familial hypokalemic periodic p.
    flaccid p.
    fleeting p.
    hyperkalemic periodic p.
    hypokalemic periodic p.
    hysterical p.
    idiopathic facial p.
    infantile p.
    Klumpke p.
    Landry type of p.
    laryngeal nerve p.
    lower lip p.
    mononeuritis with p.
    muscle p.
    nerve p.
    obstetrical p.
    oculofacial p.
    phrenic nerve p.
    poliomyelitis-like p.
    postictal p.
    recurrent laryngeal nerve p.
    respiratory p.
    sleep p.
    spastic p.
    sphincter p.
    p. of superior laryngeal nerve
    tick p.
    Todd p.
    total muscle p.
    unilateral lower lip p.
    vocal cord p.
    Werdnig-Hoffmann p.
paralytic
    p. hypotonia
    p. idiocy
    p. ileus
    p. poliomyelitis
    p. rabies

    p. shellfish poisoning
    p. strabismus
parameningeal infection
paramesonephric
parameter
    growth p.
paramethadione
paramyoclonus multiplex
paramyotonia congenita
paramyxovirus
paranasal sinus
paraneoplastic syndrome
Paranit shampoo
paranoid
    p. ideation
    p. personality disorder
paraparesis
    acute spastic p.
    areflexic p.
    flaccid p.
    HTLV-I associated
      myelopathy/tropical spastic p.
      (HAM/TSP)
    nonspastic p.
    spastic p.
    tropical spastic p. (TSP)
parapertussis
    Bordetella p.
parapharyngeal lymph node
paraphasia
paraphimosis
Paraplatin
paraplegia
    familial spastic p. (FSP)
    flaccid p.
    hereditary spastic p.
    spastic p.
paraplegic
paraplegin
parapneumonic pleural effusion
parapodium
    Toronto p.
paraprofessional
parapsilosis
    Candida p.
parapsoriasis
paraquat
    p. ingestion
    p. lung
parasagittal
    p. cerebral injury
    p. cortical infarction
parasite
    ova and p.'s (O&P)
parasitemia
parasitic
    p. gastroenteritides
    p. organism

parasitized cecal pouch
parasomnia
> NREM arousal p.
> REM p.

parasternal
> p. lift
> p. short-axis view

parasuicide
parasympathetic
> p. fiber
> p. neuron
> p. tone

parasympatholytic drug
parasympathomimetic drop
paratesticular tumor
parathyroid
> p. gland
> p. gland immaturity
> p. hormone (PTH)

parathyroidectomy
Paratrol shampoo
paratropicalis
paratyphi
> *Salmonella p.*

paratyphoid fever
paraurethral cyst
paravertebral abscess
paraxial
> p. fibular hemimelia
> p. tibial hemimelia

parched mucous membrane
parecetamol, paracetamol
> p. suppository

paregoric
parenchyma
> liver p.
> medullary p.
> patchy infiltration of medullary p.

parenchymal
> p. abscess
> p. brain lesion
> p. cyst
> p. lung disease
> p. lung morphogenesis
> p. nodule

parenchymatous
> p. cerebral cysticercosis
> p. congenital syphilis
> p. form

parent
> p. child
> P.'s Choice formula

> p. effectiveness training (PET)
> p. guidance work
> P. and Teacher Conners Scale

Parental Stress Index (PSI)
parenteral
> p. alimentation
> p. aqueous penicillin G
> p. nutrition (PN)
> p. nutrition-associated cholestatic (PNAC)
> p. nutrition-associated cholestatic liver disease

parenting
> attachment p.
> P. Stress Index (PSI)

parent-professional partnership
Parepectolin
paresis
> apparent p.
> asymmetric palatal p.
> congenital suprabulbar p.
> flaccid p.
> laryngeal p.
> ocular p.
> oculosympathetic p.
> palatal p.
> spastic p.
> suprabulbar p.
> Todd p.

paresthesia
Pari
> P. LC Plusjet nebulizer
> P. Proneb Turbo compressor

parietal
> p. bone
> p. bulge
> p. cell antibody
> p. cell hyperplasia
> p. encephalocele
> p. foramina
> p. pericardiectomy
> p. shunt

parietooccipital region
Parinaud
> P. oculoglandular syndrome
> P. sign

parity
park
> hemoglobin M Hyde P.

Parkinson-Cowan dry gas meter
Parkinson disease

NOTES

P

parkinsonian
> p. movement disorder
> p. rigidity

parkinsonian-like
parkinsonism
Parkland formula
Parks-Weber syndrome
paromomycin
paronychia
> candidal p.

parotid gland
parotitis
> acute p.
> bacterial p.
> epidemic p.
> suppurative p.

paroxetine
paroxysm
> febrile p.

paroxysmal
> p. atrial tachycardia (PAT)
> p. blinking
> p. coughing
> p. depolarization shift (PDS)
> p. dystonia
> p. emotional state
> p. hypercyanotic attack
> p. hypoxic spell
> p. kinesigenic choreoathetosis
> p. nocturnal dyspnea (PND)
> p. nocturnal hemoglobinuria (PNH)
> p. torticollis
> p. vertigo

parrot
> P. atrophy
> P. atrophy of newborn
> p. fever
> pseudoparalysis of P.
> P. syndrome

Parry-Romberg syndrome
PARS
> Personal Adjustment and Role Skills
> PARS III questionnaire

pars interarticularis
partial
> p. agenesis
> p. agenesis of vermis
> p. anomalous pulmonary venous return
> p. auxiliary orthotopic liver transplantation
> p. complex epilepsy
> p. complex seizure
> p. DiGeorge anomaly
> p. DiGeorge syndrome
> p. epileptogenic discharge
> p. external biliary diversion (PEBD)

> p. gonadal dysgenesis
> p. hepatectomy
> p. (incomplete) androgen insensitivity (PAI)
> p. lipodystrophy
> p. liquid ventilation (PLV)
> p. oculocutaneous albinism
> p. pressure
> p. pressure alveolar oxygen (PaO$_2$)
> p. pressure arterial oxygen (PaO$_2$)
> p. pressure of carbon dioxide in arterial gas (PaCO$_2$)
> p. status epilepticus
> p. thrombin time
> p. thromboplastin time (PTT)
> p. trisomy 10q syndrome
> p. villus atrophy
> p. zonal dissection (PZD)

partially
> p. duplicated ureter
> p. sighted

partial-syndrome eating disorder
partial-thickness burn
particle
> Dane p.

partition of energy metabolism
partnership
> parent-professional p.

parts per million (ppm)
parturition
parvoviral infection
parvovirus
> p. B19
> p. B19 red cell aplasia
> human p. (HPV)

parvula
> *Veillonella p.*

parvum
> *Cryptosporidium p.*

PAS
> periodic acid Schiff

passage of meconium
passive
> p. head-up tilt test
> p. immunization
> p. range of motion
> p. supination
> p. venous congestion

passivity
paste
> Bipp p.
> butt p.
> nitroglycerin p.
> Triple P.
> zinc oxide p.

Pasteurella
> *P. canis*

P. multocida
P. multocida osteomyelitis
Pastia
    P. line
    P. sign
PAT
  paroxysmal atrial tachycardia
  preventive allergy treatment
Patanol
Patau syndrome
patch
    atrophic p.
    bovine pericardium p.
    corporal cavernosal p.
    Deponit P.
    EMLA p.
    fentanyl p.
    hair p.
    hairy p.
    herald p.
    MacCallum p.
    Minitran P.
    Nitrodisc P.
    Nitro-Dur P.
    PediaPatch Transdermal P.
    pericardium p.
    Peyer p.
    salmon p.
    shagreen p.
    spontaneous atrophic p.
    transdermal fentanyl p.
    Transdermal-NTG P.
    Transderm-Nitro P.
    Trans-Plantar Transdermal P.
    Trans-Ver-Sal Transdermal P.
    p. unroofing
    p. unroofing of outflow tract
patching
patchy
    p. infiltration
    p. infiltration of medullary
      parenchyma
patella, pl. **patellae**
    absent p.
    bipartite p.
    chondromalacia p.
    congenital dislocation of p.
    dislocated p.
    dislocating p.
    hypoplastic p.
    kissing p.

    sleeve fracture of p.
    subluxating p.
patellar
    p. fracture
    p. ligament
    p. reflex
    p. tendinitis
patellofemoral
    p. malalignment
    p. malalignment pain
    p. pain syndrome (PFPS)
    p. stress syndrome
patent
    p. ductus arteriosis coil
      embolization
    p. ductus arteriosus (PDA)
    p. ductus venosus
    p. foramen ovale
    p. urachus
paternal uniparenteral isodisomy
path
    migratory p.
pathergy sign
Pathocil
pathogen
    blood-borne p.
pathogenesis
pathogenic
pathogenicity
pathognomonic
    p. Koplik spot
    p. symptom
pathologic
    p. apnca
    p. fracture
    p. reflex
pathological
    p. apnea
    p. cavus
    p. gynecomastia
pathologist
    speech-language p.
pathology
    anaplastic p.
    speech p.
    speech-language p.
pathophysiology
pathotropic
pathway
    Embden-Meyerhof p.
    neural reflex p.
    pericardial p.

NOTES

P

pathway *(continued)*
    postchiasmal visual p.
    reflex p.
    visual p.
patient
    CMV-seronegative transplant p.
    transplant p.
patient-controlled analgesia (PCA)
patient-triggered ventilation
patter
    cocktail party p.
pattern
    abnormal respiratory p.
    abnormal vasculature flow p.
    age-to-dose p.
    android p.
    apple p.
    behavior p.
    bimodal p.
    biphasic temperature p.
    BL p.
    borderline lepromatous p.
    borderline tuberculoid p.
    branching p.
    breathing p.
    BT p.
    burst-suppression p.
    capillary p.
    central fat distribution p.
    characteristic
      electroencephalogram p.
    chessboard p.
    Christmas tree p.
    complete suppression p.
    diastolic overload p.
    distribution p.
    eggbeater running p.
    extensor thrust p.
    fat distribution p.
    flow p.
    fracture p.
    gynecoid fat distribution p.
    gyral p.
    heliotrope p.
    herringbone p.
    hyperkinetic behavior p.
    hypsarrhythmic p.
    interweaving p.
    Le Fort fracture p.
    linear branching p.
    marking time p.
    menstrual p.
    motor p.
    mucopolysaccharide p.
    munching p.
    overload p.
    pear p.
    persistent primitive reflex p.

    primitive reflex p.
    prosodic p.
    reflex p.
    respiratory p.
    reticulonodular p.
    skin ridge p.
    subpleural reticulonodular p.
    sun-seeking p.
    systolic overload p.
    temperature p.
    temporospatial p.
    tonic neck p.
    urinary mucopolysaccharide p.
    vasculature flow p.
patterned breathing
patterning therapy
pauciarticular
    p. juvenile chronic arthritis
    p. juvenile rheumatoid arthritis
pauciarticular-onset
    p.-o. arthritis
    p.-o. JRA
Pauci-immune glomerulonephritis
paucity
    bile duct p.
    p. of gas
    intrahepatic bile duct p.
    nonsyndromic bile duct p.
    syndromic p.
Paul-Bunnell
    P.-B. antibody test
    P.-B. reaction
Paul-Bunnell-Davidsohn test
Pavabid
Pavatine
Pavlik harness
PAVM
    pulmonary arteriovenous malformation
pavor
    p. diurnus
    p. nocturnus
Pavulon
PAX3 gene
Paxil
Pazo Hemorrhoid
PBC
    periodic breathing cycle
    plasma bilirubin concentration
    primary biliary cirrhosis
PBF
    percent body fat
PBMC
    peripheral blood mononuclear cell
PBSC
    peripheral blood stem cell
PBZ
    pyribenzamine

p.c.
  post cibum (after meals)
PCA
  patient-controlled analgesia
  postconceptional age
PCC
  Poison Control Center
PCC-R
  Percentage of Consonants Correct-
    Revised
PCD
  primary ciliary dyskinesia
PCDAI
  Paediatric Crohn Disease Activity Index
PCEC
  purified chick embryo cell culture
    PCEC vaccine
PC formula
PC-IOL
  posterior chamber intraocular lens
PCNSL
  primary central nervous system
    lymphoma
PCO
  polycystic ovary
PCO₂
  pressure of carbon dioxide
  pressure of CO_2
PCOD
  polycystic ovarian disease
PCOS
  polycystic ovary syndrome
PCP
  phencyclidine
  Pneumocystis carinii pneumonia
PCR
  polymerase chain reaction
PCr
  phosphocreatine
PCT
  procalcitonin
    serum PCT
PCV7
  pneumococcal 7-valent conjugate vaccine
PCVC
  percutaneous central venous catheter
PCWP
  pulmonary capillary wedge pressure
P450 cytochrome
PD
  peritoneal dialysis

personality disorder
postural drainage
PDA
  patent ductus arteriosus
P.D. Access with Peel-Away needle introducer
PDD
  pervasive developmental disorder
PDD-NOS
  pervasive developmental disorder not
    otherwise specified
PDE
  personality disorder examination
PDE5
  cyclic guanosine monophosphate-specific
    phosphodiesterase 5
PdE
  pediatric endocrinology
PDI
  phosphodiesterase inhibitor
  psychiatric diagnostic interview
  psychomotor development index
PDMS
  Peabody Developmental Motor Scale
PDP
  positive distending pressure
PDS
  paroxysmal depolarization shift
PE
  pressure equalization
  pulmonary embolism
    PE tube
Peabody
  P. Developmental Motor Activity
    Cards
  P. Developmental Motor Scale
    (PDMS)
  P. Picture Vocabulary
  P. Picture Vocabulary Test (PPVT)
  P. Picture Vocabulary Test-Revised
    (PPVT-R)
peak
  p. admittance
  p. end-expiratory pressure
  p. expiratory flow rate (PEFR)
  p. flow measurement
  p. flow meter (PFM)
  p. flow meter monitor
  p. flow rate
  p. growth velocity
  p. inspiratory pressure (PIP)
  p. instantaneous gradient

NOTES

P

peak *(continued)*
> p. level
> p. and trough
> p. and trough levels
> Webb-McCall p.

peaked T wave

pearl
> epithelial p.
> Epstein p.

pear pattern

Pearson
> P. correlation
> P. correlation coefficient
> P. marrow-pancreas syndrome
> P. syndrome

peau d'orange

pebbly skin lesion

PEBD
> partial external biliary diversion

PEC
> protein-induced eosinophilic colitis

pecorum
> *Chlamydia* p.

pectin
> kaolin and p.

pectinate line

pectoriloquy
> whispered p.

pectus
> p. bar
> p. carinatum
> p. excavatum

peculiar facies

PED
> pediatric emergency department
> prenatally exposed to drugs

pedaling movement

pedal pulse

Pedersen speculum

PEDI
> Pediatric Evaluation of Disability Inventory

PediaCare
> P. Cough-Cold
> P. Fever
> P. Night Rest
> P. Oral

Pediaflor

Pedialyte
> P. formula
> P. oral electrolyte maintenance solution

Pediamist

PediaPatch Transdermal Patch

Pediapred Oral

Pediaprofen

PediaSure with Fiber formula

pediatric, paediatric
> p. acquired immunodeficiency syndrome
> P. Acute Admission Severity (PAAS)
> P. Acute Admission Severity classification
> p. advanced life support (PALS)
> p. aphakia
> P. Asthma Quality of Life Questionnaire (PAQLQ)
> p. autoimmune-mediated neuropsychiatric disorders associated with streptococcus
> p. autoimmune neuropsychiatric disorders associated with streptococcus (PANDAS)
> p. balloon
> Benylin p.
> p. bone rongeur
> p. bulldog clamp
> p. dermatology
> p. dosing information
> P. Early Elemental Examination (PEEX)
> p. emergency department (PED)
> p. emergency medicine (PEM)
> p. endocrinology (PdE)
> P. Evaluation of Disability Inventory (PEDI)
> P. Examination at Three (PEET)
> P. Examination of Educational Readiness (PEER)
> p. gonococcal conjunctivitis
> p. gonococcal infection
> p. hypertension
> p. intensive care unit (PICU)
> P. Liver Transplant-Specific Scale (PLTSS)
> p. lung surgery
> p. lupus nephropathy
> p. myelodysplasia
> p. neurocritical care
> p. neurologist
> P. Oncology Group
> p. public health
> p. pulmonary medicine
> p. radiologist
> P. Risk of Mortality
> P. Risk of Mortality Score (PRISM)
> Robitussin p.
> Rynatan p.
> p. sedation
> p. sedation unit (PSU)
> p. self-retaining retractor
> P. Spectrum of Disease (PSD)
> P. Symptom Checklist (PSC)

p. thyroid carcinogenesis
P. Trauma Score (PTS)
P. Triban
p. tuberculosis
p. vascular clamp
p. viral diarrhea
Vivonex p.
pediatrician
P. infant dietary supplement
pediatrics, paediatrics
American Academy of p. (AAP)
Pediazole
Pedi-Boro
Pedi-cap detector
pedicle
renal p.
pediculiasis
pediculosis
p. corporis
p. palpebrum
p. pubis
Pediculus
P. *humanus*
P. *humanus corporis*
P. *humanus var capitis*
Pedi-Dri Topical
PediOtic Otic
Pedi PEG tube
Pedi-Pro Topical
pedis
dorsalis p.
tinea p.
pedodontist
Pedte-Pak-5
Pedtrace-4
peduncle
cerebral p.
inferior p.
middle cerebellar p.
pedunculated molluscum fibrosum
PedvaxHIB vaccine
PEEP
positive end-expiratory pressure
PEER
Pediatric Examination of Educational
Readiness
peer
p. conformity inventory
p. relation
PEET
Pediatric Examination at Three

PEEX
Pediatric Early Elemental Examination
pefloxacin
PEFR
peak expiratory flow rate
PEG
percutaneous endoscopic gastrostomy
PEG tube
peg
rete p.
PEG-ADA
polyethylene glycol-ADA
polyethylene glycol-modified adenosine
deaminase
pegademase bovine
pegaspargase
pegboard
Groover P.
peglike teeth
peg-shaped upper central incisor
Pelargon formula
Pel-Ebstein fever
peliosis
bacillary p.
p. hepatis
Pelizaeus-Merzbacher disease (PMD)
pellagra
pellagra-like skin rash
pellet
Muse p.
Testopel P.
Pellizzi syndrome
pellucida
zona p. (ZP)
pellucidum
cavum septi p.
septum p.
pelves (*pl. of* pelvis)
pelvic
p. appendicitis
p. band
p. inflammatory disease (PID)
p. kidney
p. lengthening osteotomy
p. organ
p. tilt
p. tumor
p. ultrasound
p. venous congestion syndrome
pelviectasis
pelvis, pl. **pelves**
dilated renal p.

NOTES

P

pelvis *(continued)*
  renal p.
  trefoil p.
PEM
  pediatric emergency medicine
Pemberton
  P. acetabuloplasty
  P. procedure
pemirolast potassium
pemoline
  P. C-IV
  magnesium p.
pemphigoid
  bullous p.
  childhood cicatricial p.
pemphigus
  p. foliaceus
  p. neonatorum
  syphilitic p.
  p. vulgaris
pen
  Epi E-Z P.
Pena
  P. midsagittal anorectoplasty
  P. procedure
Pena-Shokeir syndrome (I, II)
penciclovir
pendelluft
Pendred syndrome
pendular nystagmus
pendulum
  molluscum fibrosum p.
Penecort Topical
Penetrak test
penetrans
  Mycoplasma p.
penetrating
  p. brain injury
  p. trauma
penetration
  anal p.
  cercarial skin p.
  skin p.
PenFil
  Novolin 70/30 P.
  Novolin N, R P.
penicillamine
penicillin
  antistaphylococcal p.
  aqueous crystalline p.
  aqueous crystalline p. G
  benzathine p.
  benzathine p. G (BPG)
  p. G
  p. G benzathine
  p. G procaine
  parenteral aqueous p. G
  procaine p.

  procaine p. G
  semisynthetic p.
  p. V potassium
  p. V, VK
penicillinase-producing gonococcus
penicillin-nonsusceptible *Streptococcus pneumoniae* **(PNSP)**
penicillin-resistant
  p.-r. *Staphylococcus* pneumonia (PRSP)
  p.-r. *Streptococcus pneumoniae* (PRSP)
penicilliosis
Penicillium marneffei
penile
  p. agenesis
  p. chordee
  p. curvature
  p. duplication
  p. dysgenesis
  p. erection
  p. flaccidity
  p. ischemia
  p. length
  p. torsion
  p. ulceration
  p. urethral meatus
  p. zipper entrapment
penis
  buried p.
  concealed p.
  fracture of p.
  hidden p.
  inconspicuous p.
  webbed p.
Pen-Jr
  Epi E-Z P.-Jr
penopubic urethral meatus
penoscrotal
  p. hypospadias
  p. transposition
Penrose drain
Pentacef
pentalogy
  p. of Cantrell
  Fallot p.
Pentam-300 Injection
pentamidine isethionate
pentane
  exhaled p.
Pentasa Oral
pentastarch
pentavalent vaccine
Pentax
  P. EG-2430 video endoscope
  P. FG 24-x video endoscope
  P. laryngoscope
pentazocine

pentobarbital
p. coma
sodium p.
Pentostam
pentosuria
essential benign p.
Pentothal Sodium
pentoxifylline
Pentrax
penumbra
Pen-Vee
Pen-Vee K
PEO
progressive external ophthalmoplegia
PEO syndrome
PEP
postexposure prophylaxis
Pepcid
P. AC Acid Controller
P. RPD
PEPCK
phosphoenolpyruvate carboxykinase
PEPCK deficiency
PEP/LVET
preejection period/left ventricular ejection time
Peptamen
P. Jr.
P. Jr. formula
peptic
p. esophagitis
p. gastritis
p. ulcer disease (PUD)
peptide
atrial natriuretic p. (ANP)
glucose-dependent insulinotropic p.
p. growth factor receptor signal
p. growth factor signaling mechanism
p. hormone
insulinotropic p.
91kD cytochrome b p.
mitogenic p.
natriuretic p.
PTH-derived p.
synthetic gliadin p.
thrombin receptor-activating p. (TRAP)
trypsin activation p. (TAP)
Pepto-Bismol
Peptococcus
Pepto Diarrhea Control

Peptostreptococcus
per
p. os (by mouth) (p.o.)
p. rectum (p.r.)
p. se
Perative formula
percent
p. body fat (PBF)
p. fractional shortening
percentage
high oxygen p. (HOPE)
Percentage of Consonants Correct-Revised (PCC-R)
percentile
perception
deficits in attention, motor control, p. (DAMP)
depth p.
light p. (LP)
motor p.
no light p. (NLP)
perceptual
p. domain
p. skill
perchlorate
Percocet
Percodan
Percodan-Demi
Percoll
percussion
abdominal p.
chest p.
costovertebral angle tenderness to p.
dullness to p.
flatness to p.
hyperresonance to p.
p. myotonia
p. therapy
percutaneous
p. adductor tenotomy
p. aspiration, instillation of hypertonic saline, respiration (PAIR)
p. catheter drainage
p. central venous catheter (PCVC)
p. cholangiography
p. cyst aspiration
p. endoscopic gastrostomy (PEG)
p. endoscopic gastrostomy tube
p. epididymal sperm aspiration (PESA)

NOTES

P

percutaneous *(continued)*
- p. femoral venous catheter
- p. lung tap
- p. multipuncture technique
- p. nephrostomy
- p. patent ductus arteriosus closure
- p. pin fixation
- p. renal biopsy
- p. Seldinger technique
- p. therapy
- p. tracheostomy
- p. transluminal angioplasty
- p. transluminal coronary rotational ablation (PTCRA)
- p. umbilical blood sampling (PUBS)

percutaneously inserted central line catheter (PICC)

Perdiem
- P. Fiber
- P. Plain

perennial
- allergic rhinitis p.
- p. allergic rhinitis
- p. asthma
- p. rye grass

Perez sign

perfectionism
- rigid p.

Perfectoderm Gel

perfluorocarbon (PFC)

perfluorocarbon-assisted gas exchange

perfluorochemical (PFC)
- p. liquid

perfluorodecaline (PFD)

perforated
- p. appendicitis
- p. eardrum
- p. tympanic membrane
- p. viscus

perforating granuloma annulare

perforation
- appendiceal p. (AP)
- biliary p.
- eardrum p.
- esophageal p.
- gastric p.
- spontaneous biliary p. (SBP)
- tympanic membrane p.

perfringens
- *Clostridium p.*

perfusion
- luxury p.
- mosaic p.
- pulmonary p.
- twin reversed arterial p. (TRAP)
- ventilation p.

Periactin

periadenitis mucosa necrotica recurrens

perianal
- p. abscess
- p. aphthosis
- p. candidosis
- p. dermatitis
- p. fistula
- p. hypopigmentation
- p. pruritus
- p. skin tag
- p. suture

perianastomotic ulceration

periappendiceal abscess

periaqueductal tumor

periarteritis nodosa

periarticular

periaxial encephalitis

peribronchial
- p. fibrosis
- p. infiltration

pericapillary inflammatory cuffing

pericardial
- p. effusion
- p. friction rub
- p. knock
- p. pathway
- p. puncture
- p. tamponade

pericardiectomy
- parietal p.
- visceral p.

pericardiocentesis

pericardiotomy

pericarditis
- acute fibrinous p.
- bacterial p.
- constrictive p.
- dry p.
- fibrinous p.
- immune complex-mediated p.
- infectious p.
- purulent p.

pericardium patch

perichondritis

perichondrium

Peri-Colace

pericoronitis
- acute p.

pericranium

pericyte

Peridex

perifascicular atrophy

Perifoam

perifollicular accentuation

perifolliculitis

perihepatitis
- gonococcal p.

perihilar
>p. infiltrate
>p. shadow

perikaryon, pl. **perikarya**
perilymph
perilymphatic fistula (PLF)
perimembranous
>p. septum
>p. VSD

perimesencephalic region
perimolysis
perinatal
>p. asphyxia
>p. cerebral hemorrhage
>p. herpes
>p. hydronephrosis
>p. hypoxemia
>p. insult
>p. lethal osteogenesis imperfecta
>p. period
>p. risk factor
>p. stroke
>p. telencephalic leukoencephalopathy

perinatally acquired HIV infection
perinatologist
perinatology
perineal
>p. desquamation
>p. fistula
>p. irritation
>p. itching
>p. resection
>p. testis

perineoscrotal hypospadias
perineum
perineurium, pl. **perineuria**
perinuclear
>p. ANCA
>p. antineutrophil cytoplasmic antibody (p-ANCA)

PerioChip
period
>incubation p.
>last menstrual p. (LMP)
>menstrual p.
>neonatal p.
>newborn p.
>perinatal p.
>postictal p.

periodic
>p. acid Schiff (PAS)
>p. breathing
>p. breathing cycle (PBC)
>p. breathing in infants
>p. fever, aphthous stomatitis, pharyngitis, cervical adenitis (PFAPA)
>p. movement disorder

periodontal disease
periodontitis
>p. Ehlers-Danlos syndrome
>juvenile p.
>localized juvenile p. (LJP)
>prepubertal p.

PerioGard
perioperative
perioptic meningioma
perioral rash
periorbital
>p. cellulitis
>p. ecchymosis
>p. edema
>p. fullness
>p. hyperpigmentation
>p. infantile myofibromatosis
>p. puffiness
>p. violaceous erythema

Perioseptic
>Orajel P.

periosteal
>p. cloaking
>p. elevation
>p. reaction
>p. stripping

periosteum
periostitis
peripheral
>p. ablative surgery
>p. acrocyanosis
>p. arterial catheter
>p. arterial disease
>p. arteriovenous fistula
>p. arthritis
>p. auditory disorder
>p. blood
>p. blood mononuclear cell (PBMC)
>p. blood smear
>p. blood stem cell (PBSC)
>p. cyanosis
>p. eosinophilia
>p. facial nerve palsy (PFNP)
>p. fractional oxygen extraction (PFOE)
>p. intravenous (PIV)

NOTES

P

peripheral (*continued*)
    p. intravenous catheter
    p. myelin protein (PMP)
    p. nerve injury
    p. neuritis
    p. neuroblastoma
    p. neuroectodermal tumor
    p. neuroepithelioma
    p. neurofibromatosis
    p. neutropenia
    p. precocious puberty
    p. primitive neuroectodermal tumor (PPNET)
    p. pulmonary stenosis
    p. pulmonic stenosis
    p. stem cell transplantation
    p. thrombophlebitis
    p. vision
peripherally
    p. inserted catheter (PIC)
    p. inserted central catheter (PICC)
periphery
peripubertal
perirectal abscess
perisphincteric factor
peristalsis
    visible p.
peristaltic wave
perisulcal topography
perisylvian
    p. abnormality
    p. syndrome
peritoneal
    p. cavity
    p. dialysis (PD)
    p. drain
    p. exudate
    p. fibrosis
    p. hernia
    p. sign
    p. tap
    p. venous shunt
    ventricular p. (VP)
peritoneum
    matted p.
peritonitis
    acute secondary localized p.
    bacterial p.
    bile p.
    infectious p.
    localized p.
    meconium p.
    primary p.
    secondary localized p.
    spontaneous bacterial p.
    tuberculous p.
peritonsillar
    p. abscess

    p. cellulitis
    p. edema
peritubular fibrosis
periungual
    p. avascularity
    p. desquamation
    p. erythema
    p. fibroma
    p. flaking
    p. wart
periurethral
perivascular
    p. calcification
    p. eosinophilic infiltrate
    p. inflammatory infiltrate
    p. polymorphonuclear infiltrate
    p. pseudorosette formation
perivasculitis
    granulomatous p.
periventricular
    p. echolucency (PVEL)
    p. encephalomalacia
    p. hemorrhage (PVH)
    p. heterotopia
    p. infarction
    p. leukomalacia (PVL)
periventricular-intraventricular hemorrhage (PIVH)
perivitelline space
Perkin
    P. Elmer rhodamine dye terminator kit
    P. line
perlèche
Perlman syndrome
perlocutionary stage
Perls iron stain
permanence
    object p.
permanent
    p. dentition
    p. molar
    p. posthemorrhagic hydrocephalus
    p. teeth
permanganate
    potassium p.
Permanone
Permapen
permeability
    intestinal p. (IP)
    vascular p.
permethrin
    p. 5% cream
    p. creme rinse
permissive hypercapnia
pernicious
    p. anemia
    p. vomiting

pernio
  lupus p.
Pernox
peroneal
  p. dislocation
  p. muscular atrophy
  p. muscular atrophy, axonal type
  p. muscular dystrophy
  p. nerve function
  p. retinaculum
  p. rupture
  p. spastic flatfoot
peroneum
peroneus brevis tendon
peroxidase
  p. defect
  eosinophil p.
  glutathione p.
peroxidation
  lipid p.
peroxidative enzyme
peroxide
  benzoyl p.
  carbamide p.
  hydrogen p.
Peroxin A5, A10
peroxisomal
  p. deficiency
  p. disease
  p. disorder
  p. ghost
peroxisome import disorder
Peroxyl
peroxynitrite
perphenazine
Per-Q-Cath catheter
Perrault syndrome
PERRLA
  pupils equal, round, reactive to light and
  accommodation
Persa-Gel
Persantine
perseveration
persistence
  p. of fetal circulation
  foramen ovale p.
persistent
  p. alkaline urine
  p. fetal circulation (PFC)
  p. hyperplastic primary vitreous
  (PHPV)
  p. neutropenia

  p. primitive reflex pattern
  p. processus vaginalis
  p. pulmonary hypertension (PPH)
  p. pulmonary hypertension of
  newborn (PPHN)
  p. pupillary membrane
  p. tachycardia
  p. trismus
  p. urachus
  p. vegetative state (PVS)
Personal Adjustment and Role Skills (PARS)
personality
  p. change
  p. disorder (PD)
  p. disorder examination (PDE)
  P. Inventory for Children (PIC)
perstans
  telangiectasia macularis eruptiva p.
persulcatus
  Ixodes p.
pertactin
pertechnetate
  technetium-99m p.
pertenue
  Treponema p.
Perthes disease
Pertofrane
pertubation
  cardiovascular p.
Pertussin ES
pertussis
  acellular p.
  Bordetella p.
  diphtheria, tetanus, p.
  diphtheria, tetanus toxoid,
  acellular p.
  diphtheria-tetanus toxoid with p.
  (DTwP)
  p. toxin (PT)
  p. toxoid (PT)
peruana
  verruca p.
pervasive
  p. developmental disorder (PDD)
  p. developmental disorder not
  otherwise specified (PDD-NOS)
  p. support
pes
  p. anserina bursitis
  p. anserinus
  p. cavus

NOTES

P

435

pes *(continued)*
    p. cavus deformity
    p. equinovarus
    p. planus
PESA
    percutaneous epididymal sperm aspiration
pessimistic
pesticide
    organochlorine p.
pestis
    Yersinia p.
pestivirus
PET
    parent effectiveness training
    positron-emission tomography
    postexposure treatment
    pressure equalization tube
petechia, pl. **petechiae**
    palatal p.
petechial
    p. hemorrhage
    p. rash
Peters anomaly
pethidine
petit
    p. mal
    p. mal attack
    p. mal epilepsy
    p. mal-like seizure disorder
    p. mal seizure
    p. mal status
    p. mal variant
peto
Petrie cast
petrolatum
    liquid p.
petroleum jelly
petrositis
petted teeth
Peutz-Jeghers
    P.-J. polyp
    P.-J. syndrome
Peyer patch
Pezzer
    P. catheter
    P. tube
PF1
    parainfluenza virus type 1
PF2
    parainfluenza virus type 2
PF3
    parainfluenza virus type 3
PF4
    parainfluenza virus type 4
Pfannenstiel incision
PFAPA
    periodic fever, aphthous stomatitis, pharyngitis, cervical adenitis

PFC
    perfluorocarbon
    perfluorochemical
    persistent fetal circulation
PFD
    perfluorodecaline
Pfeiffer syndrome
PFGE
    pulsed field gel electrophoresis
PFIC
    progressive familial intrahepatic cholestasis
Pfizerpen
Pfizerpen-AS
PFK
    phosphofructokinase
    PFK deficiency
PFM
    peak flow meter
    TruZone PFM
PFNP
    peripheral facial nerve palsy
PFOE
    peripheral fractional oxygen extraction
PFP
    purified fusion protein
    PFP vaccine
PFPS
    patellofemoral pain syndrome
PFS
    Adriamycin PFS
    Tarabine PFS
    Vincasar PFS
PFT
    placentofetal transfusion
    pulmonary function test
pfu
    plaque-forming unit
PG
    phosphatidylglycerol
P/G
    Fulvicin P/G
P&G
    Procter and Gamble
PGD
    preimplantation genetic diagnosis
PGK
    phosphoglycerate kinase
PGS
    prolapse gastropathy syndrome
PH-1
    primary hyperoxaluria type 1
pH
    hydrogen in concentration
    endoesophageal pH
    intracellular pH
    intragastric pH
    neutral pH

pH probe
scalp pH
umbilical arterial pH
venous pH

PHA
phytohemagglutinin

PHACE
posterior fossa malformation,
hemangiomas, arterial anomalies,
coarctation of aorta and cardiac defects,
eye abnormalities
PHACE syndrome

phagocyte
mononuclear p.
polymorphonuclear p.

phagocytic

phagocytophilia
Ehrlichia p.

phagocytosis
poor p.

phakoma

phakomatosis, pl. **phakomatoses**

phalangectomy

phalanx, pl. **phalanges**
delta p.

phalloides
Amanita p.

phalloidin

phallometric assessment

phallus

Phanatuss

phantom limb

pharaonic circumcision

pharmacodynamic response

pharmacokinetic

pharmacokinetics

pharmacologically induced hypomania

pharmacologic immunosuppression

pharmacotherapy
stand-alone p.

Pharmaflur

Pharsight
P. Trial Designer
P. Trial Designer simulation
program

pharyngeal
p. diphtheria
p. gonorrhea
p. incompetence
p. mirror
p. muscle
p. space

pharynges (*pl. of* pharynx)

pharyngitis
acute lymphonodular p.
exudative p.
GABHS p.
group C p.
lymphonodular p.
nonstreptococcal p.
purulent p.
streptococcal p.
viral p.

pharyngoconjunctival fever

pharyngoplasty

pharyngotonsillitis

pharynx, pl. **pharynges**

phase
p. advance treatment
deep tendon reflex delayed
relaxation p.
p. delay chronotherapy
delayed relaxation p.
p. delay treatment
icteric p.
immune p.
Korotkoff p.
late p.
polyuric p.
pre-pulseless p.
prolonged expiratory p.
pulseless p.
stance p.
viremic p.

phase-contrast microscopy

phased array probe

Phazyme infant drops

PHC
primary hepatocellular carcinoma

PHCO₃
plasma bicarbonate

PHE
phenylalanine
blood PHE
serum PHE

phenacetin

Phenadex Senior

Phenazine Injection

phenazopyridine

phencyclidine (PCP)

Phendry Oral

phenelzine

Phenerbel-S

NOTES

P

Phenergan
  P. Injection
  P. Oral
  P. Rectal
  P. VC
  P. VC With Codeine
Phenetron Oral
phenobarbital
  hyoscyamine, atropine,
    scopolamine, p.
phenocopy
phenolphthalein
phenomenology
phenomenon, pl. **phenomena**
  Ashman p.
  clasp-knife p.
  crankshaft p.
  dissociative p.
  doll's eye p.
  intrapsychic p.
  Kasabach-Merritt p.
  Köbner p.
  near-miss p.
  no-reflow p.
  pseudo-Köbner p.
  Raynaud p. (RP)
  ritualistic p.
  Schwartzman p.
  Somogyi p.
  squatting p.
  steal p.
  sunburst p.
  tension-discharging p.
  trigger p.
  Wenckebach phenomena
phenothiazine intoxication
phenotype
  body p.
  Bombay erythrocyte p.
  cardiac abnormality, T-cell deficit,
    clefting, hypocalcemia p.
  CATCH p.
  fibroblast growth factor-10 null p.
  hemoglobin SC, SS p.
  hemoglobin SS p.
  hemoglobin S-Thal p.
  Hunter-Hurler p.
  MASS p.
  Potter p.
  Turner p.
phenotypic female
phenoxybenzamine
phenylacetate
  sodium p.
phenylacetic acid
phenylacetylglutamine
phenylalanine (PHE)

  p. dehydroxylase
  p. hydroxylase (PAH)
phenylalaninemia
  malignant p.
  non-PKU p.
phenylbutazone
phenylbutyrate
  sodium p.
phenylephrine
  guaifenesin, phenylpropanolamine, p.
    (ULR)
  promethazine and p.
phenylethylamine
phenylketonuria (PKU)
  p. test
phenylpropanolamine
  brompheniramine and p.
phenylpyruvic acid
phenytoin
  p. encephalopathy
  p. therapy
phenytoin-associated adenopathy
phenytoin-induced gingival overgrowth
pheochromocytoma
Pherazine With Codeine
PHH
  posthemorrhagic hydrocephalus
PHI
  Prehospital Index
pHi
  intracellular hydrogen ion concentration
Phialophora
Philadelphia
  P. chromosome
  P. collar
Philip gland
Philips SensorTouch temple
  thermometer
Phillips' Milk of Magnesia
philtrum
  hypoplastic p.
  short p.
  smooth p.
phimosis
  secondary p.
phimotic ring
pHisoHex bath
phlebectasia
  congenital generalized p.
  generalized p.
phlebitis
  infective p.
  syphilitic p.
phlebotomum
  Bunostomum p.
phlebotomus fever
phlebotomy
phlegmon

phlyctenule
PHMB
    polyhexamethyl biguanide
PHN
    public health nurse
phobia
    fever p.
    school p.
    simple p. (SPh)
    social p.
    specific p.
phobic avoidance
phocomelia syndrome
pholcodine
phonation
    abnormal p.
phoneme segmentation task
phonemic awareness task
phonetics
phonological
    p. coding
    p. development
    p. disorder
phonologic-syntactic syndrome
phonology
phonophobia
phoria
Phos-Ex
Phos-Flur
phosphatase
    acid p.
    alkaline p. (ALP)
    bone-specific alkaline p.
    tyrosine p.
phosphate
    Aralen P.
    calcium p.
    chloroquine p.
    p. enema
    nicotinamide adenine dinucleotide p.
        (NADPH)
    plasma p.
    polyribosylribitol p. (PRP)
    primaquine p.
    pyridoxal p.
    sodium hydrogen p.
    p. supplement
    p. toxicity
    p. wasting
phosphate-buffered
    p.-b. saline
    p.-b. saline solution

phosphatidylcholine
    dipalmitoyl p.
    unsaturated p.
phosphatidylethanolamine
phosphatidylglycerol (PG)
    p. level
phosphatidylinositol
phosphaturia
phosphene
5-phospho-alpha-d-ribosyl pyrophosphate
    (PRPP)
phosphocreatine (PCr)
phosphodiesterase
    p. 5
    cGMP-specific p.
    cGMP-specific p. 5
    cyclic guanosine monophosphate-
        specific p. 5 (PDE5)
    p. inhibitor (PDI)
phosphoenolpyruvate
    p. carboxykinase (PEPCK)
    p. carboxykinase deficiency
phosphofructokinase (PFK)
    congenital defect of p.
    p. deficiency
phosphoglycerate kinase (PGK)
phosphokinase
    creatine p.
    creatinine p. (CPK)
phospholipase
phospholipid
    egg p.
phosphoribosylpyrophosphate synthetase
    superactivity
phosphoribosyltransferase
    adenine p.
phosphorus
    p. magnetic resonance imaging (^{31}P
        MRI)
    p. MRS
phosphoryl
phosphorylase
    p. kinase deficiency
    nucleoside p.
    purine nucleoside p. (PNP)
phosphorylated drug form
phosphorylation
    mitochondrial oxidative p.
    oxidative p. (OXPHOS)
Phospho-Soda
    Fleet P.-S.
photic stimulation

NOTES

P

photoallergic reaction
photobilirubin
photocoagulation
    laser p.
photodistributed lesion
photogenic seizure
photometabolism
photometric analysis
photometry
    scanning p.
photophobia
photophobic iritis
photoplethysmography
    near infrared p. (NIRP)
    red p.
Photoplex
photoscreening
photosensitive
    p. dermatitis
    p. epilepsy
    p. porphyria
    p. seizure
photosensitivity
phototesting
phototherapy
    double-bank p.
    fiberoptic p. (FO-PT)
    halogen spotlight p.
    intensive p.
    maximum-intensive p.
    psoralen and ultraviolet A p.
photothermolysis
phototoxic reaction
PHPV
    persistent hyperplastic primary vitreous
phrenic
    p. nerve
    p. nerve pacing
    p. nerve palsy
    p. nerve paralysis
phrenoesophageal ligament
phthalate
    dimethyl p.
PHVD
    posthemorrhagic ventricular dilation
PHVM
    posthemorrhagic ventriculomegaly
Phyllocontin
Phyllodes tumor
physeal
    p. arrest
    p. bridge
    p. closure
    p. destruction
    p. fracture
    p. injury
    p. separation
physical therapy (PT)

physician
    medical control p. (MCP)
physiologic
    p. addiction/abstinence syndrome
    p. anemia
    p. delay
    p. delay of puberty
    p. flatfoot
    p. genu valgum
    p. genu varum
    p. hypogammaglobulinemia
    p. jaundice
    p. leukorrhea
    p. reflex
    p. reflux
    p. regurgitation
    p. salt solution (PSS)
    P. Stability Index (PSI)
    p. transient hypoparathyroidism
    p. tumescence
physiological
    p. bowleg
    p. cavus
    p. gynecomastia
physiologically corrected transposition
physiology
    Eisenmenger p.
    Score for Neonatal Acute P.
    (SNAP)
physiopathologic
physiotherapist
physiotherapy
physis
    bridging p.
    broad p.
    radial p.
    serpiginous cephalad curved p.
physostigmine
phytanic
    p. acid
    p. acid oxidation disorder
phytobezoar
phytohemagglutinin (PHA)
phytonadione
phytophotodermatitis
phytosterol (PS)
PI
    ponderal index
    present illness
    protease inhibitor
Pi
    protease inhibitor
    Pi type
pial thickening
pia mater
PIC
    peripherally inserted catheter
    Personality Inventory for Children

PICA
Pictorial Instrument for Children and Adolescents

pica

PICC
percutaneously inserted central line catheter
peripherally inserted central catheter

pickettii
Burkholderia p.
Ralstonia p.

pickwickian syndrome

picky eater

picornavirus

PICP
carboxyterminal propeptide of type 1 procollagen

picrotoxin

pictorial
p. anticipatory guidance (PAG)
P. Instrument for Children and Adolescents (PICA)

picture
p. chart
p. completion test
postencephalitic parkinsonian p.

PICU
pediatric intensive care unit

PID
pelvic inflammatory disease
primary immune deficiency

PIE
pulmonary infiltrate with eosinophilia
pulmonary interstitial emphysema

piebaldism

piercing
cartilage p.

Pierre
P. Robin sequence
P. Robin syndrome

Piers-Harris Children's Self-Concept Scale

piezoelectric PVDF detector

pigeon
p. breast
p. toe

pigeontoed

Pigg-O-Stat

pigment
bile p.
melanin-like p.
p. stone

pigmentary stage

pigmentation
black p.
contiguous p.
mucocutaneous p.
reticulated p.

pigmented
p. melanocyte
p. nevus
p. nodular adrenal hyperplasia

pigmenti
Block-Sulzberger incontinentia p.
incontinentia p.

pigmentosa
congenital bullous urticaria p.
neuropathy, ataxia, retinitis p. (NARP)
retinitis p.
urticaria p.
xeroderma p.

pigmentosum
xeroderma p.

pigtail catheter

PIH
pregnancy-induced hypertension

Pilagan Ophthalmic

pilar cyst

pilaris
keratosis p.
pityriasis rubra p. (PRP)

pili (*pl. of* pilus)

pill
Carter's Little P.'s
emergency contraceptive p.
Levlen contraceptive p.
Lo/Ovral contraceptive p.
Nordette contraceptive p.
oral contraceptive p. (OCP)
Ovral contraceptive p.
Ovrette contraceptive p.
progestin-only p.
Tri-Levlen contraceptive p.
Triphasil contraceptive p.

Pilocar Ophthalmic

pilocarpine
p. iontophoresis
p. iontophoresis method

pilocytic fibrillary astrocytoma

piloid tumor

pilomatricoma

pilonidal
p. cyst

NOTES

P

441

pilonidal *(continued)*
    p. dimple
    p. sinus
Pilopine HS Ophthalmic
Piloptic Ophthalmic
pilosebaceous
    p. duct
    p. gland
    p. gland of Zeis
Pilostat Ophthalmic
Pilot audiometer
pilus, pl. **pili**
    pili annulati
    pili torti
    pili trianguli et canaliculi
Pima
pimozide
pincer grasp
pindolol
pineal
    p. body
    p. germinoma
    p. tumor
pinealoblastoma
pinealoma
    ectopic p.
pineoblastoma
ping-pong
    p.-p. ball deformity
    p.-p. ball depression
    p.-p. fracture
pinguecula
pinhole
    p. collimated scan
    p. collimation
    p. test
pink
    p. disease
    p. tetralogy of Fallot
pinked up
pinkeye
pinna, pl. **pinnae**
    displaced p.
    malformed p.
pinning
    in situ p.
pinpoint hemorrhage
Pin-Rid
pin tract
pinworm infestation
Pin-X
PIP
    peak inspiratory pressure
pipecolic acidemia
piperacillin
    p. sodium
    p. and tazobactam
piperacillin/tazobactam

piperazine
pipiens
    Culex p.
PIPP
    Premature Infant Pain Profile
Pipracil
piracetam
pirbuterol
piriform aperture stenosis
piriformis syndrome
piroxicam
pit
    commissural lip p.
    congenital lip p.
    lip p.
    preauricular p.
pitch
pitcher's elbow
Pitocin
Pitressin
pitted keratolysis
pitting
    digital p.
    p. edema
    nail p.
pituitary
    p. adenoma
    p. dwarfism
    p. gigantism
    p. gland
    p. gland gumma
    p. necrosis
pituitary-adrenal function
Pi-type ZZ defect
pityriasis
    p. alba
    p. lichenoides
    p. lichenoides et chronica (PLC)
    p. lichenoides et varioliformis acuta
      (PLEVA)
    p. rosea
    p. rubra pilaris (PRP)
    p. versicolor
Pityrosporum
    P. disease
    P. orbiculare
    P. ovale
PIV
    parainfluenza virus
    peripheral intravenous
      PIV catheter
PIVH
    periventricular-intraventricular
    hemorrhage
PIVKA
    protein-induced vitamin K absence
pivoting
    prone p.

pixel
PK
  pyruvate kinase
    PK activity
    PK factor
Pk
  Synsorb Pk
PKD
  polycystic kidney disease
    infantile PKD
PKDL
  post-kala azar dermal leishmaniasis
PKU
  phenylketonuria
    PKU test
placebo
placebo-controlled study
placement
  categorical p.
  gastrostomy tube p.
  intraosseous line p.
  irregular tooth p.
  line p.
  noncategorical p.
  open gastrostomy tube p.
  stent p.
  tooth p.
  tube p.
placenta, pl. **placentae**
  abruptio placentae
  p. abruptio
  circummarginate p.
  circumvallate p.
  p. previa
  velamentous p.
placental
  p. abruption
  p. blood flow
  p. edema
  p. insufficiency
  p. maturity index
  p. mosaicism
  p. mosaicism for triploidy
  p. pallor
  p. profusion
  p. progesterone deficiency
  p. transfer
  p. transfusion
placentation
  abnormal p.

placentitis
  coccidioidal p.
placentofetal transfusion (PFT)
Placidyl
placing
  p. reflex
  p. response
PL-ADOS
  prelinguistic autism diagnostic
  observation
plagiocephaly
  deformational occipital p.
  frontal p.
  p. headband
  p. helmet
  occipital p.
  unilateral occipital p.
plague
plain
  p. abdominal radiograph
  Agoral P.
  Perdiem P.
plan
  Individualized Family Service P.
  (IFSP)
  multimodal treatment p.
  transition p.
plana
  coxa p.
  verruca p.
  vertebra p.
planar bone scan
plane
  equatorial p.
  fat p.
  median p.
  soft-tissue fat p.
planning
  motor p.
  poor motor p.
planovalgus
  flexible pes p.
plantar
  p. dermatosis
  p. eccrine bromhidrosis
  p. fascia
  p. fasciitis
  p. grasp reflex
  p. imaging
  p. response
  p. wart

NOTES

P

plantarflexion
> p. osteotomy

plantaris
> keratosis palmaris et p.
> pustulosis palmaris et p.
> verruca p.

plantarum
> *Lactobacillus p.*

plantigrade

plant thorn synovitis

planum temporale

planus
> acute eruptive lichen p.
> eruptive lichen p.
> hypermobile pes p.
> lichen p.
> pes p.

plaque
> acuminate p.
> bacterial p.
> calcified bacterial p.
> confluent p.
> erythematous confluent p.
> filiform p.
> honey-crusted p.
> hyperpigmented lichenified p.
> lichenified p.
> p. of nummular eczema
> p. radiotherapy
> sclerose en p.
> p. of thrush
> uncalcified bacterial p.
> verrucous p.
> white p.
> white-yellow p.

plaque-forming unit (pfu)

plaquelike rash

Plaquenil Sulfate

plaque-type psoriasis

Plasbumin

plasma
> p. amino acid concentration
> p. aminogram
> p. ammonia
> p. arginine
> p. bicarbonate ($PHCO_3$)
> p. bilirubin concentration (PBC)
> p. cell
> p. cell infiltrate
> p. citrulline
> p. coagulation factor VIII, IX
> p. cortisol
> p. exchange
> p. factor
> fresh frozen p. (FFP)
> p. histamine concentration
> p. inorganic pyrophosphate
> p. lactate

> p. lactoferrin
> p. linoleic acid
> p. membrane
> p. nitrite
> p. noradrenaline
> p. oncotic pressure
> p. ornithine level
> p. phosphate
> p. phosphate concentration
> platelet-poor p. (PPP)
> platelet-rich p. (PRP)
> p. protein
> p. renin activity
> p. retinol concentration
> p. surfactant protein-B
> p. theophylline concentration
> p. thromboplastin
> p. thromboplastin antecedent
> p. TPO
> p. very-long-chain fatty acid
> p. viral load
> p. viremia
> p. vitamin A concentration

plasma-free iron

plasmapheresis

plasmin

plasminogen
> p. activator inhibitor (PAI)
> p. activator inhibitor deficiency
> p. level

Plasmodium
> chloroquine-resistant *P. falciparum*
> chloroquine-sensitive *P. falciparum*
> *P. falciparum*
> *P. malariae*
> *P. ovale*
> *P. vivax*

plaster
> Mediplast P.
> Sal-Acid P.
> urea p.

Plastibell

plastic
> p. blanket
> p. bronchitis
> p. deformation fracture
> p. heat shield
> p. obturator
> p. pleurisy

plasticity

plasty
> labioscrotal Y-V p.

plate
> agar p.
> *Brucella agar* p.
> chorionic p.
> cribriform p.
> epiphyseal growth p.

p. fracture
glanduloplasty and in situ
  tubularization of urethral p.
  (GITUP)
growth p.
hemineural p.
neural p.
tarsal p.
tubularized incised p. (TIP)
urethral p.
vaginal p.
widened growth p.
plateau encephalopathy
platelet (PLT)
p. abnormality
p. adhesion
p. aggregation
p. calmodulin level
p. concentration
p. count
p. membrane
p. plugging
TRAP-activated neonatal p.
p. trapping
platelet-antigen incompatibility
platelet-poor plasma (PPP)
platelet-rich plasma (PRP)
platelet-type von Willebrand disease
platform
wedge-shaped p.
Platinol
Platinol-AQ
platybasia
platypnea
play
p. activity
imitative p.
oral p.
parallel p.
p. therapy
vocal p.
PLC
pityriasis lichenoides et chronica
pleconaril
pledget
cotton p.
pleiotropia
pleocytosis
cerebrospinal fluid p.
CSF p.
CSF lymphocytic p.
eosinophilic p.

lymphocytic p.
mononuclear p.
neutrophilic p.
pleomorphic
p. cellular infiltrate
p. gram-negative rod
p. spindle cell tumor
pleomorphism of hepatocyte
Plesiomonas shigelloides
plethora
plethysmograph
face-out, whole-body p.
plethysmography
finger p.
respiratory inductive p. (RIP)
Respitrace inductance p.
venous occlusion p.
pleura, pl. **pleurae**
stripping of p.
pleural
p. biopsy
p. decortication
p. effusion
p. fluid analysis
p. friction rub
pleurectomy
pleurisy
dry p.
plastic p.
serofibrinous p.
pleuritis
pleuroamniotic shunt
pleurocentesis
pleurodesis
chemical p.
pleurodynia
epidemic p.
pleuropericardial
pleuroperitoneal fold
pleuropulmonary
p. blastoma (PPB)
p. involvement
pleuroscopy
PLEVA
pityriasis lichenoides et varioliformis
acuta
plexectomy
plexi (*pl. of* plexus)
plexiform neurofibroma
plexopathy
brachial p.
plexus, pl. **plexi**

NOTES

445

plexus *(continued)*
    Auerbach p.
    brachial p.
    choroid p.
    Kiesselbach p.
    Meissner p.
    myenteric p.
    pampiniform p.
PLF
    perilymphatic fistula
PLH
    pulmonary lymphoid hyperplasia
plicamycin
plicata
    lingua p.
plication
    p. of diaphragm
    diaphragmatic p.
    fundal p.
plosive
PLP
    proteolipid protein
PLT
    platelet
PLTSS
    Pediatric Liver Transplant-Specific Scale
plucked chicken skin lesion
plug
    anorectal p.
    colonic p.
    intraluminal p.
    keratinous p.
    meconium p.
    mucus p.
plugged toilet sign
plugging
    follicular p.
    platelet p.
plumbism
plus
    Cenafed P.
    Diocto-K P.
    Dioctolose P.
    DSMC P.
    D-S-S P.
    Duramist P.
    Ensure P.
    Genasoft P.
    Kalcinate Cal P.
    Lorcet P.
    Neonate One P.
    ophthalmoplegia p.
    Pro-Sof P.
    Sudafed P.
1-plus
    ALGO 1-p.
Plutchik Impulsivity Scale

PLV
    partial liquid ventilation
PM
    polymyositis
PM-60/40 formula
PMD
    Pelizaeus-Merzbacher disease
PM/DM
    polymyositis/dermatomyositis
PMI
    point of maximum impulse
PML
    progressive multifocal
      leukoencephalopathy
PMN
    polymorphonuclear
PMP
    peripheral myelin protein
^{31}P MRI
    phosphorus magnetic resonance imaging
PMS
    premenstrual syndrome
PMS-Amantadine
Pm-Scl antigen
PMT
    point of maximum tenderness
PN
    parenteral nutrition
PNAC
    parenteral nutrition-associated cholestatic
      PNAC liver disease
PncD vaccine
PNCRM7 vaccine
PncT vaccine
PnCV
    nonvalent pneumococcal conjugate
      vaccine
PND
    paroxysmal nocturnal dyspnea
    postnatal depression
pneogaster
PNET
    primitive neuroectodermal tumor
PNET/MB
    primitive neuroectodermal
      tumor/medulloblastoma
pneumatic
    p. cell
    p. dilation
    p. otoscopy
pneumatocele formation
pneumatosis intestinalis
pneumocapillary infusion pump
pneumocardiogram
pneumocele
pneumocephalus
    tension p.

pneumococcal
    p. conjugate vaccine
    p. facial cellulitis
    p. mastoiditis
    p. meningitis
    p. pneumonia
    p. polysaccharide vaccine
    p. protein conjugate vaccine
    p. sepsis
    p. 7-valent conjugate vaccine
      (PCV7)
pneumococcus, pl. **pneumococci**
    cephalosporin-resistant p.
    latex test for *P.*
    resistant p.
Pneumocystis
    P. carinii
    P. carinii pneumonia (PCP)
pneumocyte
    type II p.
pneumoencephalography
pneumogram
    2-channel p.
pneumomediastinum
Pneumomist
pneumonia
    acquired p.
    adenoviral p.
    p. alba
    aspiration p.
    bacteremia-associated
      pneumococcal p. (BAPP)
    bacterial p.
    bronchiolitis obliterans organizing p.
      (BOOP)
    chemical p.
    chlamydial p.
    Chlamydia trachomatis p.
    congenital p.
    desquamative interstitial p.
    Enterobacter p.
    eosinophilic p.
    exogenous lipoid p. (ELP)
    fulminant early-onset neonatal p.
    giant cell p.
    gram-negative p.
    group B streptococcal p.
    herpes simplex p.
    hydrocarbon p.
    hypostatic p.
    lipoid p.
    lobar p.

    measles p.
    Mycoplasma p.
    necrotizing p.
    neonatal p.
    nosocomial p.
    penicillin-resistant *Staphylococcus* p.
      (PRSP)
    pneumococcal p.
    Pneumocystis carinii p. (PCP)
    postinfluenza p.
    postviral p.
    respiratory syncytial virus p.
    rheumatic p.
    staphylococcal p.
    streptococcal p.
    Streptococcus p.
    suppurative p.
    thrush p.
    tuberculous p.
    vaccine-associated p.
    ventilator-associated p. (VAP)
    viral p.
pneumoniae
    Chlamydia p.
    Diplococcus p.
    drug-resistant *Streptococcus* p.
      (DRSP)
    Klebsiella p.
    Mycoplasma p.
    Optochin-resistant *Streptococcus* p.
      (ORSP)
    penicillin-nonsusceptible
      Streptococcus p. (PNSP)
    penicillin-resistant *Streptococcus* p.
      (PRSP)
    Streptococcus p.
pneumonic
    p. consolidation
    p. tularemia
pneumonitis
    acute p.
    chemical p.
    desquamative interstitial p. (DIP)
    hypersensitivity p.
    interstitial p.
    lipoid interstitial p. (LIP)
    lymphocytic interstitial p. (LIP)
    lymphoid interstitial p. (LIP)
    radiation p.
    RSV p.
    secondary p.
    varicella p.

NOTES

P

pneumootoscope
pneumoparotiditis
pneumopericardium
pneumoperitoneum
pneumophila
  Legionella p.
pneumotachygraph
pneumotaxic center
PNEUMOTEST kit
pneumothorax, pl. **pneumothoraces (PTX)**
  catamenial p.
  iatrogenic p.
  nontension p.
  spontaneous p.
  tension p.
  traumatic p.
Pneumovax
  P. 23
PNH
  paroxysmal nocturnal hemoglobinuria
pnomenusa
  Pandoraea p.
PNP
  purine nucleoside phosphorylase
    PNP deficiency
PNSP
  penicillin-nonsusceptible *Streptococcus*
    pneumoniae
Pnu-Imune 23
PO$_2$
  pressure of oxygen
    simultaneous preductal-postductal
      PO$_2$
p.o.
  by mouth (per os)
  per os (by mouth)
    p.o. feeding
POAH
  posterior occipitoatlantal hypermobility
Pocketpeak peak flow meter
POD
  polycystic ovary disease
Pod-Ben-25
Podocon-25
podocyte
podofilox
Podofin
podophyllin
  topical p.
podophyllotoxin
  purified p.
podophyllum resin
POE
  prone on elbows
    POE position
Pogosta virus
poikilocyte
  fragmented p.

poikilocytosis
poikiloderma
  p. congenitale
  infantile p.
point
  p. biserial correlation
  hypothalamic set p.
  infection p.
  lead p.
  p. of maximum impulse (PMI)
  p. of maximum tenderness (PMT)
  McBurney p.
  pressure p.
  set p.
  p. tenderness
pointer
  hip p.
pointes
  torsade de p.
point-spread artifact
Point-Two
Poison Control Center (PCC)
poisoning
  acute iron p.
  aflatoxin p.
  amensic shellfish p.
  antidepressant p.
  arsenic p.
  carbon monoxide p.
  ciguatera fish p.
  cobalt p.
  cyclic antidepressant p.
  diarrheal shellfish p.
  fish p.
  food p.
  heavy metal p.
  histamine fish p.
  iron p.
  lead p.
  mercury vapor p.
  metal p.
  monosodium glutamate p.
  neurologic shellfish p.
  neurotoxic shellfish p.
  niacin p.
  organic mercury p.
  paralytic shellfish p.
  rodenticide p.
  salt p.
  scombroid p.
  shellfish p.
  tetrodotoxin p.
  thallium p.
  vapor p.
poke weed mitogen (PWM)
Poland
  P. anomalad

P. anomaly
P. syndrome
Polaroid glasses
pole
kidney p.
polio
poliomyelitis
polio immunization
vaccine-associated paralytic polio (VAPP)
poliodystrophy
polioencephalitis
bulbar p.
poliomyelitis (polio)
abortive p.
bulbar p.
bulbospinal p.
inapparent p.
nonparalytic p.
paralytic p.
pure bulbar p.
spinal paralytic p.
vaccine-associated paralytic p. (VAPP)
poliomyelitis-like
p.-l. paralysis
p.-l. syndrome
poliosis
poliovirus
p. hominis
inactivated p.
p. vaccine
vaccine-acquired p.
Politano-Leadbetter technique
Politzer
method of P.
pollakiuria
pollen
p. allergy
birch tree p.
grass p.
ragweed p.
tree p.
pollen-induced rhinitis
pollical ray
pollicization of index finger
pollinosis
seasonal p.
pollution
air p.
polyacrylamide gel electrophoresis

polyarteritis
microscopic p.
p. nodosa (PAN)
p. nodosa group
polyarthritis
migratory p.
p., RF negative
RF-negative juvenile p.
p., RF positive
polyarticular
p. JRA
p. juvenile chronic arthritis
p. juvenile rheumatoid arthritis
polychotomous
polychromasia
polychromatophilia
Polycillin
Polycillin-N
Polycitra
P. K
Polycitra-LC
polyclonal
p. antiendotoxin anticore antibody
p. B cell activation
p. cryoglobulin
p. hypergammaglobulinemia
Polycose
P. liquid formula
P. powder
P. powder formula
polycystic
p. encephalomalacia
p. kidney
p. kidney disease (PKD)
p. ovarian disease (PCOD)
p. ovary (PCO)
p. ovary disease (POD)
p. ovary syndrome (PCOS, POS)
polycythemia
neonatal p.
primary p.
relative p.
secondary p.
p. vera
polycythemia-hyperviscosity syndrome
polydactylism
polydactyly
Majewski short rib p.
postaxial p.
Saldino-Noonan short rib p.
short rib p. (type I, II)

NOTES

P

polydipsia
    neurogenic p.
    primary p.
    psychogenic p.
polydysplasia
    hereditary ectodermal p.
polydystrophy
    pseudo-Hurler p.
polyethylene
    p. catheter
    p. feeding tube
    p. glycol
    p. glycol-ADA (PEG-ADA)
    p. glycol-electrolyte solution
    p. glycol-modified adenosine
      deaminase (PEG-ADA)
    p. glycol solution
Polygam S/D
Polygelin colloid solution
polygenic mode
polyglandular autoimmune disease (type I, II)
polyglutamate
    folyl p.
polyglutamation
polyglutamine-expanded Huntington
polygonal papule
polygraphy
polyhexamethyl biguanide (PHMB)
Poly-Histine CS, DM
Poly-Histine-D
polyhydramnios
polymastia
polymenorrhea
polymer
    sodium polyacrylate p.
polymerase
    p. chain reaction (PCR)
    DNA p.
    DNA-directed p.
    DNA-directed RNA p.
    viral DNA p.
polymeric diet
polymicrogyria
    syndrome of symmetric parasagittal
      parietooccipital p.
polymicrogyric
polymorpha
    Mima p.
polymorphism
    genetic p.
    restriction fragment length p.
      (RFLP)
polymorphonuclear (PMN)
    p. infiltrate
    p. leukocyte
    p. leukocyte storage pool

    p. lymphocyte
    p. phagocyte
polymorphous
    p. exanthem
    p. light eruption
    p. rash
Polymox
polymyositis (PM)
    juvenile p.
polymyositis/dermatomyositis (PM/DM)
polymyxin
    p. B, E
    neomycin and p. B
polyneuritiformis
    heredopathia atactica p.
polyneuritis
    acute infectious p.
    infantile p.
    infectious p.
    mixed sensory p.
    purely sensory p.
    relapsing infectious p.
    sensory p.
polyneuropathy
    acute inflammatory demyelinating p.
      (AIDP)
    chronic inflammatory
      demyelinating p. (CIDP)
    erythredema p.
    spinal p.
polynomial
polyomavirus JC
polyostotic fibrous dysplasia
polyp
    adenomatous p.
    allergic p.
    antral choanal p.
    aural p.
    charcoal p.
    cobblestone sessile p.
    colonic p.
    diffuse intestinal p.
    fundic gland p.
    gastrointestinal p.
    hyperplastic p.
    inflammatory p.
    intestinal p.
    juvenile colonic p.
    multiple gastrointestinal p.'s
    nasal p.
    Peutz-Jeghers p.
    prolapsing p.
    retention p.
    sessile p.
    umbilical p.
polypeptide
    gastric inhibitory p. (GIP)

small nuclear ribonucleoprotein-associated p. (SNRPN)
polyphagia
    Acanthamoeba p.
polypharmacy
polyphonic
    p. wheeze
    p. wheezing
polyposis
    adenomatous colonic p.
    colonic p.
    familial adenomatous p.
    intestinal p.
    nasal p.
    small bowel intestinal p.
    p. syndrome
Poly-Pred Liquifilm
polyradiculoneuritis
    epidemic motor p.
polyradiculoneuropathy
    chronic inflammatory demyelinating p. (CIDP)
    chronic relapsing p.
    chronic unremitting p.
polyribose phosphate polysaccharide vaccine
polyribosylribitol phosphate (PRP)
polysaccharide (PS)
    anti-O-specific p.
    p. group-specific antigen
    meningococcal p.
    purified p.
polyserositis
    idiopathic p.
polysomnogram (PSG)
polysomnographic
polysomnography (PSG)
    ambulatory p.
polyspike discharge
polysplenia syndrome
Polysporin
    P. ointment
    P. Ophthalmic
    P. Topical
polystotic
Polytar shampoo
polytef
polythelia
polytherapy
polytrauma
polyunsaturate
polyunsaturated fatty acid (PUFA)

polyuria
polyuric phase
polyvalent
    antivenin (crotalidae) p.
Poly-Vi-Flor
polyvinyl chloride
polyvinylidene fluoride (PVDF)
polyvinylpyrrolidone
Poly-Vi-Sol
pommel
pomona
    Leptospira p.
Pompe glycogen storage disease (type I, II)
pompholyx
ponderal index (PI)
pond fracture
pons
Ponstel
Pontiac fever
pontile hypertrophy
pontis
    basis p.
Pontocaine
pontocerebellar hypoplasia
pontomedullary junction
pontosubicular neuron necrosis (PSN)
pool
    polymorphonuclear leukocyte storage p.
    vaginal p.
pooling
    dependent p.
    venous p.
poor
    p. adaptability
    p. attention span
    p. caloric intake
    p. capillary refill
    p. convergence
    p. coordination
    p. dental hygiene
    p. feeding
    p. feeding interaction
    p. head control
    p. linear growth
    p. motor planning
    p. muscle tone
    p. opsonization
    p. oral intake
    p. phagocytosis

NOTES

poor *(continued)*
    p. suck
    p. weight gain
pop
    Revital-Ice rehydrating freezer p.
popcorn
    p. formation
    p. metaphysis
Pope
    P. night splint
    P. Oto-wick
popliteal
    p. angle
    p. cyst
    p. space
pop-off valve
popping
    eye p.
    skin p.
popsicle
    p. injury
    p. panniculitis
population
poractant alfa
porcine
    p. surfactant
    p. valve
porencephalic
    p. cyst
    p. diverticulum
porencephaly
    central p.
    p. cortical dysplasia
pork
    P. NPH
    P. Regular Iletin II
    p. tapeworm
PORN
    progressive outer retinal necrosis
porokeratosis of Mibelli
porphyria
    acute intermittent p. (AIP)
    congenital erythropoietic p. (CEP)
    congenital photosensitive p.
    p. cutanea tarda
    cutaneous hepatic p.
    erythropoietic p.
    hepatic p.
    hepatoerythropoietic p. (HEP)
    intermittent p.
    mixed p.
    photosensitive p.
    p. variegata
    variegate p. (VP)
porphyrin
    stool p.
Porphyromonas
port

Port-A-Cath catheter
Portagen formula
Portage project
porta hepatis
portal
    p. fibrosis
    p. hypertension
    p. inflammation
    p. pyelophlebitis
    p. system
    p. vein obstruction (PVO)
    p. vein sepsis
    p. venous pressure
Porta-Lung noninvasive extrathoracic ventilator
Portland hemoglobin
portoaortal shunt
portocaval shunt
portoenterostomy
    Kasai p.
portosystemic shunt
port-wine
    p.-w. mark
    p.-w. nevus
    p.-w. stain
    p.-w. stained angioma
POS
    polycystic ovary syndrome
POSIT
    Problem-Oriented Screening Instrument for Teenagers
position
    Adam p.
    antigravity p.
    breech p.
    cock-robin p.
    equinus p.
    fencing p.
    four-point p.
    half-kneeling p.
    hands-feet p.
    intrauterine p.
    knee-chest p.
    kneel-stand p.
    left lateral decubitus p. (LLDP)
    neutral p.
    POE p.
    prone on elbows p.
    prone sleep p.
    puppy p.
    scissored p.
    scrotal p.
    semi-Fowler p.
    sleep p.
    sniffing p.
    supine sleep p.
    supranormal scrotal p.
    swimming p.

three-point p.
Trendelenburg p.
tripod p.
tripod-supporting p.
wearing p.
withdrawal p.
W sitting p.

positional
    p. airways obstruction
    p. clubfoot
    p. nystagmus

positioner
    head p.

positioning

positive
    p. airway pressure
    p. antinuclear antibody (ANA)
    Coombs p.
    p. distending pressure (PDP)
    p. end-expiratory pressure (PEEP)
    false p.
    polyarthritis, RF p.
    p. reinforcement
    p. support reflex

positive-pressure ventilation (PPV)

positron

positron-emission tomography (PET)

postalveolar cleft

postanginal sepsis

postanoxic dystonic syndrome

postasphyxial
    p. apoptosis
    p. cerebral edema
    p. change
    p. encephalopathy
    p. seizure

postauricular
    p. ecchymosis
    p. nerve

postaxial
    p. hexadactyly
    p. polydactyly

postchiasmal visual pathway

post cibum (after meals) (p.c.)

postcoartectomy syndrome

postcoital contraception

postconceptional age (PCA)

postconcussion syndrome

postconvulsive hemiparesis

postdiphtheritic neuropathy

postdose serum

postductal coarctation

postencephalitic parkinsonian picture

postenteritis arthritis

posterior
    p. chamber intraocular lens (PC-IOL)
    p. column sensory deficit
    p. cranial fossa
    p. embryotoxon
    p. fontanelle
    p. fossa anaplastic ependymoma
    p. fossa arachnoid cyst
    p. fossa arachnoiditis
    p. fossa hemorrhage
    p. fossa malformation, hemangiomas, arterial anomalies, coarctation of aorta and cardiac defects, eye abnormalities (PHACE)
    p. fossa malformation, hemangiomas, arterial anomalies, coarctation of the aorta and cardiac defects, eye abnormalities syndrome
    p. fossa tumor
    p. fourchette
    p. iliac crest
    p. knee capsulotomy
    p. lenticonus
    p. leukoencephalopathy syndrome
    p. nasal packing
    p. neural tube closure
    p. occipitoatlantal hypermobility (POAH)
    p. pharyngeal laceration
    p. pharyngeal pseudodiverticulum
    p. pharyngeal wall elevation
    p. rectal wall resection
    p. rhizotomy
    p. sagittal anorectoplasty
    p. segmental fixation instrumentation
    p. splenium
    p. superior iliac spine
    p. synechia
    p. talofibular ligament (PTFL)
    p. tibial pulse
    p. ureteral valve
    p. urethra
    p. urethral valve
    p. uveitis

Posterisan ointment

posteroanterior (PA)

NOTES

P

posterolateral
posteromedial
    p. articular depression
    p. bow
    p. bow of tibia
    p. tibial bowing
postexchange transfusion syndrome
postexposure
    p. prophylaxis (PEP)
    p. treatment (PET)
postextubation stridor
postganglionic acetylcholine release
postgastroenteritis malabsorption syndrome
posthemorrhagic
    p. hydrocephalus (PHH)
    p. ventricular dilation (PHVD)
    p. ventriculomegaly (PHVM)
posthepatic aplastic anemia
postherpetic neuralgia
postictal
    p. confusion
    p. depression
    p. lethargy
    p. paralysis
    p. period
    p. weakness
postinfectious
    p. abducens palsy
    p. arthritis
    p. cerebellitis
    p. encephalitis
    p. encephalomyelitis
    p. glomerulonephritis
    p. immune response
    p. nephritis
    p. secondary lactase deficiency
postinfluenza
    p. pneumonia
    p. vaccination encephalitis
postingestion
postirradiation myelopathy
post-kala azar dermal leishmaniasis (PKDL)
postlumbar puncture headache
postmature
    p. fetus
    p. infant
postmeasles encephalitis
postmenstrual
postmigrainous stroke hemiplegia
postmortem lividity
postnasal drip
postnatal
    p. age
    p. bacterial meningitis
    p. depression (PND)
    p. factor

    p. gonadotropin surge
    p. penicillin prophylaxis (PPP)
    p. septicemia
postnecrotic cirrhosis
postneonatal mortality
postoperative
    p. apnea
    p. sudden death
postpartum
postperfusion syndrome
postpericardiotomy syndrome (PPS)
postphlebitic syndrome (PPS)
postpolio syndrome
postprandial plasma cholecystokinin
postpubescent
postrabies vaccine encephalomyelitis
postrenal ARF
postrheumatic valve disease
postscabetic syndrome
poststeroid panniculitis
poststreptococcal glomerulonephritis
postsynaptic fiber
postthoracotomy pulmonary edema
posttranslational
    p. modification
    p. modification of mRNA
posttransplant
    p. lymphoproliferative disease (PTLD)
    p. lymphoproliferative disorder (PTLD)
posttraumatic
    p. amnesia
    p. epilepsy
    p. hyperemia
    p. signs or symptoms (PTSS)
    p. stress disorder (PTSD)
    p. stress syndrome
posttreatment
posttussive
    p. apnea
    p. emesis
postural
    p. drainage (PD)
    p. orthostatic tachycardia syndrome (POTS)
    p. proteinuria
    p. reaction
    p. reflex
    p. round-back
    p. scoliosis
posture
    bipedal p.
    extensor leg p.
    frogleg p.
    hemiparetic p.
    scissoring p.

surrender p.
waiter tip p.
posturing
athetotic p.
decerebrate p.
decorticate p.
dystonic p.
opisthotonic p.
transient dystonic p.
postvaccinal encephalopathy
postvagotomy dumping syndrome
postviral
p. encephalitis
p. pneumonia
p. subacute thyroiditis
postvoid residual
potable
Potasalan
potassium (K)
p. chloride (KCl)
p. chloride stain
clavulanate p.
extracellular plasma p.
p. hydroxide (KOH)
p. hydroxide preparation
p. iodide
P. Iodide Enseals
pemirolast p.
penicillin V p.
p. permanganate
p. supplement
ticarcillin and clavulanate p.
total body p. (TBK)
potassium-sparing diuretic
potbelly
potent
potential
auditory evoked p. (AEP)
brainstem auditory evoked p.
(BAEP)
brief, small, abundant motor-unit
action p. (BSAP)
event-related p. (ERP)
evoked p.
fibrillation p.
insertion p.
motor evoked p. (MEP)
p. renal solute load (PRSL)
somatosensory evoked p. (SSEP)
visual evoked p. (VEP)

POTS
postural orthostatic tachycardia syndrome
POTS syndrome
Pott
P. disease
P. puffy tumor
Potter
P. disease
P. facies
P. oligohydramnios sequence
P. phenotype
P. syndrome
Potts shunt
potty-train
potty-trained
potty-training
pouce flottant
pouch
branchial p.
cecal p.
colon p.
Morison p.
parasitized cecal p.
rectal p.
right colon p.
sigmoid p.
utriculovaginal p.
vulvovaginal p.
wallaby p.
pouchitis
Pourcelot index
poverty of content
povidone-iodine solution
Powassan encephalitis
powder
Casec p.
cocaine hydrochloride p.
Fiberall P.
fluticasone propionate inhalation p.
Polycose p.
salicylic sugar p.
salmeterol p.
talcum p.
Zeasorb p.
zinc stearate p.
powdered
p. casein
p. milk formula
power spectral analysis (PSA)
POWSBP
pulse oximetry waveform systolic blood
pressure measurement

NOTES

P

pox
Poxviridae family
PP
    precocious pubarche
PPB
    pleuropulmonary blastoma
PPD
    primary peritoneal drainage
    purified protein derivative
PPH
    persistent pulmonary hypertension
PPHN
    persistent pulmonary hypertension of
      newborn
PPI
    proton pump inhibitor
ppm
    parts per million
PPNET
    peripheral primitive neuroectodermal
      tumor
PPP
    platelet-poor plasma
    postnatal penicillin prophylaxis
PPROM
    preterm premature rupture of membranes
    prolonged premature rupture of
      membranes
PPS
    postpericardiotomy syndrome
    postphlebitic syndrome
PPSH
    pseudovaginal perineoscrotal hypospadias
PPV
    positive-pressure ventilation
PPVT
    Peabody Picture Vocabulary Test
PPVT-R
    Peabody Picture Vocabulary Test-
      Revised
p.r.
    per rectum
    by way of rectum
practice
    Advisory Committee on
      Immunization P.'s (ACIP)
    best p.
    P. Parameters for the Assessment
      and Treatment of Anxiety
      Disorders
practitioner
    general p.
    National Association of Pediatric
      Nurse Associates and P.'s
      (NAPNAP)
Prader
    P. bead

    P. gonadometer
    P. orchidometer
Prader-Labhart-Willi syndrome
Prader-Willi
    P.-W. syndrome (PWS)
    P.-W. syndrome critical region
      (PWSCR)
praecox
    familial lymphedema p.
    lymphedema p.
pragmatics
pragmatic and semantic-pragmatic
  deficits
pralidoxime
Pratt
    sigmoid pouch of P.
praxis
praziquantel
prazosin
PRBC
    packed red blood cell
preadolescent
prealbumin
PreAptamil
preauricular
    p. adenopathy
    p. nerve
    p. pit
    p. tag
precapillary
PreCare Conceive
Prechtl test
precipitate delivery
precipitous
    p. delivery
    p. labor
precise finger opposition
precocious
    p. pubarche (PP)
    p. puberty
precocity
    isosexual p.
    sexual p.
precordial
    p. bulge
    p. thump
precordium
    hyperdynamic p.
    quiet p.
    silent p.
precox
    pubertas p.
precursor
    cell p.
    neurotransmitter p.
Pred
    P. Forte Ophthalmic

Liquid P.
P. Mild Ophthalmic
Predalone 50 Injection
Pred-G
Predicort-50
predigested formula
predisposition
Prednicen-M
prednisolone
p. and gentamicin
neomycin, polymyxin B, p.
p. sodium
Prednisol TBA Injection
prednisone
cyclophosphamide, doxorubicin
(Adriamycin), Oncovin
(vincristine), p.
cyclophosphamide,
hydroxydaunorubicin,
methotrexate, p. (CHOP)
cyclophosphamide, Oncovin,
methotrexate, p. (COMP)
mechlorethamine, Oncovin,
procarbazine, p.
mechlorethamine, Oncovin
(vincristine), procarbazine, p.
(MOPP)
vincristine, actinomycin-D,
methotrexate, p. (VAMP)
predominance
predominant
lymphocyte p.
preductal coarctation
preeclampsia
preeclamptic state
**preejection period/left ventricular
ejection time (PEP/LVET)**
preemie
premature
preemie nipple
preexcitation syndrome
preference
hand p.
prefilled disposable bottle
Prefrin Ophthalmic Solution
prefrontal
Pregestimil formula
pregnancy
abdominal p.
acute fatty liver of p. (AFLP)
ectopic p.

hemolytic uremia syndrome
associated with p.
pruritic urticarial papules and
plaques of p. (PUPPP)
rhinitis of p.
toxemia of p.
**pregnancy-associated plasma protein A
(PAPP-A)**
pregnancy-induced hypertension (PIH)
Pregnyl
prehension
Prehn sign
Prehospital Index (PHI)
preicteric stage
preimplantation genetic diagnosis (PGD)
prekallikrein deficiency
preleukemic syndrome
prelingual deafness
**prelinguistic autism diagnostic
observation (PL-ADOS)**
preload
LV p.
ventricular p.
Prelone Oral
PREM
Prematurity Risk Evaluation Measure
PREM score
Premarin
Prematil formula
premature (preemie)
p. adrenarche
p. aging
p. atrial contraction (PAC)
p. closure
p. closure of coronal suture
p. infant
P. Infant Pain Profile (PIPP)
p. labor
p. lung
p. placental separation
pulmonary insufficiency of p.
p. rupture of membranes (PROM)
p. senility
p. thelarche
prematurity
anemia of p.
anetoderma of p.
apnea of p. (AOP)
high oxygen percentage in
retinopathy of p. (HOPE-ROP)
hypothyroxinemia of p. (HOP)
idiopathic apnea of p.

NOTES

P

457

prematurity *(continued)*
 pulmonary insufficiency of p.
 retinopathy of p. (ROP)
 P. Risk Evaluation Measure
  (PREM)
 P. Risk Evaluation Measure score
 spontaneous atrophic patch of p.
 Supplemental Therapeutic Oxygen
  for Prethreshold Retinopathy
  of P. (STOP-ROP)
premenarchal girl
premenstrual
 p. dysphoric disorder
 p. syndrome (PMS)
premethrin
**Premier Platinum HpSA enzyme
 immunoassay, The**
premutation
prenatal
 p. asphyxia
 p. cytomegalovirus
 p. diagnosis
 p. factor
 p. fibroelastosis
 p. growth retardation
 p. history
 p. hydronephrosis
 p. infection
 p. stroke
 p. surgery
 p. ultrasound
prenatally exposed to drugs (PED)
Prentif cavity-rim cap
prenylamine
preoperational stage
preorthognatic surgery manipulation
prep
 Tczank p.
preparation
 P. H
 hemorrhoidal p.
 improper formula p.
 LE cell p.
 potassium hydroxide p.
 sickle cell p.
**preparticipation sports examination
 (PSE)**
prepartum
prepatellar bursitis
Pre-Pen
prepenile testis
prepubertal
 p. depression
 p. mania
 p. periodontitis
 p. testicular tumor
prepubertal-onset bipolarity
prepubescent vagina

prepuce
pre-pulseless phase
preputial flap
prereading stage
prerenal
 p. ARF
 p. azotemia
 p. insufficiency
presacral fascia
preschool
**preschool-age psychiatric assessment
 (PAPA)**
preschooler
 Miller Assessment for P.'s
prescription (Rx)
preseizure state
presence
 family member p. (FMP)
present
 p. episode
 p. illness (PI)
presentation
 breech p.
 brow p.
 face p.
 fetal p.
 isomorphic p.
 nonisomorphic p.
 shoulder p.
 vertex p.
preseptal cellulitis
presinusoidal
 p. hypertension
 p. obstruction
preslip
 p. SCFE
pressure
 airway opening p. (P_{ao})
 airway transmural p.
 ambulatory blood p. (ABP)
 aortic blood p.
 arterial p.
 arterial blood p. (ABP)
 auto-positive end-expiratory p.
 bilevel positive airway p. (BiPAP)
 bladder p.
 blood p. (BP)
 p. of carbon dioxide (PCO_2)
 carotid sinus p.
 central venous p. (CVP)
 cerebral perfusion p. (CPP)
 constant positive airway p. (CPAP)
 continuous distending p. (CDP)
 continuous negative extrathoracic p.
  (CNEP)
 continuous positive airway p.
  (CPAP)

crying, requirement for oxygen supplementation, increases in heart rate and blood p.
diastolic arterial p. (DAP)
diastolic blood p.
distending p.
elevated intracranial p.
p. equalization (PE)
p. equalization tube (PET)
erratic blood p.
p., facial expression, sleeplessness
fetal hydrostatic p.
finger arterial blood p. (FABP)
p. gradient
high bladder p.
hydrostatic p.
increased intracranial p.
inspiratory p.
intracranial p. (ICP)
intraluminal p.
intraocular p. (IOP)
intravascular oncotic p.
left arterial p.
LES p.
p. load
p. mapping
mean airway p. (MAP)
mean aortic p.
mean arterial p. (MAP)
mean arterial blood p. (MABP)
mean left atrial p.
mean pulmonary artery p.
mean right atrial p.
nasal continuous positive airway p. (n-CPAP)
nasal prong continuous positive airway p. (NP-CPAP)
negative inspiratory p.
net ultrafiltration p.
normal blood p.
p. of CO_2 (PCO_2)
p. of O_2
oncotic p.
osmotic p. (Op)
p. of oxygen (PO_2)
PA p.
p. palsy
partial p.
peak end-expiratory p.
peak inspiratory p. (PIP)
plasma oncotic p.
p. point

portal venous p.
positive airway p.
positive distending p. (PDP)
positive end-expiratory p. (PEEP)
pulmonary artery occluded p. (PAOP)
pulmonary artery wedge p.
pulmonary capillary wedge p. (PCWP)
right atrial p.
p. support mode
systolic arterial p. (SAP)
systolic blood p.
p. transducer
transpulmonary p.
p. urticaria
venous p.
wide pulse p.
zero end-expiratory p.
pressured speech
presternal edema
PreSun
presyncope
presystolic
    p. murmur
    p. thrill
preterm
    p. delivery
    p. formula
    p. infant
    p. premature rupture of membranes (PPROM)
    p. spontaneous rupture of membranes (PSROM)
prethickened formula
pretibial skin dimple
Pretz
prevaccination
Prevacid
prevalence
Prevalite
Preven
prevention
    Centers for Disease Control and P.
preventive
    p. allergy treatment (PAT)
    p. antibiotic
Preveon
previa
    placenta p.
Prevident
Prevnar pneumococcal vaccine

NOTES

P

459

Prevotella multocida
priapism
    idiopathy p.
prickly heat
prick test
prilocaine
    lidocaine and p.
Prilosec
Primacor
primaquine phosphate
primary
    p. acquired urticaria
    p. adrenal insufficiency
    p. amebic meningoencephalitis
    p. amenorrhea
    p. anastomosis
    p. angiitis of CNS (PACNS)
    p. antiphospholipid antibody
      syndrome
    p. aqueductal stenosis
    p. atelectasis
    p. bile acid malabsorption
    p. biliary cirrhosis (PBC)
    p. bullous disorder
    p. cardiac arrhythmia
    p. caregiver
    p. caretaker
    p. carnitine deficiency
    p. central nervous system
      lymphoma (PCNSL)
    p. chondrodystrophy
    p. ciliary dyskinesia (PCD)
    p. circular reaction
    p. cleft palate repair
    p. closure
    p. congenital glaucoma
    p. craniosynostosis
    p. dentition
    p. dysmenorrhea
    p. dystonia
    p. EFE
    p. generalized epilepsy
    p. generalized seizure
    p. headache
    p. hepatocellular carcinoma (PHC)
    p. herpetic gingivostomatitis
    p. hyperoxaluria
    p. hyperoxaluria type 1 (PH-1)
    p. hypersomnia
    p. hypoalphalipoproteinemia
    p. hypochondriasis
    p. hypomagnesemia
    p. hypophosphatemic rickets
    p. hypothyroidism
    p. immune deficiency (PID)
    p. immunodeficiency
    p. infection
    p. insomnia
    p. intraocular tumor
    p. lactic acidosis
    p. lactose intolerance
    p. lung bud formation
    p. lymphedema
    p. macrodactyly
    p. macular atrophy
    p. megalencephaly
    p. microcephaly
    p. molar
    p. nasal mastocytosis
    p. nephrotic syndrome
    p. neuraminidase deficiency
    p. nocturnal enuresis
    p. oxalosis
    p. PAP
    p. peritoneal drainage (PPD)
    p. peritonitis
    p. polycythemia
    p. polydipsia
    p. prophylaxis
    p. pulmonary hemosiderosis
    p. pulmonary tuberculosis
    p. repair of esophageal atresia
    p. sclerosing cholangitis
    p. snoring
    p. syphilis
    p. teeth
    p. testicular failure
    p. tracheal tumor
    p. tracheomalacia
    p. vesicoureteral reflux
    p. writing tremor
    p. xanthomatosis
Primatene Mist
Primaxin
Primedic-Mobicard-type ECG instrument
primidone
primigravida
priming
    p. dose
    gastrointestinal p.
primitive
    p. lipoblastoma
    p. neuroectodermal tumor (PNET)
    p. neuroectodermal
      tumor/medulloblastoma (PNET/MB)
    p. reflex
    p. reflex pattern
primordial
    p. cephalization
    p. follicle
primordium, pl. **primordia**
    choroid plexus primordia
    esophagotracheal p.
primrose
Primsol solution

primum
    foramen p.
    ostium p.
    septum p.
Principen
principle
    Fick p.
    Fontan p.
Prinivil
PR interval
prion disease
priority
Priscoline
PRISM
    Pediatric Risk of Mortality Score
prism
    optical p.
Privine Nasal
p.r.n.
    pro re nata (as the occasion arises)
proaccelerin
proanthocyanidin
Probalan
proband
Pro-Banthine
probe
    dedicated Doppler p.
    DNA p.
    Doppler p.
    in-line p.
    linear p.
    nucleic acid p.
    Ohmeda SoftProbe p.
    pH p.
    phased array p.
probenecid
probiotic
problem
    attention-distractibility p.
    chronic behavior p.
    feeding p.
    internalizing p.
    occlusal p.
    sensory p.
    p. solving
    speech p.
    V code rational p.'s
Problem-Oriented Screening Instrument for Teenagers (POSIT)
Probst
    bundle of P.
procainamide

procaine
    p. penicillin
    penicillin G p.
    p. penicillin G
procalcitonin (PCT)
    cerebrospinal fluid p.
    serum p.
Pro-Cal-Sof
procarbazine
Procardia XL
procaterol
procedural sedation and analgesia (PSA)
procedure (*See also* operation)
    antegrade continence enema p.
    anterior cricoid split p.
    arterial switch p.
    atrial inversion p.
    atrial septoplasty p.
    atrial septostomy p.
    atrial switch p.
    bidirectional Glenn p.
    Bishop-Koop p.
    Blalock-Hanlon atrial septostomy p.
    Blalock-Taussig shunt p.
    Boix-Ochoa p.
    bowel lengthening p.
    Chiari p.
    Cohen p.
    cricoid split p.
    cyclodestructive p.
    Damus-Kaye-Stansel p.
    Delorme p.
    diagnostic p.
    diverting colostomy with pull-through p.
    double-switch p.
    drainage p.
    Duhamel p.
    enema p.
    fetal surgical p.
    Fontan p.
    GITUP p.
    glans-cavernosal p.
    heel-stick p.
    Hegman p.
    hemi-Fontan p.
    Heyman-Herndon clubfoot p.
    Hoffer p.
    Ilizarov limb-lengthening p.
    Jatene arterial switch p.
    Jones p.

NOTES

P

procedure *(continued)*
    Kasai p.
    Kimura p.
    Koyanagi p.
    Ladd p.
    MacIndoe p.
    Magpi p.
    Mantel-Haenszel p.
    Mikulicz p.
    mini-Pena p.
    modified Fontan p.
    Mustard atrial switch p.
    Mustardé p.
    neobladder diversion p.
    Norwood p.
    palliative p.
    Pemberton p.
    Pena p.
    pull-through p.
    Rashkind atrial septostomy p.
    Rastelli p.
    Ravitch p.
    Ross p.
    Rotazyme diagnostic p.
    Salter p.
    Senning atrial switch p.
    Seton p.
    Soave p.
    split p.
    Steele p.
    Sting p.
    Sugiura p.
    surgical p.
    Sutherland p.
    Swenson p.
    three-stage Norwood-Fontan p.
    Tompkins p.
    Tonnis p.
    Torkildsen p.
    van Ness p.
    ventricular shunt p.
    Waterston-Cooley p.
    Waterston shunt p.
    Whipple p.
    Winter glans-cavernosal p.
process
    acromion p.
    antenatal disease p.
    attaching p.
    cleft premaxillary p.
    grieving p.
    inflammatory p.
    latching-on p.
    lateralization p.
    mastoid p.
    microangiopathic p.
    neuritic cytoplasmic p.
    odontoid p.

    short p.
    tapering cytoplasmic p.
processing
    slow cognitive p.
    visuoperceptual/simultaneous
      information p.
process-oriented measure
processus vaginalis
prochlorperazine
procoagulant protein
procollagen
    carboxyterminal propeptide of type
      1 p. (PICP)
    serum type III p.
proconvertin
Procrit
Procter and Gamble (P&G)
proctitis
    HSV2 p.
Proctocort Rectal
Proctofoam
proctography
    evacuation p.
proctoscopy
proctosigmoidoscopy
procyonis
    Baylisascaris p.
Prodium
prodromal
    p. illness
    p. symptom
prodrome, prodroma, pl. **prodromata**
    viral p.
product
    advanced oxidation protein p.
      (AOPP)
    fibrin degradation p.
    fibrinogen degradation p. (FDP)
    fibrinogen fibrin degradation p.
    fibrinogen split p.
    fibrin split p. (FSP)
    unpasteurized milk p.
production
    ketone p.
    speech p.
    in vitro antibody p. (IVAP)
productivity
Profasi HP
Profiber formula
proficiency
    Bruininks-Oseretsky Test of
      Motor P.
profilaggrin
Profilate-HP
profile
    acylcarnitine p.
    Alpern-Boll Developmental P.
    anatomic p. (AP)

biophysical p. (BPP)
fatty acid p.
Hawaii Early Learning P. (HELP)
neuropsychological p.
Premature Infant Pain P. (PIPP)
rectilinear p.
torsional p.
Profile-II
Developmental P.-II (DP-II)
Profilnine Heat-Treated
profound mental retardation
profunda
tinea p.
profundus
lupus erythematosus p.
profusa
lentiginosis p.
profusion
placental p.
progenitor
erythroid p.
progeria
adult p.
p. syndrome
progeroid facies
Progestasert
progesterone
progestin-only
p.-o. contraceptive
p.-o. pill
Proglycem Oral
prognathism
mandibular p.
prognosis
Prograf
program
Bridge Reading P.
Children's Health Insurance P.
(CHIP)
chronic hypertransfusion p.
Early Childhood Special
Education P.
early intervention p. (EIP)
Early and Periodic Screening,
Diagnosis, and Treatment p.
Epidemiologic Catchment P.
Individualized Education P. (IEP)
infant development p.
infant stimulation p.
Lovaas p.
Merrill p.

New England Regional Infant
Cardiac P. (NERICP)
Office of Special Education P.'s
(OSEP)
Pharsight Trial Designer
simulation p.
residential p.
Special Supplemental Nutrition P.
SRA Basic Reading P.
State Children's Health
Insurance P. (SCHIP)
The Injury Prevention P. (TIPP)
universal newborn hearing
screening p. (UNHSP)
Women, Infants, and Children P.
(WIC)
progressiva
fibrodysplasia ossificans p. (FOP)
myositis ossificans p.
progressive
p. biliary cirrhosis
p. bulbar palsy
p. bulbar palsy with epilepsy
p. bulbar paralysis of childhood
p. central nervous system failure
p. deforming osteogenesis
imperfecta
p. encephalitis
p. encephalopathy
p. external ophthalmoplegia (PEO)
p. facial hemiatrophy
p. familial intrahepatic cholestasis
(PFIC)
p. granuloma
p. hydronephrosis
p. labyrinthitis
p. multifocal leukoencephalopathy
(PML)
p. myoclonic epilepsy
p. obesity
p. obliterative cholangiopathy
p. outer retinal necrosis (PORN)
p. primary pulmonary tuberculosis
p. renal failure
p. rubella panencephalitis
proguanil hydrochloride
ProHIBIT vaccine
prohormone
proinflammatory cytokine
project
Fort Bragg evaluation p. (FBEP)
Portage p.

NOTES

P

463

project *(continued)*
    P. TEACCH
    P. Treatment and Education of
      Autistic and Related
      Communication-Handicapped
projectile vomiting
projection
    bony p.
    red cell spiny p.
projective assessment
prokaryotic reaction
Prokine
prokinetic agent
prolactin
    serum p.
prolactinoma
Prolamine
prolapse
    aortic cusp p.
    complete rectal p.
    concealed rectal p.
    cord p.
    p. gastropathy syndrome (PGS)
    incomplete rectal p.
    mitral valve p. (MVP)
    rectal p.
    urethral p.
    valve p.
prolapsed
    p. cord
    p. ectopic ureterocele
prolapsing
    p. apex
    p. apex of intussusception
    p. polyp
prolidase deficiency
proliferating hemangioma
proliferation
    epithelial cell p.
    mesangial cell p.
proliferative
    p. glomerulonephritis
    p. lesion
    p. lupus nephritis
    p. retinitis
    p. vasculopathy
    p. zone (PZ)
proline hydroxyproline
prolongation
    QTc p.
prolonged
    p. bradycardia
    p. capillary refill
    p. EEG monitoring
    p. expiratory phase
    p. indirect hyperbilirubinemia
    p. jaundice
    p. partial asphyxia

    p. premature rupture of membranes
      (PPROM)
    p. QT interval
    p. QT interval syndrome
    p. regard
    p. rupture of membranes
    p. unconjugated hyperbilirubinemia
Proloprim
PROM
    premature rupture of membranes
promax rotation
Prometa
Prometh
    P. Injection
    P. VC Plain Liquid
promethazine
    p. hydrochloride
    p. and phenylephrine
    p., phenylephrine, codeine
    P. VC Plain Syrup
    P. VC Syrup
Promil formula
prominence
    calcaneal p.
prominent
    p. ear
    p. heart sound
    p. mandible
    p. maxillary incisor
    p. nose
    p. skin discoloration
    p. skin discoloration of coast of
      Maine
Pro-Mix formula
ProMod formula
promoter
    chicken ovalbumin upstream p.
      (COUP)
Promote with Fiber formula
prompt
promyelocyte cell
promyelocytic leukemia
pronate
pronated foot
pronation
pronator sign
prone
    p. board
    p. extension test
    p. on elbows (POE)
    p. on elbows position
    p. pivoting
    p. sleep position
    p. stander
pronephros
Pronestyl
Pronestyl-SR

prong
  binasal p.'s
  Hudson p.'s
  n-CPAP p.'s
pronormoblast cell
PROP
  propranolol
Propacet
Propac formula
Propadrine
propagation
Propagest
propamidine
propantheline
Propaq Encore vital signs monitor
proparacaine
propeptide
  carboxyterminal p.
properdin
  p. deficiency
  p. factor B
property, pl. **properties**
  teratogenic properties
prophylactic
  p. antibiotic
  p. therapy
  p. treatment
prophylaxis
  antibiotic p.
  antimicrobial p.
  Credé p.
  drug p.
  intrapartum antibiotic p. (IAP)
  postexposure p. (PEP)
  postnatal penicillin p. (PPP)
  primary p.
  rabies p.
  secondary p.
  tetanus p.
  trimethoprim-sulfamethoxazole p.
Propine
propionate
  beclomethasone p.
  clobetasol p.
  fluticasone p.
Propionibacterium
  P. acnes
  P. propionicus
propionic acidemia
propionicus
  Propionibacterium p.

propionyl CoA carboxylase deficiency
Proplex SX-T
Proplex T
propofol
propoxyphene and acetaminophen
propping
  bottle p.
  p. reflex
2-propranol
propranolol (PROP)
  p. hydrochloride
propria
  lamina p.
  substantia p.
proprioception
proprioceptive
  p. input
  p. sensation
proprioceptor
  muscle p.
proptosis
Propulsid
propulsion
  decreased p.
propylene glycol
propylthiouracil
pro re nata (as the occasion arises) (p.r.n.)
Prorex Injection
prosencephalon
ProSobee formula
prosocial behavior scale
prosodic pattern
prosody
Pro-Sof Plus
prostacyclin
  nebulized p.
prostacyclin-stimulating factor (PSF)
prostaglandin
  p. D_2
  p. E
  p. E_1
  p. endoperoxide synthase
  p. F
  p. I_2
  serum p.
Prostaphlin
prostate
  absent p.
  high-riding p.
  hypoplastic p.

NOTES

P

prosthesis
  NeuroCybernetic p.
  ocular p.
prosthetic
  p. attachment
  p. graft implantation
  p. patch aortoplasty
prosthodontist
Prostigmin
Prostin VR
protamine sulfate
protease
  p. inhibitor (PI, Pi)
  p. inhibitor-induced lipodystrophy
  p. inhibitor type
protease-3
  neutrophil p.-3
ProtectaCap cap
protection
  p. and advocacy (P & A)
  airway p.
protective
  p. colostomy
  p. extension
  p. protein
  p. service agency
protein
  accessory p.
  agouti p.
  bactericidal/permeability-increasing p. (BPI)
  bcl-2 p.
  Bence Jones p.
  p. binding
  binding p.
  p. C
  cartilage oligomeric matrix p. (COMP)
  p. C coagulation inhibitor
  p. C concentrate
  chimeric p.
  Clara cell 16 p.
  congenital absence of iron-binding p.
  cow's milk p.
  C-reactive p. (CRP)
  p. C, S deficiency
  cystic fibrosis transmembrane conductance regulator p.
  deficiency of C4-binding p.
  Ensure High P.
  eosinophilic cationic p. (ECP)
  FK binding p. (FKBP)
  fragile X mental retardation p. (FMRP)
  G p.
  glial fibrillary acidic p. (GFAP)

gp120 viral p.
growth hormone-binding p. (GHBP)
H p.
p. hydrolysate
p. hydrolysate formula
hydrolyzed p.
insulinlike growth factor-binding p. (IGFBP)
p. intolerance
iron-binding p.
p. kinase C
LIM1 p.
p. loss
macrophage inflammatory p. (MIP)
major basic p. (MBP)
p. maxima
membrane p.
methyl-CpG-binding p. 2 (MeCP2)
p. minima
mucopolysaccharide p.
outer surface p. (Osp)
outer surface p. A (OspA)
P p.
peripheral myelin p. (PMP)
plasma p.
pregnancy-associated plasma p. A (PAPP-A)
procoagulant p.
protective p.
proteolipid p. (PLP)
pulmonary surfactant p.
purified fusion p. (PFP)
recombinant outer surface p. A (rOspA)
retinol-binding p.
p. S
p. S antithrombin
p. S coagulation inhibitor
steroidogenic acute regulatory p. (StAR)
T p.
thrombus precursor p.
thyroid-specific enhancer binding p. (T4/ebp-1)
urinary excretion of p. (UEP)
protein-1
  sphingolipid activator p.-1 (SAP1)
protein-3
  insulinlike growth factor-binding p.-3 (IGFBP-3)
protein-A
  surfactant p.-A (SP-A)
proteinaceous subretinal fluid
proteinase
  p. factor
  p. K
  serine p.

protein-B
plasma surfactant p.-B
surfactant p.-B (SP-B)
protein-C
surfactant p.-C (SP-C)
protein-calorie malnutrition
protein-conjugated vaccine
protein-energy malnutrition
protein-induced
p.-i. eosinophilic colitis (PEC)
p.-i. vitamin K absence (PIVKA)
protein-losing enteropathy
proteinosis
alveolar p.
congenital alveolar p.
lipoid p.
pulmonary alveolar p. (PAP)
protein-sparing
p.-s. modified fast (PSMF)
p.-s. modified fast diet
proteinuria
glomerular p.
idiopathic low molecular weight p.
LMW p.
low molecular weight p.
orthostatic p.
overflow p.
postural p.
renal p.
selective p.
treatment-resistant p.
tubular p.
proteinuric
proteobacteria
alpha p.
proteolipid protein (PLP)
proteolysis
cellular p.
Proteus
P. mirabilis
P. syndrome
P. syndrome myopathy
Prothazine-DC
prothrombic tendency
prothrombin
p. gene mutation
p. time (pro-time, PT)
p. time coagulation test
prothrombokinase
Protilase
pro-time
prothrombin time

protirelin
protocol
ACTG 076, 316 p.
AIDS Clinical Trials Group p.
chemotherapy p.
MOPP chemotherapy p.
Reese Clark p.
wean-and-feed p.
protocoproporphyria
protodiastolic gallop
protodyssomnia
proton
p. MRS
p. MR spectroscopy
p. pump antagonist
p. pump inhibitor (PPI)
protooncogene
Protopam
Protopic
protoporphyria
erythrohepatic p.
erythropoietic p. (EPP)
protoporphyrin
free erythrocyte p. (FEP)
tin p. (SnPP)
protoporphyrin/heme
zinc p./h. (ZPP/H)
Protozoa
protracted
p. depressive episode
p. diarrhea
p. diarrhea of infancy
protraction
Protropin Injection
protruding tongue
protrusio acetabuli
protrusion
reduction of p.
protuberant step deformity
Proventil HFA
Provera Oral
provisional calcification
provocation
bronchial p.
epinephrine p.
mucous membrane p.
p. test
provocative bronchial challenge testing
prowazekii
Rickettsia p.
proxetil
cefpodoxime p.

NOTES

Proxigel Oral
proximal
- p. bowel
- p. convoluted tubule
- p. enterostomy
- p. femoral epiphysis
- p. focal femoral deficiency
- p. humeral derotation osteotomy
- p. humeral stress fracture
- p. hypospadias
- p. jejunum
- p. pattern weakness
- p. pulmonary artery
- p. pulmonary artery banding
- p. row carpectomy
- p. RTA
- p. splenorenal shunt
- p. tibial epiphysis
- p. transverse septum
- p. tubulopathy
- p. white subungual onychomycosis

proxy
- factitious disorder by p. (FDP)
- Münchausen disease by p.
- Münchausen syndrome by p. (MSBP, MSP)
- Victa Ludorum by p.

Prozac
PRP
- pityriasis rubra pilaris
- platelet-rich plasma
- polyribosylribitol phosphate

PRPP
- 5-phospho-alpha-d-ribosyl pyrophosphate
- PRPP synthetase superactivity

PRSL
- potential renal solute load

PRSP
- penicillin-resistant *Staphylococcus* pneumonia
- penicillin-resistant *Streptococcus pneumoniae*

prune belly
prune-belly syndrome
pruning
- synaptic p.

prurigo
- actinic p.

pruritic
- p. rash
- p. urticarial papules and plaques of pregnancy (PUPPP)
- p. vesiculopapular eruption

pruritus
- anal p.
- p. ani
- perianal p.

Prussian blue

PS
- pancreas sufficient
- phytosterol
- polysaccharide
- pulmonic stenosis

PSA
- power spectral analysis
- procedural sedation and analgesia

PSC
- Pediatric Symptom Checklist

PSD
- Pediatric Spectrum of Disease

PSE
- preparticipation sports examination
- Lactulose PSE

Pseudallescheria boydii
pseudarthrosis
- congenital p.

pseudoacanthosis nigricans
pseudoachondroplasia
- p. syndrome

pseudoaddiction
pseudoappendicitis
pseudoappendicular syndrome
pseudoarthrosis
- congenital p.
- p. of tibia
- tibial p.

pseudoautomony
pseudoautosome
pseudobulbar palsy
pseudocholinesterase deficiency
pseudochylous milky fluid
pseudocoagulopathy
pseudocoloboma
- macular p.

pseudocyesis
pseudocyst
- pancreatic p.

pseudodiverticulum
- posterior pharyngeal p.

pseudoencapsulated lesion
pseudoephedrine
- carbinoxamine and p.
- triprolidine and p.

pseudoepitheliomatous hyperplasia
pseudoesotropia
pseudoexstrophy
pseudo-genu varum
pseudoglandular
- p. stage
- p. stage of lung development
- p. synovial sarcoma

pseudogynecomastia
pseudohermaphroditism
- female p.
- male p. (MPH)

pseudo-Hurler
    p.-H. deformity
    p.-H. polydystrophy
    p.-H. syndrome
pseudohypertrophic muscular dystrophy
pseudohypertrophy
pseudohypha
    nonbranching p.
pseudohypoaldosteronism
pseudohyponatremia
pseudohypoparathyroidism (type I, Ia, II)
pseudohypopyon
pseudoinfarction
pseudointestinal obstruction
pseudo-Köbner phenomenon
pseudolithiasis
    reversible biliary p.
pseudolobular cirrhosis
pseudomallei
    Burkholderia p.
    Pseudomonas p.
pseudomembrane
    adherent p.
pseudomembranous
    p. colitis
    p. conjunctivitis
Pseudomonas
    P. aeruginosa
    P. cepacia
    P. fluorescens
    P. pseudomallei
    P. septic arthritis
pseudoobstruction
    chronic intestinal p.
    intestinal p.
pseudopapilledema
pseudoparalysis of Parrot
pseudoperoxidation
    iron-catalyzed p.
pseudophedrine
pseudopili annulati
pseudoporencephalic cyst
pseudoporphyria
pseudopuberty
pseudorabies
pseudoreaction
pseudoscleroderma
pseudosclerosis
pseudoscurvy
pseudoseizure
pseudostrabismus

pseudosubluxation
pseudothalidomide syndrome
pseudotropicalis
    Candida p.
pseudotruncus
pseudotuberculosis
    Yersinia p.
pseudotumor
    p. cerebri
    inflammatory p. (IPT)
    retinal p.
pseudo-Turner syndrome
pseudovaginal perineoscrotal hypospadias (PPSH)
pseudovertigo
pseudo-von Willebrand disease
pseudo-Wernicke syndrome
pseudoxanthoma elasticum
PSF
    prostacyclin-stimulating factor
PSG
    polysomnogram
    polysomnography
PSI
    Parental Stress Index
    Parenting Stress Index
    Physiologic Stability Index
psittaci
    Chlamydia p.
psittacosis
PSMF
    protein-sparing modified fast
    PSMF diet
PSN
    pontosubicular neuron necrosis
psoas
    p. abscess
    p. margin
    p. sign
psoralen and ultraviolet A phototherapy
Psorcon
psoriasiform lesion
psoriasis
    classic plaque p.
    generalized pustular p.
    guttate p.
    plaque-type p.
    p. vulgaris
    vulvar p.
psoriasis-associated arthritis
psoriatic
    p. arthritis

NOTES

P

psoriatic (*continued*)
    p. dermatitis
    p. diaper rash
PsoriGel
Psorion Topical
PSROM
    preterm spontaneous rupture of
      membranes
PSS
    physiologic salt solution
P&S Shampoo
PSU
    pediatric sedation unit
psychedelic drug
psychiatric diagnostic interview (PDI)
psychiatrist
    child and adolescent p.
psychiatry
    American Academy of Child and
      Adolescent P. (AACAP)
    child and adolescent forensic p.
psychodynamic
    p. psychotherapy
    p. therapy
psychogenic
    p. arthralgia
    p. cough
    p. cough tic
    p. limp
    p. pain
    p. polydipsia
    p. seizure
psychological comorbidity
psychologic nonneuropathic bladder
psychologist
psychometric test
psychometrist
psychomotor
    p. development index (PDI)
    p. epilepsy
    p. retardation
    p. seizure
    p. status
psychopathology
    offspring p.
psychopharmacogenetic
psychopharmacological intervention
psychopharmacology
psychoses (*pl. of* psychosis)
psychosexual dysfunction
psychosine
psychosis, pl. **psychoses**
    brief reactive p.
    reactive p.
    symbiotic p.
psychosocial
    p. development
    p. dwarfism

psychosomatic complaint
psychostimulant medication
psychotherapy
    cognitive-behavioral p.
    nondirective supportive p.
    psychodynamic p.
    supportive p.
psychotic depression
psychotropic drug (PTD)
psyllium
PT
    pertussis toxin
    pertussis toxoid
    physical therapy
    prothrombin time
      PT coagulation test
PTA
    pure-tone average
PTC
    pulmonary tissue concentration
PTCRA
    percutaneous transluminal coronary
      rotational ablation
PTD
    psychotropic drug
P.T.E.-4, -5
pteridine ring compound
pterin
    synthetic p.
    urinary p.
pteroylglutamic acid
pterygium coli
pterygoid ulcer
PTFL
    posterior talofibular ligament
PTH
    parathyroid hormone
PTH-derived peptide
Pthirus pubis
PTLD
    posttransplant lymphoproliferative
      disease
    posttransplant lymphoproliferative
      disorder
ptosis, pl. **ptoses**
    bilateral congenital p.
    Marcus Gunn jaw-winking p.
    unilateral congenital p.
    upside-down p.
PTS
    Pediatric Trauma Score
PTSD
    posttraumatic stress disorder
PTSS
    posttraumatic signs or symptoms
PTT
    partial thromboplastin time

PTX
 pneumothorax
pubarche
 precocious p. (PP)
pubertal
 p. arrest
 p. delay
 p. gynecomastia
pubertas precox
puberty
 central precocious p. (CPP)
 delayed p.
 familial male precocious p.
 idiopathic precocious p.
 isosexual precocious p.
 peripheral precocious p.
 physiologic delay of p.
 precocious p.
pubescent
pubic
 p. louse
 p. ramus stress fracture
 p. tubercle
pubis
 mons p.
 osteitis p.
 pediculosis p.
 Pthirus p.
 symphysis p.
 widened symphysis p.
public
 p. health nurse (PHN)
 P. Law 93-247
 P. Law 94-142
 P. Law 99-457
 P. Law 101-336
puborectalis sling
PUBS
 percutaneous umbilical blood sampling
PUD
 peptic ulcer disease
puddle sign
pudendal neurogram
puerorum
 hydroa p.
puerperium
PUFA
 polyunsaturated fatty acid
puffiness
 periorbital p.
puff-of-smoke disease
puffy skin

pullback
 catheter p.
pull-down
 testicular p.-d.
pulled elbow
pulling
 hair p.
pull-through
 endorectal p.-t.
 ileoanal p.-t.
 p.-t. procedure
 retrorectal transanal p.-t.
 p.-t. surgery
 p.-t. technique
pull-up
 gastric p.-u.
Pulmicort
 P. Respules
 P. Turbuhaler
Pulmo-Aide
 P.-A. nebulizer
 P.-A. ventilator
Pulmocare formula
PulmoMate nebulizer
pulmonale
 cor p.
pulmonary
 p. acinar aplasia
 p. alveolar microlithiasis
 p. alveolar proteinosis (PAP)
 p. alveolus
 p. arterial banding
 p. arterial flow
 p. arterial oxygen content
 p. arterial trunk
 p. arteriogram
 p. arteriole
 p. arteriovenous malformation
  (PAVM)
 p. artery (PA)
 p. artery angioplasty
 p. artery atresia
 p. artery banding
 p. artery occluded pressure (PAOP)
 p. artery pressure monitoring
 p. artery sling
 p. artery wedge pressure
 p. ascariasis
 p. aspiration
 p. atresia with intact ventricular
  septum (PAIVS)
 p. bleb

NOTES

P

pulmonary *(continued)*
  p. blood flow
  p. bud
  p. capillary wedge pressure (PCWP)
  p. compliance
  p. cryptococcosis
  p. cyanosis
  p. dysplasia
  p. edema
  p. ejection click
  p. ELF
  p. embolism (PE)
  p. embolus
  p. eosinophilia
  p. fat embolism
  p. function
  p. function test (PFT)
  p. function testing
  p. hemangiomatosis
  p. hemorrhage
  p. hemosiderosis
  p. histoplasmosis
  p. hypertension
  p. hypertension of newborn
  p. hypoplasia
  p. immaturity
  p. infarction
  p. infiltrate
  p. infiltrate with eosinophilia (PIE)
  p. infiltrate with eosinophilia syndrome
  p. insufficiency
  p. insufficiency of premature
  p. insufficiency of prematurity
  p. interstitial emphysema (PIE)
  p. interstitial fibrosis
  p. lavage
  p. leukostasis
  p. lymphangiectasia
  p. lymphoid hyperplasia (PLH)
  p. medicine
  p. mucormycosis
  p. murmur
  p. overcirculation
  p. parenchymal disease
  p. perfusion
  p. porcine valve
  p. sequestration
  p. shunt
  p. sound
  p. stenosis
  p. suppuration
  p. surfactant
  p. surfactant protein
  p. thermodilution catheter
  p. tissue concentration (PTC)
  p. toilet
  p. tuberculosis
  p. tularemia
  p. undervascularity
  p. valve stenosis
  p. vascular congestion
  p. vascular development
  p. vascular marking
  p. vascular resistance (PVR)
  p. vascular tone
  p. vasodilation
  p. vein
  p. venoocclusive disease
  p. venous obstruction
  p. venous oxygen content
  p. venous return
  p. ventilation
pulmonic
  p. murmur
  p. stenosis (PS)
  p. valve
pulmonicola
  Pandoraea p.
Pulmozyme
pulp
  digital p.
  p. necrosis
pulpal degeneration
pulpectomy
pulsatile
  p. air jet
  p. fontanelle
pulsatility index
pulsating exophthalmos
pulse
  apical p.
  bounding p.
  p. dexamethasone
  dorsalis pedis p.
  p. interval
  jugular venous p.
  p. methylprednisolone
  p. oximeter
  p. oximeter sensor N-25 and I-20
  p. oximetry
  p. oximetry waveform systolic blood pressure measurement (POWSBP)
  paradoxical p.
  pedal p.
  posterior tibial p.
  p. steroid therapy
  thready p.
  p. width
pulsed
  p. field gel electrophoresis (PFGE)
  p. intervention
  p. ultrasound
  p. wave Doppler

pulseless
  p. disease
  p. phase
pulsion theory
pulsus
  p. alternans
  p. bisferiens
  p. paradoxus
pulvinar
Pulvule
  Ilosone P.'s
  Seromycin P.'s
pump
  infusion p.
  Kangaroo enteral feeding p.
  Lactina Select breast p.
  low-pressure breast p.
  MasterFlex fetal perfusion p.
  Medela breast p.
  Na⁺ p.
  pneumocapillary infusion p.
  Pump In Style breast p.
punched-out lytic lesion
punctata
  chondrodysplasia p.
  dysplasia epiphysealis p.
  rhizomelic chondrodysplasia p.
    (RCDP)
punctate
  p. epiphyseal dysplasia
  p. epithelial keratitis
  p. hyperkeratosis
  p. lenticular opacity
  recessive X-linked
    chondrodysplasia p.
  p. wheal
puncture
  bone marrow p.
  cisternal p.
  lumbar p. (LP)
  pericardial p.
  subdural p.
  transparenchymal needle p.
  ventricular p.
pupil
  Adie p.
  Argyll Robertson p.
  cat's eye p.
  conjugate p.
  p.'s equal, round, reactive to light
    and accommodation (PERRLA)
  keyhole p.

  Marcus Gunn p.
  p. reaction
  white p.
pupillae
  ectopia lentis et p.
pupillary
  p. change
  p. membrane
  p. syndrome
puppetlike appearance
PUPPP
  pruritic urticarial papules and plaques of
    pregnancy
puppy position
pure
  p. bulbar poliomyelitis
  p. esophageal atresia
  p. red cell aplasia
pureed diet
Puregon
purely sensory polyneuritis
pure-tone average (PTA)
Purge
purging
purified
  p. chick embryo cell culture
    (PCEC)
  p. chick embryo cell culture
    vaccine
  p. fusion protein (PFP)
  p. fusion protein vaccine
  p. gamma globulin
  p. podophyllotoxin
  p. polysaccharide
  p. protein derivative (PPD)
purine
  p. metabolism
  p. nucleoside phosphorylase (PNP)
  p. nucleoside phosphorylase
    deficiency
Purinethol
Purkinje
  P. cell
  P. cell tumor
  P. fiber
purple
  p. hallux
  p. hue
Purpose cream
purpura
  alloimmune thrombocytopenic p.
  anaphylactic p.

NOTES

P

purpura *(continued)*
    anaphylactoid p.
    childhood idiopathic
      thrombocytopenic p.
    p. fulminans
    p. hemorrhagica
    Henoch-Schönlein p. (HSP)
    idiopathic thrombocytopenic p.
      (ITP)
    immune thrombocytopenic p. (ITP)
    neonatal alloimmune
      thrombocytopenic p. (NATP)
    palpable p.
    Schönlein-Henoch p.
    thrombocytopenic p.
    thrombotic p.
    thrombotic thrombocytopenic p.
      (TTP)
    wet p.
purpuric
    p. light eruption
    p. rash
purse-string mouth
Purtscher retinopathy
purulent
    p. arthritis
    p. conjunctivitis
    p. meningitis
    p. nasal discharge
    p. pericarditis
    p. pharyngitis
    p. rhinitis
    p. sputum
    p. venous thrombosis
pus
    p. burrow
    sterile p.
pustular
    p. melanosis
    p. varicella
pustule
    satellite p.
pustulosa
    varicella p.
pustulosis
    infantile p.
    Malassezia furfur p.
    nonfollicular p.
    palmar p.
    p. palmaris
    p. palmaris et plantaris
    palmoplantar p.
    staphylococcal p.
putamen
PVDF
    polyvinylidene fluoride
PVEL
    periventricular echolucency

PVH
    periventricular hemorrhage
PVL
    periventricular leukomalacia
      cystic PVL
PVO
    portal vein obstruction
PVR
    pulmonary vascular resistance
PVS
    persistent vegetative state
P-wave axis
PWM
    poke weed mitogen
PWS
    Prader-Willi syndrome
PWSCR
    Prader-Willi syndrome critical region
Pycnogenol
pyelogram
    intravenous p. (IVP)
pyelography
    intravenous p.
    retrograde p.
pyelonephritis
    acute p.
    nonobstructive p.
    xanthogranulomatous p.
pyelophlebitis
    portal p.
pyeloplasty
pyelostomy
    cutaneous p.
pyknocyte
pyknocytosis
    infantile p.
pyknodysostosis syndrome
pyknoepilepsy
pyknotic cell
Pyle disease
pylephlebitis
pylori
    Campylobacter p.
    Helicobacter p.
pyloric
    p. atresia
    p. mass
    p. nitric oxide synthase
    p. olive
    p. sphincter relaxation
    p. stenosis
pyloromyotomy
    Ramstedt p.
    Ramstedt-Fredet p.
pyloroplasty
    Heineke-Mikulicz p.
pyoderma
    p. alopecia

blastomycosis-like p.
p. gangrenosum
streptococcal p.
p. vegetans
pyoderma-associated nephritis
pyogenes
Actinomyces p.
Staphylococcus p.
Streptococcus p.
pyogenic
p. bacteria
p. granuloma
p. infection
p. lymphadenitis
p. mediastinitis
p. meningitis
p. osteomyelitis
pyogranulomatous response
pyomyositis
tropical p.
pyopneumothorax
iatrogenic p.
pyramidal
p. cerebral palsy
p. lesion
p. tract
p. tract disease
p. tract sign
pyrantel pamoate
pyrazinamide (PZA)
pyrethroid
pyrethrum extract
pyrexia
pyribenzamine (PBZ)
Pyridiate
pyridinoline
Pyridium
pyridostigmine bromide
pyridoxal
p. phosphate
p. 5-phosphate

pyridoxine
p. deficiency
p. dependency
pyridoxine-dependency syndrome
pyridoxine-dependent seizure
pyridoxine-refractory sideroblastic anemia
pyrimethamine
sulfadoxine and p.
pyrimethamine-sulfadoxine
pyrimidine
pyrogenic exotoxin A, B, C factor
pyrogenicity
pyrophosphate
5-phospho-alpha-d-ribosyl p. (PRPP)
plasma inorganic p.
pyropoikilocytosis
hereditary p. (HPP)
pyrosis
pyrroloporphyria
pyruvate
p. dehydrogenase
p. dehydrogenase complex deficiency
p. dehydrogenation
p. kinase (PK)
p. kinase deficiency
p. kinase factor
pyruvic acid
6-pyruvoyl tetrahydropteridine synthetase
pyuria
amicrobic p.
sterile p.
PZ
proliferative zone
PZA
pyrazinamide
PZD
partial zonal dissection

NOTES

P

Q

    Q angle
    Q fever
    Q wave

Q10

    coenzyme Q10

22q11

    microdeletion of chromosome 22q11

q.

    every (*See also* q.q.)

q.d.

    quaque die (every day)

qEEG

    quantitative electroencephalography

q.h.

    quaque horo (every hour)

q.i.d.

    quater in die (four times a day)

q.n.s.

    quantity not sufficient

q.o.d.

    quaque altera die (every other day)

q.q.

    each
    every (*See also* q.)

QRS

    QRS axis
    QRS complex
    QRS duration
    QRS interval
    QRS morphology

QRS-T deflection

QS

    quiet sleep
    QS complex

q.s.

    quantum satis
    sufficient quantity

Qs/Qt

    intrapulmonary shunt fraction
    intrapulmonary shunt ratio
    right-to-left shunt ratio

QT

    QT corrected for heart rate (QTc)
    QT interval

QTc

    QT corrected for heart rate
    QTc prolongation

Qtest Strep test

QTL

    quantitative trait loci

quadrant

    q. assessment
    left lower q. (LLQ)
    left upper q. (LUQ)
    right lower q. (RLQ)
    right upper q. (RUQ)

quadrate hepatic lobe

quadratus labiae superioris muscle

quadriceps femoris muscle biopsy

quadrigemina

    corpora q.

quadriparesis

    flaccid q.
    spastic q.

quadriplegia

    spastic q.
    transient q.

quadriplegic

quadruped

quai

    dong q.

qualitative

    q. developmental assessment
    q. urine screen

quality-of-life

    health-related q.-o.-l. (HRQOL)

Quality of Upper Extremities Test (QUEST)

quantification

Quantikine IVD

quantitative

    q. analysis of fat content
    q. beta hCG level
    q. Bethesda assay
    q. electroencephalography (qEEG)
    q. immunoglobulin
    q. intradermal skin test
    q. serum drug assay
    q. trait loci (QTL)
    q. ultrasound (QUS)

quantity

    q. not sufficient (q.n.s.)
    sufficient q. (q.s.)

quantum satis (q.s.)

quaque

    q. altera die (every other day) (q.o.d.)
    q. die (every day) (q.d.)

quarantine

quarter-strength formula

quasi-experimental research approach

quater in die (four times a day) (q.i.d.)

Queckenstedt test

Queensland tick typhus

Quelicin

query fever

QUEST
Quality of Upper Extremities Test
questionnaire
Achenbach q.
Ages and Stages Q. (ASQ)
ANSWER System Q.
autism spectrum screening q. (ASSQ)
child health q. (CHQ)
childhood trauma q. (CTQ)
Conners Abbreviated Parent Q.
Denver Home Screening Q.
Dominic-R q.
Family APGAR q.
Harter self-esteem q.
health-related quality-of-life q.
HRQOL q.
human health and behavior q. (HBQ)
Q. for Identifying Children with Chronic Conditions (QuICCC)
Inflammatory Bowel Disease Q. (IBDQ)
Jag Tycker Jag Är self-esteem q.
Multidimensional Personality Q. (MPQ)
PARS III q.
Pediatric Asthma Quality of Life Q. (PAQLQ)
Reynolds suicide ideation q.
Seasonal Pattern Assessment Q. (SPAQ)
Terry q.
Wolraich q.
Questran Light
Quetelet body mass index
quetiapine fumarate
Quibron-T
Quibron-T/SR
QuICCC
Questionnaire for Identifying Children with Chronic Conditions

QuickVue In-Line One-Step Strep A test
quiescent
Quiess Injection
quiet
q. alertness
q. and alert state
q. precordium
q. sleep (QS)
Quikheel lancet
quinacrine
Quinaglute Dura-Tabs
Quinalan
Quinamm
Quinidex Extentabs
quinidine gluconate
quinine
q. dihydrochloride
q. sulfate
quinolinic acid
quinolone
Quinora
quinquefasciatus
Culex q.
Quinsana Plus Tropical
quinsy
quintana
Bartonella q.
quinupristin
Quiphile
quotidian fever
quotient
developmental q. (DQ)
developmental motor q. (DMQ)
Griffith General Q.
intelligence q. (IQ)
mean developmental q.
respiratory q.
QUS
quantitative ultrasound
Q-vel

R_{AW}
    regional gas exchange
R_{int}
    intrinsic flow resistance
R_{rs}
    respiratory system resistance
RA
    rheumatoid arthritis
RA27/3 rubella strain
RAA
    right aortic arch
Raaf catheter
RABA
    radioantigen-binding assay
rabbit
    r. infectivity testing
    r. nose
rabies
    r. immune globulin (RIG)
    paralytic r.
    r. prophylaxis
    r. vaccine
    r. vaccine, absorbed (RVA)
Rabson-Mendenhall syndrome
raccoon
    r. eyes
    r. eyes sign
racemic epinephrine
racemose form
rachischisis
    craniospinal r.
rachitic
    r. bone deformity
    r. change
    r. metaphysis
    r. rosary
radial
    r. aplasia-thrombocytopenia syndrome
    r. artery
    r. artery catheter
    r. artery catheterization
    r. clubhand
    r. digital grasp
    r. dysplasia
    r. epiphysis
    r. head dislocation
    r. head fracture
    r. head osteochondritis
    r. head subluxation (RHS)
    r. neck fracture
    r. nerve block
    r. palmar grasp
    r. physis

    r. ray aplasia
    r. ray defect
radial-femoral delay
radiant warmer
radiata
    corona r.
radiation
    r. carcinogenesis
    r. encephalopathy
    r. exposure
    IF r.
    involved-field r.
    r. necrosis
    r. pneumonitis
    r. syndrome
    r. therapy (RT)
radiation-induced
    r.-i. heart disease (RIHD)
    r.-i. physeal injury
radical
    free r.
    hydroxyl r. (OH)
    intrarenal venous r.
    oxygen-free r.
    r. posteromedial and plantar release (RPMPR)
    superoxide r.
    venous r.
radicular neuropathy
radiculitis
radiculomyelitis
    acute ascending r.
    ascending r.
radiculoneuritis
    Lyme r.
radii (*pl. of* radius)
radioallergosorbent
    r. test (RAST)
radioantigen-binding assay (RABA)
radiocisternography
radiodermatitis
radiofrequency
radiogram
    sinus r.
radiograph
    abdominal r.
    cephalometric r.
    chest r.
    flat abdominal r.
    frogleg lateral r.
    intercondylar r.
    lateral r.
    Lauenstein lateral r.
    oblique r.
    occlusal r.

R

radiograph *(continued)*
    panoramic r.
    plain abdominal r.
    scout r.
    sinus r.
    skyline view r.
    stress view r.
    upright abdominal r.
radiographic bone strength index (RBSI)
radiography
    digital r.
    stereotactic r.
    tunnel-view r.
radioimmunoassay (RIA)
    Raji cell r.
radioimmunoprecipitation assay (RIPA)
radioiodine ablative therapy
radioisotope
    r. angiography
    r. cisternography
    r. milk scan
radioisotopic reperfusion and excretion study
radiolabeled
    r. fibrinogen
    r. white blood cell scan
radiologic stigmata
radiologist
    pediatric r.
radiolucent
    r. circular shadow in bladder
    r. line
radionuclide
    r. bone scan
    r. cineangiography
    r. heart scan
    r. imaging
    r. scanning
    r. scintigraphy
radiopaque marker
radioreceptor-guided surgery
radiosurgery
    stereotactic r.
radiotherapy
    fractionated sterotactic r.
    hyperfractionated r.
    plaque r.
    split-course hyperfractionated r.
radiotracer
radioulnar synostosis
radius, pl. **radii**
    absent r.
    hypoplastic r.
    thrombocytopenia-absent r. (TAR)
    thrombocytopenia with absent r. (TAR)
RAG1 deficiency

RAG2 deficiency
rage
    violent r.
ragged
    r. red fiber (RRF)
    r. red myopathy
ragweed pollen
raided raspberry-like papilloma
railroad
    r. nystagmus
    r. track line
Raimondi catheter
raised
    r. lesion
    r. red-black telangiectasia
Raji
    R. cell
    R. cell assay
    R. cell radioimmunoassay
rale
Ralstonia pickettii
rami (*pl. of* ramus)
ramosum
    Clostridium r.
Ramsay Hunt syndrome
Ramstedt
    R. disease
    R. operation
    R. pyloromyotomy
Ramstedt-Fredet pyloromyotomy
ramus, pl. **rami**
    superior r.
rancid butter syndrome
random
    r. regression model
    r. X inactivation
randomized
range
    r. loss
    r. of motion (ROM)
ranitidine
RANS
    retinal arterial narrowing and straightening
Ranson criteria
RANTES
    regulated upon activation, normal T-cell expressed and secreted
ranula
RAO
    right anterior oblique
RAP
    recurrent abdominal pain
RAPA
    rapamycin
rapamycin (RAPA)
rape

raphe
> fused r.
> r. of scrotum

rapid
> r. acquisition with resolution enhancement (RARE)
> r. alternating movement
> r. antigen detection test
> r. blinking
> r. dissolution formula (RDF)
> r. eye movement (REM)
> r. eye movement sleep
> r. filter testing
> r. filter testing for bacteriuria
> r. plasma reagin (RPR)
> r. rehydration
> r. sequence induction
> r. sequence intubation (RSI)
> R. Strep screen
> r. succession movement

rapidly progressive glomerulonephritis
rapid-onset dystonia-parkinsonism
Rapp-Hodgkin ectodermal dysplasia syndrome
RARE
> rapid acquisition with resolution enhancement

rarefaction
rarefying osteitis
RARS
> refractory anemia with ring sideroblasts

RAS
> renin-angiotensin system

rasa
> tabula r.

rash
> allergic diaper r.
> ampicillin r.
> angiectatic skin r.
> atopic diaper r.
> blueberry muffin r.
> butterfly r.
> candidal diaper r.
> collarette of r.
> r. crop
> diaper r.
> diffuse morbilliform r.
> discoid r.
> drug-induced r.
> ECM r.
> eczematoid skin r.
> erythema chronicum migrans r.

> erythematous r.
> evanescent maculopapular r.
> friction diaper r.
> heliotrope r.
> irritation diaper r.
> macular r.
> maculopapular r.
> malar r.
> monilial diaper r.
> morbilliform skin r.
> nonvesicular r.
> papular r.
> pellagra-like skin r.
> perioral r.
> petechial r.
> plaquelike r.
> polymorphous r.
> pruritic r.
> psoriatic diaper r.
> purpuric r.
> roseola r.
> salmon-pink r.
> sandpaper r.
> scarlatiniform r.
> seborrheic diaper r.
> skin r.
> slapped cheek r.
> truncal r.

Rashkind
> R. atrial septostomy procedure
> R. balloon atrial septostomy

Rasmussen
> R. encephalitis
> R. syndrome

raspberry-like papilloma
raspberry tongue
RAST
> radioallergosorbent test

Rastelli
> R. operation
> R. procedure
> R. repair

rat-bite fever
rate
> aldosterone excretion r.
> basal metabolic r. (BMR)
> erythrocyte sedimentation r. (ESR)
> glomerular filtration r. (GFR)
> glucose production r. (GPR)
> growth r.
> heart r. (HR)
> nipple flow r.

R

NOTES

rate *(continued)*
   peak expiratory flow r. (PEFR)
   peak flow r.
   QT corrected for heart r. (QTc)
   resting metabolic r. (RMR)
   sedimentation r.
rating
   sexual maturity r. (SMR)
ratio
   arterial to alveolar oxygen tension r. (AaPO$_2$)
   cardiothoracic r.
   CD4:CD8 r.
   expiratory to inspiratory r.
   FEV$_1$/FVC r.
   hypoxanthine/creatinine r.
   I/E r.
   inspiratory to expiratory r. (I/E, I:E)
   international normalized r. (INR)
   intrapulmonary shunt r. (Qs/Qt)
   I/T r.
   LA:Ao r.
   lecithin to sphingomyelin r.
   L/S r.
   myeloid to erythroid r.
   odds r. (OR)
   right lung-to-head circumference r. (LHR)
   right-to-left shunt r. (Qs/Qt)
   risk-benefit r.
   testosterone to dihydrotestosterone r.
   triene-to-tetraene r.
   U/C r.
   U/L r.
   umbilical artery pulsatility index to middle cerebral artery pulsatility index r. (U/C)
   upper body segment to lower body segment r. (U/L)
   waist-hip r. (WHR)
   zinc protoporphyrin/heme r.
   ZPP/H r.
rationalize
Raven
   R. IQ
   R. Progressive Matrices (RPM)
Ravitch procedure
raw score
ray
   intercalary defect of pollical r.
   pollical r.
Rayleigh-Tyndall scattering
Raynaud
   R. disease
   R. phenomenon (RP)
   R. sign
   R. syndrome

RBBB
   right bundle branch block
RBC
   red blood cell
     RBC adenosine deaminase level
     fresh-packed RBCs
     RBC P antigen
RBF
   renal blood flow
RBSI
   radiographic bone strength index
RCCA
   right common carotid artery
RCDP
   rhizomelic chondrodysplasia punctata
RCF
   Ross carbohydrate-free
     RCF formula
RCM
   restrictive cardiomyopathy
RCMAS
   Revised Children's Manifest Anxiety Scale
RDA
   recommended daily allowance
   recommended dietary allowance
   right ductus arteriosus
RDEB
   recessive dystrophic epidermolysis bullosa
RDF
   rapid dissolution formula
     Adriamycin RDF
RDFC
   recurring digital fibroma of childhood
RDS
   respiratory distress syndrome
     neonatal RDS
reabsorption
reactant
   acute-phase r.
reaction
   acute transfusion r.
   adverse drug r. (ADR)
   adverse food r.
   anaphylactic r.
   Arthus r.
   association r.
   automatic movement r.
   balance r.
   biphasic anaphylactic r.
   bullous r.
   chain r.
   circular r.
   coccidioidin r.
   conversion r.
   delayed transfusion r.
   dermatophytid r.

R

diazo r.
dysphoric r.
equilibrium r.
febrile nonhemolytic transfusion r.
Felix-Weil r.
ferric chloride r.
fetomaternal transfusion r.
fungal id r.
gliotic r.
Gomori trichrome r.
graft-versus-leukemia r.
GVL r.
hypersensitivity r.
id r.
immediate hypersensitivity r.
insect sting r.
Jarisch-Herxheimer r.
Koebner r.
leukemoid r.
ligase-chain r. (LCR)
linear Koebner r.
Mitsuda r.
modified Gomori trichrome r.
neonatal leukemoid r.
nonhemolytic r.
paradoxical pupil r.
Paul-Bunnell r.
periosteal r.
photoallergic r.
phototoxic r.
polymerase chain r. (PCR)
postural r.
primary circular r.
prokaryotic r.
pupil r.
reverse transcription polymerase
    chain r. (RT-PCR)
righting r.
secondary circular r.
serum sickness-like r.
stranger r.
stress r.
transfusion r.
twin-to-twin transfusion r.
urine ligase chain r.
van den Bergh r.
Weil-Felix r.
wheal-and-flare r.
reactivation tuberculosis
reactive
r. airway
r. airway disease

r. arthritis
r. attachment disorder of infancy
    or early childhood
r. epilepsy
r. oxygen species (ROS)
r. perforating collagenosis (RPC)
r. psychosis
reactivity
skin test r. (STR)
substance P immune r.
reactogenicity
readiness
Pediatric Examination of
    Educational R. (PEER)
reading disability
reagent
antiimmunoglobulin r.
r. strip
TRIZOL r.
reagin
rapid plasma r. (RPR)
real-time echocardiography
rearfoot
r. valgus
r. varus
rebelliousness
rebound
r. hypertension
r. tenderness
receiver operating characteristic (ROC)
receptive
r. aphasia
r. language
r. language development
Receptive-Expressive
R.-E. Emergent Language Scale
    (REEL)
R.-E. Emergent Language Scale,
    Second Edition (REEL-2)
receptor
alpha-adrenergic r.
alpha-chemokine r.
AT1, AT2 r.
beta-adrenergic r.
beta-chemokine r.
complement r. (CR1)
cough r.
epidermal growth factor r. (EGFR)
fibroblast growth factor r. (FGFR)
fibronectin r.
granulocyte colony-stimulating
    factor r. (G-CSF-R)

NOTES

receptor *(continued)*
    growth hormone r. (GHR)
    H_1 r.
    r. for hyaluronan-mediated motility (RHAMM)
    iC3b r.
    interleukin-2 r. (IL 2R)
    irritant r.
    keratinocyte growth factor r. (KGFR)
    leptin r.
    Notch r.
    soluble tumor necrosis factor r.
    transferrin r. (TfR)
receptor-mediated endocytosis
recess
    epitympanic r.
    suprapineal r.
recession
    sternal r.
recessive
    autosomal r. (AR)
    r. disorder defect
    r. dystrophic epidermolysis bullosa (RDEB)
    r. gene
    r. inheritance
    X-linked r. (XLR)
    r. X-linked chondrodysplasia punctate
recidivism
reciprocal movement
reciprocating
    r. gait
    r. gait orthosis (RGO)
Recklinghausen disease
recognition
    facial affect r.
recognizable viral syndrome (RVS)
recombinant
    r. enzyme
    r. enzyme replacement therapy
    r. factor VIIA (rFVIIa)
    r. follicle-stimulating hormone (rFSH)
    r. hepatitis B vaccine
    r. human erythropoietin (r-EPO, rHuEPO, rHuEpo)
    r. human growth hormone (rhGH)
    r. human insulin-like growth factor-1 (rhIGF-1)
    r. human MIP-1 alpha (MIP-1 alpha)
    r. human superoxide dismutase (rhSOD)
    r. immunosorbent assay (RIBA)
    r. K29 antigen
    r. OspA
    r. outer surface protein A (rOspA)
recombinase activating gene
recombination
Recombivax
    R. HB
    R. HB immunization
    R. vaccine
recommended
    r. daily allowance (RDA)
    r. dietary allowance (RDA)
reconstitute
reconstitution
reconstruction
    cleft lip-nasal r.
    Dibbell cleft lip-nasal r.
    laryngotracheal r.
    right ventricular outflow tract r.
    umbilicus r.
    ventricular outflow tract r.
record
    Infant Behavior R. (IBR)
recorder
    Digitrapper portable pH r.
    VitaGuard 1000 event r.
recording
    closed-circuit video r.
    gastroesophageal reflux-reflex apnea r.
recovered memory
recovery
    fluid-attenuated inversion r. (FLAIR)
recrudescence of fever
recrudescent typhus
recruitment
    alveolar r.
    lung r.
rectal
    A-Caine R.
    r. administration
    r. balloon manometry
    r. examination
    r. fissure
    Fleet Babylax R.
    Hemet R.
    R. Medicone
    Phenergan R.
    r. pouch
    Proctocort R.
    r. prolapse
    RMS R.
    Rowasa R.
    r. sensation
    r. stump
    r. suppository
    r. swab
    Tebamide R.

r. temperature
T-Gen R.
Tigan R.
Trimazide R.
r. vault
r. wall resection
rectal-fourchette fistula
recti
diastasis r.
rectilinear profile
rectoanal reflex
rectocolonic saline enema
rectopexy
abdominal r.
anterior resection r.
rectoscopy
rectosphincteric
r. reflex
r. reflux
rectourethral fistula
rectum
aganglionic r.
by way of r. (p.r.)
rectus
r. femoris
r. femoris muscle
r. palsy
recumbent infant board
recurrens
periadenitis mucosa necrotica r.
recurrent
r. abdominal pain (RAP)
r. ADEM
r. affective disorder
r. angioedema
r. aphthous stomatitis
r. bacterial meningitis
r. blister
r. cholangitis
r. coarctation
r. convulsive seizure
r. epistaxis
r. fungal meningitis
r. genital aphthous ulcer
r. gross hematuria (RGH)
r. headache
r. hemolytic uremia syndrome
r. hernia formation
r. ITP
r. Japanese encephalitis virus
r. laryngeal nerve paralysis
r. myoglobinuria

r. nonconvulsive seizure
r. otitis media
r. purulent meningitis
r. pyogenic lymphadenitis
r. respiratory papillomatosis (RRP)
r. sinusitis
r. staphylococcal infection
recurrentis
Borrelia r.
recurring digital fibroma of childhood (RDFC)
recurvatum
r. deformity
genu r.
recycling
medullary r.
red
r. blood cell (RBC)
r. blood cell cast
r. blood cell membrane defect
r. blood cell sickling
r. blood cell transfusion
r. cell antigen
r. cell membrane
r. cell spiny projection
r. cell tagged scan
r. desaturation
r. fundus
r. glass test
r. nucleus
r. photoplethysmography
r. reflex
r. reflex test
r. strawberry tongue
red-black telangiectasia
redirection
intraatrial r.
Redisol
RediTab
Claritin R.
reduced
r. bladder capacity
r. liver transplant (RLT)
reduced-size liver transplant (RSLT)
reducer
Axid AR Acid R.
reducing substance
reductase
dihydropteridine r.
methylene tetrahydrofolate r.
reduction
air r.

R

NOTES

reduction *(continued)*
    failed r.
    fracture r.
    hydrostatic r.
    manual r.
    multifetal pregnancy r. (MFPR)
    r. of protrusion
    in utero r.
redundant skin
REE
    resting energy expenditure
Reed-Sternberg cell
Reed syndrome
REEL
    Receptive-Expressive Emergent
    Language Scale
REEL-2
    Receptive-Expressive Emergent
    Language Scale, Second Edition
reentrant
    r. supraventricular tachycardia
reentry tachycardia
Reese Clark protocol
Reese-Ellsworth classification
Reese's Pinworm Medicine
reexperiencing
refeeding
reference
    ambiguous r.
referential cohesion
refill
    capillary r.
    poor capillary r.
    prolonged capillary r.
reflectance pulse oximetry (RPO)
reflectometry
    acoustic r.
    spectral gradient acoustic r.
    (SGAR)
reflex
    acoustic blink r.
    r. anoxic seizure
    asymmetric tonic neck r. (ATNR)
    automatic r.
    autonomic walking r.
    axon r.
    Babinski r.
    Bezold-Jarisch r.
    biceps r.
    bite r.
    blink r.
    bowing r.
    brachioradialis r.
    cat's eye r.
    conditioned orientation r. (COR)
    cremasteric r.
    crossed adductor r.
    darkened r.

    deep tendon r. (DTR)
    delayed deep tendon r.
    diving r.
    doll's eye r.
    ejection r.
    embrace r.
    r. epilepsy
    extrusion r.
    flexion r.
    forced grasp r.
    gag r.
    Galant r.
    gastrocolic r.
    Gemini red r.
    Gordon r.
    grasp r.
    Hering-Breuer inflation r. (HBIR)
    Hoffmann r.
    knee jerk r.
    labyrinthine r.
    Landau r.
    laryngeal adductor r. (LAR)
    laryngeal vagal r.
    macular light r.
    markedly decreased r.
    McCarthy r.
    milk ejection r.
    Moro r.
    r. myoclonus
    near gaze r.
    neck r.
    neck-righting r.
    obligatory primitive r.
    obligatory tonic neck r.
    oculocephalic r.
    Oppenheim r.
    oral r.
    palmar grasp r.
    palpebral r.
    parachute r.
    patellar r.
    pathologic r.
    r. pathway
    r. pattern
    physiologic r.
    placing r.
    plantar grasp r.
    positive support r.
    postural r.
    primitive r.
    propping r.
    rectoanal r.
    rectosphincteric r.
    red r.
    rhinobronchial r.
    righting r.
    rooting r.
    Rossolimo r.

R

startle r.
r. stepping
stepping r.
suckling r.
support r.
swallow r.
swallowing r.
swimming r.
symmetrical tonic neck r. (STNR)
r. sympathetic dystrophy (RSD)
r. syncope
tendon stretch r.
tongue protrusion r.
tonic labyrinthine r.
tonic neck r. (TNR)
triceps r.
truncal incurvation r.
walking r.
white pupillary r.
reflex-placing response
reflux
acid r.
r. of air
alkaline r.
complicated gastroesophageal r.
contralateral r.
dilating r.
esophageal r.
r. esophagitis
gastroesophageal r. (GER)
gastrointestinal r.
intrarenal r.
nasopharyngeal r. (NPR)
r. nephropathy
r. neuropathy
physiologic r.
primary vesicoureteral r.
rectosphincteric r.
secondary vesicoureteral r.
silent gastroesophageal r.
vesicoureteral r. (grade I–V)
   (VUR)
refraction
refractive error
refractory
r. anemia with ring sideroblasts
   (RARS)
r. ascites
r. Crohn disease
r. depressive symptom
r. dyserythropoietic anemia
r. epistaxis

r. hypoglycemia
r. sprue
r. status epilepticus (RSE)
Refsum
R. disease
R. syndrome
Regan-Lowe medium
regard
prolonged r.
visual r.
regeneration
aberrant r.
regimen
COMP drug r.
conditioning r.
hypertransfusion r.
region
breakpoint cluster r. (bcr)
bulbo ponto mesencephalic r.
hilar r.
parietooccipital r.
perimesencephalic r.
Prader-Willi syndrome critical r.
   (PWSCR)
subependymal r.
subpial r.
zygomaticofrontal r.
regional
r. enteritis
r. gas exchange (R$_{AW}$)
r. ileitis
r. lymphadenitis
r. nerve block
r. perinatal intensive care center
   (RPICC)
r. wall motion abnormality
register
high-risk r. (HRR)
registered nurse (RN)
registry
cord blood r. (CBR)
National Pediatric Trauma R.
   (NPTR)
Reglan
Regonol Injection
regression
Regulace
regular
R. (Concentrated) Iletin II U-500
R. Iletin I, II
R. Iletin II U-500

NOTES

regular *(continued)*
    r. immune globulin
    R. Purified Pork Insulin
regulated upon activation, normal T-cell expressed and secreted (RANTES)
regulation
    arginine vasopressin r.
    Baby Doe R.'s
    cellular r.
    molecular r.
regulator
    cystic fibrosis transmembrane r. (CFTR)
    cystic fibrosis transmembrane conductance r. (CFTR)
Regulax SS
Reguloid
regurgitant fraction
regurgitate
regurgitation
    aortic r.
    effortless r.
    gastric r.
    nasal r.
    physiologic r.
Regutol
rehabilitate
rehabilitation cookie swallow
Rehydralyte formula
rehydration
    rapid r.
Reifenstein syndrome
Reilly granule
reimplant
    common sheath r.
reimplantation
    extravesical ureteral r.
    r. of ureter
    ureteral trigonal r.
reinforcement
    contingent r.
    negative r.
    positive r.
Reissner membrane
Reiter syndrome
reject
    zero r.
rejecting
rejection
    accelerated r.
    acute r.
    allograft r.
    chronic r.
    hyperacute r.
relapse
    bone marrow r.
    testicular r.

relapsing
    r. fever
    r. infectious polyneuritis
    r. iridocyclitis
    r. nodular nonsuppurative panniculitis
related services
relation
    peer r.
relationship
    blood r.
    depth r.
    spatial r.
relative
    r. afferent defect
    blood r.
    r. macroglossia
    r. polycythemia
    r. vascular resistance (RVR)
Relaxadon
relaxant
    muscle r.
relaxation
    pyloric sphincter r.
    r. volume
release
    Acutrim Precision R.
    complete subtalar r. (CSTR)
    hip adduction r.
    increased renin r.
    myofascial r.
    postganglionic acetylcholine r.
    radical posteromedial and plantar r. (RPMPR)
    Sever r.
    soft tissue r.
Relefact TRH
Relenza
reliability
relief
    Fleet R.
    R. Ophthalmic Solution
religiosity
REM
    rapid eye movement
    REM latency
    REM parasomnia
    REM sleep
    REM sleep behavior disorder
remifentanil
remineralization
remission
    spontaneous r.
remnant
    omphalomesenteric duct r.
    tracheobronchial r.

remodeling
    bone r.
    fracture r.
removal
    surgical r.
remyelination
Renaissance spirometry system
renal
    r. agenesis
    r. aminoaciduria
    r. artery stenosis
    r. blastema
    r. blood flow (RBF)
    r. calculus
    r. calyx
    r. candidiasis
    r. cortex
    r. cortex cyst
    r. cortical necrosis
    r. cortical nephropathy
    r. cystic disease
    r. dysfunction
    r. dysgenesis
    r. electrolyte wasting
    r. failure
    r. Fanconi syndrome
    r. fungus ball
    r. hypercalciuria
    r. hypodysplasia
    r. insufficiency
    r. interstitium
    r. loss
    r. medullary carcinoma
    r. medullary dysplasia
    r. mycetoma
    r. myofibromatosis
    r. obstruction
    r. osteodystrophy
    r. pedicle
    r. pelvis
    r. proteinuria
    r. reserve filtration capacity (RRFC)
    r. rickets
    r. salt wasting
    r. scarring
    r. scintigraphy
    r. solute load (RSL)
    r. tract
    r. tuberculosis
    r. tubular acidosis (RTA)
    r. tubular bicarbonate wasting
    r. tubular crystalluria
    r. tubular epithelial cell
    r. tubular Fanconi syndrome
    r. tubular pituitary syndrome
    r. tubule
    r. ultrasound
    r. vasculitis
    r. vein
    r. vein thrombosis
Rendu-Osler-Weber
    R.-O.-W. disease
    R.-O.-W. syndrome
renin
    elevated r.
renin-angiotensin system (RAS)
Renografin
renogram
    MAG-3 diuretic r.
renography
    diuretic r.
renovascular
reossification
reossify
Reoviridae
Reovirus (type 1–3)
reoxygenation
repair
    Cantwell-Ransley r.
    CDH r.
    clawhand deformity r.
    cleft palate r.
    delayed r.
    hypospadias r.
    imperforate anus r.
    intraatrial r.
    palate r.
    primary cleft palate r.
    Rastelli r.
    Snodgrass hypospadias r.
    staged r.
    Tennison-Randall r.
    transannular patch r.
    Zancolli clawhand deformity r.
repeated partial seizure
reperfusion injury
replacement
    esophageal r.
    gamma globulin r.
    r. therapy
    volume r.
replicate
replication

NOTES

Replogle
  R. suction catheter
  R. sump tube
r-EPO
  recombinant human erythropoietin
repolarization
reporter
  mandated r. (of child abuse)
repositioning
  scapular r.
representation
  internal r.
  symbolic r.
reproductive toxin
Repronex
reptilase time
requirement
  minimum daily r. (MDR)
RER
  rough endoplasmic reticulum
Rescriptor
rescue
  r. breathing
  r. dose
  r. medication
  r. surfactant
  r. therapy
Research Network
resection
  atretic extrahepatic bile duct r.
  bile duct r.
  bowel loop r.
  bowel segment r.
  dilated bowel loop r.
  distal dilated bowel segment r.
  duodenal r.
  en bloc r.
  extrahepatic bile duct r.
  gallbladder r.
  pancreatic head r.
  perineal r.
  posterior rectal wall r.
  rectal wall r.
  in utero r.
Resectisol Irrigation Solution
reseeding
reserpine
reserve
  coronary flow r. (CFR)
  r. zone (RZ)
reservoir
  catheter r.
  ileal r.
  Ommaya r.
  subcutaneous ventricular catheter r.
resident
residential program

residual
  r. coarctation
  r. hearing
  postvoid r.
  r. vision
  r. volume (RV)
residuum, pl. **residua**
resin
  cholestyramine r.
  podophyllum r.
resistance
  airway r.
  androgen r.
  antiretroviral r.
  fetal pulmonary vascular r.
  increased vascular r.
  insulin r.
  intrinsic flow r. (R_{int})
  lithium r.
  multidrug r. (MDR)
  pulmonary vascular r. (PVR)
  relative vascular r. (RVR)
  respiratory system r. (R_{rs})
  systemic vascular r. (SVR)
  tissue insulin r.
  total peripheral r. (TPR)
  vascular r.
resistant
  ampicillin r.
  drug r.
  r. pneumococcus
resisted abduction
resolve
  adaptability, partnership, growth, affection, r. (APGAR)
resorption
  r. atelectasis
  bone r.
resource
  R. Just for Kids formula
  R. Plus formula
  r. specialist
  R. Standard formula
Respa-DM
Respa-GF
Respbid
Resp-EZ piezoelectric sensor
RespiGam
Respihaler
  Decadron R.
Respinol-G
respiration
  artificial r.
  Cheyne-Stokes r.
  gasping r.
  grunting r.
  Kussmaul r.
  paradoxic r.

R

percutaneous aspiration, instillation
  of hypertonic saline, r. (PAIR)
sighing r.
respirator
Ambu r.
BABYbird r.
Babylog 8000 r.
Bird r.
cuirass r.
mechanical r.
Med-Neb r.
Merck r.
Monaghan r.
Morch r.
Morsch-Retec r.
Moynihan r.
negative-pressure r.
Sanders jet r.
Stephan HF 300 r.
respiratory
r. acidosis
r. alkalosis
r. arrest
r. burst assay
r. chamber
r. cycle
r. depression
r. distress
r. distress syndrome (RDS)
r. distress syndrome of newborn
r. drive
r. embarrassment
r. epithelium
r. failure
r. index score (RIS)
r. inductive plethysmography (RIP)
r. insufficiency
r. movement
r. papilloma
r. papillomatosis
r. paralysis
r. pattern
r. quotient
r. sinus arrhythmia
r. suction
r. suctioning
r. syncytial virus (RSV)
r. syncytial virus antigen
r. syncytial virus bronchiolitis
  (RSVB)
r. syncytial virus immune globulin
  (RSVIG, RSV-IG)

r. syncytial virus immunoglobulin
  (RSVIG, RSV-IG)
r. syncytial virus intravenous
  immunoglobulin (RSV-IVIG)
r. syncytial virus pneumonia
r. system elastance (E_{dyn})
r. system resistance (R_{rs})
Taiwan acute r. (TWAR)
r. therapist
r. therapy
r. therapy pack
r. toilet
r. tract infection
Respirgard II nebulizer
respite care
Respitrace inductance plethysmography
Respivir
response
acute insulin r.
age-related pharmacodynamic r.
anamnestic immune r.
antistreptolysin O r.
asthmatic r.
auditory brainstem r. (ABR,
  ABSR)
auditory evoked r. (AER)
automated auditory brainstem r.
  (AABR, A-ABR)
Babinski r.
biphasic r.
Bobath r.
brainstem auditory evoked r.
  (BAER, BSAER)
brainstem evoked r. (BSER)
buttress r.
characteristic emotional r.
chronotropic r.
clasp-knife r.
r. cost
cremasteric r.
CTL r.
cytotoxic lymphocyte r.
doll's eye r.
early asthmatic r. (EAR)
emotional r.
evoked r.
fall-away r.
fetal inflammatory r.
fight-and-flight r.
glabellar r.
immune r.
inflammatory r.

NOTES

response *(continued)*
    r. inhibition
    insulin r.
    Koebner r.
    Landau r.
    late asthmatic r. (LAR)
    r. latency
    local inflammatory r.
    metabolic r.
    Moro r.
    neck r.
    neuroendocrine r.
    parachute r.
    pharmacodynamic r.
    placing r.
    plantar r.
    postinfectious immune r.
    pyogranulomatous r.
    reflex-placing r.
    righting r.
    sound-field r.
    staircase r.
    startle r.
    stepping r.
    thermogenic r.
    thermoregulatory r.
    tonic neck r.
    Treppe r.
    vagally mediated r.
    visual evoked r. (VER)
Respules
    Pulmicort R.
rest
    ectopic pancreatic r.
    gut r.
    r., ice, compress, elevate
    r., ice, compression, elevation
      (RICE)
    intralobar r.
    nephrogenic r.
    PediaCare Night R.
resting
    r. calorimetry
    r. energy expenditure (REE)
    r. metabolic rate (RMR)
restless
    r. legs syndrome
    r. sleep
restlessness
    motor r.
restraint
    child r.
restriction
    fetal growth r. (FGR)
    fluid r.
    r. fragment length polymorphism
      (RFLP)

    r. fragment length polymorphism
      analysis
    intrauterine growth r. (IUGR)
restrictive
    r. cardiomyopathy (RCM)
    r. lung disease
    r. respiratory disease
restructuring
resuscitate
resuscitation
    bag-and-mask r.
    cardiopulmonary r. (CPR)
    cerebral r.
    fluid r.
    mouth-to-mouth r.
    mouth-to-nose/mouth r.
    neonatal r.
retained fetal lung fluid (RFLF)
retardate
    Screening Tests for Young
      Children and R.'s (STYCAR)
    Sheridan Tests for Young Children
      and R.'s (STYCAR)
retardation
    American Association on
      Mental R. (AAMR)
    deafness, onychodystrophy,
      osteodystrophy, mild to severe
      mental r. (DOOR)
    growth r.
    r. of growth and deafness
    head-sparing intrauterine growth r.
    intrauterine growth r. (IUGR)
    linear growth r.
    mental r.
    mild mental r.
    moderate mental r.
    nonspecific mental r.
    prenatal growth r.
    profound mental r.
    psychomotor r.
    severe mental r.
    Wilms tumor, aniridia, genitourinary
      malformations, mental r. (WAGR)
retarded
    specific reading r. (SRR)
rete
    r. peg
    r. ridge elongation
retention
    carbon dioxide r.
    r. polyp
    sodium r.
    stool r.
rethrombosis
reticula (*pl. of* reticulum)
reticular
    r. dysgenesia

R

r. dysgenesis
r. reflex myoclonus
reticularis
livedo r.
zona r.
reticulata
substantia nigra pars r.
reticulated
r. hyperpigmentation
r. pigmentation
reticulocyte count
reticulocytopenia
reticulocytosis
reticuloendothelial
r. cell
r. sequestration
r. system
reticuloendotheliosis
reticulonodular pattern
reticulum, pl. **reticula**
rough endoplasmic r. (RER)
sarcoplasmic r.
stellate r.
Retin-A
retina
dragging of r.
embryonic neural r.
mottled r.
neural r.
retinaculum, pl. **retinacula**
peroneal r.
retinae
commotio r.
retinal
r. angioma
r. arterial narrowing and
straightening (RANS)
r. change
r. detachment
r. dysplasia
r. edema
r. hemorrhage
r. infiltrate
r. pigmentary degeneration
r. pigment epithelium (RPE)
r. pseudotumor
r. vasculitis
r. venous dilation and tortuosity
(RVDT)
r. vessel telangiectasia
retinitis
CMV r.

indolent granular CMV r.
r. pigmentosa
proliferative r.
retinoblast
retinoblastoma
bilateral r.'s
hereditary r.
trilateral r.
retinoblastoma-mental retardation
syndrome
retinoic
r. acid
r. acid embryopathy
retinoid therapy
retinol
retinol-binding protein
retinopathy
diabetic r.
Keith-Wagener r.
r. of newborn
nonproliferative diabetic r.
r. of prematurity (ROP)
Purtscher r.
retinoschisis
congenital hereditary r.
hereditary r.
juvenile X-linked r.
X-linked r.
retractile testis
retraction
accessory muscle r.
intercostal r.
substernal r.
supraclavicular r.
retractive nystagmus
retractor
Aufricht nasal r.
Desmarres r.
nasal r.
pediatric self-retaining r.
retractorius
nystagmus r.
retransposition
arterial r.
retroambiguus
nucleus r.
retroauricular
retrobulbar neuritis
retrocallosal
retrocaval ureter
retrocecal hernia
retrocerebellar arachnoidal cyst

NOTES

retrochiasmatic
retrocollis
retroesophageal abscess
retrognathism
retrograde
r. amnesia
r. axoplasmic flow
r. pyelography
retrolental fibroplasia (RLF)
retroperitoneal fibrosis
retropharyngeal
r. abscess
r. cellulitis
r. lymph node
retroplacental hematoma
retrorectal transanal pull-through
retrosternal
r. chest pain
r. hernia
retrotonsillar abscess
retrotorsion
retroversion
femoral r.
Retrovir
retroviral syndrome
retrovirus
retrusion
Rett
R. disorder
R. syndrome
return
anomalous pulmonary venous r.
intraatrial redirection of venous r.
partial anomalous pulmonary
venous r.
pulmonary venous r.
supracardiac total anomalous
pulmonary venous r.
systemic caval r.
total anomalous pulmonary
venous r. (TAPVR)
venous r.
revacuolization
duodenal r.
revascularization
revenge fantasy
reversal
role r.
reverse
r. genetics
r. last shoe
r. Marcus Gunn sign
r. 3 sign
r. transcriptase inhibitor (RTI)
r. transcription polymerase chain
reaction (RT-PCR)
reversible
r. biliary pseudolithiasis

r. obstructive airway
r. posterior leukoencephalopathy
syndrome (RPLS)
Reversol
review
annual r.
r. of symptoms (ROS)
r. of systems (ROS)
revised
R. Children's Manifest Anxiety
Scale (RCMAS)
Gesell Adaptive and Personal
Behavior Domain, R.
Gesell Developmental Schedules, R.
Gesell Gross Motor Domain, R.
R. Gesell Language Domain
r. Jones criteria
r. Jones criteria for diagnosis of
acute rheumatic fever
R. Tests of Cognitive Ability
R. Trauma Score (RTS)
revision
lip scar r.
shunt r.
Revital-Ice rehydrating freezer pop
rewarming
extracorporeal r.
Reye
R. hepatic encephalopathy
R. syndrome
Reye-like syndrome
Reynell
R. Developmental Language Scale
R. Language Developmental Scale
(RLDS)
R. Verbal Comprehension Test
Reynolds
R. Child Depression Scale
R. number
R. suicide ideation questionnaire
RF
rheumatoid factor
RFA
right femoral artery
RFLF
retained fetal lung fluid
RFLP
restriction fragment length polymorphism
RFLP analysis
RF-negative juvenile polyarthritis
RF-seropositive
rFSH
recombinant follicle-stimulating hormone
rFVIIa
recombinant factor VIIa
R-Gel
R-Gene

RGH
  recurrent gross hematuria
RGO
  reciprocating gait orthosis
Rh
  Rhesus
    Rh complex
    Rh disease of newborn
    Rh factor
    Rh incompatibility
    Rh isoimmune hemolytic disease
    Rh isoimmunization
    Mini-Gamulin Rh
    Rh null cell
rhabdoid tumor
rhabdomyoblast
rhabdomyolysis
  copper-induced r.
  hyperthermic r.
  malignant hyperthermic r.
rhabdomyoma
  cardiac r.
rhabdomyosarcoma (RMS)
  r. retinoblastoma
  undifferentiated r.
rhagas, pl. **rhagades**
RHAMM
  receptor for hyaluronan-mediated motility
rhamnosus
  Lactobacillus r.
RhD immunoglobulin
Rheaban
rhegmatogenous detachment
Rheomacrodex
rheometer
Rhesonativ
Rhesus (Rh)
  R. factor
  R. rotavirus tetravalent (RRV-TV)
  R. rotavirus tetravalent vaccine
rheumatic
  r. carditis
  r. exanthema
  r. fever
  r. pneumonia
  r. valvular heart disease
rheumatism
  desert r.
  European League Against R.
    (EULAR)
  International League Against R.
    (ILAR)

rheumatogenic
  r. strain
  r. streptococcus
rheumatoid
  r. arthritis (RA)
  r. factor (RF)
  r. granuloma
  r. nodule
  r. spondylitis
rheumatology
Rheumatrex Oral
rhGH
  recombinant human growth hormone
rhIGF-1
  recombinant human insulin-like growth
    factor-1
Rhinall Nasal Solution
Rhindecon Rhinocaps
rhinencephalon
rhinitis
  allergic r.
  eosinophilic nonallergic r.
  erosive r.
  infectious r.
  r. medicamentosa
  neutrophilic r.
  nonallergenic perineal r.
  nonallergic r.
  perennial allergic r.
  pollen-induced r.
  r. of pregnancy
  purulent r.
  seasonal allergic r.
  serosanguineous r.
  r. sicca
  vasomotor r.
rhinobronchial reflex
rhinobronchitis
Rhinocaps
  Rhindecon R.
rhinocerebral
  r. infection
  r. mucormycosis
rhinoconjunctivitis
  allergic r.
Rhinocort
  R. Aqua nasal spray
  R. Turbuhaler
rhinorrhea
  cerebrospinal fluid r.
  CSF r.
rhinoscopy

R

NOTES

rhinosinusitis
    bacterial r.
Rhinosyn-DMX
Rhino Triangle brace
rhinovirus
rhizomelic
    r. chondrodysplasia
    r. chondrodysplasia punctata
      (RCDP)
    r. dwarfism
rhizotomy
    dorsal r.
    functional posterior r.
    posterior r.
    selective dorsal r. (SDR)
    selective posterior r.
Rh-negative mother
rhodamine
rhodamine-auramine stain
Rhodesian trypanosomiasis
Rho(D) immune globulin
Rhodococcus equi
RhoGAM
rhombencephalitis
rhombencephalosynapsis
rhombomere segmentation
rhonchorous cough
rhonchus, pl. **rhonchi**
RHS
    radial head subluxation
rhSOD
    recombinant human superoxide dismutase
rHuEPO, rHuEpo
    recombinant human erythropoietin
Rhulicaine
rhus dermatitis
rhusiopathiae
    Erysipelothrix r.
rhysodes
    Acanthamoeba r.
rhythm
    circadian r.
    escape r.
    gallop r.
    junctional r.
rhythmic movement disorder
RIA
    radioimmunoassay
rib
    cervical r.
    r. hump
    r. notching
    r. rotation
    r. splitting
RIBA
    recombinant immunosorbent assay

ribavirin
    aerosolized r.
    intraventricular r.
Ribbing skeletal abnormality
ribbonlike stool
riboflavin deficiency
Ribomunyl
ribonucleic acid (RNA)
ribonucleoprotein antigen
ribosome
ribosuria
ribotide
    succinyl aminoimidazole
      carboxamide r. (SAICAR)
RICE
    rest, ice, compression, elevation
    RICE sequence
Rice-Lyte
rich
    calcium r.
Richner-Hanhart syndrome
Richter hernia
ricinus
    Ixodes r.
rickets
    familial hypophosphatemic r.
    hypophosphatemic r.
    nonnutritional r.
    nutritional r.
    oncogenous r.
    primary hypophosphatemic r.
    renal r.
    vitamin D-dependent r.
    vitamin D-resistant r.
    X-linked hypophosphatemic r.
    (XLHR)
rickettsemia
Rickettsia
    R. africae
    R. akari
    R. australis
    R. conorii
    R. felis
    R. honei
    R. japonica
    R. prowazekii
    R. rickettsii
    R. siberica
    R. typhi
rickettsiae
rickettsial
    r. agglutination
    r. disease
    r. infection
rickettsialpox
rickettsii
    Rickettsia r.
rickettsiosis

RID
> R. gel
> R. liquid
> R. Mousse
> R. shampoo

Rid-A-Pain
Ridaura
Ridenol
ride-on toy
ridge
> alveolar r.
> apical ectodermal r.
> ectodermal r.
> hyperkeratotic r.

Riedel lobe
Rieger
> R. anomaly
> R. syndrome

rifabutin
Rifadin
rifampin
rifamycin
rifapentine
> 25-desacetyl r.

Rift Valley fever
RIG
> rabies immune globulin

Riga-Fede disease
right
> r. anterior oblique (RAO)
> r. aortic arch (RAA)
> r. atrial hypertrophy
> r. atrial pressure
> r. axis deviation
> r. bundle branch block (RBBB)
> r. colon pouch
> r. common carotid
> r. common carotid artery (RCCA)
> r. ductus arteriosus (RDA)
> r. femoral artery (RFA)
> r. hepatectomy
> r. lower quadrant (RLQ)
> r. lung hypoplasia
> r. lung-to-head circumference ratio (LHR)
> r. middle lobe syndrome
> r. sit
> termination of parental r.'s
> r. upper quadrant (RUQ)
> r. ventricle (RV)
> r. ventricular dysplasia
> r. ventricular hypertrophy
> r. ventricular infundibulum
> r. ventricular outflow tract (RVOT)
> r. ventricular outflow tract obstruction
> r. ventricular outflow tract reconstruction

righting
> head r.
> r. reaction
> r. reflex
> r. response

right-left discrimination
right-sided
> r.-s. heart failure
> r.-s. lesion

right-to-left
> r.-t.-l. shunt
> r.-t.-l. shunting
> r.-t.-l. shunt ratio (Qs/Qt)

rigid
> r. cerebral palsy
> r. clubfoot
> r. open-tube endoscope
> r. perfectionism
> r. spine syndrome
> r. supination deformity

rigidity
> chest wall r.
> decerebrate r.
> muscle r.
> nuchal r.
> parkinsonian r.

rigidus
> hallux r.

Rigiflex balloon
rigor
RIHD
> radiation-induced heart disease

Riley-Day syndrome
Riley-Shwachman syndrome
Riley-Smith syndrome
Rimactane
rimantadine
ring
> constriction r.
> r. constriction
> division of pancreatic r.
> Falope r.
> r. finger
> Kayser-Fleischer r.
> pancreatic r.
> phimotic r.

NOTES

ring *(continued)*
  Saturn r.
  r. sideroblast (RS)
  vascular r.
  visual tracking of red r.
  Waldeyer r.
  Wimberger r.
Ringer's
  R. lactate
  R. solution
ringworm
  beard r.
  black dot r.
  body r.
  groin r.
  nail r.
  scalp r.
rinse
  Nix Creme R.
  permethrin creme r.
Riobin
Riopan
RIP
  respiratory inductive plethysmography
RIPA
  radioimmunoprecipitation assay
rippling muscle disease
RIS
  respiratory index score
risedronate
risk
  r. behavior
  biological r.
  direct suicide r. (DSR)
  environmental r.
  established r.
  haplotype relative r. (HRR)
  high r.
  neonatal mortality r. (NMR)
risk-benefit ratio
risk-taking behavior
Risperdal
risperidone
Risser
  R. brace
  R. classification
  R. curve
  R. localizer cast
  R. sign
ristocetin cofactor activity
risus sardonicus
Ritalin
Ritalin-SR
Rite Time
RIT 4385 mumps strain
ritonavir (RTV)
Ritter disease

ritualism
ritualistic phenomenon
RLDS
  Reynell Language Developmental Scale
RLF
  retrolental fibroplasia
RLQ
  right lower quadrant
RLT
  reduced liver transplant
RMR
  resting metabolic rate
RMS
  rhabdomyosarcoma
    alveolar RMS
    embryonal RMS
    RMS Rectal
RMSF
  Rocky Mountain spotted fever
RN
  registered nurse
RNA
  ribonucleic acid
    RNA electrophoresis
    serum HCV RNA
Robafen AC, DM
Robaxin
Roberts-SC phocomelia syndrome
Robicillin VK
Robinow
  R. mesomelic dysplasia
  R. syndrome
Robins and Guze validation strategy
Robin syndrome
Robinul Forte
Robitet Oral
Robitussin
  R. A-C
  R. Cough Calmers
  R. Pediatric
Robitussin-DM
  R.-D. infant drops
Robomol
ROC
  receiver operating characteristic
Rocaltrol
Rocephin
Rochalimaea henselae
Roche Amplicor Monitor assay
Rochester
  R. criteria
  R. HKAFO
rocker-bottom
  r.-b. foot
  r.-b. foot deformity
rocking
  body r.

Rocky
    R. Mountain spotted fever (RMSF)
    R. Mountain wood tick
rocuronium
rod
    gram-negative r. (GNR)
    Harrington r.
    intramedullary r.
    Küntscher r.
    nemaline r.
    pleomorphic gram-negative r.
Rodby Electronik AB braked cycle ergometer
rodenticide poisoning
Roenigk
    R. classification scale
    R. grade
roentgenogram
roentgenograph
roentgenographic examination
roentgenography
    chest r.
Roferon-A
Rogaine Topical
Roger
    maladie de R.
Rohrer index
Rohypnol
Rokitansky-Küster-Hauser syndrome
rolandic
    r. epilepsy
    r. seizure
role reversal
roll
    therapy r.
Rollator
rolling
    segmental r.
ROM
    range of motion
Romaña sign
Romano-Ward long QT syndrome
Romazicon
    R. Injection
Romberg test
Rondec
    R. Drops
    R. Filmtab
    R. Syrup
Rondec-DM
Rondec-TR

rongeur
    pediatric bone r.
    Tobey ear r.
roof
    acetabular r.
    flat acetabular r.
rooftop incision
room air
rooming in
root
    aortic r.
    broad nasal r.
    mesenteric r.
    nasal r.
rooting reflex
ROP
    retinopathy of prematurity
ropelike filum terminale
rope sign
Rorschach test
ROS
    reactive oxygen species
    review of symptoms
    review of systems
rosacea
    acne r.
Rosai-Dorfman disease
rosary
    rachitic r.
    scorbutic r.
rosea
    pityriasis r.
Rosenberg Self-Esteem Scale (RSES)
Rosenthal fiber
roseola
    r. infantum
    r. rash
roseola-like illness
rose spot
rosette
    Homer Wright r.
    mucosal r.
rosettelike blister
ROSNI
    round spermatid nuclei injection
rOspA
    recombinant outer surface protein A
    rOspA Lyme disease vaccine
Ross
    R. carbohydrate-free (RCF)
    R. carbohydrate-free formula
    R. growth chart

R

NOTES

Ross *(continued)*
R. operation
R. procedure
R. pulmonary porcine valve
R. River virus
Ro/SSA antigen
Ross-Konno operation
Ross-Konno-Switch operation
Rossolimo reflex
rostral
r. direction
r. ventromedial medulla
rostrocaudal
rostrum
Rotacaps
Ventolin R.
Rotadisk
Flovent R.
Rotamune
rotary
r. atlantoaxial luxation
r. chewing
r. subluxation
RotaShield rotavirus vaccine
rotation
external r.
hip r.
lateral r. (LR)
lateral hip r.
medial r. (MR)
medial hip r.
r. movement
neutral r.
promax r.
rib r.
r. of spine
trunk r.
varimax r.
rotational
r. malalignment
r. osteotomy
rotationplasty
rotatory
r. displacement
r. subluxation
rotavirus (Rv)
r. enteritis
r. gastroenteritis
infantile diarrhea r.
r. vaccination
r. vaccine
Rotazyme
R. diagnostic procedure
R. test
rote memory
Rothmund syndrome
**Rothmund-Thomson cancer
predisposition syndrome**

Roth spot
Rotor
R. disease
R. syndrome
Rotter Sentence Completion Test
rough endoplasmic reticulum (RER)
rough-feeling skin
round
r. back deformity
r. cell tumor
r. iliac bone
r. moon face
r. spermatid nuclei injection
(ROSNI)
r. window electrocochleography
(RWECochG)
round-back
postural r.-b.
roundworm
Roussy-Lévy
R.-L. disease
R.-L. syndrome
route of delivery
routine wound management
Roux-en-Y
R.-e.-Y anastomosis
R.-e.-Y choledochojejunostomy
Rowasa Rectal
Roxanol SR Oral
Roxicet 5/500
Roxicodone
Roxilox
Roxiprin
roxithromycin
RP
Raynaud phenomenon
RPC
reactive perforating collagenosis
RPD
Pepcid RPD
RPE
retinal pigment epithelium
RPICC
regional perinatal intensive care center
RPLS
reversible posterior leukoencephalopathy
syndrome
RPM
Raven Progressive Matrices
RPMPR
radical posteromedial and plantar release
RPO
reflectance pulse oximetry
RPO oximeter
RPR
rapid plasma reagin
RRF
ragged red fiber

RRFC
 renal reserve filtration capacity
R-R interval
RRP
 recurrent respiratory papillomatosis
RRV-TV
 Rhesus rotavirus tetravalent
  RRV-TV vaccine
RS
 ring sideroblast
RS-61443
 mycophenolate mofetil
RSD
 reflex sympathetic dystrophy
RSE
 refractory status epilepticus
RSES
 Rosenberg Self-Esteem Scale
RSI
 rapid sequence intubation
RSL
 renal solute load
RSLT
 reduced-size liver transplant
RSV
 respiratory syncytial virus
  RSV antigen
  RSV bronchiolitis
  RSV immunoglobulin for
   intravenous administration (RSV-
   IGIV)
  RSV nasal wash
  RSV pneumonitis
RSVB
 respiratory syncytial virus bronchiolitis
RSVIG, RSV-IG
 respiratory syncytial virus immune
  globulin
 respiratory syncytial virus
  immunoglobulin
RSV-IGIV
 RSV immunoglobulin for intravenous
  administration
RSV-IVIG
 respiratory syncytial virus intravenous
  immunoglobulin
RT
 radiation therapy
RTA
 renal tubular acidosis
  distal RTA
  hyperkalemic RTA

  mineralocorticoid-deficiency RTA
  proximal RTA
  type IV RTA
RTI
 reverse transcriptase inhibitor
RT-PCR
 reverse transcription polymerase chain
  reaction
RTS
 Revised Trauma Score
RTV
 ritonavir
rub
  friction r.
  pericardial friction r.
  pleural friction r.
rubber bleb nevus
rubella
  congenital r.
  r. infection
  measles, mumps, r. (MMR)
  r. panencephalitis
  r. scarlatinosa
  r. syndrome
  third disease r.
  r. virus
rubeola
  r. scarlatinosa
  r. titer
Rubex
Rubinstein syndrome
Rubinstein-Taybi syndrome
Rubin tube
Rubivirus
rubor
rubra
  miliaria r.
Rubramin-PC
rubroolivocerebellorubral loop
rubrum
  tinea r.
  Trichophyton r.
Rudiger syndrome
rudimentary
  r. testis syndrome
  r. vagina
rudimentary-type digit
3-way Rudolph valve
Rud syndrome
Rufen
rugated vaginal mucosa
rugger jersey spine

NOTES

R

rule
    10% r.
    r. of nines
    Ottawa Ankle R.'s (OAR)
    Trauma Triage R. (TTR)
Rumack-Matthew nomogram
rumble
    middiastolic r.
rumbling murmur
rumination disorder
Rum-K
runoff
    aortic r.
rupture
    aortic arch r.
    arterial r.
    cardiac r.
    neural tube r.
    ovarian r.
    peroneal r.
    testicular r.
    ureteral r.
ruptured
    r. appendicitis
    r. bronchiole
    r. globe
    r. sinus of Valsalva aneurysm
RUQ
    right upper quadrant
Rusch bag
rush immunotherapy
Russell
    R. sign
    R. syndrome
    R. traction
Russell-Silver dwarf syndrome
Russian spring-summer encephalitis

rust-colored sputum
ruthenium
Rutledge syndrome
Rutter mean score
Ruvalcaba-Myhre-Smith syndrome
Ru-Vert-M
RV
    residual volume
    right ventricle
Rv
    rotavirus
      Rv vaccine
RVA
    rabies vaccine, absorbed
RVDT
    retinal venous dilation and tortuosity
RVOT
    right ventricular outflow tract
RVPaque cream
RVR
    relative vascular resistance
RVS
    recognizable viral syndrome
R wave
RWECochG
    round window electrocochleography
Rx
    prescription
      Rx medibottle
Ryan agar
Rye classification
Ryna-C
Ryna-CX
Ryna Liquid
Rynatan Pediatric
RZ
    reserve zone

S-26
    S-26 formula
    S-26 LBW formula
S-29 formula
S-44 formula
SA
    sinoatrial node
saber shin
Sabin
    S. OPV
    S. vaccine
Sabin-Feldman dye test
sabot
    coeur en s.
Sabourad dextrose media
sabre
    scleroderma en coup de s.
    s. shin deformity
Sabril
sac
    nasolacrimal s.
    yolk s.
SACA
    Service Assessment for Children and
    Adolescents
saccade
saccharate
    dextroamphetamine s.
Saccharomyces
    S. boulardii
    S. cerevisiae
saccharopinuria
saccular
    s. dilation
    s. stage
    s. stage of lung development
sacral
    s. agenesis
    s. dimple
    s. meningomyelocele
sacrococcygeal teratoma
sacroiliac (SI)
sacroiliitis
sacrosidase
sacrum
SAD
    seasonal affective disorder
    separation anxiety disorder
saddle
    s. anesthesia
    s. nose
saddleback
    s. fever
    s. temperature curve

saddle-nose deformity
S-adenosylhomocysteine (SAH)
sadness
Saethre-Chotzen syndrome
Safe Tussin 30
saginata
    Taenia s.
sagittal
    s. craniosynostosis
    s. sinus
    s. sinus thrombosis
    s. suture
    s. synostosis
sagrada
    cascara s.
SAH
    S-adenosylhomocysteine
SAICAR
    succinyl aminoimidazole carboxamide
    ribotide
sail sign
Saizen Injection
Sakati-Nyhan syndrome
salaam seizure
Salacid Ointment
Sal-Acid Plaster
Salagen Oral
salbutamol
Saldino-Noonan
    S.-N. short rib polydactyly
    S.-N. syndrome
Saleto-200
Saleto-400
salicylate intoxication
salicylic
    s. acid
    s. acid ointment
    s. sugar powder
salicylism
saline
    extrarenal s.
    heparinized s.
    hypotonic s.
    iced s.
    s. infusion sonography (SIS)
    isotonic s.
    s. lavage
    normal s.
    s. nose drop
    phosphate-buffered s.
    s. solution
SalineX
saliva
salivarius
    Streptococcus s.

S

salivary
>s. adenitis
>s. amylase
>s. cortisol
>s. cortisol assay
>s. gland

Salk
>S. IPV
>S. vaccine

Salla disease
salmeterol
>s. powder
>s. xinafoate

Salmonella
>S. bacteria
>S. *choleraesuis*
>S. *dublin*
>S. *enteritidis*
>S. gastroenteritis
>S. *heidelberg*
>S. *hirschfeldii*
>S. meningitis
>S. *newport*
>non-typhi *S.* (NTS)
>nontyphoidal *S.*
>S. *oranienburg*
>S. *oranienburg* sepsis
>S. osteomyelitis
>S. *paratyphi*
>S. *schottmuelleri*
>S. *typhi*
>S. *typhimurium*

salmonellosis
Salmonine
salmon patch
salmon-pink rash
salpingitis
salt
>bile s.
>calcium s.
>s. craving
>s. frosting of skin
>gold s.
>guanidine s.
>inorganic mercury s.
>s. poisoning
>s. wasting

salt-and-pepper appearance
Salter
>S. injury (type I–IV)
>S. procedure

Salter-Harris
>S.-H. classification
>S.-H. classification of epiphyseal plate injury
>S.-H. classification of fracture
>S.-H. epiphyseal fracture
>S.-H. fracture (type I–V)

salt-losing adrenogenital syndrome
salt-wasting adrenogenital syndrome
saltwater near drowning
salute
>allergic s.

salvage
>s. chemotherapy
>s. laparotomy
>limb s.

sample
>blood s.
>citrate blood s.
>cord blood s.
>midstream urine s.
>urine s.

sampling
>blood s.
>chorionic villus s. (CVS)
>fetal scalp blood s.
>percutaneous umbilical blood s. (PUBS)
>umbilical blood s.
>venous blood s.

San
>S. Joaquin fever
>S. Luis Valley syndrome

Sanders jet respirator
Sandhoff
>S. disease
>S. GM_2 gangliosidosis (type I, II)

Sandifer syndrome
Sandimmune
Sandoglobulin
Sandostatin LAR Depot
sandpaper rash
Sanfilippo A, B syndrome
SangCya
sanguinis
>*Gemella s.*

Sani-Supp Suppository
SANS
>schedule for negative symptoms

Santavuori
>S. disease
>muscle-eye-brain disease of S.

S 100 antibody
Santulli-Blanc enterostomy
Santulli enterostomy
SAO
>Southeast Asian ovalocytosis

SAP
>systolic arterial pressure

SAP1
>sphingolipid activator protein-1

saphenous
>s. nerve entrapment
>s. vein

Sapporo virus

saprophytic
saprophyticus
    Staphylococcus s.
SAPS
    schedule for positive symptoms
    simplified acute physiology score
saquinavir (SQV)
sarcoid
    alveolar s.
sarcoidosis
    nervous system s.
    ocular s.
    subcutaneous s.
sarcolemma
sarcoma
    alveolar soft part s.
    blue-cell s.
    s. botryoides
    Burkitt s.
    chordoid s.
    clear cell s.
    Ewing s.
    extraosseous Ewing s.
    granulocytic s.
    immunoblastic s.
    Kaposi s. (KS)
    Kaposi varicelliform s.
    neurogenic s.
    nonrhabdomyogenic soft tissue s.
    nonrhabdomyomatous s.
    nonrhabdomyosarcoma soft tissue s.
      (NRSTS)
    osteogenic s.
    pseudoglandular synovial s.
    soft-tissue s.
    synovial s.
    tenosynovial s.
    vaginal s.
sarcomatous tumor
sarcomere
sarcomeric filament
sarcoplasmic reticulum
sarcoptic mange
sarcosinemia
sardonic smile
sardonicus
    risus s.
sargramostim
Sarna lotion
Sarnat
    S. encephalopathy
    S. score

Saskatoon
    hemoglobin M S.
Sastid Plain Therapeutic Shampoo and Acne Wash
satellite
    s. lesion
    s. melanocytic nevus
    s. papule
    s. pustule
satellitosis
satiety
    early s.
sativa
    Cannabis s.
saturated solution of potassium iodide (SSKI)
saturation
    O_2 s.
    oxygen s.
    oxyhemoglobin s.
    transferrin s.
Saturn ring
Sauflon PW contact lens
Saunders disease
sausage digit
sausage-shaped bulla
Save-A-Tooth
sawtoothed flutter wave
S-beta-thal
SBFE
    Stanford-Binet Fourth Edition
SBHC
    school-based health center
SBM
    selective broth medium
SBP
    spontaneous biliary perforation
SBS
    short bowel syndrome
SBT
    serum bactericidal titer
SC
    hemoglobin SC
SCA
    spinocerebellar ataxia (type 1)
Scabene
scabicide
scabies
    animal s.
    canine s.
    crusted s.
    human s.

S

NOTES

scabies *(continued)*
    s. mite
    neonatal s.
    Norwegian s.
    s. scraping
SCAD
    short-chain acyl coenzyme A
    dehydrogenase
    SCAD deficiency
scala tympani
scalded skin syndrome (SSS)
scalding injury
scale
    Abnormal Involuntary Movement S.
      (AIMS)
    Alberta Infant Motor S. (AIMS)
    Albert Einstein Neonatal
      Developmental S.
    anxiety-withdrawal s.
    Attention Deficit Disorders
      Evaluation S.
    attrition rate s.
    BAMO s.
    Barnes Akathisia S. (BAS)
    Bayley Developmental S.
    Bayley Mental S.
    Behavioral and Emotional
      Rating S. (BERS)
    Behavior Rating S. (BRS)
    Bieri s.
    Brazelton Neonatal Assessment S.
      (BNAS)
    Brazelton Neonatal Behavioral
      Assessment S. (BNBAS)
    broad-band s.
    Canadian Acute Respiratory Illness
      and Flu S. (CARIFS)
    Carey Temperament S.
    Cattell Infant Intelligence S.
    CGI s.
    Child and Adolescent Functional
      Assessment S. (CAFAS)
    Childhood Autism Rating S.
      (CARS)
    S. for Children and Adolescents
    Children's Depression S.
    Children's Depression Rating S.-
      Revised (CDRS-R)
    Children's Global Assessment S.
      (CGAS)
    Children's Manifest Anxiety S.
    Clinical Adaptive Test/Clinical
      Linguistic and Auditory
      Milestone S. (CAT/CLAMS)
    Clinical Global Impairment s.
    Clinical Global Impressions s.
    Clinical Global Improvement s.

    Clinical Linguistic and Auditory
      Milestone S. (CLAMS)
    color analog s.
    Columbia Impairment S.
    Conners Rating S. (CRS)
    CRIES Neonatal Postoperative
      Pain S.
    depression rating s.
    Depression Self-Rating S.
    Disruptive Behavior Disorder S.
    Dyadic Adjustment S.
    Dyskinesia Identification System:
      Condensed User S. (DISCUS)
    Early Language Milestone s.
    Edinburgh Postnatal Depression S.
      (EPDS)
    Einstein Neonatal Neurobehavioral
      Assessment S. (ENNAS)
    electronic s.
    ELM s.
    Emotionality Activity Sociability S.
      (EAS)
    Externalizing Behavior S.
    Family Adaptability and Cohesion
      Evaluation S. (FACES)
    Family Adaptability and
      Cohesion S.-III
    Family Environment S.
    FLACC s.
    Flint Infant Security S.
    Functional Assessment S.
    Gesell Child Development Age S.
      (GCDAS)
    Gesell Developmental S. (GDS)
    Gesell Infant S.
    Glasgow Coma S. (GCS)
    gray s.
    Griffiths Mental Developmental S.
      (GMDS)
    Hamilton Depression S. (HAMD)
    HOME s.
    Home Observation for Measurement
      of the Environment s.
    HSC S.
    Internalizing Behavior S.
    IPAT Depression S.
    Kent Infant Development S.
    Leiter International Performance S.
    Likert s.
    linear visual analog s.
    Locus of Control S.
    McCarthy Memory S.
    McGrath s.
    mental s.
    motor s.
    Multidimensional Student Life
      Satisfaction S. (MSLSS)

Neonatal Behavioral Assessment S.
  (NBAS)
Neonatal Infant Pain S. (NIPS)
Newborn Behavior Assessment S.
  (NBAS)
NIMH global s.
Oucher s.
Parent and Teacher Conners S.
Peabody Developmental Motor S.
  (PDMS)
Pediatric Liver Transplant-
  Specific S. (PLTSS)
Piers-Harris Children's Self-
  Concept S.
Plutchik Impulsivity S.
prosocial behavior s.
Receptive-Expressive Emergent
  Language S. (REEL)
Revised Children's Manifest
  Anxiety S. (RCMAS)
Reynell Developmental Language S.
Reynell Language Developmental S.
  (RLDS)
Reynolds Child Depression S.
Roenigk classification s.
Rosenberg Self-Esteem S. (RSES)
shyness s.
Simpson-Angus rating s.
standardized observation s.
Stanford-Binet Intelligence S.
Tanner Developmental S.
Toddler Temperament S.
Toronto Alexithymia S. (TAS)
Vineland Adaptive Behavior S.
Vineland Social Maturity S.
visual analog s. (VAS)
Wechsler Memory S.
Wender Utah Rating S. (WURS)
Wong-Baker Faces Pain Rating S.
Yale-Brown Obsessive
  Compulsive S. (YBOCS)
Yale Global Tic Severity S.
  (YGTSS)
Yale Observation S.
scalene muscle
scaling
  brawny s.
  s. bulla
  keratotic s.
  Organ Injury S. (OIS)
  oval s.
scalloped temporalis muscle

scalloping
scalp
  s. electrode
  s. intravenous
  s. IV
  s. pH
  s. ringworm
  s. seborrheic dermatitis
  s. vein catheter
  s. vein catheterization
Scalpicin Topical
scaly dermatitis
SCAN
  suspected child abuse or neglect
scan
  bone s.
  computed tomography s.
  computerized tomographic s.
  CT s.
  DEXA s.
  diethylenetetramine pentaacetic acid
    radionuclide s.
  double-contrast CT s.
  DTPA s.
  dual-energy x-ray absorptiometry s.
  expiratory s.
  gallium s.
  gallium-67 s.
  helical s.
  indium-labeled leukocyte s.
  Meckel s.
  MIBG s.
  milk s.
  MUGA s.
  pinhole collimated s.
  planar bone s.
  radioisotope milk s.
  radiolabeled white blood cell s.
  radionuclide bone s.
  radionuclide heart s.
  red cell tagged s.
  spiral s.
  Tc HMPAO leukocyte s.
  technetium bone s.
  technetium
    hexamethylpropyleneamine oxime
    leukocyte s.
  technetium-99m bone s.
  testicular flow s.
  ventilation-perfusion s.
  xenon CT s.
ScandiShake

S

NOTES

scanner
Acuson 128/XP10 s.
scanning
CAT s.
computerized tomography s.
CT s.
Doppler s.
gated blood pool s.
isotope s.
s. photometry
radionuclide s.
spectrophotometric s.
ultrasound s.
scaphocephalism
scaphocephaly
scaphoid
s. abdomen
s. pad
s. scapula
scapula, pl. **scapulae**
scaphoid s.
scapular
s. fracture
s. repositioning
s. winging
scapularis
Ixodes s.
scapulohumeral muscular dystrophy
scapuloperoneal dystrophy
scapulothoracic motion
scar
depressed s.
hypertrophic s.
s. tissue
scare
vaccine-autism s.
SCARED
Screen for Child Anxiety-Related
Emotional Disorders
scarf sign
scarlatina antitoxin
scarlatiniform
s. eruption
s. erythema
s. rash
scarlatinosa
rubella s.
rubeola s.
scarlet
s. fever
s. fever exanthem
SCARMD
severe childhood autosomal recessive
muscular dystrophy
scarring
corneal s.
renal s.
Scatchard analysis

scattered scores
scattering
Rayleigh-Tyndall s.
SCD
sickle cell disease
Scepter system
SCFA
short-chain fatty acid
SCFE
slipped capital femoral epiphysis
acute on chronic SCFE
chronic SCFE
Preslip SCFE
SCHAD
short-chain hydroxyacyl-coenzyme A
dehydrogenase
schedule
S. for Affective Disorders and
Schizophrenia for School-Age
Children (K-SADS)
S. for Affective Disorders and
Schizophrenia for School-Age
Children-Epidemiologic Version
(K-SADS-E)
S. for Affective Disorders and
Schizophrenia for School-Age
Children-Present Episode (K-
SADS-P)
agglomeration s.
Autism Diagnostic Observation S.
(ADOS)
child assessment s. (CAS)
Gesell Developmental S.'s
life events and difficulties s.
(LEDS)
s. for negative symptoms (SANS)
s. for positive symptoms (SAPS)
Scheibe
S. anomaly
S. aplasia
Scheie syndrome
schema
TNM s.
schenckii
Sporothrix s.
Scheuermann
S. disease
S. juvenile kyphosis
Scheuer score
Scheuthauer-Marie-Sainton syndrome
Schiff
periodic acid S. (PAS)
S. test
Schilder
S. disease
S. encephalitis
Schilling test
Schimke immunoosseous dysplasia

Schindler disease
Schinzel-Giedion syndrome
Schinzel-type acrocallosal syndrome
SCHIP
> State Children's Health Insurance
> Program
> SCHIP evaluation tool

schistocyte
schistocytic hemolytic anemia
Schistosoma
> S. *haematobium*
> S. *intercalatum*
> S. *japonicum*
> S. *mansoni*
> S. *mekongi*

schistosomal myelopathy
schistosomiasis
> acute s.
> cerebral s.
> chronic s.

schistosomula
schistothorax
schizencephaly
schizoaffective disorder
schizoid personality disorder
schizont
schizophasia
schizophrenia
> childhood s.
> childhood-onset s. (COS)
> early-onset s. (EOS)
> very early onset s. (VEOS)

schizophrenic
schizophreniform disorder
schizotypal
schizotypy
Schlemm canal
Schmid-like metaphyseal chondrodysplasia
Schmid metaphyseal dysplasia
Schmidt-Lantermann incisure
Schmidt syndrome
Schmorl node
Schober test
Schofield
> S. weight-based resting energy expenditure prediction equation
> S. weight- and height-based resting energy expenditure prediction equation

Schönlein-Henoch purpura

school
> s. avoidance
> s. failure hypothesis
> s. phobia
> S. Sleep Habits Survey

school-based
> s.-b. health center (SBHC)
> s.-b. intervention

school, home, activities, depression/self-esteem, substance
schottmuelleri
> *Salmonella s.*

Schuco nebulizer
Schuknecht
> S. classification
> S. classification of congenital aural atresia (type A–D)

Schwann cell
schwannian differentiation
schwannoma
> acoustic s.
> malignant s.

Schwartz-Jampel
> S.-J. disease
> S.-J. syndrome

Schwartzman phenomenon
Schwarz measles strain
sciatic nerve
SCID
> severe combined immunodeficiency
> severe combined immunodeficiency disease

SCIDS
> severe combined immunodeficiency syndrome

science
> Statistical Package for Social S.'s (SPSS)

scimitar syndrome
scintigram
scintigraphy
> cortical s.
> dipyridamole myocardial s.
> hepatobiliary s.
> radionuclide s.
> renal s.
> somatostatin receptor s.
> thyroid s.

scintillating scotoma
scintillation
scintography
> gallium s.

S

NOTES

509

scissored position
scissoring posture
SCIWORA
  spinal cord injury without radiographic
    abnormality
    SCIWORA syndrome
sclera, pl. sclerae
  blue s.
scleral icterus
scleredema
  s. adultorum
  s. of Buschke
  s. neonatorum
sclerema neonatorum
sclerocornea
sclerodactyly
scleroderma
  s. en coup de sabre
  focal s.
  limited systemic s.
  linear s.
  localized s.
  morphea s.
  s. renal crisis
  secondary s.
  systemic s.
scleroderma-like syndrome
sclerodermatomyositis antigen
scleromyxedema
sclerosant
sclerose en plaque
sclerosing
  s. cholangitis
  s. osteomyelitis
  s. panencephalitis
sclerosis, pl. scleroses
  Ammon horn s.
  amyotrophic lateral s.
  arterial fibrosing s.
  bone s.
  childhood progressive systemic s.
  concentric s.
  diffuse glomerular s.
  diffuse mesangial s. (DMS)
  disseminated s.
  endocardial s.
  focal segmental glomerular s.
  glomerular s.
  hippocampal s.
  isolated diffuse mesangial s.
    (IDMS)
  juvenile amyotrophic lateral s.
  lobar s.
  mantle s.
  mesangial s.
  mesial temporal s. (MTS)
  metaphysical s.
  multiple s. (MS)

  myelinoclastic diffuse cerebral s.
  nodular cortical s.
  sudanophilic cerebral s.
  sudanophilic diffuse s.
  systemic s. (SS)
  tuberous s.
sclerosis-hyalinosis
  focal and segmental glomerular s.-
    h.
sclerotherapy
  endoscopic s.
  endoscopic variceal s. (EVS)
  injection s.
sclerotome
SCM
  split cord malformation
  sternocleidomastoid
  SCM muscle
SCMI
  single central maxillary incisor
SCN
  severe chronic neutropenia
scoliometer
scoliosis
  adolescent s.
  adolescent idiopathic s. (AIS)
  compensatory s.
  congenital s.
  Dwyer correction of s.
  s. film
  idiopathic s.
  infantile idiopathic s.
  juvenile idiopathic s.
  mild s.
  neuromuscular s.
  postural s.
  secondary s.
scombroid
  s. intoxication
  s. poisoning
scooter board
Scop
  Transderm S.
scopolamine
scorbutic rosary
score
  acute change clinical s. (ACCS)
  Akaike s.
  Apgar s.
  Ashworth s.
  Asthma Severity S. (ASS)
  Ballard s.
  Ballard Assessment S. (BAS)
  Bayley Motor S.
  Berlin s.
  bilirubin-induced neurologic
    dysfunction s.
  BIND s.

birth weight Z s.
Boix-Ochoa s. (BOS)
CRIB s.
Croup S.
developmental assessment s.
Downes s.
Dubowitz s.
EDIN behavioral s.
Euler and Byrne s.
externalizing s.
global seasonality s.
Herson-Todd s.
home cognitive s.
I antigen s.
injury severity s. (ISS)
internalizing s.
Kaufman Factor S.
Methods for the Epidemiology of
  Child and Adolescent Disorders
  T s.
Modified Injury Severity S. (MISS)
Neonatal Abstinence S. (NAS)
S. for Neonatal Acute Physiology
  (SNAP)
S. for Neonatal Acute Physiology-
  Perinatal Extension
Neonatal Skin Assessment S.
New Ballard S. (NBS)
Nursery Neurobiological Risk S.
  (NBRS)
optimality s.
Pediatric Risk of Mortality S.
  (PRISM)
Pediatric Trauma S. (PTS)
PREM s.
Prematurity Risk Evaluation
  Measure s.
raw s.
respiratory index s. (RIS)
Revised Trauma S. (RTS)
Rutter mean s.
Sarnat s.
scattered s.'s
Scheuer s.
Shwachman s.
Shwachman-Kulczycki s.
simplified acute physiology s.
  (SAPS)
SNAP s.
standard deviation s. (SDS)
Stanford-Binet s.
Vineland standard s.'s

WDL asthma s.
WISC-III factor s.'s
Wood-Downes asthma s.
Wood-Downes-Lecks asthma s.

SCOT
  succinyl CoA:3-ketoacid CoA transferase
  SCOT deficiency
Scotch tape slide test
scotoma, pl. **scotomata**
  facultative s.
  scintillating s.
scotopic sensitivity syndrome
Scot-Tussin
  S.-T. DM Dough Chasers
  S.-T. Senior Clear
Scotty dog
scout radiograph
SCPUFA
  short-chain polyunsaturated fatty acid
scrapie
scraping
  conjunctival s.
  scabies s.
  skin s.
screaming
screen
  S. for Child Anxiety-Related
    Emotional Disorders (SCARED)
  Monospot s.
  qualitative urine s.
  Rapid Strep s.
  serum lysosomal enzyme s.
  suicide risk s. (SRS)
  Supplemental Newborn S.
  TORCH s.
  toxicology s.
  triple s.
  universal bilirubin s.
  universal hearing s.
  urine toxicology s.
screener
  Algo newborn hearing s.
  Oregon Adolescent Depression
    Project-Conduct Disorder S.
    (OADP-CDS)
screening
  AABR hearing s.
  amino acid s.
  automated auditory brainstem
    response hearing s.
  s. culture
  Denver II s.

S

NOTES

screening *(continued)*
  FA s.
  s. test
  S. Tests for Young Children and Retardates (STYCAR)
screw
  cannulated s.
screw-tipped intraosseous needle
scrofula
scrofulaceum
  Mycobacterium s.
scrofuloderma
scrofulosorum
  lichen s.
scrotal
  s. edema
  s. mass
  s. orchiopexy
  s. position
  s. testis
  s. tongue
scrotum, pl. **scrota, scrotums**
  bifid s.
  raphe of s.
scrub
  Exidine S.
  s. typhus
SCT
  stem cell transplantation
scurvy
  hemorrhagic s.
  infantile s.
scybala
S/D
  Gammagard S/D
  Polygam S/D
SDH
  subdural hematoma
SDR
  selective dorsal rhizotomy
SDS
  standard deviation score
SE
  signed English
  status epilepticus
se
  per s.
SEA
  seronegativity, enthesopathy, arthropathy spondylitis, enthesitis, arthritis
  SEA syndrome
seabather's eruption
sea-blue histiocyte
seallike cough
seam
  osteoid s.
  urethral s.
SeaMist

searching toe
seasonal
  s. affective disorder (SAD)
  s. allergic rhinitis
  s. asthma
  S. Pattern Assessment Questionnaire (SPAQ)
  s. pollinosis
seat
  bath s.
  s. belt sign
  s. belt syndrome
SEB
  staphylococcal enterotoxin B
sebacceous hyperplasia
sebaceous
  s. collar
  s. duct
  s. gland
  s. gland lobule
  s. miliaria
  s. nevus
  s. nevus syndrome
sebaceum
  adenoma s.
seborrhea
  adolescent s.
  infantile s.
seborrheic
  s. blepharitis
  s. dermatitis
  s. diaper rash
  s. eczema
seborrheic-like facies
seborrheic-looking skin lesion
Sebulex
sebum secretion
Sebutone shampoo
Seckel syndrome
secobarbital
Seconal
second
  s. bicuspid
  s. branchial cleft cyst
  forced expiratory volume in 1 s. (FEV$_1$)
  s. heart sound
  s. impact syndrome
  S. National Incidence Study (NIS-2)
  s. permanent molar
  s. primary molar
secondary
  s. adrenal hypoplasia
  s. alopecia
  s. amenorrhea
  s. amyloidosis
  s. apnea

s. carnitine deficiency
s. circular reaction
s. closure
s. craniosynostosis
s. dystonia
s. enuresis
s. epilepsy
s. headache
s. hematoma
s. hyperoxaluria
s. hypochondriasis
s. intention
s. localized peritonitis
s. lymphedema
s. macrodactyly
s. macular atrophy
s. microcephaly
s. moyamoya disease
s. nail dystrophy
s. nephrotic syndrome
s. osteosarcoma
s. PAP
s. phimosis
s. pneumonitis
s. polycythemia
s. prophylaxis
s. scleroderma
s. scoliosis
s. seizure
s. solar urticaria
s. syphilis
s. teeth
s. tracheomalacia
s. vesicoureteral reflux
s. viremia
second-degree
s.-d. burn
s.-d. heart block
s.-d. hypospadias
second-hand smoking
secretagogue
secrete
secretin
Secretin-Ferring
secretion
dysregulated insulin s.
excessive acid s.
excessive insulin s.
inappropriate antidiuretic
hormone s.
insulin s.

sebum s.
SIADH s.
secretively
secretory
s. diarrhea
s. otitis media
section
cesarean s.
secundum
s. ASD
foramen s.
ostium s.
secure attachment
SED
serious emotional disturbance
spondyloepiphyseal dysplasia
late-onset SED
sedation
chloral hydrate s.
conscious s.
ketamine s.
Observer Assessment of Alertness
and S. (OAAS)
pediatric s.
sedative
sedentary
sediment
urine s.
sedimentation rate
sedlakii
Citrobacter s.
SEE
signed exact English
seed
vitreous s.
seeding
hematogenous s.
single tumor with s.
tumor s.
vitreous s.
seeking
food s.
seesaw
s. breathing
s. nystagmus
SEF
spectral edge frequency
segment
upper body s.
segmental
s. amyoplasia
s. aneuploidy

NOTES

S

513

segmental *(continued)*
  s. dystonia
  s. edema
  s. hypoplasia
  s. mesangial hypercellularity
  s. neurofibromatosis
  s. rolling
  s. spinal instrumentation
segmentation
  rhombomere s.
segmentectomy
segmented
  s. neutrophil
  s. neutrophil cell
segregation
Seip-Lawrence syndrome
Seitelberger disease
seizure
  absence s.
  afebrile s.
  akinetic s.
  anoxic s.
  apneic s.
  astatic s.
  atonic s.
  atypical absence s.
  atypical petit mal s.
  autonomic s.
  benign familial neonatal s.
  bicuculline-induced s.
  brief tonic s.
  clonic s.
  complex febrile s.
  complex partial s. (CPS)
  convulsive s.
  s. disorder
  drop s.
  epilepsy s.
  familial neonatal s.
  febrile s.
  focal motor s.
  generalized tonic-clonic s.
  grand mal s.
  hypocalcemic s.
  hypoglycemic s.
  hyponatremic s.
  hysteric s.
  hysterical s.
  idiopathic s.
  infantile monoclonic s.
  infantile myoclonic s.
  jackknife s.
  jacksonian s.
  local s.
  localization-related epilepsy s.
  major motor s.
  minor motor s.
  monoclonic s.

  motor s.
  multifocal clonic s.
  myoclonic s.
  myoclonic-astatic s.
  neonatal s.
  nonconvulsive s.
  nonepileptic s.
  nonphotogenic s.
  partial complex s.
  petit mal s.
  photogenic s.
  photosensitive s.
  postasphyxial s.
  primary generalized s.
  psychogenic s.
  psychomotor s.
  pyridoxine-dependent s.
  recurrent convulsive s.
  recurrent nonconvulsive s.
  reflex anoxic s.
  repeated partial s.
  rolandic s.
  salaam s.
  secondary s.
  sensory s.
  severe s.
  simple febrile s.
  simple partial s. (SPS)
  subtle s.
  sylvian s.
  temporal lobe s.
  tetanic s.
  tonic s.
  tonic-clonic s.
  versive s.
  vertiginous s.
  vestibular s.
  vestibulogenic s.
Seldane
Seldinger technique
selective
  s. angiography
  s. aplasia
  s. aplasia of vermis
  s. broth medium (SBM)
  s. dorsal rhizotomy (SDR)
  s. IgA deficiency
  s. intrapartum chemoprophylaxis (SIC)
  s. mutism
  s. neuronal necrosis
  s. posterior rhizotomy
  s. proteinuria
  s. pulmonary arteriography
  s. reading disability
  s. renal vein renin determination
  s. right ventriculography

S

s. serotonin reuptake inhibitor (SSRI)
Select joint
selenium sulfide
Sele-Pak
Selepen
Selestoject Injection
self
self-comforting behavior
self-concept
self-control
self-deprecation
self-esteem
self-harm
self-reported s.-h. (SRSH)
self-harming act
self-help domain
self-induced vomiting
self-injectable epinephrine
self-injurious behavior (SIB)
self-limited
self-mutilating behavior
self-mutilation
compulsive s.-m.
self-report
youth s.-r. (YSR)
self-reported self-harm (SRSH)
self-statement
coping s.-s.
self-stimulation
self-worth
sella, pl. **sellae**
J-shaped s.
tuberculum s.
s. turcica
Sellick maneuver
Selsun Blue Shampoo
selvagem
Fogo s.
SEM
skin, eye, mucocutaneous
systolic ejection murmur
SEM infection
semantic-pragmatic disorder
semantics
semiallogenic
semicircular canal
semiclemental casein hydrolysate formula
semifluid diet
semi-Fowler position
semilobar holoprosencephaly

semilunar
s. valvular stenosis
semimembranosus muscle
seminiferous
s. tubule
s. tubule dysgenesis
seminoma
semistructured psychiatric interview (SSI)
semisynthetic penicillin
semitendinosus muscle
Sengers
S. cardiomyopathy
S. mitochondrial myopathy
S. syndrome
Sengstaken-Blakemore tube
senility
premature s.
senior
Phenadex S.
Senior-Loken syndrome
senna
Senna-Gen
sennetsu
Ehrlichia s.
s. ehrlichiosis
Senning
S. atrial switch procedure
S. operation
Senokot
Senolax
sensation
impaired rectal s.
integrate s.
proprioceptive s.
rectal s.
sense
vibration s.
sensitivity
chemoreceptor s.
culture and s. (C&S)
gluten s.
sensitization
contact s.
food-antigen s.
utero s.
sensor
acoustic respiratory motion s. (ARMS)
multiparameter intraarterial s. (MPIAS)
Resp-EZ piezoelectric s.

NOTES

515

Sensorcaine
Sensorcaine-MPF
sensorimotor integration
sensorineural
    s. deafness
    s. hearing impairment
    s. hearing loss (SNHL)
sensorium
    altered s.
    clouding of s.
    depressed s.
Sensormedic 3100A 8000 oscillator
sensory
    s. arthropathy
    s. impairment
    s. information
    s. integration
    s. integration therapy
    s. loss
    s. nerve
    s. nerve conduction velocity
    s. neuropathy
    s. overload
    s. polyneuritis
    s. problem
    s. seizure
    s. stimulation
    s. threshold
sensory-motor stage
sentence
    five-word s.
sentinel loop
separation
    s. anxiety
    s. anxiety disorder (SAD)
    commissural s.
    decreased commissural s.
    Ficoll s.
    physeal s.
    premature placental s.
separation-reunion experience
Sephardic Jew
Sep-Pak
sepsis
    bacterial s.
    Chlamydia s.
    early-onset s.
    Escherichia coli s.
    fulminant s.
    group B streptococcal s.
    late-onset s.
    Listeria monocytogenes s.
    neonatal s.
    nosocomial s.
    pneumococcal s.
    portal vein s.
    postanginal s.
    Salmonella oranienburg s.

    s. syndrome
    s. workup
sepsis/shock syndrome
septa (*pl. of* septum)
septal
    s. defect
    s. deviation
    s. panniculitis
Septata intestinalis
septate vagina
septation
    aorticopulmonary s.
    cardiac s.
    tracheoesophageal s.
    ventricular s.
Septa Topical Ointment
septectomy
    atrial s.
    surgical s.
septi (*gen. of* septum)
septic
    s. arthritis
    s. bursitis
    s. embolus
    s. encephalitis
    s. joint
    s. meningitis
    s. shock
    s. thrombophlebitis
septicemia
    clostridia s.
    gonococcal s.
    meningococcal s.
    postnatal s.
septicum
    Clostridium s.
Septisol
septooptic dysplasia
septooptic-pituitary dysplasia
septophilic
septophobic
septostomy
    atrial s.
    balloon s.
    balloon atrial s. (BAS)
    catheter s.
    echo-guided balloon atrial s.
    Rashkind balloon atrial s.
Septra DS
septum, gen. septi, pl. septa
    anterior nasal s.
    conotruncal s.
    deviated s.
    interventricular s.
    membranous s.
    midvaginal transverse s.
    muscular ventricular s.
    nasal s.

nucleus accumbens septi
orbital s.
outlet s.
s. pellucidum
perimembranous s.
s. primum
proximal transverse s.
pulmonary atresia with intact
   ventricular s. (PAIVS)
Swiss cheese s.
trabecular muscular s.
tracheoesophageal s.
transverse vaginal s.
s. transversum
vaginal s.
ventricular s.
sequel
   Diamox S.'s
sequela, pl. **sequelae**
   cardiovascular s.
   delayed neuropsychological s.
   (DNS)
   neurodevelopmental s.
   subtle neurologic s.
sequence
   amniotic band disruption s.
   breech deformation s.
   cephalocaudal s.
   Pierre Robin s.
   Potter oligohydramnios s.
   RICE s.
sequencing
   temporal s.
   verbal s.
sequential
   s. memory
   s. peak flow measurement
sequestered
   s. lobe
   s. lung
sequestra (*pl. of* sequestrum)
sequestration
   acute splenic s.
   bile acid s.
   bronchopulmonary s. (BPS)
   s. crisis
   extralobar s.
   intralobar s.
   pulmonary s.
   reticuloendothelial s.
   splenic s.

sequestrative
sequestrum, pl. **sequestra**
   s. formation
   pancreatic s.
sera (*pl. of* serum)
Serentil
Serevent
   S. Diskus
   S. Diskus inhaler
serial
   s. casting
   s. neurologic examination
series
   eight-drugs-in-one-day treatment s.
   Kell s.
   treatment s.
   upper gastrointestinal s.
serine proteinase
serious emotional disturbance (SED)
sermorelin acetate
seroconversion illness
seroconverting
serofibrinous pleurisy
serogroup B meningococcus
serological marker
serology
   C-urea s.
seroma
   auricular s.
Seromycin Pulvules
seronegative
   s. enthesopathy and arthropathy
     syndrome
   s. neonate
   s. spondyloarthropathy
seronegativity, enthesopathy, arthropathy
(SEA)
seropositive
   ANA s.
seroprevalence
Seroquel
seroreverter
serosa
serosanguineous rhinitis
serositis
serostatus
Serostim Injection
serotonergic
   s. dysfunction
   s. function
   s. reuptake blockade
   s. system

S

NOTES

serotonin
   s. deficiency
   s. hypothesis
   s. receptor antagonist
   s. receptor blockade
   s. reuptake blocker
   s. reuptake inhibitor (SRI)
   s. syndrome
   s. transporter 5-HTT
serotype
serous
   s. form
   s. form of tuberculous meningitis
   s. otitis media
   s. retinal detachment
serpiginosa
   elastosis perforans s.
serpiginous
   s. border
   s. cephalad curved physis
Serratia
   S. marcescens
   S. marcescens infection
Sertoli cell
sertraline hydrochloride
serum, pl. **sera**
   s. acetaminophen level
   acute sera
   s. albumin concentration
   s. amino acid
   s. amino acid concentration
   s. aminotransferase
   s. ammonia
   s. amylase level
   s. anticonvulsant level
   s. antienterocyte antibody
   antilymphocyte sera
   antirabies s.
   s. apolipoprotein
   s. bactericidal titer (SBT)
   s. bile salt level
   s. bilirubin
   s. bilirubin-binding capacity
   s. carotene level
   s. complement
   convalescent sera
   convalescent s.
   s. copper
   s. copper level
   s. cortisol level
   s. digoxin level
   s. erythropoietin
   s. ferritin
   s. ferritin concentration
   s. glucose
   s. glutamic-oxalacetic
   s. glutamic-oxaloacetic transferase (SGOT)

   s. glutamic-pyruvic transaminase (SGPT)
   s. HCV RNA
   s. hepatitis
   hereditary erythroblastic multinuclearity with positive acidified s. (HEMPAS)
   s. hexosaminidase A
   s. hexosaminidase assay
   s. histamine level
   s. immunoglobulin G anti-*Toxoplasma*
   s. inhibit B concentration
   s. inhibitory titer (SIT)
   s. ketoacid
   s. lactate dehydrogenase concentration
   s. lead level
   s. leptin level
   s. lysosomal enzyme screen
   s. melatonin concentration
   s. osmolality
   s. osteocalcin
   s. PCT
   s. PHE
   postdose s.
   s. procalcitonin
   s. prolactin
   s. prostaglandin
   s. protease inhibitor
   s. protein concentration
   s. sickness
   s. sickness-like reaction
   s. sickness-like syndrome
   s. test
   s. thyrotropin
   s. type III procollagen
   s. urea nitrogen (SUN)
   s. uric acid
   s. zinc
Serutan
service
   S. Assessment for Children and Adolescents (SACA)
   Child, Adolescent, and Family Mental Health S. (CAFMHS)
   Child Protective S.'s (CPS)
   children's s.
   s. coordinator
   Crippled Children's S.'s (CCS)
   Department of Children and Family S.'s (DCFS)
   Department of Children's S.'s (DCS)
   Department of Public Social S.'s (DPSS)
   related s.'s
   support s.'s

S. Utilization and Risk Factors
(SURF)
servocontrolled homeothermy
Servo 900C ventilator
sessile polyp
sestamibi
set
Neo-Sert umbilical vessel catheter
insertion s.
s. point
Seton procedure
setting
fire s.
setting-sun sign
Sever
S. disease
S. release
severe
s. childhood autosomal recessive
muscular dystrophy (SCARMD)
s. chronic neutropenia (SCN)
s. combined immunodeficiency
(SCID)
s. combined immunodeficiency
disease (SCID)
s. combined immunodeficiency
syndrome (SCIDS)
s. congenital neutropenia
s. dehydration
s. gastrointestinal bleeding (SGIB)
s. growth failure
s. ketoacidosis
s. megaloblastic anemia
s. mental retardation
s. micrognathia
s. myoclonic epilepsy
s. myoclonic epilepsy in infancy
(SMEI)
s. myopia
s. refractory hypoglycemia
s. respiratory compromise
s. seizure
severity
Pediatric Acute Admission S.
(PAAS)
sevoflurane
sex
s. chromosome
s. cord-stromal tumor
s. hormone-binding globulin
(SHBG)

s. steroid
s. steroid add-back therapy
sexarche
sex-linked disorder
sexual
s. abuse
s. ambiguity
s. infantilism
s. intercourse
s. maturation
s. maturity rating (SMR)
s. precocity
sexuality
sexualization
traumatic s.
sexually transmitted disease (STD)
SF-1
steroidogenic factor-1
SFA
subclavian flap aortoplasty
S-F Kaon
S-14 formula
SGA
small for gestational age
SGAR
spectral gradient acoustic reflectometry
SGBS
Simpson-Golabi-Behmel syndrome
SGH
subgaleal hematoma
SGIB
severe gastrointestinal bleeding
SGLT1
sodium/glucose co-transporter-1
SGLT1 gene
SGOT
serum glutamic-oxaloacetic transferase
SGPT
serum glutamic-pyruvic transaminase
SGS
short gut syndrome
SH
short hydrophobic
sitting height
sulfhydryl
shadow
cardiothymic s.
double-bubble gas s.
heart s.
perihilar s.
thymic s.

NOTES

519

shaft
  clavicular s.
shagreen
  s. patch
  s. spot
Shah permanent tube
Shah-Waardenburg syndrome
shaken
  s. baby syndrome
  s. impact syndrome
  s. infant syndrome
shake test
shaking wrist
shallow
  s. acetabulum
  s. ulcer
  s. ulceration
shampoo
  Barc s.
  Exsel s.
  Ionil-T s.
  Kwell s.
  lindane s.
  Paranit s.
  Paratrol s.
  Polytar s.
  P&S S.
  RID s.
  Sebutone s.
  Selsun Blue S.
  T/Gel s.
  Triple X s.
shaping
Shapiro-Wilk test
sharing
  United Network for Organ S. (UNOS)
sharp facial features
sharp-wave
  s.-w. discharge
  s.-w. transient
SHBG
  sex hormone-binding globulin
shear
  s. fracture
  s. stress
shearing
  s. of catheter
  s. force
shear-strain deformation
sheath
  abdominal s.
  7-French s.
  Mullins long transseptal s.
  myelin s.
  optic nerve s.
shedding
  fecal s.

  s. of nails
  viral s.
Sheehan syndrome
Sheehy syndrome
sheep cell agglutinin titer
sheepskin glove
sheeting
  silicon gel s.
shell
  body s.
  s. shock
  s. vial culture
shellfish poisoning
shelter
Shenton line
shepherd crook deformity
Sheridan-Gardiner cards
Sheridan Tests for Young Children and Retardates (STYCAR)
shield
  Lea s.
  plastic heat s.
shield-shaped chest
shift
  biobehavioral s.
  midline s.
  ontogenetic s.
  paroxysmal depolarization s. (PDS)
shifting
  s. dullness
  weight s.
Shiga
  S. lipopolysaccharide
  S. toxin (Stx)
  S. toxin-producing *Escherichia coli* (STEC)
Shiga-like toxin
Shigella
  S. bacteria
  S. *dysenteriae* (type 1)
  S. dysentery
  S. *flexneri*
  S. *flexneri* 2b
  S. *sonnei*
  S. vaginitis
shigelloides
  Plesiomonas s.
shigellosis
Shimada-Chatten histology
Shimada criteria
shin
  saber s.
  s. splint
shiner
  allergic s.
shingles
shinsplints
shipyard conjunctivitis

SHMF
Similac Human Milk Fortifier
shock
anaphylactic s.
anaphylactoid s.
bacteremic s.
cardiogenic s.
cardiovascular s.
compensated s.
cool s.
distributive s.
endotoxic s.
gram-negative endotoxic s.
gram-negative endotoxin-induced s.
hemorrhagic s.
hypovolemic s.
insulin s.
s. liver
s. lung
septic s.
shell s.
spinal s.
s. stage
uncompensated s.
warm s.

shoe
s. contact dermatitis
reverse last s.
straight last s.
s. wedge
Shohl solution
Shone syndrome
short
s. attention span
s. axis
s. beaked nose
s. bowel syndrome (SBS)
s. gut syndrome (SGS)
s. hydrophobic (SH)
s. leg walking cast
s. limb
s. maxilla
s. metacarpal bone
S. Michigan Alcoholism Screening
Test (SMAST)
s. neck
s. philtrum
s. PR interval
s. process
s. process of malleus
s. rib polydactyly (type I, II)
s. small bowel (SSB)

s. stature (SS)
s. stature homeobox (SHOX)
s. vagina
short-acting beta-2 agonist bronchodilator
short-axis view
short-bevel 21-gauge needle
short-chain
s.-c. acyl coenzyme A
dehydrogenase (SCAD)
s.-c. fatty acid (SCFA)
s.-c. hydroxyacyl-coenzyme A
dehydrogenase (SCHAD)
s.-c. polyunsaturated fatty acid
(SCPUFA)
shortening
acromelic s.
s. dorsal wedge radial osteotomy
s. fraction
fractional s.
mesomelic s.
metacarpal s.
metatarsal s.
percent fractional s.
short-limb dwarfism
short-rib polydactyly syndrome
short-segment stenosis
short-stay ward (SSW)
shot
cardiogenic s.
shotty cervical lymphadenopathy
shoulder
s. dystocia
Little League s.
s. presentation
s. sign
s. subluxation
swimmer's s.
SHOX
short stature homeobox
Shprintzen-Goldberg syndrome
Shprintzen velocardiofacial syndrome
shuddering
s. attack
s. spell
Shulman syndrome
shunt
aortic-to-pulmonary s.
aortopulmonary s.
atrial s.
bidirectional Glenn s.
Blalock-Taussig s.

S

NOTES

shunt *(continued)*
s. blockage
B-T s.
central s.
Clatworthy mesocaval s.
congenital portosystemic venous s.
Cordis-Hakim s.
cutaneous s.
cystoperitoneal s.
Delta s.
distal splenorenal s.
double-bubble ventriculoperitoneal s.
Drapanas mesocaval s.
ductal s.
end-to-side portocaval s.
enterohepatic s.
extracardiac s.
Glenn s.
intracardiac s.
intrapulmonary s.
jugular s.
Kasai peritoneal venous s.
left-to-right s.
LeVeen s.
lumboperitoneal s.
s. malfunction
mesocaval s.
modified Blalock-Taussig s.
s. nephritis
neurosurgical s.
OPV s.
palliative s.
parietal s.
peritoneal venous s.
pleuroamniotic s.
portoaortal s.
portocaval s.
portosystemic s.
Potts s.
proximal splenorenal s.
pulmonary s.
s. revision
right-to-left s.
side-to-side portocaval s.
side-to-side splenorenal s.
single-reservoir, single-pump s.
splenorenal s.
subdural-peritoneal s.
synthetic portoaortal s.
s. tap
transjugular intrahepatic
  portosystemic s. (TIPS)
VA s.
ventricular s.
ventriculoatrial s.
ventriculoexternal s.
ventriculojugular s.
ventriculoperitoneal s. (VPS)

ventriculopleural s.
ventriculovascular s.
vesicoamniotic s.
VP s.
Warren s.
Waterston s.
Y s.
shunt-dependent hydrocephalus
shunted hydrocephalus
shunting
bidirectional s.
ductal s.
enterohepatic s.
intrapulmonary s.
left-to-right s.
right-to-left s.
ventriculoperitoneal s.
Y s.
shuttle
cortisol-cortisone s.
Shwachman
S. score
S. syndrome
Shwachman-Diamond syndrome
Shwachman-Kulczycki score
Shy-Drager syndrome
shy-inhibited temperament
shyness scale
SI
sacroiliac
syncytium inducing
SIADH
syndrome of inappropriate antidiuretic
  hormone
syndrome of inappropriate secretion of
  antidiuretic hormone
  SIADH secretion
sialadenitis
sialadenosis
sialidosis
sialoglycoprotein
glomerular s.
sialogram
sialography
sialomucin
sialophorin
sialuria
sialyl
s. Lewis X
s. Lewis X determinant
Siamese twin
SIB
self-injurious behavior
siberica
Rickettsia s.
Siblin
sibling

SIC
    selective intrapartum chemoprophylaxis
sicca
    s. complex
    keratitis s.
    keratoconjunctivitis s.
    rhinitis s.
    s. syndrome
sick
    s. euthyroid syndrome
    s. sinus node syndrome
sickle
    s. beta-thalassemia
    s. cell
    s. cell anemia
    s. cell crisis
    s. cell dactylitis
    s. cell disease (SCD)
    s. cell-hemoglobin C disease
    s. cell-hemoglobin D disease
    s. cell hemoglobinopathy
    s. cell nephropathy
    s. cell preparation
    s. cell sludging
    s. cell thalassemia
    s. cell-thalassemia disease
    s. cell trait
    s. hemoglobin
    s. hepatopathy
Sickledex test
sickling
    s. crisis
    s. disorder
    intravascular s.
    red blood cell s.
sickness
    car s.
    falling s.
    Jamaican vomiting s.
    motion s.
    mountain s.
    serum s.
    sleeping s.
side
    s. effect
    s. lyer
    s. sitting
side-port adapter
sideroblast
    refractory anemia with ring s.'s
      (RARS)
    ring s. (RS)

sideroblastic anemia
siderophilic
siderosis
    myocardial s.
side-to-end anastomosis
side-to-side
    s.-t.-s. portocaval shunt
    s.-t.-s. splenorenal shunt
sideways walking
SIDS
    sudden infant death syndrome
    near-miss SIDS
Siegel otoscope
Siemens Servo 300, 900C ventilator
sift
    fluid s.
sighing respiration
sighted
    partially s.
SigmaStat
    S. software
sigmoid
    s. pouch
    s. pouch of Pratt
    s. sinus
sigmoidoscopy
sign
    3 s.
    apprehension s.
    Auspitz s.
    Babinski s.
    banana s.
    Barlow s.
    Barré s.
    Battle s.
    bilateral pyramidal tract s.'s
    Blanche s.
    blue dot s.
    Brudzinski s.
    candlestick s.
    Chadwick s.
    Chvostek s.
    cock-robin s.
    Comby s.
    Corrigan s.
    cracked-pot s.
    Crowe s.
    Cullen s.
    curtsey s.
    cutoff s.
    Dalrymple s.
    Dance s.

S

NOTES

sign *(continued)*
    Darier s.
    double-bubble s.
    double-tract s.
    E s.
    extrapyramidal s.
    eye-of-the-tiger s.
    false localizing s.
    falx s.
    figure 3 s.
    flag s.
    Gage s.
    Galeazzi s.
    Goodell s.
    Gower s.
    Gower s. C
    Grey-Turner s.
    Hegar s.
    Hennebert s.
    Hertoghe s.
    Higoumenakis s.
    Homans s.
    Kernig s.
    Kernohan s.
    Kussmaul s.
    s. language
    lateralizing s.
    Lhermitte s.
    localizing s.
    long-tract s.
    Macewen s.
    Marcus Gunn s.
    Marfan s.
    McMurray s.
    meningeal s.
    milkmaid's s.
    motor neuron s.
    Munson s.
    Murphy s.
    neonatal abstinence s.
    Nikolsky s.
    nuchal-spinal s.
    obturator s.
    oromotor s.
    Ortolani s.
    palmar-plantar s.
    palpable spongy mass s.
    Parinaud s.
    Pastia s.
    pathergy s.
    Perez s.
    peritoneal s.
    plugged toilet s.
    Prehn s.
    pronator s.
    psoas s.
    puddle s.
    pyramidal tract s.

    raccoon eyes s.
    Raynaud s.
    reverse 3 s.
    reverse Marcus Gunn s.
    Risser s.
    Romaña s.
    rope s.
    Russell s.
    sail s.
    scarf s.
    seat belt s.
    setting-sun s.
    shoulder s.
    silk s.
    snowman s.
    soft s.
    steeple s.
    Stellwag s.
    Sternberg s.
    string s.
    thumb s.
    thymic wave s.
    Trendelenburg s.
    tripod s.
    Trousseau s.
    Uhthoff s.
    umbrella s.
    upper motor neuron s.
    vital s.'s
    von Graefe s.
    W s.
    Wartenberg s.
    water lily s.
    Weill s.
    Wimberger s.

signal
    extracellular matrix s.
    s. extraction pulse oximetry
    peptide growth factor receptor s.
    specific growth factor s.

signaling

signed
    s. English (SE)
    s. exact English (SEE)

signing

Siker laryngoscope

Siladryl Oral

Silafed

Silain

Silapap

Silastic
    S. catheter
    S. spring-loaded silo
    S. tube intubation

silence
    electrocortical s.

silent
    s. carrier

s. celiac disease
s. DVT
s. gastroesophageal reflux
s. myocarditis
s. precordium
s. stroke

Silfedrine
Children's S.

silhouette
cardiac s.

silibinin

silica

silicon
arsenic nickel s.
s. gel sheeting

silicone catheter

silk
s. sign
s. tie

SILL
subischial leg length

Sillence classification of osteogenesis imperfecta (type I, IA, IB, II, III, IV, IVA, IVB)

silliness
hebephrenic s.

silo
s. decompression
s. filler's disease
Silastic spring-loaded s.

Silon tent

Silphen
S. Cough
S. DM

Silsoft extended wear contact lens

Siltussin DM

Silvadene

silver
s. fork deformity
s. nitrate
s. nitrate administration
s. nitrate conjunctivitis
s. nitrate drops
s. nitrate solution
s. nitrate stick
s. stain
s. sulfadiazine
s. sulfadiazine cream
S. syndrome
s. thermal hat

Silverman-Handmaker dyssegmental dysplasia

Silverman and Nelles Anxiety Disorders Interview Schedule for Children

Silver-Russell syndrome

silver-wire appearance

Sim
S. SC-20 formula
S. SC-24 formula
S. SC-40 formula

simethicone

simian
s. B virus
s. crease

Similac
S. 24 formula
S. Human Milk Fortifier (SHMF)
S. Natural Care formula
S. NeoCare formula
S. PM 60/40 Low Iron formula
S. Special Care with Iron 20 formula
S. Special Care with Iron 24 formula
S. with Iron

similarities test

Simkania
S. negevensis
S. negevensis strain Z

Simon focus

simple
s. central anisocoria
s. coarctation
s. ectopia lentis
s. epispadias
s. febrile seizure
s. meconium ileus
s. metatarsus adductus
s. motor tic
s. partial seizure (SPS)
s. phobia (SPh)
s. squamous blepharitis
s. syndactyly
s. TGA
s. ureterocele
s. vocal tic

simplex
Dowling Meara epidermolysis bullosa s.
epidemic keratoconjunctivitis herpes s.
epidermolysis bullosa s.
herpes s. (HS)

S

NOTES

simplex *(continued)*
> herpetiformis epidermolysis
>   bullosa s.
> s. infection
> Koebner epidermolysis bullosa s.
> lichen s.
> neonatal herpes s.
> nevus s.
> s. virus
> Weber-Cockayne epidermolysis
>   bullosa s.

simplified acute physiology score
  (SAPS)
simplistic method
Simpson-Angus rating scale
Simpson-Golabi-Behmel
> S.-G.-B. fetal overgrowth syndrome
> S.-G.-B. syndrome (SGBS)

Simron
simultaneous
> s. preductal-postductal PO_2
> S. Technique for Acuity and
>   Readiness Testing (STAR)

SIMV
> synchronized intermittent mandatory
>   ventilation

Sinarest 12 Hour Nasal Solution
Sindbis virus
Sinding-Larsen-Johansson syndrome
Sinding-Larsen lesion
sinensis
> *Clonorchis s.*

Sinequan Oral
Sinex Long-Acting
single
> s. central maxillary incisor (SCMI)
> s. collecting system
> s. ring-enhancing mass lesion
> s. transverse palmar crease
> s. tumor
> s. tumor with seeding
> s. ventricle

single-isotope tracer technique
single-photon
> s.-p. emission computed
>   tomography (SPECT)
> s.-p. emission tomography

single-reservoir, single-pump shunt
single-suture craniosynostosis
singleton
single-walled incubator
Singulair
singultus
sinister
> oculus s. (left eye) (o.s., OS)

SinNombre virus
sinoatrial
> s. block

> s. conduction time
> s. node (SA)
> s. node artery

Sinografin
sinopulmonary
> s. tract infection

Sinumist-SR Caplets
sinus
> s. arrest
> s. arrhythmia
> s. bradycardia
> branchial cleft s.
> cavernous s.
> cervical s.
> complex unroofed coronary s.
>   (CUCS)
> coronary s.
> s. cycle length
> dermal s.
> endodermal s.
> ethmoid s.
> external branchial s.
> s. fistula
> high urogenital s.
> s. histiocytosis
> internal branchial s.
> lumbosacral s.
> marginal s.
> maxillary s.
> s. node dysfunction (SND)
> s. node function
> open dermal s.
> paranasal s.
> pilonidal s.
> s. radiogram
> s. radiograph
> sagittal s.
> sigmoid s.
> straight s.
> superior sagittal s.
> s. surgery
> s. tachycardia
> s. thrombophlebitis
> s. thrombosis
> s. tumor
> unroofed coronary s.
> urogenital s.
> Valsalva s.
> s. of Valsalva
> s. venosus
> s. venosus defect

sinusitis
> acute s.
> allergic s.
> bacterial s.
> cavernous s.
> chronic s.
> idiopathic cavernous s.

invasive s.
recurrent s.
sinusoid
coronary s.
hepatic s.
sinusoidal channel
Sinusol-B
siphon effect
Sipple syndrome
sirenomelia syndrome
sirolimus
SIRS
systemic inflammatory response
syndrome
SIS
saline infusion sonography
Sistrunk operation
SIT
serum inhibitory titer
sit
right s.
site
Luer lock s.
venipuncture s.
sitosterol
sitosterolemia
sitting
s. height (SH)
long leg s.
side s.
tailor s.
situ
in s.
situated learning
situs
s. ambiguus
s. indeterminus
s. inversus
organ s.
s. solitus
visceral s.
visceroatrial s.
sitz bath
sivelestat
sixth disease
size
abnormal head s.
appropriate blood pressure cuff s.
blood pressure cuff s.
body s.
cardiac s.
head s.

infant s. (IS)
small body s.
small head s.
tongue s.
Sjögren-Larsson syndrome
Sjögren syndrome
skeletal
s. anomaly
s. arthrogryposis
s. defect
s. dysplasia
s. mineralization
s. survey
s. traction
skewfoot
skier's thumb
skill
attending s.
basic s.
decreased attending s.
Kaufman Survey of Early
Academic and Language S.'s (K-
SEALS)
meal-time s.
motor s.
perceptual s.
Personal Adjustment and Role S.'s
(PARS)
thinking s.
skin
s. cyst
s. defect
s. discoloration
doughy s.
dry s.
s. end-point titration
s., eye, mucocutaneous (SEM)
s., eye, or mucocutaneous infection
s. flora
s. fold
s. graft
hyperextensile s.
hyperkeratotic dry s.
s. hyperlaxity
s. lesion
mitral valve, aorta, skeleton, s.
(MASS)
Oxy-5 Advanced Formula for
Sensitive S.
Oxy-10 Advanced Formula for
Sensitive S.
s. penetration

NOTES

S

skin *(continued)*
 s. popping
 s. prick test
 puffy s.
 s. rash
 redundant s.
 s. ridge pattern
 rough-feeling s.
 salt frosting of s.
 s. scraping
 staphylococcal scalded s.
 s. suture
 s. tag
 s. temperature
 s. tenting
 s. test conversion
 s. test reactivity (STR)
 thin vulvar s.
 s. traction
 vagabond s.
 s. vesicle
skin-covered lipomyelomeningocele
skinfold
 s. caliper technique
 infarction of s.
 s. thickness
skip lesion
skull
 thickened base of s.
SKY
 spectral karyotyping
skyline view radiograph
S/L
 A-Spas S/L
slant
 antimongoloid eye s.
 eye s.
 mongoloid s.
 palpebral s.
slapped
 s. cheek rash
 s. cheek syndrome
slapped-cheek appearance
slapping storklike gait
slate-gray cyanosis
SLE
 St. Louis encephalitis
 systemic lupus erythematosus
 SLE 2000 ventilator
sleep
 active s. (AS)
 s. apnea
 s. apnea syndrome
 s. architecture
 s. attack
 s. bruxism
 s. cystogram
 s. debt

 deep s.
 delta s.
 s. disturbance
 s. efficiency
 s. epoch
 S. Guardian foam pad
 s. hygiene
 indeterminate s.
 s. latency
 s. myoclonus
 narcoleptic s.
 s. paralysis
 s. position
 quiet s. (QS)
 rapid eye movement s.
 REM s.
 restless s.
 s. start
 s. study
 s. talking
 s. terror
 s. terror disorder
 s. with rapid eye movement
sleep-disordered
 s.-d. breathing
 s.-d. breathing syndrome
Sleep-eze 3 Oral
Sleepinal
sleep-induced dyskinesia
sleeping
 difficulty s.
 excessive s.
 s. sickness
sleepless
 crying, requires, increased,
  expression, s. (CRIES)
sleeplessness
 facial expression and s.
 pressure, facial expression, s.
sleep-related headache
sleeptalking
sleep-wake transition disorder
sleepwalking disorder
Sleepwell 2-nite
sleeve
 s. fracture
 s. fracture of patella
sliding hiatal hernia
Slim-Mint
sling
 s. anomaly
 s. baby
 puborectalis s.
 pulmonary artery s.
slipped
 s. capital femoral epiphysis (SCFE)
 s. epiphysis
 s. upper femoral epiphysis (SUFE)

slit-lamp
    s.-l. biomicroscopy
    s.-l. examination
slit ventricle syndrome
SLO
    Smith-Lemli-Opitz
    SLO syndrome
Slo-bid Gyrocaps
Slo-Niacin
Slo-Phyllin Gyrocaps
Slosson Oral Reading Test-Revised (SORT-R)
sloughing
    mucosal s.
slow
    s. channel syndrome
    s. cognitive processing
    S. FE
    s. growth
    s. rate of learning
slowing
    bilateral s.
    generalized s.
Slow-K
Slow-Mag
sludging
    sickle cell s.
slurry
    DE s.
    diatomaceous earth s.
Sly
    S. disease
    S. syndrome
SMA
    spinal muscular atrophy
S-M-A formula
small
    s. body size
    s. bowel atresia
    s. bowel biopsy
    s. bowel dysmotility
    s. bowel enteroscopy
    s. bowel intestinal polyposis
    s. bowel overgrowth
    s. bowel transplantation
    s. cell cleaved lymphoma
    s. cell osteosarcoma
    s. for dates
    s. for gestational age (SGA)
    s. head size
    s. intestine
    s. intestine stasis

    s. jaw
    s. left colon syndrome
    s. maxillary bone
    s. noncleaved cell lymphoma (SNCCL)
    s. nuclear ribonucleoprotein-associated polypeptide (SNRPN)
    s. premature infant
    s. round blue cell tumor of childhood
    s. stature
smallpox
Sm antigen
smart
    street s.
SMAST
    Short Michigan Alcoholism Screening Test
smear
    acid-fast sputum s.
    blood s.
    nasal s.
    Pap s.
    Papanicolaou s.
    peripheral blood s.
    s. positive
    sputum s.
    thick blood s.
    Tzanck s.
    vaginal s.
    Wright-stained s.
smegma
SMEI
    severe myoclonic epilepsy in infancy
smile
    Cheshire cat s.
    sardonic s.
Smith-Lemli-Opitz (SLO)
    S.-L.-O. syndrome
Smith-Magenis syndrome
SMO
    supramalleolar orthosis
smoke
    cigarette s.
    environmental tobacco s. (ETS)
smokeless tobacco
smoking
    maternal s.
    second-hand s.
smooth
    s. chorion
    s. muscle hamartoma

NOTES

S

529

smooth *(continued)*
    s. philtrum
    s. tongue
SMR
    sexual maturity rating
snakebite envenomation
SNAP
    Score for Neonatal Acute Physiology
       SNAP score
snap
Snaplets-FR
snapping
    s. hip
    s. knee syndrome
SNCCL
    small noncleaved cell lymphoma
SND
    sinus node dysfunction
Snellen
    S. acuity chart
    S. test
SNHL
    sensorineural hearing loss
sniffing
    s. position
    toluene s.
SNIPPV
    synchronized nasal intermittent positive-
       pressure ventilation
S-nitrosoglutathione
Sn-mesoporphyrin (SnMP)
SnMP
    Sn-mesoporphyrin
    tin mesoporphyrin
Snodgrass hypospadias repair
snoring
    habitual s.
    primary s.
Snow
    S. Mountain agent
    S. Mountain virus
snowman sign
SNP
    sodium nitroprusside
SnPP
    tin protoporphyrin
SNRPN
    small nuclear ribonucleoprotein-
       associated polypeptide
snuffbox tenderness
snuffles
soap
    Alpha Keri s.
    Basis s.
    Lowila s.
    Oilatum s.
soap-bubble appearance
Soave procedure

sober
sociability
social
    s. anxiety disorder
    s. deprivation
    s. development
    s. isolation
    s. maturity
    s. phobia
    S. Security Disability Insurance
       (SSDI)
    S. Support Scale for Children test
    s. withdrawal
    s. worker
social/emotional
    s./e. developmental area
    s./e. domain
social-emotional learning disability
social-evaluative fear
social-occupational dysfunction
social-pragmatic teaching
society
sociocultural stressor
sociodemographic data
socioeconomic
sock
    verruca s.
socket
    dry s.
sodium (Na)
    s. acetate
    s. bicarbonate ($NaHCO_3$)
    Brevital S.
    cefazolin s.
    cefoperazone s.
    cefotaxime s.
    ceftriaxone s.
    cefuroxime s.
    cephalothin s.
    s. channelopathy
    s. chloride
    s. cromoglycate
    cromolyn s.
    dantrolene s.
    Diphenylan S.
    divalproex s.
    s. docusate
    s. excess
    fractional excretion of s. (FeNa)
    heparin s.
    s. hydrogen phosphate
    s. hydroxide
    s. hyposulfite
    methicillin s.
    mezlocillin s.
    nafcillin s.
    nedocromil s.
    nitroprusside s.

s. nitroprusside (SNP)
olsalazine s.
oxacillin s.
s. pentobarbital
Pentothal S.
s. phenylacetate
s. phenylacetate and sodium benzoate
s. phenylbutyrate
piperacillin s.
s. polyacrylate polymer
s. polystyrene sulfonate
prednisolone s.
s. retention
S. Sulamyd
thiopental s.
s. thiosulfate
total body s.
s. wasting
sodium-free formula
sodium/glucose
s./g, co-transporter-1 (SGLT1)
s./g, co-transporter gene
soft
s. Boston orthosis
Modane S.
s. palate
s. sign
s. spot
s. tissue
s. tissue balancing
s. tissue release
s. tissue syndactyly
Softgel
DC 240 S.
DOS S.
soft-tissue
s.-t. density
s.-t. fat plane
s.-t. sarcoma
software
EsopHogram s.
SigmaStat s.
Sohval-Soffer syndrome
soilage
bacterial s.
Solarcaine Topical
solar urticaria
Solatene
Solbar
sole crease

Solenopsis
S. invecta
S. xyloni
soleus
accessory s.
Solfoton
Solganal
solid
s. organ transplantation (SOT)
s. rod segmental construct
s. tumor
solid-phase
s.-p. enzyme-linked immunospot (ELISPOT)
s.-p. enzyme-linked immunospot assay
solitarius
nucleus tractus s.
solitary
s. bone cyst
s. bone lesion
s. kidney
s. renal myofibromatosis
solitus
situs s.
solium
Taenia s.
soluble tumor necrosis factor receptor
Solu-Cortef Injection
Solumbra 30+ SPF fabric
Solu-Medrol Injection
Soluprick skin prick test
Solurex LA Injection
Soluspan
Celestone S.
solute diuresis
solution
Afrin Nasal S.
AK-Dilate Ophthalmic S.
AK-Nefrin Ophthalmic S.
Alamast ophthalmic s.
Alconefrin Nasal S.
Allerest 12 Hour Nasal S.
aluminum acetate s.
Anestacon Topical S.
arterial line flush s.
Atrovent Inhalation S.
Bronkosol Inhalation S.
Burow s.
cardioplegic s.
chlorhexidine s.
Chlorphed-LA Nasal S.

S

NOTES

solution *(continued)*
    Ciloxan ophthalmic s.
    Condylox s.
    crystalloid s.
    Dey-Drop Ophthalmic S.
    Doktors Nasal S.
    Domeboro s.
    Dristan Long Lasting Nasal S.
    Duration Nasal S.
    Freezone S.
    Fungoid Topical S.
    gum arabic rehydration s.
    Hanks balanced salt s. (HBSS)
    hypertonic saline s.
    iodine povidone s.
    I-Phrine Ophthalmic S.
    Isopto Frin Ophthalmic S.
    isotonic electrolyte s.
    Mucomyst s.
    Mydfrin Ophthalmic S.
    nedocromil sodium ophthalmic s.
    neomycin-polymycin combination
      otic s.
    Neo-Synephrine 12 Hour Nasal S.
    Neo-Synephrine Ophthalmic S.
    normal saline s. (NSS)
    Norvir oral s.
    Nostril Nasal S.
    NTZ Long Acting Nasal S.
    Ocuflox ophthalmic s.
    oral rehydration s. (ORS)
    Pedialyte oral electrolyte
      maintenance s.
    phosphate-buffered saline s.
    physiologic salt s. (PSS)
    polyethylene glycol s.
    polyethylene glycol-electrolyte s.
    Polygelin colloid s.
    povidone-iodine s.
    Prefrin Ophthalmic S.
    Primsol s.
    Relief Ophthalmic S.
    Resectisol Irrigation S.
    Rhinall Nasal S.
    Ringer's s.
    saline s.
    Shohl s.
    silver nitrate s.
    Sinarest 12 Hour Nasal S.
    St. Joseph Measured Dose
      Nasal S.
    TOBI Inhalation S.
    tobramycin s.
    trimethoprim HCl oral s.
    Twice-A-Day Nasal S.
    Tyrode's s.
    Verukan S.
    Vicks Sinex Nasal S.

    4-Way Long Acting Nasal S.
    Xopenex inhalation s.
    Xylocaine Topical S.
    Zenker s.
solvent
solving
    means-end problem s. (MEPS)
    problem s.
somatic
    s. complaint
    s. growth measurement
    s. mosaicism
somatization disorder
somatoform disorder
somatomedin
    s. C
somatosensory
    s. aura
    s. evoked potential (SSEP)
    s. impairment
somatostatinergic
somatostatin receptor scintigraphy
somatotropic
somatrem
somatrope
somatropin
    s. of rDNA origin
    s. (rDNA origin) for injection
Sominex Oral
somite
somnambulism
somniloquy
somnolence syndrome
somnolent
Somogyi phenomenon
Somophyllin
Somophyllin-CRT
Sones catheter
Sonic hedgehog
Sonksen-Silver visual acuity card
sonnei
    Shigella s.
sonogram
sonography
    s. blood dyscrasia
    saline infusion s. (SIS)
sonohysterography
sonometer
    Bruel and Kjaer s.
SOP
    Lacri-Lube SOP
sorbitol
    Actidose with S.
sore
    canker s.
    oriental s.
    s. throat
Sorensen Transpac transducer

Sorsby syndrome
sorting
    cell s.
SORT-R
    Slosson Oral Reading Test-Revised
SOS
    speed of sound
SOT
    solid organ transplantation
Sotos syndrome
sound
    abnormally wide splitting of
      second heart s.
    adventitial pulmonary s.
    ambient s.
    bilabial speech s.
    bowel s.
    breath s.
    bronchial breath s.
    bronchovesicular breath s.
    cracked-pot s.
    decreased breath s.
    first heart s.
    first Korotkoff s.
    fourth heart s.
    heart s.
    high-pitched bowel s.
    Korotkoff s.
    labiodental speech s.
    muffled heart s.
    prominent heart s.
    pulmonary s.
    second heart s.
    speech s.
    speed of s. (SOS)
    third heart s.
    tibial speed of s.
    vesicular breath s.
    vowel s.
sound-field response
soup kid facies
South
    S. African tick fever
    S. American blastomycosis
Southeast Asian ovalocytosis (SAO)
SOX9 gene
Soyacal
Soyalac formula
soy-based protein isolate formula
soy milk
SPA
    sperm penetration assay

SP-A
    surfactant protein-A
    SP-A protein of lungs
space
    antecubital s.
    apophyseal s.
    s. blanket
    Bowman s.
    cranial s.
    dead s.
    intercostal s.
    intersphincteric s.
    intracranial cystic s.
    mechanical dead s.
    obliteration of apophyseal s.
    perivitelline s.
    pharyngeal s.
    popliteal s.
    subaponeurotic cranial s.
    Virchow-Robin s.
space-occupying lesion
spaciness
spacing
    third s.
span
    arm s.
    attention s.
    liver s.
    s. of liver dullness
    poor attention s.
    short attention s.
Span-FF
SPAQ
    Seasonal Pattern Assessment
    Questionnaire
sparfloxacin
sparing
    brain s.
    fetal brain s.
sparse hair
Spaslin
spasm
    adductor s.
    arterial s.
    carpopedal s.
    ciliary s.
    cryptogenic infantile s.
    diffuse esophageal s.
    esophageal s.
    glottic s.
    hemifacial s.
    infantile s.

S

NOTES

spasm *(continued)*
  laryngeal s.
  mixed infantile s.
  myoclonic s.
  symptomatic s.
  tetanic s.
spasmodic
  s. croup
  s. dysphonia
  s. torticollis
Spasmoject Injection
Spasmolin
Spasmophen
spasmus nutans
Spasquid
spastic
  s. abductor hallucis
  s. ataxia
  s. cerebral palsy
  s. colon
  s. diplegia
  s. diplegia syndrome
  s. dysphonia
  s. hemiparesis
  s. hemiplegia
  s. levator ani
  s. monoplegia
  s. paralysis
  s. paraparesis
  s. paraplegia
  s. paresis
  s. quadriparesis
  s. quadriplegia
  s. synergy
spasticity
  Ashworth score of s.
  bilateral s.
spatial
  s. cognition
  s. memory
  s. orientation
  s. relationship
SP-B
  surfactant protein-B
  SP-B protein of lungs
SP-C
  surfactant protein-C
  SP-C protein of lungs
SPEA
  streptococcal exotoxin-A
spearing
Spearman
  S. coefficient
  S. correlation
  S. rank correlation test
spear tackling
special
  s. education

  s. needs
  S. Supplemental Nutrition Program
specialist
  development s.
  infant development s.
  mobility s.
  resource s.
species
  Klebsiella-Enterobacter s.
  reactive oxygen s. (ROS)
specific
  s. growth factor signal
  s. immune globulin
  s. phobia
  s. reading disability
  s. reading retarded (SRR)
  s. transcription factor
specified
  pervasive developmental disorder
    not otherwise s. (PDD-NOS)
speckled lentiginous nevus
SPECT
  single-photon emission computed
    tomography
Spec-T
spectacle
  s. correction
  s. treatment
Spectazole
spectophotometrical
spectral
  s. edge frequency (SEF)
  s. gradient acoustic reflectometry
    (SGAR)
  s. karyotyping (SKY)
  orthogonal polarization s. (OPS)
  s. power analysis
spectrin
spectrofluorometric
spectrometer
  atomic absorption s.
  mass s.
spectrometry
  electrospray ionization mass s.
    (ESIMS)
  gas chromatography-mass s.
  mass s. (MS)
  tandem mass s.
spectrophotometer
  narrow band s.
spectrophotometric scanning
spectrophotometry
spectroscopy
  gas chromatography-mass s. (GC-
    MS)
  longitudinal proton MR s.
  magnetic resonance s. (MRS)
  medical optical s. (MOS)

near-infrared s.
nuclear magnetic resonance s.
optical s.
proton MR s.

spectrum
faccioauriculovertebral s. (FAVS)

speculum
ear s.
s. examination
nasal s.
Pedersen s.

Spee
curve of S.

speech
cued s.
s. delay
s. development
s. disorder
dysarthritic s.
dysfluent s.
hypernasal s.
hyponasal s.
s. lesson
motherease s.
parallel s.
s. pathology
pressured s.
s. problem
s. production
s. reception threshold
s. recognition threshold (SRT)
s. sound
s. therapist
s. therapy

speech-language
s.-l. pathologist
s.-l. pathology

speechreading

speed
s. of sound (SOS)
tibial s.

Speed-Vac

spell
blue s.
breath-holding s.
cyanotic breathholding s.
hypercyanotic s.
hypoxic s.
pallid breathholding s.
paroxysmal hypoxic s.
shuddering s.
staring s.

syncopal s.
tet s.

spelt wheat

sperm
s. aspiration
s. penetration assay (SPA)
subzonal injection of s.
s. surface antibody

spermatic cord

spermatocele

spermatogenesis

sperm-containing cyst

spermicide

SpermMAR mixed antiglobulin reaction test

SPh
simple phobia

sphenoid
s. bone
s. dysplasia

spherical congruent hips

spherocytic
s. HE
s. hereditary elliptocytosis
s. red blood cell

spherocytosis
congenital s.
hereditary s.

sphincter
anal s.
esophageal s.
external anal s.
incompetent lower esophageal s.
lower esophageal s. (LES)
s. musclc
s. paralysis
s. tone
urinary s.
vertiginous external anal s.
voluntary urinary s.

sphincteric incompetence

sphingolipid
s. activator protein-1 (SAP1)
s. activator protein deficiency
s. storage disease

sphingolipidosis
infantile cerebral s.

Sphingomonas

sphingomyelin
lecithin to s. (L/S)

sphingosine

S

NOTES

sphygmomanometer
Tycos aneroid s.
spica
s. cast
panty s.
s. splint
spiculated red cell
spider
s. angioma
black widow s.
brown recluse s.
s. nevus
vascular s.
Spielberger
S. State-Trait Anxiety Inventory
(STAI)
S. State-Trait Inventory
Spielmeyer-Vogt
S.-V. disease
S.-V. neural ceroid lipofuscinosis
S.-V. type
S.-V. type of late infantile and
juvenile amaurotic idiocy
spike
benign partial epilepsy with
centrotemporal s. (BPEC)
centrotemporal s.
interictal s.
multifocal s.
spiked P wave
spillage
tumor s.
spilus
nevus s.
spina, pl. **spinae**
s. bifida
s. bifida cystica
s. bifida occulta
spinal
s. arachnoiditis
s. column
s. concussion
s. cord
s. cord compression
s. cord dysfunction
s. cord glioma
s. cord injury without radiographic
abnormality (SCIWORA)
s. cord tethering
s. cord tumor
s. defect
s. dysraphism
s. epidural abscess
s. fusion
s. muscle atrophy
s. muscular atrophy (SMA)
s. muscular dystrophy
s. needle

s. neurofibromatosis
s. optosis
s. osteomyelitis
s. paralytic poliomyelitis
s. polyneuropathy
s. shock
s. subarachnoid block
s. tap
s. tuberculosis
spindle
s. cell
s. cell epithelioid nevus
s. cell tumor
spine
anterior superior iliac s.
bamboo s.
curvature of s.
iliac s.
lateral curvature of s.
posterior superior iliac s.
rotation of s.
rugger jersey s.
superior iliac s.
spin-echo
half-Fourier acquisition single-shot
turbo s.-e. (HASTE)
Spinhaler
spinigerum
Gnathostoma s.
spinning top deformity
spinocerebellar
s. ataxia (type 1) (SCA)
s. degeneration
s. syndrome
spinothalamic sensory deficit
spinulosus
lichen s.
spiral
Curschmann s.
s. endometrial artery
s. scan
s. tibial fracture
spiralis
Trichinella s.
spiramycin
spirillary rat-bite fever
Spirillum minus
spirochetal infection
spirochete
spiroforme
Clostridium s.
spirometric test
spirometry
Spironazide
spironolactone
hydrochlorothiazide and s.
Spirozide
spit fistula

Spitz nevus
splanchnic
splash burn
SPLATT
    split anterior tibial tendon transfer
splayfoot
spleen
    accessory s.
    fetal s.
splenectomized
splenectomy
splenic
    s. Fc blockade
    s. flexure
    s. sequestration
    s. sequestration crisis
    s. vein
splenium, pl. splenia
    posterior s.
splenocyte
splenomegaly
splenoportography
splenorenal shunt
splenorrhaphy
splint
    abduction s.
    acrylic s.
    ankle stirrup s.
    clubfoot s.
    Denis Browne clubfoot s.
    Denis Browne night s.
    dorsal extension s.
    dynamic s.
    Fillauer night s.
    Freidman s.
    Frejka pillow s.
    Lorenz night s.
    malleable s.
    night s.
    opponens s.
    Orthoglass s.
    Pope night s.
    shin s.
    spica s.
    static s.
    sugar-tong s.
    talipes hobble s.
    thumb spica s.
    triangular s.
    volar s.
splinter hemorrhage

splinting
    night s.
splint/stent
    kidney internal s./s. (KISS)
split
    anterior cricoid s. (ACS)
    s. anterior tibial tendon transfer (SPLATT)
    s. cord malformation (SCM)
    cricoid s.
    s. flexor hallucis longus tendon
    s. procedure
    s. spinal cord malformation (SSCM)
split-course hyperfractionated radiotherapy
splittable needle
splitting
    rib s.
split-virus vaccine
spondylitis
    ankylosing s.
    s., enthesitis, arthritis (SEA)
    juvenile ankylosing s. (JAS)
    rheumatoid s.
    tuberculous s.
spondyloarthropathy, pl. spondyloarthropathies
    ankylosing s.
    seronegative s.
spondylocostal dysplasia syndrome
spondyloepiphyseal
    s. dysplasia (SED)
    s. dysplasia congenita
    s. dysplasia congenita syndrome
    s. dysplasia tarda
spondylolisthesis
spondylolysis
spondylometaphyseal dysplasia
spondylothoracic dysplasia syndrome
spongiform encephalopathy
spongiosis
spongiosum
    corpus s.
spongiosus
    status s.
spongy
    s. degeneration
    s. degeneration of white matter
    s. mass
spontaneous
    s. abortion

NOTES

S

spontaneous *(continued)*
    s. atrophic patch
    s. atrophic patch of prematurity
    s. bacterial peritonitis
    s. biliary perforation (SBP)
    s. descent
    s. descent of testis
    s. nystagmus
    s. periodic breathing
    s. pneumothorax
    s. remission
    s. thymic involution
spoon-shaped nail
sporadic
    s. aniridia
    s. Burkitt lymphoma
    s. Creutzfeldt-Jakob disease
    s. myoglobinuria
Sporanox
spore
    mold s.
Sporothrix schenckii
sporotrichoid appearance
sporotrichosis
    cutaneous s.
    extracutaneous s.
sport
    wheelchair s.
sporulation enterotoxin
spot
    ash-leaf s.
    Bitot s.
    black s.
    blood s.
    Brushfield s.
    café-au-lait s.
    cherry-red macular s.
    cotton-wool s. (CWS)
    Forchheimer s.
    Fordyce s.
    Koplik s.
    macular cherry-red s.
    Mongolian s.
    pathognomonic Koplik s.
    rose s.
    Roth s.
    shagreen s.
    soft s.
    s. test
spotted
    s. fever
    s. fever group
spotty necrosis
S-pouch
spousal abuse
sprain
spray
    Astelin Nasal S.

    Atrovent Nasal S.
    CaldeCort Anti-Itch Topical S.
    DDAVP nasal s.
    desmopressin acetate nasal s.
    Dristan Saline S.
    hair s.
    intranasal s.
    Itch-X s.
    Merthiolate s.
    Miacalcin Nasal S.
    midazolam nasal s.
    mometasone furoate aqueous
      nasal s. (MFNS)
    Nasarel Nasal S.
    Nitrolingual Translingual S.
    Rhinocort Aqua nasal s.
    sumatriptan nasal s.
    Tri-Nasal S.
    Xylocaine Topical S.
spread
    centripetal s.
spreading factor
Sprengel
    S. anomaly
    S. deformity
sprinkle
    Depakote s.
    Humibid S.
    Theo-Dur S.
sprouting
    mossy fiber s.
sprue
    celiac s.
    refractory s.
    tropical s.
SPS
    simple partial seizure
SPSS
    Statistical Package for Social Sciences
spun
    s. glass hair
    s. hematocrit
spur
    bony s.
spurt
    growth s.
Spurway syndrome
sputorum
    Campylobacter s.
    Pandoraea s.
sputum, pl. **sputa**
    carbonaceous s.
    clear mucoid s.
    cloudy s.
    s. culture
    s. eosinophilia
    mucoid s.
    purulent s.

rust-colored s.
s. smear
squamous metaplasia
square
chi s.
squatting phenomenon
squeezing
eyelid s.
SQUIDS
superconducting quantum interference
device susceptometer
squint
convergent s.
SQV
saquinavir
SR
Calan SR
Cardizem SR
Indocin SR
Isoptin SR
Mag-Tab SR
S-R
stimulus-response
Sr.
EpiPen Sr.
SRA Basic Reading Program
SRI
serotonin reuptake inhibitor
SRR
specific reading retarded
SRS
suicide risk screen
SRSH
self-reported self-harm
SRT
speech recognition threshold
SS
short stature
systemic sclerosis
hemoglobin SS
Regulax SS
Uroplus SS
SSB
short small bowel
SSCM
split spinal cord malformation
SSD
SSD AF
SSD Cream
SSDI
Social Security Disability Insurance

SSEP
somatosensory evoked potential
S-shaped curve
SSI
semistructured psychiatric interview
Supplemental Security Income
SSKI
saturated solution of potassium iodide
SSNS
steroid-sensitive idiopathic nephrotic
syndrome
SSPE
subacute sclerosing panencephalitis
SSRI
selective serotonin reuptake inhibitor
SSS
scalded skin syndrome
SSS syndrome
SSSS
staphylococcal scalded skin syndrome
SSVC
systemic venous collateral
SSW
short-stay ward
St.
St. Anthony's fire
St. Joseph Aspirin-Free Cold
Tablets for Children
St. Joseph Cough Suppressant
St. Joseph Measured Dose Nasal
Solution
St. Jude Children's Research
Hospital staging system
St. Jude Research Hospital
St. Louis encephalitis (SLE)
St. Vitus dance
STA analyzer
stability
ankle s.
collateral ligament s.
joint s.
stabilizer
mast cell s.
stabilizing bar
stable
s. factor
s. microbubble test
staccato
s. cough
s. voiding
staccato-like cough

NOTES

S

539

Stachybotrys
   S. atra
   S. chartarum
stacked-coin appearance
Staclot test
stadiometer
   Harpenden s.
   Holtain height s.
   neonatal s.
stage
   s. A, B, C, N infection
   acceptance s.
   alveolar s.
   anger s.
   bargaining s.
   s. C
   canalicular s.
   decoding s.
   denial s.
   depression s.
   hemolymphatic s.
   hyperirritable s.
   illocutionary s.
   intermediate dystonic s.
   locutionary s.
   Marshall and Tanner pubertal s.
   meningoencephalitic s.
   Norwood s.
   perlocutionary s.
   pigmentary s.
   preicteric s.
   preoperational s.
   prereading s.
   pseudoglandular s.
   saccular s.
   sensory-motor s.
   shock s.
   Tanner developmental s.
   Tanner genital s.
   Tanner maturation s.
   Theiler s.
   transitional reader s.
   understanding s.
staged repair
Stagesic
staging
   Marshall and Tanner pubertal s.
   Tanner s. (I–V)
stagnant loop syndrome
STAI
   Spielberger State-Trait Anxiety Inventory
   State-Trait Anxiety Inventory
stain
   acetylcholinesterase histochemical s.
   acid-fast s.
   acridine orange s.
   auramine-rhodamine s.
   Betke s.

   Brown-Hopp tissue Gram s.
   calcofluor white s.
   Csaba s.
   Dieterle s.
   direct fluorescent antibody s.
   eosin s.
   fluorescein s.
   Giemsa s.
   Golgi s.
   Gomori methenamine-silver s.
   Gomori trichrome s.
   Gram s.
   Hansel s.
   H&E s.
   hematoxylin and eosin s.
   immunoperoxidase s.
   India ink s.
   Kinyoun acid-fast s.
   Kinyoun carbol fuchsin s.
   Kleihauer s.
   Kleihauer-Betke s.
   Lugol iodine s.
   Luna-Parker acid fuscin s.
   macular s.
   methenamine silver s.
   modified Dieterle s.
   modified Kinyoun acid-fast s.
   modified trichrome s.
   Perls iron s.
   port-wine s.
   potassium chloride s.
   rhodamine-auramine s.
   silver s.
   Sudan s.
   supravital s.
   toluidine blue s.
   trichrome s.
   Warthin-Starry silver s.
   Warthin-Starry tissue Gram s.
   Wayson s.
   Wright s.
   Ziehl-Neelsen s.
stained
   meconium s.
staining
   acid-Schiff s.
   DFA s.
   direct fluorescent antibody s.
   direct immunofluorescent s.
   direct immunohistochemical s.
   endomysial s.
   meconium s.
staircase
   s. approach
   s. response
stalk
   mesenteric s.
   narrow mesenteric s.

stammering
Stamm gastrostomy
stance
    horse-riding s.
    s. phase
stand
    warming s.
    s. x-ray
stand-alone pharmacotherapy
standard
    s. deviation
    s. deviation score (SDS)
standardization
standardized
    s. observation scale
    s. reading inventory
    s. test
stander
    prone s.
standstill
    cardiac s.
Stanford-Binet
    S.-B. Fourth Edition (SBFE)
    S.-B. Intelligence Scale
    S.-B. Intelligence Scale for
      Children
    S.-B. Intelligence Scale, Fourth
      Edition
    S.-B. Intelligence Test
    S.-B. L-M
    S.-B. Memory Scale, 4th Edition
    S.-B. score
Stanford Diagnostic Reading Test
stanozolol
stapes
Staphcillin
staphylococcal
    s. blepharitis
    s. furuncle
    s. furunculosis
    s. impetigo
    s. infection
    s. pneumonia
    s. pustulosis
    s. scalded skin
    s. scalded skin syndrome (SSSS)
    s. scarlet fever
    s. toxic shock syndrome
staphylococcal enterotoxin B (SEB)
Staphylococcus
    S. aureus
    S. aureus molluscum

    coagulase-negative *S.*
    coagulase-positive *S.*
    S. epidermidis
    S. epidermidis folliculitis
    S. intermedius
    S. pyogenes
    S. saprophyticus
staphylococcus, pl. **staphylococci**
Staphylococcus **epidermis**
staple anastomosis
stapler
    TL-90 Ethicon s.
stapling
    epiphyseal s.
    gastric s.
    unilateral s.
STAR
    Simultaneous Technique for Acuity and
      Readiness Testing
StAR
    steroidogenic acute regulatory protein
star chart
starch malabsorption
STARFlex device
Stargardt disease
staring spell
Starling
    S. force
    S. mechanism
start
    Head S.
    sleep s.
startle
    s. disease
    s. epilepsy
    s. reflex
    s. response
starvation ketosis
stasis, pl. **stases**
    bile s.
    bowel s.
    colonic s.
    gallbladder s.
    large bowel s.
    small intestine s.
    urinary s.
state
    active and intense crying s.
    s. of alertness
    awake and active s.
    behavioral s.

S

NOTES

state *(continued)*
S. Children's Health Insurance Program (SCHIP)
emotional s.
hyperammonemic s.
hypercoagulable s.
hyperosmolar s.
intense emotional s.
paroxysmal emotional s.
persistent vegetative s. (PVS)
preeclamptic s.
preseizure s.
quiet and alert s.
steady s.
transient insulinopenic s.
uremic s.

State-Trait
S.-T. Anxiety Inventory (STAI)
S.-T. Anxiety Inventory for Children

static
s. admittance
s. deformity
s. elastance (E_{st})
s. encephalopathy
s. splint

Staticin
O-V S.

Statistical Package for Social Sciences (SPSS)

stature
constitutional short s.
familial short s.
idiopathic short s. (ISS)
non-growth hormone-deficient short s. (NGHD-SS)
short s. (SS)
small s.

status
absence s.
s. asthmaticus
circumcision s.
s. dysmyelinatus
s. epilepticus (SE)
s. loss
s. marmoratus
petit mal s.
psychomotor s.
s. spongiosus
visceral protein s.

stavudine (d4T)
ST change
S-T Cort Topical
STD
sexually transmitted disease
steady state

steal
s. phenomenon
subclavian s.
stearin-lanolin cream
steatocystoma multiplex
steatohepatitis
nonalcoholic s. (NASH)
steatorrhea
idiopathic s.
steatosis
microvesicular s.
STEC
Shiga toxin-producing *Escherichia coli*
Steele
Blanche sign of S.
S. procedure
steeple sign
Steinert disease
Stein-Leventhal syndrome
Stelazine
stellate
s. cell
s. ganglion ablation
s. iris
s. reticulum
stellatoides
Candida s.
Stellwag sign
stem
s. cell
s. cell bone marrow transplantation
s. cell therapy
s. cell transplantation (SCT)
stenosis, pl. **stenoses**
acute subglottic s.
annular s.
anorectal s.
antral s.
aortic s. (AS)
aortic valve s.
aqueductal s.
bile duct s.
choanal s.
chronic subglottic s.
congenital aortic s.
congenital esophageal s.
congenital hypertrophic pyloric s.
congenital nasal pyriform aperture s. (CNPAS)
congenital tracheal s.
critical aortic s.
critical pulmonic s.
discrete subaortic s. (DSS)
duodenal s.
esophageal s.
s. of esophagus
hypertrophic s.
hypertrophic pyloric s. (HPS)

idiopathic hypertrophic subaortic s. (IHSS)
infantile hypertrophic pyloric s. (IHPS)
infundibular s.
lacrimal duct s.
laryngeal s.
laryngotracheal s. (LTS)
long-segment congenital tracheal s. (LSCTS)
meatal s.
mild pulmonic s.
mitral s.
nasal pyriform aperture s.
peripheral pulmonary s.
peripheral pulmonic s.
piriform aperture s.
s. post intubation
primary aqueductal s.
pulmonary s.
pulmonary valve s.
pulmonic s. (PS)
pyloric s.
renal artery s.
semilunar valvular s.
short-segment s.
subaortic s.
subglottic s.
supravalvular aortic s.
supravalvulvar pulmonary s.
s. of trachea
tracheal s.
tricuspid s.
valvular pulmonic s.

stenotic
s. hymen
s. nasolacrimal duct

Stenotrophomonas
S. *maltophilia*
S. *maltophilia* infection

Stensen duct
stent
Aboulker s.
endoluminal s.
expandable esophageal s. (EES)
Palmaz s.
pancreatic duct s.
s. placement

stenting
endoluminal s.

stepdown therapy
Stephan HF 300 respirator

Stephanie 8000 oscillator
stepoff
stepping
reflex s.
s. reflex
s. response

stepwise antiinflammatory therapy
Sterapred
stercoralis
Strongyloides s.

stereoacuity
stereognosis
stereotactic
s. radiography
s. radiosurgery
s. thalamotomy

stereotypical
s. movement
s. movement disorder

stereotypic behavior
stereotypy, pl. **stereotypies**
sterile
s. pus
s. pyuria
s. water gastric drip (SWGD)

sterna (*pl. of* sternum)
sternal
s. fracture
s. recession

Sternberg sign
sternochondral junction
sternocleidomastoid (SCM)
s. fibroma

sternomastoid
s. foramen
s. tumor

sternotomy
sternum, pl. **sterna**
fissure of s.

steroid
s. acne
anabolic androgenic s.
androgenic s.
antenatal s.
gonadal s.
inhaled s.
s. inhaler
sex s.
s. sulfatase (STS)
s. sulfatase deficiency
s. sulfate (STS)
systemic s.

S

NOTES

steroid *(continued)*
    s. therapy
    s. treatment
steroid-dependent colitis
steroid-induced myopathy
steroidogenic
    s. acute regulatory protein (StAR)
    s. factor-1 (SF-1)
steroid-sensitive
    s.-s. idiopathic nephrotic syndrome (SSNS)
    s.-s. nephrotic syndrome
stertor
stethoscope
    bell s.
Stevens-Johnson syndrome
stick
    arterial s.
    heel s.
    Kinney S.'s
    silver nitrate s.
Sticker disease
Stickler
    S. dysplasia
    S. syndrome
sties *(pl. of* sty)
stiff-baby syndrome
stiff-man syndrome
stiff neck
stiffness
    lead pipe s.
stigma, pl. **stigmata**
    Down stigmata
    radiologic stigmata
    Ulrich-Turner stigmata
stigmasterol
stigmatization
stilbestrol
Still
    S. disease
    S. murmur
stillbirth
stillborn
Stilling-Türk-Duane syndrome
Stimate
stimulant drug
stimulation
    direct s.
    electrical s.
    electrophrenic s.
    enterochromaffin cell s.
    labyrinthine s.
    laryngopharyngeal sensory s. (LPSS)
    oral s.
    photic s.
    sensory s.
    sympathetic s.
    tactile s.
    transcranial magnetic s. (TMS)
    transcutaneous electrical nerve s. (TENS)
    vagal nerve s.
    vestibular s.
stimulator
    long-acting thyroid s. (LATS)
stimulus
    amblyogenic s.
    antigenic s.
    click s.
    congenital amblyogenic s.
    high-intensity click s.
    neonatal amblyogenic s.
    nociceptive s.
    tactile s.
stimulus-response (S-R)
Sting procedure
stippled epiphysis
stippling
    basophilic s.
    corneal s.
    s. of epiphyses
stirrup
STNR
    symmetrical tonic neck reflex
stocking-glove sensory loss
Stock-Spielmeyer-Vogt syndrome
Stokes-Adams
    S.-A. attack
    S.-A. syndrome
stoma, pl. **stomas, stomata**
    ileal s.
stomach
    s. ache
    herniated s.
    infarction of herniated s.
Stomahesive
stomas *(pl. of* stoma)
stomata *(pl. of* stoma)
stomatitis
    angular s.
    aphthous s.
    fusospirillary gangrenous s.
    gangrenous s.
    herpes s.
    herpetic s.
    recurrent aphthous s.
    vesiculoulcerative s.
    Vincent s.
stomatocyte
stomatocytosis
    hereditary s.
stone
    cholesterol s.
    cystine s.
    kidney s.

pigment s.
struvite s.
uric acid s.

stool

acholic s.
s. antigen test
s. colonization
currant jelly s.
electron microscopy of s.
greasy s.
grossly bloody s.
guaiac-negative s.
guaiac-positive s.
heme-negative s.
heme-positive s.
72-hour s. collection
milk s.
pale s.
s. porphyrin
s. retention
ribbonlike s.
transition s.

stooling
stool-reducing substance
stopcock

three-way s.

STOP-ROP

Supplemental Therapeutic Oxygen for
Prethreshold Retinopathy of Prematurity
STOP-ROP trial

storage

abnormal glucosylceramide s.
s. disease
s. disorder

STORCH

syphilis, toxoplasmosis, other agents,
rubella, cytomegalovirus, herpes
simplex virus

storiform-pleomorphic histologic subtype
stork bite
storm

affective s.
thyroid s.

story-stem

new MacArthur emotion s.-s.'s

Storz infant bronchoscope
STR

skin test reactivity

strabismic amblyopia
strabismus

comitant s.
s. concomitans

constant s.
convergent s.
divergent s.
incomitant s.
intermittent s.
nonparalytic s.
paralytic s.
s. syndrome

straddle injury
straddling atrioventricular valve
strae vascularis
straight

s. last shoe
s. sinus

straight-back syndrome
straightening

retinal arterial narrowing and s.
(RANS)

straight-leg immobilizer
straight-line graph method
strain

compression-rarefaction s.
Enders Edmonston measles s.
impetigo s.
Jeryl Lynn mumps s.
macrophage-tropic s.
M-tropic s.
non-syncytium-inducing s.
NSI s.
Oka s.
RA27/3 rubella s.
rheumatogenic s.
RIT 4385 mumps s.
Schwarz measles s.
Simkania negevensis s. Z
T cell-tropic syncytium-inducing s.
T-tropic SI s.

stranger

s. anxiety
s. reaction

strangulating obstruction
strap

figure-of-eight clavicle s.

strapping

figure-of-eight s.

Strassman metroplasty
strategy

maladaptive coping s.
Robins and Guze validation s.

stratum corneum
Strauss method

NOTES

S

strawberry
    s. cervix
    s. hemangioma
    s. mark
    s. nevus
    s. tongue
streak
    s. gonad
    marbled hypopigmented s.
Streeter dysplasia
street smart
strength
    Allerest Headache S.
    Allerest Maximum S.
    Anbesol Maximum S.
    Biotin Forte Extra S.
    Clocort Maximum S.
    double s. (XX)
    Kaopectate Maximum S.
    Maalox Plus Extra S.
    Orajel Maximum S.
    Tylenol Extra S.
    Vanceril Double S.
strep
    s. breath
    s. throat
Streptase
Streptex
Streptobacillus moniliformis
streptococcal
    s. antibody
    s. antigen panel
    s. bacteremia
    s. cellulitis
    s. exotoxin-A (SPEA)
    s. gangrene
    s. group
    group A beta-hemolytic s.
    s. infection
    s. meningitis
    s. pharyngitis
    s. pneumonia
    s. pyoderma
    s. tonsillitis
    s. tonsillopharyngitis
    s. toxic shock syndrome
streptococci (*pl. of* streptococcus)
streptococcosis
Streptococcus
    S. agalactiae
    S. aureus
    S. bacteria
    S. bovis
    S. constellates
    S. milleri
    S. mutans
    S. pneumonia

    S. pneumoniae
    S. pyogenes
    S. salivarius
    S. viridans
streptococcus, pl. **streptococci**
    anaerobic s.
    group A beta-hemolytic s.
    (GABHS)
    group B s. (GBS)
    group C s.
    group G s.
    pediatric autoimmune-mediated
    neuropsychiatric disorders
    associated with s.
    pediatric autoimmune
    neuropsychiatric disorders
    associated with s. (PANDAS)
    streptococci rapid antigen detection
    test
    rheumatogenic s.
    viridans s.
streptogene
    erythema s.
streptogramin
streptokinase factor
Streptomyces griseus
streptomycin
Streptozyme test
stress
    adrenocortical s.
    behavioral s.
    clastogenic s.
    cold s.
    end-systolic s. (ESS)
    end-systolic wall s.
    s. erythrocytosis
    s. erythropoiesis
    s. fracture
    s. incontinence
    s. injury
    neonatal s.
    s. neonate
    s. oximetry
    s. reaction
    shear s.
    s. test
    thermal s.
    s. view radiograph
stress-associated ulcer
stress-induced syncope
stressor
    sociocultural s.
stress-related peptic ulcer disease
stretched
    s. penile length
    s. phallic length
stretch and hair groomer's syncope

stretching
    bladder s.
stria, pl. **striae**
    striae atrophicae
    striae cutis distensae
    Haab s.
    Wickham s.
striata
    osteopathia s.
striatal toe
striate
    s. body
    s. hyperkeratosis
striation
    dense s.
    longitudinal dense s.
    transverse dense s.
    vertical s.
striatothalamic junction
striatum
striatus
    lichen s.
stricto
    Borrelia burgdorferi sensu s.
stricture
    colonic s.
    esophageal s.
    midureteral s.
stricturoplasty
stride
stridor
    audible s.
    congenital laryngeal s.
    inspiratory s.
    laryngeal s.
    postextubation s.
stridulous breathing
strike
    heel s.
string
    egg on a s.
    s. sign
strip
    Dextrostix reagent s.
    DiaScreen reagent s.
    reagent s.
    s. test
stripping
    apical pleural s.
    periosteal s.
    s. of pleura

stroke
    mitochondrial encephalopathy, lactic
      acidosis, s.
    perinatal s.
    prenatal s.
    silent s.
stroma, pl. **stromata**
    cellular desmoplastic s.
    fibromyxoid s.
stromal tumor
strong virilization
Strongyloides stercoralis
strongyloidiasis
strongyloidosis
Stroop test
structural integration
structure
    limbic s.
struvite stone
strychnine
STS
    steroid sulfatase
    steroid sulfate
    STS deficiency
ST-segment
    ST-s. abnormality
    ST-s. elevation
ST-T wave abnormality
Stuart-Power factor
stuck
    s. twin gestation
    s. twin syndrome
Student t-test
study
    Bogalusa Heart S. (BHS)
    breath hydrogen s.
    child behavioral s. (CBS)
    Childhood Cancer Survivor S.
    CHIME s.
    clinical cohort s.
    coagulation s.
    cohort s.
    Collaborative Home Infant
      Monitoring Evaluation s.
    Collaborative Perinatal S. (CPS)
    Diagnostic Interview for Genetic S.
      (DIGS)
    DONALD s.
    Doppler flow s.
    Dortmund Nutritional and
      Anthropometrical Longitudinally
      Designed s.

S

NOTES

study *(continued)*
    double-blind s.
    Dunedin longitudinal s.
    electroencephalographic sleep s.
    embryonic organ culture s.
    epidemiological s.
    gene s.
    high oxygen percentage in
      retinopathy of prematurity s.
    HOPE-ROP s.
    immunofluorescence s.
    large-volume blood s.
    longitudinal s.
    MacArthur Longitudinal Twin S.
    MECA s.
    methodology s.
    mineral balance s.
    molecular genetic s.
    Multicenter AIDS Cohort S.
      (MACS)
    National Acute Spinal Cord
      Injury S.
    nerve conduction s.
    neuroimaging s.
    North American Collaborative
      Crohn Disease S. (NCCDS)
    placebo-controlled s.
    radioisotopic reperfusion and
      excretion s.
    Second National Incidence S. (NIS-
      2)
    sleep s.
    videofluoroscopic swallowing s.
      (VFSS)
    videourodynamic s.
    Women and Infants
      Transmission S. (WITS)
stuff
    Numby S.
stump
    appendiceal s.
    inverted appendiceal s.
    rectal s.
    umbilical s.
stun
    cardiac s.
stunned myocardium
stunning
    myocardial s.
stunting
    growth s.
stupor
stuporous
Sturge-Kalischer-Weber syndrome
Sturge syndrome
Sturge-Weber
    S.-W. disease
    S.-W. syndrome (SWS)

stuttering
    medication-induced s.
    neurogenic s.
Stx
    Shiga toxin
sty, stye, pl. **sties, styes**
STYCAR
    Screening Tests for Young Children and
      Retardates
    Sheridan Tests for Young Children and
      Retardates
Stycar graded balls
stye *(var. of* sty)
styes *(pl. of* sty)
style
    learning s.
stylomastoid foramen
subacute
    s. bacterial endocarditis
    s. combined degeneration
    s. encephalitis
    s. fetal hypoxia
    s. myeloopticoneuropathy
    s. necrotizing encephalomyopathy
    s. necrotizing encephalopathy
    s. neuritis
    s. neuronopathic Gaucher disease
    s. osteomyelitis
    s. sclerosing panencephalitis (SSPE)
    s. thyroiditis
    s. tracheitis
subaortic
    s. conus
    s. hypertrophic cardiomyopathy
    s. membrane
    s. stenosis
subaponeurotic cranial space
subarachnoid
    s. bolt
    s. hemorrhage
subareolar tissue
subaverage intelligence
subcapsular hepatic hematoma
subclavian
    s. artery
    s. artery defect
    s. flap aortoplasty (SFA)
    s. steal
subclinical
subconjunctival hemorrhage
subcoronal hypospadias
subcortical laminar heterotopia
subcostal
    s. incision
    s. view
subcutanea
    lipogranulomatosis s.

subcutaneous
- s. calcification
- s. desferrioxamine therapy
- s. emphysema
- s. fat necrosis
- s. granuloma annulare
- s. neurofibroma
- s. nodule
- s. sarcoidosis
- s. tunnel
- s. ventricular catheter reservoir

subdiaphragmatic air
subdural
- s. abscess
- s. effusion
- s. empyema
- s. hematoma (SDH)
- s. hemorrhage
- s. puncture
- s. tap

subdural-peritoneal shunt
subendocardial
subependymal
- s. bleeding
- s. cryptic angioma
- s. germinal matrix hemorrhage
- s. germinolysis
- s. heterotopia
- s. region

subepidermal
- s. blister
- s. keratin cyst

subfibulare
- os s.

subgaleal
- s. hematoma (SGH)
- s. hemorrhage

subglottic
- s. edema
- s. stenosis

subhyaloid hemorrhage
subiculum
subischial leg length (SILL)
subitum
- exanthum s.

sublamina densa
Sublimaze Injection
sublingual
- s. gland
- s. hematoma
- Nitrostat S.

- s. onychomycosis
- s. thyroid

subluxating patella
subluxation
- atlantoaxial s.
- cervical spine s.
- s. dislocation
- habitual shoulder s.
- radial head s. (RHS)
- rotary s.
- rotatory s.
- shoulder s.

subluxed hip
submaxillary gland
submental
- s. hematoma
- s. lymphadenitis
- s. lymphadenopathy

submentovertex view
submersion
- iced saline s.
- s. injury

submucosal arterial malformation
submucous
- s. cleft
- s. cleft palate

subnormal
- s. growth velocity
- s. temperature

subonychomycosis
suborbital edema
subperiosteal
- s. abscess
- s. aspiration

subphrenic
- s. abscess
- s. gas collection

subpial region
subpleural reticulonodular pattern
subpulmonic area
subretinal
- s. exudate
- s. fluid

subsalicylate
- bismuth s.

subscale
subscapular skinfold thickness
subsegmental atelectasis
substance
- s. abuse
- s. abuse, sexuality, safety
  assessment

NOTES

substance *(continued)*
    illegal s.
    s. P immune reactivity
    reducing s.
    school, home, activities,
      depression/self-esteem, s.
    stool-reducing s.
    thiobarbituric acid-reacting s.
      (TBARS)
    urine-reducing s.
    s. use disorder (SUD)
substance-induced psychotic disorder
substantia
    s. gelatinosa
    s. nigra
    s. nigra pars reticulata
    s. propria
substernal retraction
substitute care
subsyndromal depressive symptom
subtalar facet
subtest
    Digit Span S.
subthalamicum
    corpus s.
subtilis
    Bacillus s.
subtle
    s. neurologic sequela
    s. seizure
subtrigonal injection
subtype
    Estren-Damashek s.
    myxoid histopathologic s.
    storiform-pleomorphic histologic s.
subungual
    s. exostosis
    s. fibroma
subureteric Teflon injection
subvalvular
subxiphoid
subzonal
    s. injection (SUZI)
    s. injection of sperm
    s. insertion
succedaneum
    caput s.
succimer
succinate
    s. dehydrogenase
    hydrocortisone sodium s.
succinyl
    s. aminoimidazole carboxamide
    ribotide (SAICAR)
    s. CoA:3-ketoacid CoA transferase
    (SCOT)
    s. CoA:3-ketoacid CoA transferase
    deficiency

succinylcholine
succumb
suck
    poor s.
    weak s.
sucking
    s. blister
    s. pad
suckling reflex
Sucraid
sucralfate
sucrase-isomaltase deficiency
Sucrets Cough Calmers
sucrose
    concentrated oral s.
    s. gradient
    s. hemolysis test
    s. pacifier
sucrosuria
suction
    nasopharyngeal s.
    open endotracheal s.
    respiratory s.
    Trach Care s.
    wall s.
suctioning
    closed endotracheal s.
    closed endotracheal tube s.
    nasopharyngeal s.
    open endotracheal s.
    respiratory s.
SUD
    substance use disorder
    sudden unexpected death
Sudafed
    S. Cough Syrup
    S. 12 Hour
    S. Plus
sudamina
    miliary s.
sudanophilic
    s. cerebral sclerosis
    s. diffuse sclerosis
Sudan stain
sudden
    s. death
    s. infant death
    s. infant death syndrome (SIDS)
    s. infant death unexplained by
    history
    s. unexpected death (SUD)
Sudeck atrophy
sudomotor dysfunction
sudoral miliaria
SUFE
    slipped upper femoral epiphysis
Sufedrin
Sufenta Injection

sufentanil
sufficient
    pancreas s. (PS)
    s. quantity (q.s.)
    quantity not s. (q.n.s.)
suffocation
    infant s.
    mechanical s.
suffusion
    conjunctival s.
sugar
    blood s.
    s. diabetes
    fasting blood s.
    s. intoxication
    low blood s.
    mannose-type s.
sugar-dipped pacifier
sugar-tong splint
Sugiura procedure
suicidal ideation
suicidality
suicide
    attempted s.
    s. gene therapy
    hospitalized attempted s. (HAS)
    s. risk screen (SRS)
suis
    Brucella s.
Sulamyd
    Sodium S.
sulbactam
    ampicillin and s.
sulcus, pl. **sulci**
    Harrison s.
Sulf-10
sulfa
sulfacetamide
sulfadiazine
    silver s.
sulfadoxine and pyrimethamine
Sulfair
Sulfalax
Sulfamethoprim
sulfamethoxazole and trimethoprim
Sulfamylon cream
sulfasalazine
sulfatase
    iduronate s. (IDS)
    steroid s. (STS)
sulfate
    abacavir s.

    amikacin s.
    amphetamine s.
    atropine s.
    chondroitin s.
    dehydroepiandrosterone s. (DHEAS)
    dermatan s.
    dextroamphetamine s.
    ferrous s.
    gentamicin s.
    heparin s.
    hexoprenaline s.
    hydrazine s.
    hydroxychloroquine s.
    keratan s.
    magnesium s.
    morphine s.
    Mycifradin S.
    neomycin s.
    Plaquenil S.
    protamine s.
    quinine s.
    steroid s. (STS)
    terbutaline s.
    trimethoprim s.
    zinc s.
sulfatide
Sulfatrim DS
sulfhydryl (SH)
sulfide
    selenium s.
sulfisoxazole
    erythromycin and s.
sulfite oxidase deficiency
sulfonamide
sulfonate
    sodium polystyrene s.
sulfonylurea
sulfur
    s. dioxide
    s. and salicylic acid
sulindac
sulprostone
sum
    cumulative s. (CUSUM)
Sumacal formula
sumatriptan nasal spray
summation gallop
Sumycin Oral
SUN
    serum urea nitrogen
sunburn
    blistering s.

S

NOTES

sunburst
    s. appearance
    s. phenomenon
sunflower
    s. cataract
    s. oil challenge test
sunken anterior fontanelle
Sunlight Omnisense ultrasound
Sunna circumcision
sunrise view
sun-seeking pattern
sunset eyes
sunsetting eyes
sunstroke
super
    S. Block
    s. blue light
    s. syringe
superabsorbent
superactivity
    phosphoribosylpyrophosphate
      synthetase s.
    PRPP synthetase s.
superconducting quantum interference
  device susceptometer (SQUIDS)
superfamily
    transforming growth factor beta s.
superfecundation
superfetation
superficial
    s. compartment
    s. ectopic testis
    s. onychomycosis
superfluous
superinfection
superior
    s. iliac crest
    s. iliac spine
    s. laryngeal nerve
    s. mediastinal syndrome
    s. mesenteric angiogram
    s. mesenteric artery syndrome
    s. mesenteric vein
    s. oblique muscle
    s. olivary nucleus
    s. olive
    s. ramus
    s. sagittal sinus
    s. vena cava (SVC)
    s. vena cava syndrome
    s. venous system
    s. vesical fissure
supernatant
supernumerary
    s. breast
    s. digit
    s. kidney
    s. nipple

superoxide
    s. dismutase-1
    s. radical
supersaturation of bile
SuperVent
supinate
supination
    passive s.
supine
    s. length
    s. sleep position
Suplena formula
supplement
    Boost nutritional s.
    dietary s.
    EleCare nutritional s.
    enzyme s.
    infant dietary s.
    iron s.
    magnesium s.
    NeoSure nutritional s.
    Nutriset s.
    nutritional s.
    Pediatrician infant dietary s.
    phosphate s.
    potassium s.
    zinc s.
Supplemental
    S. Newborn Screen
    S. Security Income (SSI)
    S. Therapeutic Oxygen for
      Prethreshold Retinopathy of
      Prematurity (STOP-ROP)
    S. Therapeutic Oxygen for
      Prethreshold Retinopathy of
      Prematurity trial
supplementation
support
    advanced cardiac life s. (ACLS)
    advanced life s. (ALS)
    advanced pediatric life s. (APLS)
    advanced trauma life s. (ATLS)
    basic life s. (BLS)
    extensive s.
    extracorporeal life s. (ECLS)
    inotropic s.
    intermittent s.
    limited s.
    medial longitudinal arch s.
    Multidimensional Scale of
      Perceived Social S. (MSPSS)
    neonatal adjuvant life s.
    pediatric advanced life s. (PALS)
    pervasive s.
    s. reflex
    s. services
    s. trust
    ventilatory s.

supportive
> s. group therapy
> s. psychotherapy

suppository
> Anusol-HC S.
> bisacodyl s.
> Cort-Dome High Potency S.
> Dilaudid S.
> glycerin s.
> intravaginal s.
> parecetamol s.
> rectal s.
> Sani-Supp S.

Supprelin

suppressant
> St. Joseph Cough S.

suppression
> adrenal s.
> bone marrow s.
> s. burst
> fetal parathyroid s.

Suppress lozenge

Supprettes
> Aquachloral S.

suppurate

suppurating sinus tract

suppuration
> intracranial s.
> joint s.
> pulmonary s.

suppurativa
> hidradenitis s.
> vulvar hidradenitis s.

suppurative
> s. arthritis
> s. bursitis
> s. cholangitis
> s. infection
> s. labyrinthitis
> s. lymphadenitis
> s. mediastinitis
> s. otitis media
> s. parotitis
> s. pneumonia
> s. thyroiditis

suprabasal blister

suprabulbar paresis

supracardiac total anomalous pulmonary venous return

supraclavicular
> s. indrawing
> s. retraction

supracondylar humeral fracture

supracristal ventricular septal defect

supraglottic
> s. aperture
> s. web

supraglottitis

supralevator
> s. abscess
> s. imperforate anus

supramalleolar orthosis (SMO)

supranormal scrotal position

supranuclear palsy

supraorbital nerve block

suprapineal recess

suprapubic
> s. aspiration of urine
> s. bladder aspiration
> s. cystostomy
> s. discomfort
> s. fat pad
> s. mass

suprasellar
> s. arachnoid cyst
> s. meningioma

suprasternal
> s. notch
> s. notch thrill
> s. view

supratentorial
> s. anaplastic ependymoma
> s. white matter

supratip nasal tip deformity

supravalvular
> s. aortic stenosis
> s. pulmonary stenosis

supraventricularis
> crista s.

supraventricular tachycardia (SVT)

supravital
> s. stain
> s. stain test

Suprax

sural nerve biopsy

767 SureTemp4 oral thermometer

SURF
> Service Utilization and Risk Factors

Surfacaine

surface
> decreased mucosal s.
> s. electromyogram
> s. furrowing
> s. furrowing of tongue

S

NOTES

553

surface *(continued)*
    hepatitis B s. (HBs)
    lingual s.
surfactant
    bovine lavage extract s. (BLES)
    s. deficiency syndrome
    exogenous s.
    heterologous s.
    homologous s.
    Infrasurf s.
    s. lavage
    porcine s.
    s. protein-A (SP-A)
    s. protein-B (SP-B)
    s. protein-C (SP-C)
    s. protein deficiency
    pulmonary s.
    s. replacement therapy
    s. replacement trial
    rescue s.
    Survanta s.
    synthetic s.
surfactant-associated protein C enhancer
surfactant-deficient lung
Surfacten
Surfak
Sur-Fast needle
Surfaxin
    dilute S.
surf test
surge
    postnatal gonadotropin s.
    TSH s.
surgeon
surgery
    ablative s.
    endoscopic sinus s.
    extraocular muscle s.
    fetal s.
    gamma knife s.
    inferior turbinate s.
    laser s.
    lung s.
    muscle s.
    open heart s.
    orthognathic s.
    palliative s.
    pediatric lung s.
    peripheral ablative s.
    prenatal s.
    pull-through s.
    radioreceptor-guided s.
    sinus s.
    thoracic s.
    video-assisted thoracic s. (VATS)
    video-assisted thoracoscopic s. (VATS)

surgical
    s. containment
    s. cricothyrotomy
    s. enucleation
    s. hemostasis
    s. mastoiditis
    s. neonate
    s. procedure
    s. removal
    s. scarlet fever
    s. septectomy
    s. tape occlusion
Surgicel
surgicopathologic staging system
surrender posture
surrogate
Survanta surfactant
surveillance colonoscopy
survey
    Juvenile Wellness and Health S. (JWHS)
    Kids Eating Disorder S.
    National Ambulatory Medical Care S. (NAMCS)
    National Educational Longitudinal S. (NELS)
    National Health and Nutrition Examination S. (NHANES)
    School Sleep Habits S.
    skeletal s.
    youth risk behavioral s. (YRBS)
survival
    decreased red cell s.
survivor guilt
susceptibility hypothesis
susceptible
susceptometer
    superconducting quantum interference device s. (SQUIDS)
suspected child abuse or neglect (SCAN)
suspension
    budesonide inhalation s. (BIS)
    Children's Advil S.
    Children's Motrin S.
    Cortisporin Ophthalmic S.
    Cortisporin Otic S.
    Curosurf intratracheal s.
    horizontal s.
    Infasurf intratracheal s.
    inhalation s.
    orciprenaline oral s.
    ventral s.
suspensory ligament laxity
Sus-Phrine
suspicion
Sustacal Plus formula
Sustagen formula

S

sustained
s. autonomic hypoarousal
s. clonus
s. ventricular tachycardia
sustained-release
s.-r. albuterol
s.-r. theophylline
Sustaire
Sustiva
Sutherland procedure
Sutilains Ointment
suture
coronal s.
cranial s.
Maxon s.
nasofrontal s.
s. penile laceration
perianal s.
premature closure of coronal s.
sagittal s.
skin s.
wide cranial s.
suxamethonium
SUZI
subzonal injection
SVC
superior vena cava
SVR
systemic vascular resistance
SVT
supraventricular tachycardia
swab
calcium alginate s.
cotton-tipped s.
nasal s.
nasopharyngeal s.
rectal s.
throat s.
umbilical s.
swallow
barium s.
modified barium s. (MBS)
s. reflex
rehabilitation cookie s.
s. syncope
swallowed
s. blood syndrome
s. maternal blood
swallowing
air s.
s. difficulty
s. reflex

Swan-Ganz catheter
Swanson, Nolan, and Pelham checklist
sway
lateral shoulder s.
swayback
sweat
s. chloride
s. chloride concentration
s. chloride determination
s. chloride level
s. chloride test
s. duct
s. gland
night s.
s. testing
sweating
anhidrotic s.
excessive s.
hypohidrotic s.
nocturnal s.
Swedish national growth chart
sweetened pacifier
Sweet syndrome
swelling
brain s.
cerebral s.
diffuse brain s. (DBS)
focal axonal s.
global brain s.
hypoosmotic s. (HOS)
Swenson procedure
SWGD
sterile water gastric drip
Swift disease
Swim-Ear water drying aid
swimmer's
s. ear
s. itch
s. shoulder
swimming
s. movement
s. pool granuloma
s. position
s. reflex
swine-flu influenza vaccine
swinging
blanket s.
s. flashlight test
Swiss cheese septum
switch
adaptive s.
venous s.

NOTES

swivel walker
swollen
    s. glomerular tuft
    s. joint
SWS
    Sturge-Weber syndrome
Swyer-James-Macleod syndrome
Swyer-James syndrome
Swyer syndrome
SX-T
    Proplex SX-T
sycosis barbae
Sydenham
    S. chorea
    S. chorea criteria
Syllact
sylvatic typhus
sylvian
    s. aqueduct syndrome
    s. epilepsy
    s. seizure
Sylvius
    aqueduct of S.
Symadine
symbiotic psychosis
symblepharon
symbolic representation
Syme amputation
symmelia
Symmetrel
symmetric
    s. demyelination
    s. IUGR
    s. progressive erythrokeratoderma
symmetrical
    s. conjoined twin
    s. movement
    s. tonic neck reflex (STNR)
sympathetic
    s. chain
    s. ganglion
    s. innervation
    s. nerve system
    s. stimulation
    s. tissue
sympatholytic drop
sympathomimetic amine
sympathovagal
symphysis
    s. pubis
    s. pubis diastasis
symptom
    B s.'s
    s. contagion
    depressive s.
    dissociative s.
    intrusion s.

    mitochondrial encephalomyelopathy, lactic acidosis, strokelike s.'s
    neurovegetative s.
    neurovegetative functioning or s.
    obstructive s.
    pathognomonic s.
    posttraumatic signs or s.'s (PTSS)
    prodromal s.
    refractory depressive s.
    review of s.'s (ROS)
    schedule for negative s.'s (SANS)
    schedule for positive s.'s (SAPS)
    subsyndromal depressive s.
    tic s.
    Uhthoff s.
    vegetative s.
    vertiginous s.
symptomatic
    s. chronic empyema
    s. dystonia
    s. epilepsy
    s. progressive hydrocephalus
    s. spasm
    s. status epilepticus
symptomatology
Synacort Topical
synactive theory
Synagis
Synalar-HP Topical
Synalar Topical
synapse
synaptic pruning
synaptogenesis
synchondrosis disruption
synchronized
    s. DC cardioversion
    s. intermittent mandatory ventilation (SIMV)
    s. nasal intermittent positive-pressure ventilation (SNIPPV)
synchronously
syncopal
    s. episode
    s. spell
syncope
    cardiac s.
    cerebral s.
    cough s.
    micturition s.
    neurally mediated s. (NMS)
    neurocardiogenic s.
    reflex s.
    stress-induced s.
    stretch and hair groomer's s.
    swallow s.
    vasopressor s.
    vasovagal s.
syncytia (*pl. of* syncytium)

syncytiotrophoblast
syncytiotrophoblastic tumor giant cell
syncytium, pl. **syncytia**
    s. inducing (SI)
syndactylism
syndactylization
syndactyly
    complex s.
    digit s.
    simple s.
    soft tissue s.
    toe s.
syndesmosis, pl. **syndesmoses**
    tibiofibular s.
syndet cleaning bar
syndrome
    AAA s.
    Aagene s.
    Aarskog s.
    Aarskog-Scott s.
    abdominal compartment s. (ACS)
    ablepharon macrostomia s. (AMS)
    absent pulmonary valve s.
    abstinence s.
    Abt-Letterer-Siwe s.
    achalasia-addisonianism-alacrimia s.
    Achard s.
    achondrogenesis s.
    achondroplasia s.
    acquired immune deficiency s.
    (AIDS)
    acquired immunodeficiency s.
    (AIDS)
    acquired inflammatory Brown s.
    acrocallosal s.
    acrodysostosis s.
    acrorenal s.
    acrorenocular s.
    acrorenomandibular s.
    acute aseptic meningitis s.
    acute chest s. (ACS)
    s. of acute hemiplegia
    acute meningoencephalitis s.
    acute radiation s.
    acute respiratory distress s.
    (ARDS)
    acute retroviral s.
    acute traumatic compartment s.
    Adair-Dighton s.
    Adams-Oliver s.
    Adams-Stokes s.
    addisonian s.

Adie chronic pupillary s.
adiposogenital s.
adrenogenital s.
afebrile pneumonia s.
aglossia-adactylia s.
Aicardi s.
airway obstruction s.
Alagille s.
Albers-Schönberg s.
Albright s.
Aldrich s.
Alice in Wonderland s.
Allemann s.
Allgrove s.
Alpers s.
Alport s.
Alström s.
Alström-Hallgren s.
amenorrhea-galactorrhea s.
amniotic band s.
amniotic infection s.
amotivational s.
Anderson s.
androgen insensitivity s.
androgen resistance s.
anemia s.
Angelman s.
angioosteohypertrophy s.
anterior chamber cleavage s.
anterior chamber dysgenesis s.
anticonvulsant hypersensitivity s.
antiphospholipid s. (APS)
antiphospholipid antibody s.
Antley-Bixler s.
Apert s.
Apert-Crouzon s.
Arnold Chiari s.
arteriomesenteric duodenal
  compression s.
arthritis-dermatitis s.
arthrochalasis multiplex congenita
  Ehlers-Danlos s.
aseptic meningitis s.
Asherman s.
Asperger s. (AS)
asphyxiating thoracic dysplasia s.
asphyxiating thoracodystrophy s.
aspiration s.
asplenia s.
atypical hemolytic uremia s.
autistic s.

S

NOTES

syndrome *(continued)*

autoimmune lymphoproliferative s. (ALPS)
autoimmune polyendocrine s.
autosomal recessive ocular Ehlers-Danlos s.
Babinski-Fröhlich s.
baby bottle s.
bacterial overgrowth s.
Ballantyne-Runge s.
Baller-Gerold s.
Bannayan s.
Bannwarth s.
Banti s.
Bardet-Biedl s.
bare lymphocyte s.
Barlow s.
Bart s.
Barth s.
Bartter s.
basal cell nevus s.
Bassen-Kornzweig s.
Bazex s.
BBB s.
Beckwith s.
Beckwith-Wiedemann s. (BWS)
Behçet s.
Berardinelli-Seip s.
Bernard-Soulier s.
Bielschowsky s.
Biemond s.
Biglieri s.
binge eating s.
biopsychosocial s.
bird-headed dwarf s.
Björnstad s.
Blackfan-Diamond s.
Bland-Garland-White s.
blepharophimosis-ptosis s.
blind loop s.
Blizzard s.
Bloch-Sulzberger s.
Bloom s.
Blount s.
blue baby s.
blueberry muffin s.
blue diaper s.
blue histiocyte s.
blue rubber bleb nevus s. (BRBNS)
bobble-head doll s.
Bonnet-Dechaume-Blanc s.
Bonnevie-Ullrich s.
Boom s.
Bosma Henkin Christiansen s.
Bowen Hutterite s.
brachioskeletal-genital s.
Brachmann-de Lange s.

bradycardia-tachycardia s.
branchial arch s.
branchiootorenal s.
Brandt s.
Brett s.
bright thalamus s.
bronze baby s.
Brown-Séquard s.
Brown superior oblique tendon sheath s.
Brugada s.
bubbly lung s.
Budd-Chiari s.
Buschke-Ollendorf s.
Byler s.
Caffey s.
Caffey-Silverman s.
Calvé-Legg-Perthes s.
camptomelic s.
Camurati-Englemann s.
cancer family s.
cancer predisposition s.
Cantrell s.
capillary leak s. (CLS)
carbohydrate-deficient glycoprotein s. (type I) (CDGS)
carcinoid s.
cardiac, abnormal facies, thymic hypoplasia, cleft palate, hypocalcemia s.
cardiac-limb s.
cardiofacial s.
cardiofaciocutaneous s.
cardiovascular/central nervous system s.
Carpenter s.
Cast s.
catatonic s.
CATCH 22 s.
cat's eye s.
cat's urine s.
cauda equina s.
caudal dysplasia s.
caudal regression s.
cavernous sinus s.
Caylor cardiofacial s.
celiac s.
central anticholinergic s. (CAS)
central cord s.
central hypoventilation s.
central nervous system/cardiovascular s.
s. of cerebral atrophy
cerebral dysfunction s.
cerebral salt-wasting s.
cerebrohepatorenal s. (CHRS)
cerebrooculofacial-skeletal s.
Chanarin-Dorfman s.

Char s.
Charcot-Marie-Tooth s.
Charcot-Marie-Tooth-Hoffmann s.
CHARGE s.
Charlevois-Saguenay s.
Chédiak-Higashi s.
cherry-red spot myoclonus s.
chest s.
Chiari-Arnold s.
Chilaiditi s.
Chinese restaurant s.
cholestatic s.
Chotzen s.
Christ-Siemens-Touraine s.
chronic aspiration s.
chronic biopsychosocial s.
chronic compartment s.
chronic fatigue s. (CFS)
chronic pupillary s.
Churg-Strauss s.
chylomicronemia s.
Clarke-Hadfield s.
cleavage s.
cleidocranial dysplasia s.
Clifford s.
clitoris tourniquet s. (CTS)
Clouston s.
cloverleaf skull s.
clumsy child s.
COACH s.
Cobb s.
Cockayne s. (A, B)
Coffin-Lowry s.
Coffin-Siris s.
COFS s.
Cogan s.
Cohen s.
Cole-Hughes macrocephaly-mental
  retardation s.
compartment s.
compensatory antiinflammatory s.
complete DiGeorge s.
congenital anemia s.
congenital central hypoventilation s.
  (CCHS)
congenital Guillain-Barré s.
congenital heart defect s.
congenital high airway
  obstruction s. (CHAOS)
congenital hypothyroidism s.
congenital LCMV s.
congenital long QT s.

congenital nephrotic s.
congenital rubella s. (CRS)
congenital varicella s.
conjunctivitis-otitis s.
Conn s.
conotruncal anomaly face s.
  (CTAFS)
conotruncal facial s.
Conradi s.
Conradi-Hünermann s.
constriction band s.
contiguous gene deletion s.
contractural arachnodactyly s.
conus medullaris s.
Cornelia de Lange s.
corpus callosum hypoplasia,
  retardation, adducted thumbs,
  spastic paraplegia,
  hydrocephalus s.
Cowden s.
Crandall ectodermal dysplasia s.
craniocarpotarsal s.
craniosynostotic s.
CRASH s.
CREST s.
Creutzfeldt-Jakob s.
cri du chat s.
Crigler-Najjar s. (type I, II)
s. of crocodile tears
Cronkhite-Canada s.
Cross s.
Cross-McKusick-Breen s.
Crouzon s.
CRST s.
cryptophthalmia s.
cryptophthalmia-syndactyly s.
cryptophthalmos s.
Cushing s.
cushingoid s.
cyclic vomiting s.
cytomegaly s.
dancing eye s.
Dandy-Walker s.
Darrow-Gamble s.
Davidenkow s.
Deal s.
Debré-Fibiger s.
Debré-Sémélaigne s.
Dejerine-Klumpke s.
Dejerine-Sottas s.
de Lange s.
delayed sleep phase s. (DSPS)

S

NOTES

syndrome *(continued)*

deletion s.
de Morsier s.
de Morsier-Gauthier s.
dengue shock s.
Denys-Drash s.
De Sanctis-Cacchione s.
de Toni-Fanconi s.
de Toni-Fanconi-Debré s.
diabetes insipidus, diabetes mellitus,
   optic atrophy, deafness s.
Diamond-Blackfan s.
diarrhea-associated hemolytic
   uremic s.
DIDMOAD s.
diencephalic s. (DS)
DiGeorge s.
digitorenocerebral s.
distal intestinal obstruction s.
disuse s.
Donahue s.
DOOR s.
double cortex s.
Down s.
Drash s.
dry eye s.
Duane retraction s.
Dubin-Johnson s.
Dubowitz s.
dumping s.
Duncan s.
duplication-deficiency s.
Dyggve-Melchior-Clausen s.
Dyke-Davidoff s.
dysfibronectinemic Ehlers-Danlos s.
dysgenesis s.
dysmorphic s.
dysmotile cilia s.
dysmotility s.
dysplasia s.
dysplastic nevus s.
dysuria-pyuria s.
Eagle-Barrett s.
Eaton-Lambert myasthenic s.
ecchymotic Ehlers-Danlos s.
ectodermal dysplasia s.
ectrodactyly-ectodermal dysplasia-
   clefting s.
Edwards s.
Edwards-Gale s.
EEC s.
Ehlers-Danlos s. (EDS)
Eisenmenger s.
Elejalde s.
elfin facies s.
Ellis-van Creveld s.
Emery-Dreifuss s.
EMG s.

empty sella s.
endovascular hemolytic-uremic s.
enterocolitis s.
eosinophilia-myalgia s.
epicomus s.
epidermal nevus s.
epileptic s.
epiphyseal s.
episodic dyscontrol s.
Erb-Goldflam s.
euthyroid sick s.
Evans s.
exomphalos, macroglossia,
   gigantism s.
extraordinary urinary frequency s.
extrapyramidal-pyramidal s.
facet s.
facial dysmorphia s.
faciodigitogenital s.
failure-to-thrive s.
familial atypical multiple mole
   melanoma s.
familial chylomicronemia s.
familial insomnia s.
familial pyridoxine-dependency s.
Fanconi-Bickel s.
Fanconi pancytopenia s.
Farber s.
fast channel s.
fatigue s.
Felty s.
fetal alcohol s. (FAS)
fetal alcohol effects s.
fetal Dilantin s.
fetal hydantoin s. (FHS)
fetal nutritional deprivation s.
fetal overgrowth s.
fetal rubella s.
fetal transfusion s.
fetofetal transfusion s.
Feuerstein-Mimms s.
FG s.
Finnish-type congenital nephrotic s.
first arch s.
floppy infant s.
flulike s.
focal dermal hypoplasia s.
food-induced enterocolitis s.
Forbes-Albright s.
fragile X mental retardation s.
Franceschetti s.
Franceschetti-Klein s.
Francois s.
Fraser s.
Freeman-Sheldon s.
frequency dysuria s.
Fried s.
Fröhlich s.

Fryn s.
functional prepubertal castrate s.
G s.
Gardner s.
Gasser s.
gastrointestinal s.
gender dysphoria s.
genitopalatocardiac s.
Gerstmann s.
Gerstmann-Sträussler-Scheinker s.
Gianotti-Crosti s.
Gilbert s.
Gilbert-Dreyfus s.
Gilles de la Tourette s.
Gitelman s.
Glanzmann s.
glossopalatine ankylosis s.
gloves and socks s.
glutaric aciduria s. (type I, II)
Goldberg s.
Goldenhar microphthalmia s.
Goltz s.
Goltz-Gorlin s.
gonadal agenesis s.
Goodman s.
Goodpasture s.
Gordon s.
Gorlin s.
Gradenigo s.
gravis Ehlers-Danlos s.
gray baby s.
gray platelet s.
Greig cephalopolysyndactyly s.
Griscelli s.
Grisel s.
Guillain-Barré s. (GBS)
Guillain-Barré-Landry s.
HAIR-AN s.
Hakim s.
Hallermann-Streiff s.
Hallervorden-Spatz s.
Hallopeau-Siemens s.
Hall-Pallister s.
Hamman-Rich s.
hand-foot-genital s.
hand-foot-mouth s.
hand-foot-uterus s.
Hand-Schüller-Christian s.
Hanhart s.
hantavirus cardiopulmonary s. (HCPS)
hantavirus pulmonary s.

happy puppet s.
HARP s.
Haw River s.
heart defect s.
heart-hand s.
Heerfordt s.
Heiner s.
HELLP s.
hematophagocytic s.
hematopoietic s.
hematuria-dysuria s. (HDS)
hemolysis, elevated liver enzymes, low platelet count s.
hemolytic uremic s. (HUS)
hemophagocytic s.
hemorrhagic fever with renal s. (HFRS)
hemorrhagic shock s.
hemorrhagic shock and encephalopathy s. (HSES)
hepatic copper overload s.
hepatitis B arthritis-dermatitis s.
hepatopulmonary s. (HPS)
hepatorenal s.
hepatotoxic s.
hereditary benign intraepithelial dyskeratosis s.
hereditary dysplastic nevus s.
Hermansky-Pudlak s.
heterotaxy s.
HHH s.
high airway obstruction s.
Hinman s.
hirsutism, androgen excess, insulin resistance, acanthosis nigricans s.
Holt-Oram s.
Hopkins s.
Horner s.
Hoyeraal-Hreidarsson s. (HHS)
Hünermann-Happle s.
Hunter s.
Hurler s.
Hurler-Scheie s.
Hutchinson s.
Hutchinson-Gilford s.
hyaline membrane s.
17-hydroxylase deficiency s.
hyperammonemia, hyperornithinemia, homocitrullinuria s.
hypercalcemia elfin-facies s.
hypereosinophilic s.
hyper-IgD s.

S

NOTES

syndrome *(continued)*

hyper-IgE s.
hyper-IgM s.
hyperimmunoglobulin E s.
hyperinsulinism/hyperammonemia s.
hyperkinetic child s.
hyperlucent lung s.
hypermobile Ehlers-Danlos s.
hypermobility s.
hyperphosphaturic s.
hyperplastic right heart s.
hyperprostaglandin E_2 s.
hyperprostaglandinuric tubular s.
hypertelorism-hypospadias s.
hyperventilation s.
hyperviscosity s.
hypocalcemia and microdeletion
    22q11 s.
hypochondroplasia s.
hypocomplementemic urticarial
    vasculitis s. (HUVS)
hypoglossia-hypodactyly s.
hypomelia, hypotrichosis, facial
    hemangioma s.
hypoplasia s.
hypoplastic congenital anemia s.
hypoplastic left heart s. (HLHS)
hypothyroidism s.
hypoventilation s.
IADH s.
ichthyosis with keratitis and
    deafness s.
idiopathic hemolytic uremia s.
idiopathic long Q-T s.
idiopathic minimal lesion
    nephrotic s. (IMLNS)
idiopathic nephrotic s. (INS)
idiopathic respiratory distress s.
idiopathic steroid-resistant
    proteinuria/nephrotic s.
IgE s.
iliotibial band friction s.
Imerslünd s.
Imerslünd-Gräsbeck s.
immotile cilia s.
immunodeficiency s.
impingement s.
s. of inappropriate antidiuretic
    hormone (SIADH)
s. of inappropriate secretion of
    antidiuretic hormone (SIADH)
incontinentia pigmenti s.
infantile respiratory distress s.
infantile tremor s.
infant respiratory distress s. (IRDS)
infection-associated
    hemophagocytic s. (IAHS)
inflammatory Brown s.

influenza-like s.
inherited hemolytic uremia s.
insomnia s.
inspissated bile s.
inspissated milk s.
intraepithelial dyskeratosis s.
irritable bowel s. (IBS)
Isaacs s.
Ivemark s.
Jackson-Weiss s.
Jacobsen s.
Jadassohn-Lewandowski s.
Jaffe-Lichtenstein s.
Jakob-Creutzfeldt s.
James s.
Jansen s.
Jansky-Bielschowsky s.
Janus s.
Janz s.
Jarcho-Levin s.
JC s.
Jensen s.
Jervell s.
Jervell-Lange-Nielsen s.
Jeune s.
Job s.
Johanson-Blizzard s.
Josephs-Diamond-Blackfan s.
Joubert s. (type B)
Juberg-Marsidi s.
Kabuki make-up s.
Kallmann s.
Kanner s.
Kartagener s.
Kasabach-Merritt s.
Kaufman s.
Kawasaki s. (KS)
Kaznelson s.
Kearns-Sayre s. (KSS)
Keipert s.
Kelley-Seegmiller s.
Kenny s.
Kenny-Caffey s.
keratitis, ichthyosis, deafness s.
KID s.
Kimmelstiel-Wilson s.
kinky-hair s.
Kinsbourne s.
kleeblattschädel s.
Kleine-Levin s.
Klein-Waardenburg s.
Klinefelter s.
Klippel-Feil s.
Klippel-Trenaunay s.
Klippel-Trenaunay-Weber s.
Kniest s.
Kocher-Debré-Sémélaigne s.
Koerber-Salus-Elschnig s.

Kostmann s.
lacrimoauriculodentodigital s.
Ladd s.
LAMB s.
Lambert-Eaton s.
Landau-Kleffner s. (LKS)
Landry-Guillain-Barré s.
Lange-Nielsen s.
Langer-Giedion s.
Laron s.
Larsen s.
laryngeal atresia s.
late luteal phase s.
Laugier-Hunziker s.
Launois-Cléret s.
Laurence-Moon-Bardet-Biedl s.
Laurence-Moon-Biedl s.
Lawrence-Seip s.
lazy bladder s.
lazy leukocyte s.
LCMV s.
Leigh s.
Leiner s.
Lemierre s.
Lemli-Opitz s.
Lennox-Gastaut s.
lentigines, electrocardiographic
  abnormalities, ocular hypertelorism,
  pulmonary stenosis, abnormalities
  of genitalia, retardation of
  growth, deafness s.
Lenz microphthalmia s.
LEOPARD s.
Lesch-Nyhan s. (LNS)
leukocyte adhesion deficiency 2 s.
leukoencephalopathy s.
Levy-Hollister s.
Lévy Roussy s.
lexical-syntactic s. (LSS)
Lhermitte-Duclos s.
LHON s.
Liddle s.
Li-Fraumeni s.
Lightwood-Albright s.
Lignac s.
limb abnormality s.
limp infant s.
LMB s.
Löffler s.
Löfgren s.
long Q-T s. (LQTS)
Louis-Bar s.

low cardiac output s.
Lowe s.
low-sodium s.
low T3 s.
Lucey-Driscoll s.
lupus anticoagulant s.
lupuslike s.
Lutembacher s.
Lyell s.
lymphoproliferative s.
Lynch s.
3M s.
Macleod s.
macrophage activation s. (MAS)
Maffucci s.
malabsorption s.
malalignment s.
Marden-Walker s.
Marfan s.
Marie s.
Marinesco-Sjögren s.
Maroteaux-Lamy s.
Marshall s.
Marshall-Smith s.
Mauriac s.
Mayer-Rokitansky-Küster-Hauser s.
McCune-Albright s.
McKusick-Kaufman s.
McLeod s.
Meckel s.
Meckel-Gruber s.
meconium aspiration s. (MAS)
meconium blockage s.
meconium plug s.
medial collateral ligament s.
medial snapping hip s.
s. of median longitudinal fasciculus
megacystis-megaureter s.
megalocystis microcolon intestinal
  hypoperistalsis s.
Meigs s.
MELAS s.
Melkersson s.
Melkersson-Rosenthal s.
Melnick-Fraser s.
Melnick-Needles s.
mendelian s.
Ménière s.
meningitis or encephalitis,
  metabolic, Reye s. (MMR)
meningoencephalitis s.
meningovascular s.

NOTES

syndrome *(continued)*
Menkes s.
mental retardation s.
MERRF s.
metabolic s. X
microangiopathic hemolytic
  uremic s.
microdeletion s.
migraine s.
Mikity-Wilson s.
Mikulicz s.
milk-alkali s.
Miller-Dieker s.
Miller-Fisher s.
MIMyCA s.
minimal change nephrotic s.
  (MCNS)
minimal lesion nephrotic s.
  (MLNS)
mirror s.
mitis Ehlers-Danlos s.
mixed antiinflammatory s. (MARS)
MMIH s.
Möbius s.
Mohr s.
mononucleosis-type s.
monosomy 7 s.
Morgagni-Adams-Stokes s.
Morquio s.
Morquio-Ullrich s.
moyamoya s.
Moynihan s.
mucocutaneous lymph node s.
  (MCLS, MLNS)
mucosal neuroma s.
multiorgan dysfunction s. (MODS)
multiple basal cell nevoid s.
s. of multiple endocrine neoplasia
multiple hamartoma s.
multiple lentigines s.
multiple neuroma s.
multiple organ dysfunction s.
  (MODS)
multiple pterygium s.
multiple X s.
Münchausen s.
musculoskeletal pain s. (MSPS)
myasthenia-like s.
myasthenic s.
myelodysplastic s. (MDS)
myeloproliferative s.
myocardial steal s.
myoclonus s.
Nager s.
nail-patella s.
NAME s.
NARP s.
neonatal abstinence s. (NAS)

neonatal Bartter s. (NBS)
neonatal Guillain-Barré s.
neonatal hepatitis s.
neonatal Marfan s.
neonatal myasthenic s.
neonatal respiratory distress s.
neonatal small left colon s.
nephrotic s.
Netherton s.
Nettleship s.
Neu-Laxova s.
neurocutaneous melanosis s.
neurofibromatosis s.
neuroleptic malignant s. (NMS)
neuromuscular scoliosis s.
nevoid basal cell carcinoma s.
newborn respiratory distress s.
Nezelof s.
Nijmegen breakage s. (NBS)
Noack s.
noncleft median face s.
nonnarcotic abstinence s.
nonprogressive hypoplastic s.
nonprogressive motor impairment s.
Noonan s.
Noonan-Ehmke s.
Norman-Wood s.
Norrie s.
nutritional deprivation s.
obesity hypoventilation s.
obstruction s.
obstructive sleep apnea s. (OSAS)
occipital horn s.
OCRL s.
oculoauriculovertebral s.
oculocerebral s.
oculocerebrorenal s.
oculodentodigital s.
oculomandibulofacial s.
OFD s., type I–III
Ollier s.
Omenn s.
Ondine-Hirschsprung s.
opercular s.
Opitz s.
Opitz-Frias s.
Opitz-Kaveggia s.
s. of opsoclonus-myoclonus
oral allergy s.
organic hyperkinetic s.
organic mental s.
orofaciodigital s.
orthostatic tachycardia s.
Osgood-Schlatter s.
Osler-Weber s.
Osler-Weber-Rendu s. (OWRS)
osteogenesis imperfecta congenita s.
osteoporosis pseudoglioma s.

otitis-conjunctivitis s.
otopalatodigital s.
otosclerosis s.
otospongiosis s.
overdose s.
overtraining s.
overuse s.
4p s.
5p s.
9p s.
pachyonychia congenita s.
Pallister-Hall s.
Pallister-Killian s.
pancytopenia s.
Papillon-Léage-Psaume s.
Papillon-Lefèvre s.
paraneoplastic s.
Parinaud oculoglandular s.
Parks-Weber s.
Parrot s.
Parry-Romberg s.
partial DiGeorge s.
partial trisomy 10q s.
Patau s.
patellofemoral pain s. (PFPS)
patellofemoral stress s.
4p deletion s.
Pearson s.
Pearson marrow-pancreas s.
pediatric acquired
  immunodeficiency s.
Pellizzi s.
pelvic venous congestion s.
Pena-Shokeir s. (I, II)
Pendred s.
PEO s.
periodontitis Ehlers-Danlos s.
perisylvian s.
Perlman s.
Perrault s.
Peutz-Jeghers s.
Pfeiffer s.
PHACE s.
phocomelia s.
phonologic-syntactic s.
physiologic addiction/abstinence s.
pickwickian s.
Pierre Robin s.
piriformis s.
Poland s.
poliomyelitis-like s.
polycystic ovary s. (PCOS, POS)

polycythemia-hyperviscosity s.
polyposis s.
polysplenia s.
postanoxic dystonic s.
postcoartectomy s.
postconcussion s.
posterior fossa malformation,
  hemangiomas, arterial anomalies,
  coarctation of the aorta and
  cardiac defects, eye
  abnormalities s.
posterior leukoencephalopathy s.
postexchange transfusion s.
postgastroenteritis malabsorption s.
postperfusion s.
postpericardiotomy s. (PPS)
postphlebitic s. (PPS)
postpolio s.
postscabetic s.
posttraumatic stress s.
postural orthostatic tachycardia s.
  (POTS)
postvagotomy dumping s.
POTS s.
Potter s.
Prader-Labhart-Willi s.
Prader-Willi s. (PWS)
preexcitation s.
preleukemic s.
premenstrual s. (PMS)
primary antiphospholipid antibody s.
primary nephrotic s.
progeria s.
prolapse gastropathy s. (PGS)
prolonged QT interval s.
Proteus s.
prune-belly s.
pseudoachondroplasia s.
pseudoappendicular s.
pseudo-Hurler s.
pseudothalidomide s.
pseudo-Turner s.
pseudo-Wernicke s.
pulmonary infiltrate with
  eosinophilia s.
pupillary s.
pyknodysostosis s.
pyridoxine-dependency s.
13q s.
18q s.
22q11.2 deletion s.
Rabson-Mendenhall s.

NOTES

syndrome *(continued)*

radial aplasia-thrombocytopenia s.
radiation s.
Ramsay Hunt s.
rancid butter s.
Rapp-Hodgkin ectodermal
 dysplasia s.
Rasmussen s.
Raynaud s.
recognizable viral s. (RVS)
recurrent hemolytic uremia s.
Reed s.
Refsum s.
Reifenstein s.
Reiter s.
renal Fanconi s.
renal tubular Fanconi s.
renal tubular pituitary s.
Rendu-Osler-Weber s.
respiratory distress s. (RDS)
restless legs s.
retinoblastoma-mental retardation s.
retroviral s.
Rett s.
reversible posterior
 leukoencephalopathy s. (RPLS)
Reye s.
Reye-like s.
Richner-Hanhart s.
Rieger s.
right middle lobe s.
rigid spine s.
Riley-Day s.
Riley-Shwachman s.
Riley-Smith s.
Roberts-SC phocomelia s.
Robin s.
Robinow s.
Rokitansky-Küster-Hauser s.
Romano-Ward long QT s.
Rothmund s.
Rothmund-Thomson cancer
 predisposition s.
Rotor s.
Roussy-Lévy s.
rubella s.
Rubinstein s.
Rubinstein-Taybi s.
Rud s.
Rudiger s.
rudimentary testis s.
Russell s.
Russell-Silver dwarf s.
Rutledge s.
Ruvalcaba-Myhre-Smith s.
Saethre-Chotzen s.
Sakati-Nyhan s.
Saldino-Noonan s.

salt-losing adrenogenital s.
salt-wasting adrenogenital s.
Sandifer s.
Sanfilippo A, B s.
San Luis Valley s.
scalded skin s. (SSS)
Scheie s.
Scheuthauer-Marie-Sainton s.
Schinzel-Giedion s.
Schinzel-type acrocallosal s.
Schmidt s.
Schwartz-Jampel s.
scimitar s.
SCIWORA s.
scleroderma-like s.
scotopic sensitivity s.
SEA s.
seat belt s.
sebaceous nevus s.
Seckel s.
secondary nephrotic s.
second impact s.
Seip-Lawrence s.
Sengers s.
Senior-Loken s.
sepsis s.
sepsis/shock s.
seronegative enthesopathy and
 arthropathy s.
serotonin s.
serum sickness-like s.
severe combined
 immunodeficiency s. (SCIDS)
Shah-Waardenburg s.
shaken baby s.
shaken impact s.
shaken infant s.
Sheehan s.
Sheehy s.
Shone s.
short bowel s. (SBS)
short gut s. (SGS)
short-rib polydactyly s.
Shprintzen-Goldberg s.
Shprintzen velocardiofacial s.
Shulman s.
Shwachman s.
Shwachman-Diamond s.
Shy-Drager s.
sicca s.
sick euthyroid s.
sick sinus node s.
Silver s.
Silver-Russell s.
Simpson-Golabi-Behmel s. (SGBS)
Simpson-Golabi-Behmel fetal
 overgrowth s.
Sinding-Larsen-Johansson s.

Sipple s.
sirenomelia s.
Sjögren s.
Sjögren-Larsson s.
slapped cheek s.
sleep apnea s.
sleep-disordered breathing s.
slit ventricle s.
SLO s.
slow channel s.
Sly s.
small left colon s.
Smith-Lemli-Opitz s.
Smith-Magenis s.
snapping knee s.
Sohval-Soffer s.
somnolence s.
Sorsby s.
Sotos s.
spastic diplegia s.
spinocerebellar s.
spondylocostal dysplasia s.
spondyloepiphyseal dysplasia
  congenita s.
spondylothoracic dysplasia s.
Spurway s.
SSS s.
stagnant loop s.
staphylococcal scalded skin s.
  (SSSS)
staphylococcal toxic shock s.
Stein-Leventhal s.
steroid-sensitive idiopathic
  nephrotic s. (SSNS)
steroid-sensitive nephrotic s.
Stevens-Johnson s.
Stickler s.
stiff-baby s.
stiff-man s.
Stilling-Türk-Duane s.
Stock-Spielmeyer-Vogt s.
Stokes-Adams s.
strabismus s.
straight-back s.
streptococcal toxic shock s.
stuck twin s.
Sturge s.
Sturge-Kalischer-Weber s.
Sturge-Weber s. (SWS)
sudden infant death s. (SIDS)
superior mediastinal s.
superior mesenteric artery s.

superior vena cava s.
surfactant deficiency s.
swallowed blood s.
Sweet s.
Swyer s.
Swyer-James s.
Swyer-James-Macleod s.
sylvian aqueduct s.
s. of symmetric parasagittal
  parietooccipital polymicrogyria
systemic inflammatory response s.
  (SIRS)
systemic vasculitis s.
tachy-brady s.
Takao s.
TAR s.
Taussig-Bing s.
Taybi s.
teratogenic s.
Terry s.
testicular feminization s.
tethered cord s.
thalidomide teratogenicity s.
Thal intermedia-like s.
thanatophoric dysplasia s.
thrombocytopenia with absent
  radius s.
Tietze s.
tin ear s.
Tolosa-Hunt s.
tooth and nail s.
TORCH s.
Tourette s.
toxemic shock s.
toxic oil s.
toxic shock s. (TSS)
toxoplasmosis, rubella,
  cytomegalovirus, herpes simplex s.
transfusion s.
transient myeloproliferative s.
transient neonatal myasthenic s.
transient respiratory distress s.
translocation Down s.
TRAP s.
traumatic compartment s.
Treacher Collins s.
Treacher Collins-Franceschetti s.
tremor s.
trichodentoosseous s.
Trichuris dysentery s.
trilateral retinoblastoma s.
triple X s.

S

NOTES

syndrome *(continued)*
    triploidy s.
    trisomy 8 s.
    trisomy 9 s.
    trisomy 13 s.
    trisomy 13-15 s.
    trisomy 16-18 s.
    trisomy 18 s.
    trisomy 21 s.
    trisomy D s.
    trisomy 4p s.
    trisomy 20p s.
    trisomy 10q s.
    Troyer s.
    tuberous sclerosis s.
    tubulopathy of Lowe s.
    tumor lysis s.
    Turcot s.
    Turner mosaic s.
    Turner XO s.
    twin reversed arterial perfusion s.
    twin-to-twin transfusion s.
    Ullrich s.
    Ullrich-Feichtiger s.
    Ullrich-Turner s.
    uncombable hair s.
    Unna-Thost s.
    unstable bladder s.
    Unverricht-Lundborg s.
    upper airway resistance s. (UARS)
    upper motor neuron s.
    uremic s.
    urethral s.
    Usher s. (type 1)
    uveomeningoencephalitic s.
    uveoparotid fever s.
    VACTERL s.
    valves, unilateral reflux,
      dysplasia s.
    van Buchem s.
    van der Hoeve s.
    van der Woude s.
    vanished testes s.
    vanishing testicle s.
    varicella s.
    vascular ring s.
    vasculitis s.
    VATER s.
    velocardiofacial s. (VCFS)
    viral s.
    visceromegaly s.
    vitamin B_6 dependence s.
    Vogt s.
    Vogt-Koyanagi s.
    Vogt-Koyanagi-Harada s.
    Vohwinkel s.
    von Hippel-Lindau s.
    vulnerable child s.

    VURD s.
    Waardenburg s.
    Waardenburg-Klein s.
    WAGR s.
    Walker-Warburg s.
    Warburg s.
    wasting s.
    Waterhouse-Friderichsen s.
    Watson-Alagille s.
    Weaver s.
    Weber-Christian s.
    Weil s.
    Weill-Marchesani s.
    Werdnig-Hoffmann s.
    Werner s.
    Wernicke s.
    Wernicke-Korsakoff s.
    West s.
    wet brain s.
    wet lung s.
    WIC s.
    Wildervanck s.
    Wilkins s.
    Williams s. (WS)
    Williams-Beuren s.
    Williams-Campbell s.
    Wilson-Mikity s.
    Winchester s.
    Winter s.
    Wiskott-Aldrich s. (WAS)
    Wolf-Parkinson-White s.
    Wolfram s.
    Women, Infants, Children s.
    Wyburn-Mason s.
    s. X
    X-linked Ehlers-Danlos s.
    X-linked lymphoproliferative s.
    X-linked recessive skeletal Ehlers-
      Danlos s.
    X-linked severe combined
      immunodeficiency s.
    XO s.
    XXY s.
    XYY s.
    yellow nail s.
    yellow vernix s.
    Young s.
    Yunis Varon s.
    Zellweger cerebrohepatorenal s.
    Ziehen-Oppenheim s.
    Zinsser-Cole-Engman s.
    Zollinger-Ellison s.

syndromic
    s. cleft
    s. craniosynostosis
    s. paucity

synechia, pl. **synechiae**

anterior s.
posterior s.
Synemol Topical
Synercid
synergism
synergistic gangrene
synergy
spastic s.
synesthesia
syngeneic
s. bone marrow transplantation
s. stem cell
Synkayvite
synkinesis
synostosis
coronal s.
lambdoid s.
radioulnar s.
sagittal s.
tribasilar s.
unilambdoid s.
synovectomy
synovial
s. biopsy
s. fluid
s. hypertrophy
s. joint
s. sarcoma
synoviocyte
fibroblastoid s.
synovioma
synovitis
monoarticular s.
plant thorn s.
toxic s.
transient monoarticular s.
villonodular s.
synovium
Synsorb Pk
syntax
synthase
cystathionine s.
prostaglandin endoperoxide s.
pyloric nitric oxide s.
synthesis, pl. **syntheses**
bile acid s.
cholesterol s.
inborn error of bile acid s.
thyroxine s.
tissue s.
synthesize

synthesizer
voice s.
synthetase
carbamoyl phosphate s. (CPS)
endothelial nitric oxide s.
holocarboxylase s. (HCS)
N-acetylglutamate s.
6-pyruvoyl tetrahydropteridine s.
synthetic
s. DNA
s. gliadin peptide
s. portoaortal shunt
s. pterin
s. surfactant
Synthroid
S. Injection
S. Oral
syphilis
congenital s.
early congenital s.
endemic s.
late congenital s.
parenchymatous congenital s.
primary s.
secondary s.
tertiary s.
s., toxoplasmosis, other agents, rubella, cytomegalovirus, herpes simplex virus (STORCH)
s., toxoplasmosis, other agents, rubella, cytomegalovirus, HSV
syphilitic
s. infection
s. keratitis
s. meningitis
s. pemphigus
s. phlebitis
Syracol-CF
syringe
Auto S.
bulb s.
super s.
tuberculin s.
syringobulbia
syringocystadenoma papilliferum
syringohydromyelia
syringoma
eruptive s.
syringomyelia
familial lumbosacral s.
syringomyelic cavity
syringopleural drainage

S

NOTES

syringosubarachnoid drainage
syrinx
syrup

    Benylin Cough S.
    Bydramine Cough S.
    Carbodec S.
    Cardec-S S.
    Claritin s.
    Decofed S.
    Dilaudid Cough S.
    Extra Action Cough S.
    Hydramyn S.
    s. of ipecac
    ipecac s.
    Karo s.
    Naldecon EX Children's S.
    Neo-Calglucon s.
    Promethazine VC S.
    Promethazine VC Plain S.
    Rondec S.
    Sudafed Cough S.
    Triaminic S.
    Tusstat S.
    Uni-Bent Cough S.
    Versed s.
    Zyrtec s.

Sysmex NE8000 cell counter
system

    Aggregate Neurobehavioral Student Health & Education Review S.
    Aladdin Infant Flow S.
    Androderm Transdermal S.
    Ann Arbor Staging S.
    ascending reticular activating s. (ARAS)
    autonomic nervous s. (ANS)
    Autoread centrifuge hematology s.
    Baby CareLink s.
    Bactec blood-culturing s.
    basolateral membrane transport s.
    Bethesda classification s.
    Biliblanket Phototherapy S.
    BioMerieux Vitek s.
    cardiovascular s.
    Cartesian s.
    central nervous s. (CNS)
    centrencephalic s.
    cerebellar-vestibular s.
    circulatory s.
    ColorMate TLc BiliTest S.
    Companion 318 Nasal CPAP S.
    cytochrome *b* s.
    dentatorubrothalamocortical s.
    Diastat Rectal Delivery S.
    dopaminergic s.
    double collecting s.
    drooping lily appearance of lower collecting s.

    dysfunctional voiding scoring s. (DVSS)
    embryonic branchial s.
    EMLA disc topical anesthetic adhesive s.
    EntriStar Gastrostomy S.
    extrapyramidal nervous s.
    Gordon diagnostic s. (GDS)
    Halo Sleep S.
    haversian s.
    hematopoietic s.
    hemorrhagic shock-encephalopathy s.
    His-Purkinje s.
    humoral immune s.
    immune s.
    INOvent delivery s.
    International Neuroblastoma Staging S. (INSS)
    International Staging S.
    kallikrein-kinin s.
    LactAid STARTrainer Nursing S.
    Lancefield typing s.
    limbic GABAergic s.
    lower collecting s.
    McAllister grading s.
    mitochondrial glycine cleavage s.
    molecular adsorbent recirculating s. (MARS)
    motion artifact rejection s. (MARS)
    neonatal facial coding s. (NFCS)
    Neotrend s.
    nervous s.
    noradrenergic s.
    portal s.
    Renaissance spirometry s.
    renin-angiotensin s. (RAS)
    reticuloendothelial s.
    review of s.'s (ROS)
    Scepter s.
    serotonergic s.
    single collecting s.
    St. Jude Children's Research Hospital staging s.
    superior venous s.
    surgicopathologic staging s.
    sympathetic nerve s.
    Tesla s.
    1.5-Tesla Siemens s.
    Testoderm Transdermal S.
    therapeutic transdermal fentanyl s.
    transdermal therapeutic s. (TTS)
    Vaccine Adverse Events Reporting S. (VAERS)
    visual magnocellular s.
    Wallaby Phototherapy S.

systemic
    s. azole therapy
    s. behavior family therapy

s. candidiasis
s. carnitine deficiency
s. caval return
s. fatty acid deficiency
s. flow
s. inflammatory response syndrome (SIRS)
s. juvenile chronic arthritis
s. lupus erythematosus (SLE)
s. mastocytosis
s. outflow obstruction
s. scleroderma
s. sclerosis (SS)
s. steroid
s. vascular resistance (SVR)

s. vasculitis syndrome
s. venous collateral (SSVC)
systemic-onset juvenile rheumatoid arthritis
systole
systolic
s. arterial pressure (SAP)
s. blood pressure
s. component
s. continuous murmur
s. ejection murmur (SEM)
s. overload
s. overload pattern
Sytobex

NOTES

T

 T cell
 T connector
 T helper
 T lymphocyte
 T protein
 T wave

T3

 triiodothyronine

T4

 thyroxine

TA

 Takayasu arteritis
 therapeutic abortion

T&A

 tonsillectomy and adenoidectomy

tab

 Meda T.

tabes

 t. dorsalis
 t. infantum
 juvenile t.

tablet

 Actifed Allergy T.
 Allerest Children's T.'s
 bisacodyl t.
 Bromatapp Relief 4 Hour T.
 Carbiset T.
 Carbiset-TR T.
 Carbodec TR T.
 Cardizem T.
 Coricidin T.'s
 Coricidin-D T.'s
 Dexone T.
 Dimetapp T.'s
 Hexadrol T.
 Metadate ER t.'s
 Nitrong Oral T.
 Triaminic Cold T.'s
 Veltane T.

tabula rasa

TAC

 tetracaine, adrenaline, cocaine
 transient aplastic crisis

Tac-3 Injection

Tac-40 Injection

tache noir

tachyarrhythmia

 atrial t.

tachy-brady syndrome

tachycardia

 aberrant supraventricular t.
 accelerated junctional ectopic t.
 atrial t.
 atrioventricular nodal reentrant t. (AVNRT)
 atrioventricular reciprocating t. (AVRT)
 automatic atrial t.
 AV nodal reentry t.
 chaotic atrial t.
 congenital paroxysmal atrial t.
 ectopic atrial t.
 fetal reentrant supraventricular t.
 intraatrial reentrant t. (IART)
 junctional t.
 junctional ectopic t. (JET)
 maternal t.
 multifocal atrial t.
 narrow complex supraventricular t.
 nodal t.
 nonsustained ventricular t.
 paroxysmal atrial t. (PAT)
 persistent t.
 reentrant supraventricular t.
 reentry t.
 sinus t.
 supraventricular t. (SVT)
 sustained ventricular t.
 ventricular t.
 wide complex t.

tachygastria

tachyphylaxis

tachypnea

 transient t.

tachypneic

tackling

 spear t.

tacrolimus (FK-506)

 t. level

tactile

 t. defensiveness
 t. discrimination
 t. fever
 t. fremitus
 t. stimulation
 t. stimulus
 t. temperature

Taenia

 T. saginata
 T. solium

taeniasis

TAF

 tracheobronchial aspirate fluid

tag

 cutaneous t.
 hymeneal t.
 perianal skin t.

tag *(continued)*
  preauricular t.
  skin t.
Tagamet
Tagamet-HB
tailor sitting
Taiwan acute respiratory (TWAR)
Takao syndrome
Takayasu
  T. arteritis (TA)
  T. disease
TAL
  tendo Achillis lengthening
talar
  t. decancellation
  t. dome fracture
  t. to first metatarsal angle
  t. tilt test
talcum powder
tali (*pl. of* talus)
talipes
  t. calcaneovalgus
  t. equinovalgus
  t. equinovarus (TEV)
  t. equinovarus deformity
  t. hobble splint
talking
  sleep t.
tall P wave
talocalcaneal (TC)
  t. angle (TCA)
  t. bar
  t. fusion
talus, pl. **tali**
  congenital vertical t.
  vertical t.
Talwin NX
Tambocor
TAME
  tosylarginine methyl ester
Tamine
tamoxifen
tampon
  nasal t.
tamponade
  balloon t.
  cardiac t.
  gastroesophageal balloon t.
  pericardial t.
tandem
  t. mass spectrometry
  t. walking
Tangier disease
tangle
  fibrillary t.
  neurofibrillary t.
Tanner
  T. Developmental Scale

  T. developmental stage
  T. genital stage
  T. maturation stage
  T. staging (I–V)
  T. and Whitehouse II bone-age
    determination method
**Tanner-Whitehouse bone age reference
  value**
tan papilloma
tantrum
TAP
  trypsin activation peptide
tap
  bladder t.
  infant subdural t.
  lung t.
  percutaneous lung t.
  peritoneal t.
  shunt t.
  spinal t.
  subdural t.
  ventricular t.
  VP shunt t.
Tapanol
Tapazole
tape
  Broselow t.
  glucose oxidase test t.
  twill t.
tapering cytoplasmic process
tapetoretinal degeneration
tapeworm
  pork t.
taping
  buddy t.
tapir
  levre de t.
  t. mouth
TAPVC
  total anomalous pulmonary venous
    connection
TAPVR
  total anomalous pulmonary venous return
Taq **I enzyme**
TAR
  thrombocytopenia-absent radius
  thrombocytopenia with absent radius
    TAR syndrome
tar
  Aqua T.
  coal t.
  DHS T.
Tarabine PFS
tarda
  hypophosphatasia t.
  lymphedema t.
  osteopetrosis t.

porphyria cutanea t.
spondyloepiphyseal dysplasia t.
tardive
    t. dyskinesia
    t. dystonia
target lesion
targetoid lesion
tarsal
    t. coalition
    t. navicular osteochondritis
    t. plate
tarsalis
    Culex t.
tarsi (*pl. of* tarsus)
tarsometatarsal mobilization
tarsorrhaphy
tarsus, pl. **tarsi**
Tarui disease
TAS
    Toronto Alexithymia Scale
task
    Continuous Performance T.
    t. load
    Paired Associate Learning T.
      (PALT)
    phoneme segmentation t.
    phonemic awareness t.
taste
    t. bud
    impaired t.
TAT
    tetanus antitoxin
taurine
Taussig-Bing
    T.-B. anomaly
    T.-B. syndrome
Tavist
Tavist-1
Taxol
taxonomic and assessment dilemma
taxonomy
Taybi syndrome
Taylor dispersion
Tay-Sachs disease
tazarotene
Tazicef
Tazidime
tazobactam
    piperacillin and t.
TB
    tuberculosis

TBARS
    thiobarbituric acid-reacting substance
TBE
    tick-borne encephalitis
TBG
    thyroid-binding globulin
    thyroxine-binding globulin
      TBG deficiency
      TBG excess
TBI
    total body irradiation
    traumatic brain injury
TBK
    total body potassium
TBMD
    thin basement membrane disease
TBSA
    total body surface area
      TBSA burned
TBW
    total body water
TC
    talocalcaneal
3TC
    lamivudine
Tc
    technetium
      Tc HMPAO leukocyte scan
TCA
    talocalcaneal angle
    trichloroacetic acid
    tricyclic antidepressant
TcB
    transcutaneous bilirubin
TCC
    transcatheter closure
TCD
    transcranial Doppler
TCE
    trichloroethanol
T-cell
    T-c. activation defect
    T-c. antibody induction therapy
    CD4 T-c.
    CD8 T-c.
    T-c. depletion
    T-c. dysfunction
    T-c. lymphoma
    T-c. trophic (T-trophic)
T-cell-depleted
    T-c.-d. graft

NOTES

T

575

T-cell-depleted *(continued)*
     T-c.-d. haploidentical bone marrow
          stem cell
T-cell-mediated disease
T-cell-tropic syncytium-inducing strain
Tc HMPAO
TC II
     transcobalamin II
TCT
     thrombin clotting time
          TCT coagulation test
Tczank prep
TD
     Tourette disorder
     traveler's diarrhea
Td
     tetanus and diphtheria
          Td toxoid vaccine
TdaP-IPV vaccine
TdaP vaccine
TDEE
     total daily energy expenditure
T/Derm
     Neutrogena T.
T-Derm body oil
TDI
     therapeutic donor insemination
     tissue Doppler imaging
Td-IPV vaccine
TDT
     transmission disequilibrium test
TE
     thromboembolic event
tea
     Chuen-Lin herbal t.
     herbal t.
TEACCH
     treatment and education of autistic and
          related communications handicapped
          children
          Project TEACCH
teacher
     infant t.
     T. Rating Form (TRF)
     T. Report Form (TRF)
teaching
     discrete-trial t.
     social-pragmatic t.
team
     interdisciplinary t.
     multidisciplinary t.
     transdisciplinary t.
tear
     absent t.'s
     t. film
     Mallory-Weiss t. (MWT)
     meniscus t.
     no t.'s

     t. overflow
     syndrome of crocodile t.'s
tear-drop vesicle
Tebamide Rectal
T4/ebp-1
     thyroid-specific enhancer binding protein-
          1
TEC
     transient erythroblastopenia of childhood
technetium (Tc)
     t. bone scan
     t. hexamethylpropyleneamine oxime
     t. hexamethylpropyleneamine oxime
          leukocyte scan
technetium-labeled red blood cell
technetium-99m
     t.-99m bone scan
     t.-99m pertechnetate
technique
     agar gel precipitation t.
     agar immunoprecipitin t.
     automated radiometric t.
     Barlow t.
     brain imaging t.
     buccal feeding t.
     capillary isoelectric focusing t.
     catheter-in-a-catheter t.
     catheter-over-needle t.
     catheter-over-wire t.
     clean-catch t.
     Cobb measurement t.
     Cohen transtrigonal t.
     dead space t.
     double-catheter t.
     double-freeze t.
     enzyme-multiplied immunoassay t.
          (EMIT)
     E-test t.
     Glenn-Anderson t.
     hyperglycemic clamp t.
     intraluminal electrical impedance t.
     labial traction t.
     Lester-Martin t.
     Lich-Gregoire t.
     Menghini t.
     Mitrofanoff t.
     multipuncture t.
     Mustard t.
     Nuss t.
     Ortolani t.
     oscillometric t.
     percutaneous multipuncture t.
     percutaneous Seldinger t.
     Politano-Leadbetter t.
     pull-through t.
     Seldinger t.
     single-isotope tracer t.
     skinfold caliper t.

thorascopic t.
toothbrush culture t.
tripod fixation t.
technology
assisted reproductive t. (ART)
assistive t. (AT)
tectal brainstem glioma
tectocerebellar dysraphia
tectum
mesencephalic t.
teddy-bear gait
Tedral
TEE
transesophageal echocardiography
teenager
Problem-Oriented Screening
Instrument for T.'s (POSIT)
teeth
baby t.
conical t.
crowded t.
deciduous t.
Hutchinson t.
hypoplastic t.
missing t.
natal t.
peglike t.
permanent t.
petted t.
primary t.
secondary t.
teething
Babee T.
Numzit T.
TEF
thermic effect of food
tracheoesophageal fistula
Teflon
Teflon-coated wire
Tega-Vert Oral
tegmen
tegmentum
Tegopen
Tegretol
Tegretol-XR
Tegrin-HC Topical
teicoplanin
Telachlor Oral
Teladar Topical

telangiectasia
calcinosis cutis, Raynaud
phenomenon, sclerodactyly, t.
(CRST)
calcinosis, Raynaud phenomenon,
esophageal dysmotility,
sclerodactyly, t. (CREST)
flat red-black t.
hemorrhagic t.
hereditary hemorrhagic t. (HHT)
intestinal t.
t. macularis eruptiva perstans
nail bed t.
nail fold t.
oculocutaneous t.
raised red-black t.
red-black t.
retinal vessel t.
telangiectasis
conjunctival t.
cutaneous t.
telangiectatic
t. granuloma
t. nevus
t. osteosarcoma
telangiectatica
cutis marmorata t.
Teldrin Oral
telecanthus
telecardiology
telemetry
telencephalic
t. neuroepithelium
t. subependymal germinal matrix
telepsychiatry
teleroentgenogram
television epilepsy
Teline Oral
telogen effluvium
telophase
TEM
therapeutic electromembrane
transmission electron microscopy
Temovate
temper
temperament
shy-inhibited t.
temperature
absolute t.
ambient t.
artificial t.
aseptic t.

NOTES

577

temperature *(continued)*
>aural t.
>axillary t.
>basal body t. (BBT)
>body t.
>core t.
>critical t.
>t. dysregulation
>ephemeral t.
>erratic t.
>eruptive t.
>maximum t.
>normal t.
>oral t.
>t. pattern
>rectal t.
>skin t.
>subnormal t.
>tactile t.
>tympanic t.

temperature-controlled isolette

temporal
>t. lobe
>t. lobe epilepsy
>t. lobe seizure
>t. sequencing

temporale
>planum t.

temporalis muscle

temporomandibular
>t. joint (TMJ)
>t. joint dysfunction

temporospatial pattern

Tempra

TEN
>titanium elastic nailing
>toxic epidermal necrolysis

tenacious

tendency
>prothrombic t.

tender enthesis

tenderness
>abdominal t.
>costovertebral angle t.
>CVA t.
>epigastric t.
>joint line t.
>point t.
>point of maximum t. (PMT)
>rebound t.
>snuffbox t.

tendinea, pl. **tendineae**
>chordae tendineae

tendinitis (*var. of* tendonitis)

tendinitis, tendonitis
>patellar t.
>triceps t.

tendo
>t. Achillis
>t. Achillis lengthening (TAL)

tendon
>Achilles t.
>bowstringing of t.
>calcaneal t.
>fat flexor hallucis longus t.
>flexor hallucis longus t.
>t. lengthening
>peroneus brevis t.
>split flexor hallucis longus t.
>t. stretch reflex
>t. transfer
>t. xanthoma

tendon-bone interface

tendonitis, tendinitis (*var. of* tendinitis)

tenesmus

Tenex

teniposide (VM-26)

Ten-K

tennis elbow

Tennison-Randall repair

Tenolin

Tenormin

tenosynovial sarcoma

tenosynovioma

tenosynovitis

tenosynovitis-dermatitis

tenotomy
>percutaneous adductor t.

TENS
>transcutaneous electrical nerve stimulation

tense
>t. ascites
>t. blister
>t. lobule

Tensilon test

tension
>alveolar oxygen t.
>arterial oxygen t.
>end-tidal CO_2 t.
>t. pneumocephalus
>t. pneumothorax

tension-discharging phenomenon

tent
>CAM t.
>face t.
>mist t.
>oxygen t.
>Silon t.

tenting
>skin t.

tentorial
>t. laceration
>t. margin
>t. opening

tentorium
tenuis
> *Dirofilaria* t.

TEOAE
> transient evoked otoacoustic emission
> TEOAE testing

tepid
terathanasia
teratocarcinoma
teratogen
> environmental t.

teratogenesis
teratogenic
> t. exposure
> t. properties
> t. syndrome

teratogenicity
teratoid tumor
teratologic dislocation
teratoma, pl. **teratomata**
> atypical t.
> benign t.
> cystic t.
> germ cell t.
> immature t. (grade 0–3)
> malignant t.
> mature t.
> mediastinal t.
> ovarian t.
> sacrococcygeal t.

teratozoospermia
terbinafine
terbutaline
> caffeine t.
> t. sulfate

ter in die (three times a day) (t.i.d.)
teres
> ligamentum t.

terfenadine
terlipressin
term
> full t. (FT)
> t. infant

terminal
> t. blush
> t. blush formation
> t. bronchiole
> t. complement component
> t. complement component
>   deficiency
> t. ileitis

> t. lung differentiation
> t. maturation

terminale
> filum t.
> ossiculum t.
> ropelike filum t.

terminalis
> lamina t.

terminate
termination of parental rights
terreus
> *Aspergillus* t.

terror
> night t.
> sleep t.

terrorizing
Terry
> T. questionnaire
> T. syndrome

Terson disease
tertiary
> t. closure
> t. hypothyroidism
> t. syphilis

Tesamone Injection
TESE
> testicular sperm extraction

1.5-Tesla Siemens system
Tesla system
TEST
> tubal embryo stage transfer

test
> ^{13}C-urea breath t.
> ^{14}C-urea breath t.
> Accu-Chek t.
> acidified serum lysis t.
> acoustic reflex t.
> ACTH stimulation t.
> activated partial thromboplastic time
>   coagulation t.
> Adams forward-bending t.
> agglutination t.
> air leak t.
> Alcohol Use Disorders
>   Inventory T. (AUDIT)
> Allen picture t.
> alternate-cover t.
> alternating breath t. (ABT)
> anterior drawer t.
> antigen detection t.
> antiglobulin t.
> Apley compression t.

T

NOTES

test *(continued)*

apprehension t.
Apt-Downey t.
APTT coagulation t.
arginine-insulin stimulation t.
arginine-insulin tolerance t.
automated reagin t. (ART)
BAER t.
Barlow and Ortolani t.
BD t.
Bender Visual Motor Gestalt T.
Benton Visual Retention T.
Berens 3-character t.
BH$_4$ loading t.
block design t.
Boston Naming T.
brainstem auditory evoked
  response t.
Bratton-Marshall t.
breath H$_2$ t.
breath hydrogen excretion t.
Breslow-Day t.
Bruininks-Oseretsky t.
Burt Word Reading T.
cAMP t.
Candida skin t.
caramel t.
carbon-14 t.
carbon-13 urea breath t.
Cattell Infant Intelligence T.
CF t.
Children of Alcoholics
  Screening T. (CAST)
chi-square t.
chromosome breakage t.
Clinical Adaptive T. (CAT)
cocaine t.
Cochran-Mantel-Haenszel t.
Color Trails T.
complement fixation t.
continuous performance t. (CPT)
contraction stress t. (CST)
Coombs t.
corneal light reflex t.
Cortrosyn stimulation t.
cover t.
criterion-referenced t.
cumulative sum t.
C-urea breath t.
CUSUM t.
cyclic adenosine monophosphate t.
deferoxamine challenge t.
Denver Developmental Screening T.
  (DDST)
Denver Developmental Screening T.
  II
dexamethasone suppression t.
Dick t.

DIF t.
differential agglutination t.
dipstick t.
direct antiglobulin t. (DAT)
direct Coombs t.
Dochez serum t.
dot ELISA t.
Draw-a-Person T.
Duncan t.
dye decolorization t.
dye disappearance t.
E t.
Eating Attitudes T.
Einstein screening t.
Elek t.
ELISA t.
epicutaneous t.
Expressive One-Word Picture
  Vocabulary T.
F t.
Fagan t.
Farber t.
Farr t.
FAST blood t.
ferric chloride t.
figure-of-four t.
finger-nose-finger t.
finger-tapping t.
fingertip number writing t.
finger-to-nose t.
Fisher exact t.
five-hop t.
fluorescence spot t.
fluorescent treponemal antibody t.
  (FTA)
fluorescent treponemal antibody
  absorption t. (FTA-ABS)
foam stability t. (FST)
forward-bending t.
free beta t.
Free Running Asthma T. (FRAST)
fructose intolerance t.
FTA t.
galactose breath t.
Gardner Expressive One-Word
  Vocabulary T.-Revised
GeneAmp PCR t.
geometric design t.
Gesell Preschool T.
Gesell School Readiness T.
Gilmore Oral Reading T. (GORT)
glucose challenge t.
glucose tolerance t. (GTT)
Goldmann perimeter visual field t.
Goodenough-Harris Drawing T.
Gordon Distractibility T.
granulocyte immunofluorescence t.
  (GIFT)

Gray Oral Reading T.
Gray Oral Reading T.-Revised
  (GORT-R)
growth hormone stimulation t.
guaiac t.
Guthrie t.
hair bulb incubation t.
halo t.
Hausman t.
heel-shin t.
heel-to-shin t.
hemagglutination t.
Hematest t.
Hemoccult t.
hemoglobin S solubility t.
HEMPAS t.
hereditary erythroblastic
  multinuclearity associated with
  positive acidified serum lysis t.
heterophile t.
HFD t.
hip rotation t.
Hirschberg corneal reflex t.
Hirschberg light reflex t.
HIV t.
Hivagen t.
homocysteine loading t.
Hotelling t.
Human Figure Drawing T.
human immunodeficiency virus t.
hyperoxia t.
hyperventilation provocative t.
ICD-p24 t.
IgA AGA t.
IgG-IFA t.
IgG indirect fluorescent antibody t.
IgM-IFA t.
IgM indirect fluorescent antibody t.
IHA t.
immunobead t. (IBT)
impingement t.
India ink t.
indirect Coombs t.
indirect hemagglutination t.
intelligence t.
intradermal t.
inversion stress tilt t.
ischemic exercise t.
Isojima t.
IVA visual consistency t.
Kahn t.
Kinyoun acid-fast staining t.

Kleihauer-Betke t.
Kremer t.
Kruskal-Wallis t.
Kurzrok-Miller t.
KW t.
Lachman t.
lactose breath hydrogen t.
lactose tolerance t.
Landau t.
latex fixation t.
latex particle agglutination t.
Leiter t.
leukocyte histamine release t.
levothyroxine t.
limulus lysate t.
Lundh t.
lysis t.
Macherey-Nagel strep t.
Mann-Whitney U t.
Mantel-Haenszel t.
Mantoux tuberculin skin t.
MAST blood t.
Matching Familiar Figures T.
McMurray t.
McNemar t.
mental arithmetic t.
metabolic t.
methemoglobin reduction t.
microhemagglutination t.
microimmunofluorescence t.
microscopic agglutination t. (MAT)
MIF t.
Monospot t.
Montenegro skin t.
mucin clot t.
Multiple Sleep Latency T. (MSLT)
multipuncture t. (MPT)
muscle enzyme t.
NAA t.
NBT dye t.
nitroblue tetrazolium dye
  reduction t.
nitrogen washout t.
nongamma Coombs t.
noninvasive t.
nonstress t. (NST)
nontreponemal t.
norm-referenced t.
nucleic acid amplification t.
object assembly t.
Optochin t.
oral glucose tolerance t.

T

NOTES

test *(continued)*
  O'Riain wrinkle t.
  orthostatic t.
  Ortolani t.
  Otis-Lennon Intelligence T.
  paced auditory serial addition t.
  passive head-up tilt t.
  Paul-Bunnell antibody t.
  Paul-Bunnell-Davidsohn t.
  Peabody Picture Vocabulary T. (PPVT)
  Peabody Picture Vocabulary T.-Revised (PPVT-R)
  Penetrak t.
  phenylketonuria t.
  picture completion t.
  pinhole t.
  PKU t.
  Prechtl t.
  prick t.
  prone extension t.
  prothrombin time coagulation t.
  provocation t.
  psychometric t.
  PT coagulation t.
  pulmonary function t. (PFT)
  Qtest Strep t.
  Quality of Upper Extremities T. (QUEST)
  quantitative intradermal skin t.
  Queckenstedt t.
  QuickVue In-Line One-Step Strep A t.
  radioallergosorbent t. (RAST)
  rapid antigen detection t.
  red glass t.
  red reflex t.
  Reynell Verbal Comprehension T.
  Romberg t.
  Rorschach t.
  Rotazyme t.
  Rotter Sentence Completion T.
  Sabin-Feldman dye t.
  Schiff t.
  Schilling t.
  Schober t.
  Scotch tape slide t.
  screening t.
  serum t.
  shake t.
  Shapiro-Wilk t.
  Short Michigan Alcoholism Screening T. (SMAST)
  Sickledex t.
  similarities t.
  skin prick t.
  Snellen t.
  Social Support Scale for Children t.
  Soluprick skin prick t.
  Spearman rank correlation t.
  SpermMAR mixed antiglobulin reaction t.
  spirometric t.
  spot t.
  stable microbubble t.
  Staclot t.
  standardized t.
  Stanford-Binet Intelligence T.
  Stanford Diagnostic Reading T.
  stool antigen t.
  streptococci rapid antigen detection t.
  Streptozyme t.
  stress t.
  strip t.
  Stroop t.
  Student t-t.
  sucrose hemolysis t.
  sunflower oil challenge t.
  supravital stain t.
  surf t.
  sweat chloride t.
  swinging flashlight t.
  talar tilt t.
  TCT coagulation t.
  Tensilon t.
  tetraiodothyronine t.
  Thayer-Martin t.
  therapeutic pulmonary function t.
  Thomas t.
  thrombin clotting time coagulation t.
  thyroid function t.'s
  thyroxine t.
  tilt-table t.
  tine t.
  Titmus stereoacuity t.
  TOH t.
  TOL t.
  Tower of Hanoi t.
  Tower of London t.
  TPI t.
  Trail Making T.
  transglutaminase antibody t.
  transmission disequilibrium t. (TDT)
  Trendelenburg t.
  Treponema pallidum immobilization t.
  triiodothyronine t.
  tuberculin t.
  tuberculin skin t. (TST)
  urea breath t. (UBT)
  urine ferric chloride t.
  Uriscreen t.

T. of Variables of Attention
(TOVA)
t. of variables of attention deficit
disorder
visual-motor integration t.
visual-perceptual t.
vocabulary t.
Wada t.
Wald t.
Watson-Schwartz t.
Weber t.
Wechsler t.
Wepman Auditory
Discrimination T.
Western blot t.
Westerner t.
whiff t.
Whitaker t.
Wide Range Assessment of
Memory and Learning T.
Wilcoxon rank sum t.
Wilcoxon signed rank t.
Wisconsin Card Sorting T.
(WCST)
Woodcock-Johnson reading t.
WRAML t.
Ziehl-Neelsen t.
ZstatFlu t.
testes (*pl. of* testis)
testicle
undescended t.
testicular
t. absence
t. appendage
t. appendage torsion
t. atrophy
t. attachment
t. descent
t. dislocation
t. dysfunction
t. feminization
t. feminization syndrome
t. flow scan
t. hematoma
t. leukemia
t. pull-down
t. relapse
t. rupture
t. sperm extraction (TESE)
t. tumor
t. volume

testing
airway reactivity t.
antimicrobial susceptibility t.
audiological t.
audiometric t.
breath t.
bronchial provocation t.
cranial nerve t.
dexamethasone suppression t. (DST)
DNA-based t.
dynamic exercise t.
filter paper blood lead t.
FP blood lead t.
genetic t.
inhalation bronchial challenge t.
Institute of Personality and
Ability T. (IPAT)
laryngopharyngeal sensory
stimulation t.
ligase-chain reaction t.
LPSS t.
methacholine provacative t.
muscle t.
mutation t.
OAE t.
otoacoustic emission t.
paracoccidioidin skin t.
provocative bronchial challenge t.
pulmonary function t.
rabbit infectivity t.
rapid filter t.
Simultaneous Technique for Acuity
and Readiness T. (STAR)
sweat t.
TEOAE t.
transient evoked otoacoustic
emissions t.
upright tilt-table t.
urodynamic t.
Weil-Felix antibody t.
testis, pl. **testes**
absent t.
acquired ascending undescended t.
annular t.
appendix t.
canalicular t.
contralateral hypertrophy of t.
cryptorchid t.
dislocated t.
dysgenetic t.
ectopic t.
endocrine nonfunctional t.

T

NOTES

testis *(continued)*
 femoral t.
 hidden t.
 high annular t.
 high scrotal t.
 intraabdominal t.
 t. migration defect
 nonpalpable t.
 perineal t.
 prepenile t.
 retractile t.
 scrotal t.
 spontaneous descent of t.
 superficial ectopic t.
 torsion of t.
 transverse scrotal t.
 true undescended t.
 t. tumor
 undescended t.
 t. within superficial inguinal pouch
  of Denis Browne
testitoxicosis
Testoderm
 T. Transdermal System
 T. TTS
 T. with Adhesive
test-of-cure culture
testolactone
Testopel Pellet
testosterone
 t. to dihydrotestosterone ratio
 free t.
 total t.
Test-Revised
 Slosson Oral Reading T.-R.
  (SORT-R)
 Wide Range Achievement T.-R.
  (WRAT-R)
TET
 tubal embryo transfer
tetani
 Clostridium t.
tetanic
 t. seizure
 t. spasm
tetanospasmin
tetanus
 t. antiserum
 t. antitoxin (TAT)
 cephalic t.
 t. and diphtheria (Td)
 t. and diphtheria toxoids vaccine
 generalized t.
 t. immune globulin
 t. immunoglobulin (TIG)
 neonatal t.
 t. neonatorum
 t. neurotoxin

 t. prophylaxis
 t. toxin
 t. toxoid (TT)
 t. toxoid and diphtheria
 t. toxoid and diphtheria vaccine
tetanus-diphtheria immunization
tetany
 hypocalcemic t.
 hypomagnesemic t.
 infantile t.
 neonatal t.
 t. of vitamin D deficiency
tethered
 t. conus medullaris
 t. cord syndrome
 t. spinal cord
tethering
 spinal cord t.
tetrabenazine
tetracaine
 t., adrenaline, cocaine (TAC)
 t., epinephrine, cocaine
 lidocaine, epinephrine, t. (LET)
Tetracap Oral
tetrachloride
 carbon t.
tetracycline
tetracycline-induced esophagitis
tetraethyl lead
tetrahydrobiopterin
 t. cofactor (BH$_4$)
 t. deficiency
tetrahydrocannabinol (THC)
tetrahydrozoline
tetraiodothyronine test
Tetralan Oral
tetralogy of Fallot (TOF)
Tetramune
tetraplegia
 flaccid t.
tetraploidy
tetravalent
 Rhesus rotavirus t. (RRV-TV)
tetrazolium
 nitroblue t. (NBT)
tetrodotoxin poisoning
tet spell
TEV
 talipes equinovarus
TEWL
 transepidermal water loss
Texacort Topical
Texas
 T. Scottish Rite Hospital (TSRH)
 T. Scottish Rite instrumentation
texture
Tf
 transferrin

TFA
thigh-foot angle
tFA
trans fatty acid
TFCC
triangular fibrocartilaginous complex
TFM
total fat mass
TFP
trifunctional protein deficiency
TfR
transferrin receptor
TG
transglutaminase
TGA
transposition of great arteries
isolated TGA
simple TGA
T/Gel
T. shampoo
T-Gen Rectal
T-Gesic
TGF-1
transforming growth factor-1
TGF-B
transforming growth factor beta
TGV
thoracic gas volume
transposition of great vessels
TH
total hydroperoxide
Thal
T. fundoplication
T. intermedia-like syndrome
thalamostriatic artery
thalamotomy
stereotactic t.
thalamus
thalassemia
alpha t.
beta t.
t. facies
homozygous t.
t. intermedia
t. major
t. minor
sickle cell t.
t. trait
transfusion-dependent t.
thalidomide
t. embryopathy
t. teratogenicity syndrome

thallium
t. imaging
t. intoxication
t. poisoning
thallium-201
THAM
thanatophoric
t. dwarfism
t. dysplasia
t. dysplasia syndrome
Thayer-Martin
T.-M. agar
T.-M. test
THC
tetrahydrocannabinol
theca
t. cell tumor
lumbar t.
Theiler
T. murine encephalomyelitis virus
T. stage
thelarche
premature t.
T-helper cell
thenar
Theo-24
Theobid
Theochron
Theoclear-80
Theoclear L.A.
Theo-Dur
T.-D. Sprinkle
T.-D. Theolair
Theolair
Theo-Dur T.
theophylline
sustained-release t.
t. toxicity
theory
birth trauma t.
crowding t.
t. of mind
pulsion t.
synactive t.
traction t.
Theo-Sav
Theospan-SR
Theostat-80
Theovent
Theo-X
Thera-Flur
Thera-Flur-N

NOTES

T

585

TheraGym exercise ball
therapeutic
- t. abortion (TA)
- t. blood level
- t. donor insemination (TDI)
- t. electromembrane (TEM)
- t. insemination, husband (THI, TIH)
- t. pulmonary function test
- t. pulmonary lavage
- t. transdermal fentanyl (TTS-fentanyl)
- t. transdermal fentanyl system

therapist
- respiratory t.
- speech t.
- vision t.

therapy
- add-back t.
- aerosol t.
- aldosterone replacement t.
- alkali t.
- amnioinfusion t.
- animal-assisted t. (AAT)
- antiangiogenic t.
- antibiotic infusion t.
- antibody induction t.
- antibody replacement t.
- anti-D t.
- antiinflammatory t.
- antileukemic t.
- antimicrobial t.
- antioxidant t.
- antipyretic t.
- antiretroviral t.
- antituberculous t.
- antiviral t.
- azole t.
- behavioral t.
- behavioral family systems t. (BFST)
- behavior family t.
- Bobath t.
- butyrate t.
- caffeine t.
- chelation t.
- chest physical t. (CPT)
- cognitive t.
- cognitive behavioral t. (CBT)
- corticosteroid t.
- deficit t.
- desferrioxamine t.
- directly observed t. (DOT)
- drainage, irrigation, fibrinolytic t. (DRIFT)
- ego-oriented individual t. (EOIT)
- electroconvulsive t. (ECT)
- empiric t.
- enzyme replacement t.
- eradication t.
- exogenous surfactant t.
- external beam radiation t.
- eye salvage t.
- family t.
- fibrinolytic t.
- flashlamp-pulsed laser t.
- gene t.
- group problem-solving t.
- helmet-molding t.
- higher-dose t.
- highly active antiretroviral t. (HAART)
- home antibiotic infusion t.
- HS-tk gene t.
- hyperbaric oxygen t. (HOBT)
- hyperfractionated radiation t.
- immunosuppressive t.
- induction t.
- interactive play t.
- interferon t.
- intracisternal t.
- intralesional steroid t.
- intraventricular fibrinolytic t.
- in utero stem cell t.
- IV anti-D t.
- light t.
- macrolide t.
- massage t.
- megavitamin t.
- milieu t.
- mist t.
- multidrug t. (MDT)
- multisystemic t. (MST)
- myoblast transfer t.
- neurodevelopment t. (NDT)
- occupational t. (OT)
- octreotide t.
- oral contraceptive t. (OCT)
- oral rehydration t. (ORT)
- orthomolecular t.
- oxygen t.
- patterning t.
- percussion t.
- percutaneous t.
- phenytoin t.
- physical t. (PT)
- play t.
- prophylactic t.
- psychodynamic t.
- pulse steroid t.
- radiation t. (RT)
- radioiodine ablative t.
- recombinant enzyme replacement t.
- replacement t.
- rescue t.
- respiratory t.

retinoid t.
t. roll
sensory integration t.
sex steroid add-back t.
speech t.
stem cell t.
stepdown t.
stepwise antiinflammatory t.
steroid t.
subcutaneous desferrioxamine t.
suicide gene t.
supportive group t.
surfactant replacement t.
systemic azole t.
systemic behavior family t.
T-cell antibody induction t.
thiamin t.
triple-drug t.
vision t.
xanthochromia t.
zinc t.
thermal
t. hat
t. injury
t. neutral environment
t. stress
Thermazene
thermic effect of food (TEF)
thermistor
3F t. wire
nasal tip t.
t. thermometer
Thermodigital thermometer
thermodilution method
thermodynamic
thermogenesis
thermogenic response
thermometer
Braun tympanic t.
Philips SensorTouch temple t.
767 SureTemp4 oral t.
thermistor t.
Thermodigital t.
Thermoscan Pro-1-Instant t.
thermoregulation
thermoregulatory response
Thermoscan Pro-1-Instant thermometer
thermotherapy
Theroxide Wash
THI
therapeutic insemination, husband

transient hypogammaglobulinemia of
infancy
thiabendazole
thiacetazone
thiaminase
thiamine deficiency
thiamine-response sideroblastic anemia
thiamin therapy
thiazide
thick
t. blood smear
t. neck
thickened
t. base
t. base of skull
thickening
bronchial wall t.
bronchiolar t.
fusiform nerve t.
intimal t.
nerve t.
nodular nerve t.
nuchal pad t.
pial t.
thickness
skinfold t.
subscapular skinfold t.
triceps skinfold t. (TSF)
Thiemann disease
Thiersch operation
thiethylperazine
thigh-foot
t.-f. angle (TFA)
t.-f. axis
thigh-leg angle (TLA)
thimerosal
t. free
vaccinal t.
thimerosal-free vaccine
thin
t. basement membrane disease
(TBMD)
t. basement membrane nephropathy
t. vaginal mucosa
t. vulvar skin
thinking
abstract t.
auditory integration t. (AIT)
t. skill
thin-layer chromatography (TLC)
thinned dermis

NOTES

thinness
　　drive for t.
thiobarbituric acid-reacting substance (TBARS)
thioctic acid
thiocyanate
thioguanine
thiomalate
　　gold sodium t.
thiopental sodium
Thioplex
thiopurine
　　t. methyltransferase (TPMT)
　　t. methyltransferase deficiency
thioridazine hydrochloride
thiosulfate
　　t. lotion
　　sodium t.
thiotepa
thiothixene
third
　　t. disease rubella
　　t. heart sound
　　t. permanent molar
　　t. space loss
　　t. spacing
　　t. spacing of fluid
　　t. ventricle fenestration
third-degree
　　t.-d. AV block
　　t.-d. burn
　　t.-d. hypospadias
Thomas
　　T. heel
　　T. test
Thompson disease
Thomsen
　　T. disease
　　T. myotonia congenita
Thomsen-Friedenreich
　　T.-F. antigen
　　T.-F. antigen assay
thoracentesis
　　needle t.
thoracic
　　t. aortogram
　　t. cavity
　　t. duct drainage
　　t. duct ligation
　　t. dystrophy
　　t. gas volume (TGV)
　　t. kyphosis
　　t. surgery
　　t. wall excursion
thoracoabdominal ectopia cordis
thoracolumbar kyphosis
thoracolumbosacral orthosis (TLSO)
thoracopagus

thoracoplasty
thoracoscope
thoracoscopic pleural débridement
thoracostomy
　　tube t.
thoracotomy
　　closed t.
thorascopic technique
thorax
　　great vessel of t.
　　milk lines of t.
Thorazine
thought
　　t. action fusion
　　t. disorder
　　t. disturbance
threadworm
thready pulse
threatened abortion
three
　　Pediatric Examination at T. (PEET)
three-day
　　t.-d. fever
　　t.-d. measles
three-point position
three-stage Norwood-Fontan procedure
three-way stopcock
threonine
threshold
　　high pain t.
　　low sensory t.
　　pain t.
　　sensory t.
　　speech reception t.
　　speech recognition t. (SRT)
thrill
　　diastolic t.
　　presystolic t.
　　suprasternal notch t.
thrive
　　failure to t. (FTT)
　　nonorganic failure to t. (NOFT, NOFTT)
throat
　　t. clearing
　　eyes, ears, nose, t. (EENT)
　　sore t.
　　strep t.
　　t. swab
　　Vicks Chloraseptic Sore T.
thrombasthenia
　　Glanzmann t.
thrombectomy
thrombi (*pl. of* thrombus)
thrombin
　　t. clotting time (TCT)
　　t. clotting time coagulation test

t. receptor-activating peptide (TRAP)
t. time
topical t.
Thrombinar
thrombocyte
thrombocythemia
essential t. (ET)
thrombocytopenia
alloimmune t.
amegakaryocytic t.
congenital amegakaryocytic t.
consumptive t.
familial dominant t.
fetomaternal alloimmune t. (FMAIT)
immune t.
immune-mediated t.
isoimmune t.
neonatal alloimmune t.
neonatal isoimmune t.
t. with absent radius (TAR)
t. with absent radius syndrome
X-linked t.
thrombocytopenia-absent radius (TAR)
thrombocytopenic purpura
thrombocytosis
thromboembolic event (TE)
thromboembolism
venous t.
Thrombogen
thrombohemolytic disease
thrombomodulin
thrombopenia
thrombophilia
genetic t.
hereditary t.
thrombophlebitis
cortical t.
diffuse cortical t.
peripheral t.
septic t.
sinus t.
venous sinus t.
thromboplastin
plasma t.
thrombopoiesis
thrombopoietin (TPO)
thrombosis, pl. **thromboses**
anal t.
arterial t.
cavernosal artery t.

cavernous sinus t.
deep venous t. (DVT)
dural sinus t.
dural venous t.
external anal t.
intracranial venous sinus t.
jugular vein t.
lateral sinus t.
mural t.
purulent venous t.
renal vein t.
sagittal sinus t.
sinus t.
venous sinus t.
Thrombostat
thrombotic
t. endocarditis
t. microangiopathy (TMA)
t. purpura
t. thrombocytopenic purpura (TTP)
thromboxane (Tx)
t. A2
thrombus, pl. **thrombi**
chorionic vessel t.
endocardial t.
fibrin t.
t. precursor protein
thrush
oral t.
plaque of t.
t. pneumonia
thrust
jaw t.
manual t.
tongue t.
thumb
broad t.
floating t.
gamekeeper's t.
hitchhiker's t.
t. hyperabduction
hypoplastic t.
indwelling t.
t. in palm deformity
t. sign
skier's t.
t. spica cast
t. spica splint
thumbing
cortical t.
thumbsucking

NOTES

T

thump
　　precordial t.
thymectomy
thymic
　　t. alymphoplasia
　　t. aphasia
　　t. hypoplasia
　　t. hypoplasia anomaly
　　t. shadow
　　t. wave sign
thymidine analog NRTI
thymine nucleotide
thymocyte
thymoma
thymus
　　t. gland
　　t. transplantation
Thypinone
Thyrel TRH
Thyro-Block
thyroglobulin
thyroglossal
　　t. duct
　　t. duct cyst
　　t. duct cyst excision
thyroid
　　t. aplasia
　　t. cancer
　　t. carcinoma
　　t. crisis
　　t. deficiency
　　ectopic t.
　　t. function tests
　　t. gland
　　t. gland dysfunction
　　t. gland malformation
　　hemigland t.
　　hypothalamic, pituitary, t. (HTP)
　　t. nodule
　　t. ophthalmopathy
　　t. and pituitary agenesis
　　t. scintigraphy
　　t. storm
　　sublingual t.
　　t. transcription factor-1 (TTF-1)
thyroid-binding
　　t.-b. globulin (TBG)
　　t.-b. globulin deficiency
thyroidectomy
thyroiditis
　　acute suppurative t.
　　autoimmune t.
　　chronic lymphocytic t.
　　Hashimoto t.
　　lymphocytic t.
　　postviral subacute t.

　　subacute t.
　　suppurative t.
thyroid-related ophthalmopathy (TRO)
thyroid-specific enhancer binding
　　protein-1 (T4/ebp-1)
thyroid-stimulating hormone (TSH)
thyrotoxic crisis
thyrotoxicosis
　　neonatal t.
thyrotropin
　　serum t.
thyrotropin-releasing hormone (TRH)
thyrotropin-secreting pituitary adenoma
thyroxine, thyroxin (T4)
　　free t.
　　t. synthesis
　　t. test
thyroxine-binding
　　t.-b. globulin (TBG)
　　t.-b. globulin deficiency
tiagabine
Tiamate
Tiazac
tibia, pl. **tibiae**
　　congenital longitudinal deficiency
　　　of t.
　　congenital pseudoarthrosis of t.
　　osteochondrosis deformans tibiae
　　posteromedial bow of t.
　　pseudoarthrosis of t.
　　t. vara
tibial
　　t. bowing
　　childhood accidental spiral t.
　　　(CAST)
　　t. epiphysis
　　t. film
　　t. hemimelia
　　t. metaphysis
　　t. pseudoarthrosis
　　t. shaft fracture
　　t. speed
　　t. speed of sound
　　t. stress fracture
　　t. torsion
　　t. tubercle
　　t. valgus osteotomy
　　t. version
tibiofibular syndesmosis
tic
　　chronic t.
　　complex motor t.
　　complex vocal t.
　　cough t.
　　t. disorder
　　maladie des t.'s
　　motor t.
　　multiple t.'s

psychogenic cough t.
simple motor t.
simple vocal t.
t. symptom
vocal t.

Ticar
ticarcillin
t. clavulanate
t. and clavulanate potassium
t. disodium
ticarcillin/clavulanic acid
tick
dog t.
t. fever
Lone Star t.
t. paralysis
Rocky Mountain wood t.
wood t.
tick-borne
t.-b. encephalitis (TBE)
t.-b. relapsing fever
t.-b. typhus
ticlopidine
Ticon Injection
t.i.d.
ter in die (three times a day)
tidal
t. breathing
t. liquid ventilation (TLV)
t. volume (TV, VT)
tide mark dermatitis
tie
silk t.
Tietze syndrome
TIG
tetanus immunoglobulin
Tigan
T. Injection
T. Rectal
tight heel cord
tightness
idiopathic heel-cord t.
TIH
therapeutic insemination, husband
Tilade Inhalation Aerosol
Tillaux
fracture of T.
T. fracture
tilt
head t.
head-up t. (HUT)
lateral head t.

pelvic t.
ulnar t.
tilted disk
tilt-table test
tiludronate
time
activated clotting t. (ACT)
activated partial thromboplastin t.
(APTT)
capillary filling t.
capillary refill t.
euglobulin clot lysis t. (ECLT)
euglobulin lysis t. (ELT)
inspiration t.
inspiratory t. (IT)
isovolumic relaxation t. (IVRT)
Lee-White clotting t.
partial thrombin t.
partial thromboplastin t. (PTT)
preejection period/left ventricular
ejection t. (PEP/LVET)
prothrombin t. (pro-time, PT)
reptilase t.
Rite T.
sinoatrial conduction t.
thrombin t.
thrombin clotting t. (TCT)
Timecelles
Timentin
time-of-flight and absorbance (TOFA)
time-out
time-resolved fluoroimmunoassay
timolol malate
Timoptic Ophthalmic
Timoptic-XE Ophthalmic
timothy grass
tin
t. car syndrome
t. mesoporphyrin (SnMP)
t. protoporphyrin (SnPP)
Tinactin
tincture
alcoholic t.
Fungoid T.
t. of iodine
opium t.
T-independent antigen
Tine
tinea
t. capitis
t. corporis
t. cruris

T

NOTES

tinea *(continued)*
    t. gladiatorum
    t. incognito
    t. manuum
    t. nigra palmaris
    t. pedis
    t. profunda
    t. rubrum
    t. unguium
    t. versicolor
tine test
tinidazole
tinnitus
tinted
    Oxy-5 T.
TINU
    tubulointerstitial nephritis
Tinver
tioconazole 6.5% ointment
TIP
    tubularized incised plate
tip
    bulbous nasal t.
    Frazier suction t.
TIPP
    The Injury Prevention Program
TIPS
    transjugular intrahepatic portosystemic
      shunt
tissue
    adipose t.
    t. anoxia
    bronchus-associated lymphoid t.
      (BALT)
    t. catabolism
    conductive t.
    connective t.
    contused t.
    t. culture-grown attenuated virus
    t. Doppler imaging (TDI)
    embryonic t.
    epipericardial connective t.
    t. expander
    t. factor
    fibrous t.
    fragile t.
    gastrointestinal-associated
      lymphoid t. (GALT)
    gut-associated lymphoid t. (GALT)
    hyperplastic lymphoid t.
    hypertrophied t.
    t. insulin resistance
    intestine-associated lymphoid t.
    larynx-associated lymphoid t.
      (LALT)
    lymphoid t.
    mucosa-associated lymphoid t.
      (MALT)

    nasopharyngeal-associated
      lymphoid t. (NALT)
    t. necrosis
    scar t.
    soft t.
    subareolar t.
    sympathetic t.
    t. synthesis
    t. transglutaminase (tTG)
    t. typing
titanium
    t. elastic nail
    t. elastic nailing (TEN)
titer
    ADB t.
    AH t.
    anti-DNase B t.
    antihyaluronidase t.
    antimycoplasma t.
    antineutrophil cytoplasmic
      antibody t.
    t. of anti-ragweed IgE antibody
    antistreptolysin t.
    ASO t.
    Forssman t.
    geometric mean t. (GMT)
    HI t.
    IgG antibody t.
    IgM t.
    IgM antibody t.
    rubeola t.
    serum bactericidal t. (SBT)
    serum inhibitory t. (SIT)
    sheep cell agglutinin t.
    TORCH t.
    virus t.
Titmus stereoacuity test
Titralac
titration
    skin end-point t.
titubation
TL-90 Ethicon stapler
TLA
    thigh-leg angle
TLC
    thin-layer chromatography
    total lung capacity
TLSO
    thoracolumbosacral orthosis
TLV
    tidal liquid ventilation
    total liquid ventilation
TMA
    thrombotic microangiopathy
    transcription-mediated amplification
    transmalleolar axis angle
      TMA assay

TMJ
temporomandibular joint
TMP-SMX
trimethoprim-sulfamethoxazole
TMS
transcranial magnetic stimulation
TND
transient neonatal diabetes
TNF
tumor necrosis factor
TNF-alpha
tumor necrosis factor-alpha
TNM
tumor, node, metastases
TNM schema
TNR
tonic neck reflex
TnT
troponin T
to-and-fro
t.-a.-f. flow
t.-a.-f. murmur
toast
bananas, rice, applesauce, tea, t.
(BRATT)
bananas, rice cereal, applesauce, t.
(BRAT)
tobacco
smokeless t.
TOBEC
total body electrical conductivity
Tobey ear rongeur
TOBI
tobramycin solution for inhalation
TOBI Inhalation Solution
TobraDex
tobramycin
t. solution
t. solution for inhalation (TOBI)
Tobrex Ophthalmic
tocolysis
tocolytic drug
tocopherol deficiency
tocotransducer
Todd
T. paralysis
T. paresis
Todd-Hewitt broth
toddler-age nodulocystic acne
toddler's
t. diarrhea
t. fracture

Toddler Temperament Scale
toe
adducted great t.
broad t.
curly t.
floating great t.
t. grasp
great t.
mallet t.
overlapping t.
overriding t.
pigeon t.
searching t.
striatal t.
t. syndactyly
t. walking
toeing
t. in
t. out
toe-in gait
toenail
ingrown t.
toe-off
toe-out gait
toewalking
TOF
tetralogy of Fallot
tracheoesophageal fistula
TOFA
time-of-flight and absorbance
Tofranil
Tofranil-PM
Togaviridae
togavirus
TOH
Tower of Hanoi
TOH test
toilet
pulmonary t.
respiratory t.
t. training
TOL
Tower of London
TOL test
tolazoline hydrochloride
tolbutamide
Tolectin DS
tolerance
glucose t.
impaired glucose t. (IGT)
Tolerex formula
tolmetin

NOTES

T

tolnaftate
Tolosa-Hunt syndrome
toluene sniffing
toluidine blue stain
Tolu-Sed DM
tomaculous neuropathy
tomogram
tomography
    computed t. (CT)
    computed axial t. (CAT)
    computer-assisted axial t. (CAAT)
    delayed-phase computed t.
    electron-beam computed t. (EBCT)
    focused computed t.
    high-resolution chest computed t.
    high-resolution computed t. (HRCT)
    optical t.
    positron-emission t. (PET)
    single-photon emission t.
    single-photon emission computed t. (SPECT)
Tompkins
    T. metroplasty
    T. procedure
tone
    anal t.
    bronchomotor t.
    decreased anal t.
    decreased sphincter t.
    flaccid t.
    flexor t.
    fluctuating t.
    high t.
    low muscle t.
    muscle t.
    parasympathetic t.
    poor muscle t.
    pulmonary vascular t.
    sphincter t.
    uterine t.
    vagal t.
    vascular t.
tongs
    Gardner-Wells t.
tongue
    t. biting
    black hairy t.
    chameleon t.
    darting t.
    t. depressor
    t. fasciculation
    fissured t.
    geographic t.
    hairy t.
    hypoplastic t.
    large t.
    protruding t.
    t. protrusion reflex

    raspberry t.
    red strawberry t.
    scrotal t.
    t. size
    smooth t.
    strawberry t.
    surface furrowing of t.
    t. thrust
    white strawberry t.
tongue-lip adhesion
tongue-tied
tonic
    t. downgaze
    t. labyrinthine reflex
    t. neck pattern
    t. neck reflex (TNR)
    t. neck response
    t. seizure
tonic-clonic
    t.-c. convulsion
    t.-c. seizure
Tonnis procedure
tonoclonic
tonometry
    gastric t.
    gut t.
tonsil
    cerebellar t.'s
tonsillar
    t. edema
    t. exudate
tonsillectomy and adenoidectomy (T&A)
tonsillitis
    acute exudative t.
    acute follicular t.
    adenoviral t.
    exudative t.
    follicular t.
    streptococcal t.
    white t.
tonsillopharyngeal exudate
tonsillopharyngitis
    streptococcal t.
tonsurans
    Trichophyton t.
tonus
tool
    Adolescent and Pediatric Pain T. (APPT)
    SCHIP evaluation t.
too-soft voice
tooth
    t. bud
    canine t.
    t. decay
    dystrophic t.
    t. loss
    t. and nail syndrome

t. placement
wisdom t.
toothbrush culture technique
Topamax
topectomy
tophus, pl. **tophi**
urate tophi
Topicaine
topical
Achromycin T.
Acticort T.
Aeroseb-HC T.
Ala-Cort T.
Ala-Scalp T.
Alphatrex T.
Anusol HC-1 T.
Anusol HC-2.5% T.
Aristocort A T.
A/T/S T.
Baciguent T.
Benadryl T.
Betalene T.
Betatrex T.
Beta-Val T.
CaldeCort T.
Caldesene T.
Cetacort T.
CortaGel T.
Cort-Dome T.
Cortef Feminine Itch T.
Cortizone-5 T.
Cortizone-10 T.
Cruex T.
Delcort T.
Delta-Tritex T.
Dermacort T.
Dermarest Dricort T.
Derma-Smoothe/FS T.
Dermolate T.
Dermtex HC with Aloe T.
DesOwen T.
Diprolene AF T.
Diprosone T.
Efudex T.
Eldecort T.
ETS-2% T.
Fluonid T.
Fluoroplex T.
Flurosyn T.
Flutex T.
FS Shampoo T.
Gynecort T.

Hi-Cor-1.0 T.
Hi-Cor-2.5 T.
Hycort T.
Hydrocort T.
Hydro-Tex T.
Hytone T.
t. imidazole
Kenalog T.
Kenonel T.
LactiCare-HC T.
Lanacort T.
Locoid T.
Lotrimin AF T.
Maxivate T.
MetroGel T.
Micatin T.
Monistat-Derm T.
Mycelex-G T.
Mycitracin T.
Neomixin T.
t. nitroglycerin
Nutracort T.
Orabase HCA T.
Pedi-Dri T.
Pedi-Pro T.
Penecort T.
t. podophyllin
Polysporin T.
Psorion T.
Rogaine T.
Scalpicin T.
Solarcaine T.
S-T Cort T.
Synacort T.
Synalar T.
Synalar-HP T.
Synemol T.
Tegrin HC T.
Teladar T.
Texacort T.
t. thrombin
Topicycline T.
Triacet T.
Triple Antibiotic T.
U-Cort T.
Undoguent T.
Uticort T.
Valisone T.
Vitec T.
Westcort T.
Topicort
Topicycline Topical

T

NOTES

topiramate
topography
    perisulcal t.
topoisomerase-1
Toradol
    T. Injection
    T. Oral
TORCH
    toxoplasmosis, other agents, rubella,
      cytomegalovirus, herpes
    toxoplasmosis, other agents, rubella,
      cytomegalovirus, herpes simplex virus
      TORCH infection
      TORCH screen
      TORCH syndrome
      TORCH titer
Torecan
Torkildsen procedure
Tornalate
Toronto
    T. Alexithymia Scale (TAS)
    T. parapodium
    T. tumor (group I–IV)
torovirus
torpedo
torque depressor
torrential pulmonary flow
torsade de pointes
torsemide
torsion
    adnexal t.
    appendage t.
    t. of appendix
    t. dystonia
    external femoral t.
    external tibial t.
    femoral t.
    t. of gut
    internal femoral t.
    internal tibial t.
    lateral femoral t. (LFT)
    lateral tibial t. (LTT)
    medial femoral t. (MFT)
    medial tibial t. (MTT)
    ovarian t.
    t. of ovary
    penile t.
    testicular appendage t.
    t. of testis
    tibial t.
torsional
    t. alignment
    t. deformity
    t. profile
torti
    pili t.
torticollis
    acquired t.

    acute t.
    benign paroxysmal t.
    congenital muscular t.
    idiopathic t.
    infantile muscular t.
    juvenile muscular t.
    muscular t.
    neonatal t.
    paroxysmal t.
    spasmodic t.
tortuosity
    retinal venous dilation and t.
      (RVDT)
tortuous capillary
Torulopsis glabrata
torus fracture
tosylarginine
    t. methyl ester (TAME)
    t. methyl ester esterase
Totacillin
Totacillin-N
total
    t. anomalous pulmonary venous
      connection (TAPVC)
    t. anomalous pulmonary venous
      return (TAPVR)
    t. bilirubin
    t. body electrical conductivity
      (TOBEC)
    t. body iron
    t. body iron content
    t. body irradiation (TBI)
    t. body potassium (TBK)
    t. body sodium
    t. body surface area (TBSA)
    t. body surface area burned
    t. body water (TBW)
    t. cavopulmonary anastomosis
    t. colonic aganglionosis
    t. communication
    t. daily energy expenditure (TDEE)
    T. Eclipse
    t. energy expenditure
    t. fat mass (TFM)
    t. hemispherectomy
    t. hemolytic complement
    t. hepatectomy
    t. hydroperoxide (TH)
    t. liquid ventilation (TLV)
    t. lung capacity (TLC)
    t. magnesium
    t. mixing lesion
    t. muscle paralysis
    t. parenteral nutrition (TPN)
    t. parenteral nutrition-associated
      cholestasis
    t. peripheral parenteral nutrition
      (TPPN)

t. peripheral resistance (TPR)
t. serum bilirubin (TSB)
t. testosterone
t. villous atrophy
totalis
alopecia universalis t.
Tourette
T. disease
T. disorder (TD)
Gilles de la T.
T. syndrome
tourniquet
hair t.
Touro Ex
TOVA
Test of Variables of Attention
Tower
T. of Hanoi (TOH)
T. of Hanoi test
T. of London (TOL)
T. of London test
toxemia of pregnancy
toxemic shock syndrome
toxic
t. alopecia
t. appearance
t. cascade
t. dynamics
t. epidermal necrolysis (TEN)
t. erythema
t. hepatitis
t. megacolon
t. myocarditis
t. neuropathy
t. oil syndrome
t. shock syndrome (TSS)
t. shock syndrome toxin-1 (TSST-1)
t. synovitis
toxicity
aluminum t.
bismuth t.
bone marrow t.
carbon monoxide t.
chronic cyanide t.
citrate t.
cognitive t.
cyanide t.
iron t.
oxygen t.
phosphate t.
theophylline t.

zinc t.
t. zone
toxicokinetics
toxicologic analysis
toxicology screen
toxicosis
copper t.
idiopathic copper t.
toxicum
erythema t.
erythema neonatorum t.
toxidrome
toxin
albumin-bound t.
botulinum t.
botulinum t. A (BTA)
botulism t.
clostridial t.
Clostridium botulinum type A t.
diphtheria t. (DT)
epidermolytic t.
epsilon t.
pertussis t. (PT)
reproductive t.
Shiga t. (Stx)
Shiga-like t.
tetanus t.
toxin-1
toxic shock syndrome t.-1 (TSST-1)
toxin-induced scarlet fever exanthem
Toxocara
T. canis
T. cati
toxocariasis
toxoid
pertussis t. (PT)
tetanus t. (TT)
Toxoplasma
T. antigen
T. encephalitis
T. gondii
T. lymphadenopathy
toxoplasmic
t. chorioretinitis
t. encephalitis
toxoplasmosis
congenital t.
ocular t.
t., other agents, rubella, CMV, HSV

NOTES

T

toxoplasmosis *(continued)*
    t., other agents, rubella, cytomegalovirus, herpes (TORCH)
    t., other agents, rubella, cytomegalovirus, herpes simplex virus (TORCH)
    t., rubella, cytomegalovirus, herpes simplex syndrome
toy
    ride-on t.
TPC
    tympanocentesis
T-Phyl
TPI
    Treponema pallidum immobilization
    triose phosphate isomerase
        TPI deficiency
        TPI test
TPMT
    thiopurine methyltransferase
        TPMT deficiency
TPN
    total parenteral nutrition
TPO
    thrombopoietin
        plasma TPO
TPPN
    total peripheral parenteral nutrition
TPR
    total peripheral resistance
TRA
    traumatic rupture of thoracic aorta
trabecular muscular septum
trabeculodysgenesis
trabeculotomy
Trace-4
trace metal
Trach Care suction
trachea
    blind t.
    stenosis of t.
tracheal
    t. aspirate
    t. atresia
    t. catheter
    t. lavage
    t. occlusion
    t. stenosis
    t. tube
    t. tumor
tracheitis
    acute t.
    bacterial t.
    subacute t.
tracheobronchial
    t. aspirate
    t. aspirate fluid (TAF)
    t. compression

    t. obstruction
    t. remnant
    t. tree
tracheobronchitis
tracheobronchomegaly
tracheocutaneous fistula
tracheoesophageal
    t. atresia
    t. fistula (TEF, TOF)
    t. septation
    t. septum
tracheomalacia
    intrathoracic t.
    primary t.
    secondary t.
tracheostomy
    flap t.
    percutaneous t.
    t. tube
    t. tube flange
tracheotomy
trachoma
trachomatis
    Chlamydia t. (CT)
tracing
track
    bear t.'s
tracker
    Breath T.
tracking
    J t.
    visual t.
Tracrium
tract
    brainstem auditory t.
    dermal sinus t.
    endomesenchymal t.
    extrapyramidal t.
    gastrointestinal t.
    genitourinary t.
    gooseneck deformity of left ventricular outflow t.
    left ventricular outflow t. (LVOT)
    Lissauer t.
    lower respiratory t.
    mesolimbic dopamine t.
    narrow pulmonary outflow t. (NPOT)
    nerve t.
    nigrostriatal t.
    outflow t.
    patch unroofing of outflow t.
    pin t.
    pyramidal t.
    renal t.
    right ventricular outflow t. (RVOT)
    suppurating sinus t.
    upper respiratory t.

urinary t.
urogenital t.
traction
90/90 t.
t. alopecia
t. apophysitis
t. apophysitis of medial epicondyle
axial t.
Bryant t.
45-degree skin t.
distal femoral skeletal t.
halo t.
t. injury
Russell t.
skeletal t.
skin t.
t. theory
t. treatment
tractional retinal detachment
traffic-light diet
tragus, pl. **tragi**
accessory t.
Trail Making Test
training
auditory t.
auditory integration t. (AIT)
forced bowel t.
parent effectiveness t. (PET)
toilet t.
trait
hereditary t.
sickle cell t.
thalassemia t.
TRALI
transfusion-associated lung injury
trampoline
Trandate
tranexamic acid
tranquilizer drug
transabdominal ultrasonography
transalar sphenoidal encephalocele
transaminase
alanine t. (ALT)
aspartate t. (AST)
elevated t.
glutamic-pyruvic t.
hepatic t.
serum glutamic-pyruvic t. (SGPT)
transannular patch repair
transcarbamylase
ornithine t. (OTC)
transcarotid balloon valvuloplasty

transcatheter
t. closure (TCC)
t. coil embolization
transcobalamin
t. II (TC II)
t. II deficiency
transcranial
t. Doppler (TCD)
t. magnetic stimulation (TMS)
transcription
transcription-mediated
t.-m. amplification (TMA)
t.-m. amplification assay
transcutaneous
t. bilirubin (TcB)
t. electrical nerve stimulation (TENS)
t. jaundice meter
t. oximetry
transdermal
Catapres-TTS T.
Climara T.
Duragesic T.
t. fentanyl patch
t. therapeutic system (TTS)
Vivelle T.
Transdermal-NTG Patch
Transderm-Nitro Patch
Transderm Scop
transdisciplinary team
transducer
pressure t.
Sorensen Transpac t.
transection
complete cord t.
cord t.
esophageal t.
lower esophageal t.
multiple subpial t. (MST)
transepidermal water loss (TEWL)
transesophageal
t. echocardiography (TEE)
t. fistula
trans fatty acid (tFA)
transfer
anterior tibialis t.
antibody transplacental t.
placental t.
split anterior tibial tendon t. (SPLATT)
tendon t.
transplacental allergen t.

NOTES

599

transfer (*continued*)
    tubal embryo t. (TET)
    tubal embryo stage t. (TEST)
transferase
    t. deficient galactosemia
    serum glutamic-oxaloacetic t.
      (SGOT)
    succinyl CoA:3-ketoacid CoA t.
      (SCOT)
transferrin (Tf)
    t. receptor (TfR)
    t. saturation
transformation
    malignant t.
transforming
    t. growth factor-1 (TGF-1)
    t. growth factor beta (TGF-B)
    t. growth factor beta superfamily
transfusion
    exchange t. (EXT)
    fetofetal t.
    fetomaternal t.
    gamma-irradiated cellular
     products t.
    granulocyte t.
    intrauterine maternofetal t.
    late complication of t.
    maternofetal t.
    neutrophil t.
    packed red blood cell t.
    placental t.
    placentofetal t. (PFT)
    t. reaction
    red blood cell t.
    t. syndrome
    t. transmitted (TT)
    t. transmitted virus
    twin-to-twin t.
    umbilical vein packed red blood
     cell t.
    umbilical vein platelet t.
transfusion-associated
    t.-a. cytomegalovirus
    t.-a. lung injury (TRALI)
transfusion-dependent thalassemia
transfusion-induced hemosiderosis
transgastric window
transgene
transgenerational analysis
transgenic
transglutaminase (TG)
    t. antibody
    t. antibody test
    t. deficiency
    tissue t. (tTG)
trans-Golgi network
transgrediens
    keratoderma palmoplantaris t.

transient
    t. amblyopia
    t. aplastic crisis (TAC)
    t. bilirubin encephalopathy
    t. candidemia
    t. cerebellar ataxia
    t. cortical blindness
    t. dystonia
    t. dystonic posturing
    t. erythroblastopenia
    t. erythroblastopenia of childhood
     (TEC)
    t. evoked otoacoustic emission
     (TEOAE)
    t. evoked otoacoustic emissions
     testing
    t. familial neonatal
     hyperbilirubinemia
    t. hemianopia
    t. hyperammonemia
    t. hypogammaglobulinemia
    t. hypogammaglobulinemia of
     infancy (THI)
    t. hypoglycemia
    t. hypothyroxinemia
    t. hypotonia
    t. insulinopenic state
    t. keratitis
    t. monoarticular synovitis
    t. mutism
    t. myeloproliferative disorder
    t. myeloproliferative syndrome
    t. neonatal cystinuria
    t. neonatal diabetes (TND)
    t. neonatal myasthenia
    t. neonatal myasthenia gravis
    t. neonatal myasthenic syndrome
    t. neonatal pustular melanosis
    t. neutropenia
    t. oliguria
    t. opsoclonus
    t. pharyngeal muscle dysfunction
    t. protein intolerance
    t. quadriplegia
    t. respiratory distress syndrome
    sharp-wave t.
    t. tachypnea
    t. tachypnea of newborn (TTN)
    t. tic disorder
    t. tyrosinemia
    t. tyrosinemia of newborn
    t. vasospasm
transiliac lengthening osteotomy
transilluminate
transillumination
transit
    abnormal t.

transition
  t. plan
  t. stool
transitional reader stage
transitory
  t. fever
  t. fever of newborn
  t. hydrocele
transjugular intrahepatic portosystemic shunt (TIPS)
translation
  anterior t.
translevator imperforate anus
translocation
  chromosomal t.
  t. Down syndrome
  t. trisomy 21
translucency
  nuchal t.
transmalleolar
  t. axis
  t. axis angle (TMA)
transmembrane glycoprotein gp41
transmesenteric hernia
transmissible spongiform encephalopathy (TSE)
transmission
  t. disequilibrium
  t. disequilibrium test (TDT)
  t. electron microscopy (TEM)
  horizontal t.
  mother-infant t.
  vertical t.
transmitted
  transfusion t. (TT)
transmucosal midazolam
transmural inflammation
transparenchymal needle puncture
transparent bulla
transpeptidase
  gamma glutamyl t.
transpericardial echocardiography
transplacental
  t. allergen transfer
  t. infection
transplant
  bone marrow t. (BMT)
  t. coronary artery disease
  haploidentical bone marrow t.
  heart t.
  liver t.
  t. patient

reduced liver t. (RLT)
reduced-size liver t. (RSLT)
Trans-Plantar Transdermal Patch
transplantation
  allogenic bone marrow t.
  allogenic stem cell t.
  autologous bone marrow t.
  autologous stem cell t.
  auxiliary orthotopic liver t.
  bone marrow t. (BMT)
  cord blood t. (CBT)
  cord stem cell marrow t.
  double-lung t.
  fetal stem cell t.
  heart t.
  hematopoietic stem cell t.
  hepatic t.
  heterotopic liver t.
  International Society for Heart T. (ISHT)
  intestinal t.
  in utero t.
  kidney t.
  liver t.
  marrow t.
  orthotopic heart t.
  orthotopic liver t. (OLTx)
  partial auxiliary orthotopic liver t.
  peripheral stem cell t.
  small bowel t.
  solid organ t. (SOT)
  stem cell t. (SCT)
  stem cell bone marrow t.
  syngeneic bone marrow t.
  thymus t.
  umbilical cord blood t.
transport
  bus t.
  fixed-wing t.
  Kid-EXB 2 child's chair for bus t.
  neonatal t.
transporter
  carbohydrate homeostasis t.
  glucose t. (GLUT)
transposition
  aortopulmonary t.
  complete t.
  t. of great arteries (TGA)
  t. of great vessels (TGV)
  penoscrotal t.
  physiologically corrected t.

NOTES

601

transpulmonary pressure
transpyloric tube feeding
transtelephonic monitoring (TTM)
transtentorial herniation
transthoracic echocardiography
transthyretin (TTR)
transtracheal
    t. aspiration
    t. catheter
    t. ventilation
transtubular potassium concentration
  gradient (TTKG)
transudate
transudative pleural effusion
transurethral
    t. ablation
    t. ablation of valve
    t. self-detachable balloon
transvaginal ultrasonography
transvalensis
    Nocardia t.
transvascular
transvenous
    t. coil embolization
    t. pacing
transversal nasal crease
Trans-Ver-Sal Transdermal Patch
transverse
    t. arch hypoplasia
    t. dense striation
    t. incision
    t. loop colostomy
    t. myelitis
    t. nail groove
    t. scrotal testis
    t. vaginal septum
transversum
    septum t.
Tranxene
TRAP
    thrombin receptor-activating peptide
    twin reversed arterial perfusion
      TRAP syndrome
trap
    Alden-Senturia collection t.
    Luekens t.
TRAP-activated neonatal platelet
trapping
    air t.
    ion t.
    platelet t.
Trasylol
trauma
    acoustic t.
    American Association for the
      Surgery of T. (AAST)
    birth t.
    blunt chest t.

chest t.
craniocerebral t.
dehydration, poisoning, t. (DPT)
dental t.
Focused Assessment by Sonography
  for T. (FAST)
forceps birth t.
head t.
penetrating t.
T. Score and Injury Severity Score
  Analysis (TRISS)
T. Symptom Checklist for Children
  (TSCC)
T. Triage Rule (TTR)
Traumacal formula
traumatic
    t. alopecia
    t. aortic injuries in children
    t. bowing
    t. brain injury (TBI)
    t. compartment syndrome
    t. glaucoma
    t. hematoma
    t. hyphema
    t. idiocy
    t. imagery
    t. labyrinthitis
    t. pneumothorax
    t. rupture of thoracic aorta (TRA)
    t. sexualization
Travase
traveler's diarrhea (TD)
trazodone
Treacher
    T. Collins-Franceschetti syndrome
    T. Collins syndrome
treadmill
treatment
    allergy t.
    antenatal corticosteroid t. (ANS)
    antibiotic t.
    anticonvulsant t.
    anti-D globulin t.
    antiinflammatory t.
    antimanic t.
    antimicrobial t.
    brace t.
    corticosteroid t.
    double diaper t.
    t. and education of autistic and
      related communications
      handicapped children (TEACCH)
    ex utero intrapartum t. (EXIT)
    immunomodulatory t.
    mutagenic t.
    neurodevelopmental t.
    Otovent negative pressure t.
    phase advance t.

phase delay t.
postexposure t. (PET)
preventive allergy t. (PAT)
prophylactic t.
t. series
spectacle t.
steroid t.
traction t.
treatment-refractory depression
treatment-resistant proteinuria
Trecator-SC
tree
bronchial t.
extrahepatic biliary t.
t. pollen
tracheobronchial t.
trefoil pelvis
Treitz
ligament of T.
trembling
hereditary chin t.
tremor
coarse t.
essential t.
familial t.
hereditary t.
intention t.
primary writing t.
t. syndrome
tremulousness
trench
t. fever
t. mouth
Trendar
Trendelenburg
T. gait
T. limp
T. position
T. sign
T. test
Trental
trephination
nail t.
Treponema
T. carateum
T. pallidum
T. pallidum immobilization (TPI)
T. pallidum immobilization test
T. pertenue
treponemal
Treppe response
tretinoin

TRF
Teacher Rating Form
Teacher Report Form
TRH
thyrotropin-releasing hormone
Relefact TRH
Thyrel TRH
Triacet Topical
triad
aspirin t.
Beck t.
Charcot t.
Currarino t.
Cushing t.
female athlete t. (FAT)
Hutchinson t.
triage
trial
Canadian Crohn Relapse
Prevention T.
Diabetes Control and
Complications T. (DCCT)
high-frequency ventilation t. (HIFT)
STOP-ROP t.
Supplemental Therapeutic Oxygen
for Prethreshold Retinopathy of
Prematurity t.
surfactant replacement t.
Triam-A Injection
triamcinolone
t. acetonide
t. acetonide ointment
t. hexacetonide
Triam Forte Injection
Triaminic
T. Allergy
T. AM Decongestant Formula
T. Chewables
T. Cold Tablets
T. Expectorant
T. Infant Drops
T. Syrup
Triaminic-DM
Triamonide Injection
triamterene
triangle
Codman t.
triangular
t. facies
t. fibrocartilaginous complex
(TFCC)
t. splint

NOTES

T

triatriatum
    cor t.
triazolam
Triban
    Pediatric T.
tribasilar synostosis
triceps
    t. reflex
    t. skinfold thickness (TSF)
    t. tendinitis
trichilemmal cyst
trichilemmoma
Trichinella spiralis
trichinosis
trichiura
    Trichuris t.
trichloroacetic acid (TCA)
trichloroethanol (TCE)
trichobezoar
trichodentoosseous syndrome
trichodysplasia
    hereditary t.
trichoepithelioma
trichomegaly
    eyelash t.
trichomonad
trichomonal
    t. infection
    t. vaginitis
Trichomonas vaginalis
trichomoniasis
trichophagia
trichophagy
Trichophyton
    T. mentagrophytes
    T. rubrum
    T. tonsurans
trichopoliodystrophy
trichorhinophalangeal dysplasia
trichorrhexis
    t. invaginata
    t. nodosa
trichoschisis
Trichosporon beigelii
trichosporonosis
trichothiodystrophy
trichotillomania
trichrome stain
trichuriasis
Trichuris
    T. dysentery syndrome
    T. trichiura
Tricosal
tricuspid
    t. atresia
    t. insufficiency

    t. stenosis
    t. valve
tricyclic antidepressant (TCA)
Tridesilon
Tridil Injection
triene-to-tetraene ratio
trientine
triethanolamine polypeptide oleate-
    condensate
triethylene tetramine dihydrochloride
trifluoperazine
trifluorothymidine
trifluridine
trifunctional protein deficiency (TFP)
trigeminal
    t. herpes zoster
    t. nerve
    t. nerve distribution
trigger
    t. digit
    t. phenomenon
triginous area
triglyceride
    t. hyperlipemia
    medium-chain t. (MCT)
    milk t.
    t. storage disease (type I)
triglycine
    mercaptoacetyl t.
trigonal hypertrophy
trigonocephaly
trigonum
    os t.
trihexose
    ceramide t.
Trihexy
trihexyphenidyl
TriHIBit vaccine
Tri-Immunol vaccine
triiodothyronine (T3)
    free t.
    t. test
Tri-K
Tri-Kort Injection
trilaminar embryonic disk
trilateral
    t. retinoblastoma
    t. retinoblastoma syndrome
trileaflet aortic valve
Tri-Levlen contraceptive pill
Trilisate
Trilog Injection
trilogy
    Fallot t.
Trilone Injection
Trimazide
    T. Oral
    T. Rectal

trimester
trimethadione
trimethaphan camsylate
trimethobenzamide hydrochloride
trimethoprim
   cotrimoxazole t.
   t. HCl oral solution
   t. sulfate
trimethoprim-sulfamethoxazole (TMP-SMX)
   t.-s. prophylaxis
trimethylaminuria
Trimox
Trimpex
Trinalin
Tri-Nasal Spray
Triofed
triopathy
triose
   t. phosphate isomerase (TPI)
   t. phosphate isomerase deficiency
Triostat Injection
Tripedia vaccine
tripelennamine
triphasic pattern blastemal cell
Triphasil contraceptive pill
triphosphatase
   adenosine t.
triphosphate
   adenosine t. (ATP)
   deoxynucleotide t.
   guanosine t. (GTP)
   lead t.
triplane fracture
triple
   T. Antibiotic Topical
   t. arthrodesis
   t. dye
   T. Paste
   T. Paste ointment
   t. screen
   T. X shampoo
   t. X syndrome
triple-drug therapy
triplegia
triple-lumen tube
triplet
triploid
triploidy
   placental mosaicism for t.
   t. syndrome

tripod
   t. fixation technique
   t. position
   t. sign
tripod-supporting position
Triposed
triprolidine and pseudoephedrine
TripTone Caplets
triradius
   distal t.
trisalicylate
   choline-magnesium t.
trisegmentectomy
triseriatus
   Aedes t.
trismus
   t. nascentium
   t. neonatorum
   persistent t.
Trisoject Injection
trisomy
   t. 2
   t. 9
   t. 13
   t. 14
   t. 15
   t. 18
   t. 19
   t. 21
   t. D syndrome
   nondisjunction t. 21
   t. 4p syndrome
   t. 20p syndrome
   t. 10q syndrome
   t. 8 syndrome
   t. 9 syndrome
   t. 13 syndrome
   t. 13-15 syndrome
   t. 16-18 syndrome
   t. 18 syndrome
   t. 21 syndrome
   translocation t. 21
TRISS
   Trauma Score and Injury Severity Score Analysis
trisulfapyrimidine
trivalent
TRIZOL reagent
TRO
   thyroid-related ophthalmopathy
Trocal

NOTES

trochanter
  greater t.
troche
  clotrimazole t.
  Mycelex T.
trochlear
  t. nerve
  t. nerve palsy
troglitazone
troleandomycin
trombiculiasis
tromethamine
  ketorolac t.
  lodoxamide t.
Tronolane
TrophAmine
trophic
  t. feed
  T-cell t. (T-trophic)
trophoblast
trophozoite
tropic
  macrophage t. (M-tropic)
tropica
  Leishmania t.
Tropicacyl
tropical
  t. ataxic neuropathy
  t. pyomyositis
  Quinsana Plus T.
  t. spastic paraparesis (TSP)
  t. spastic paraparesis/HTLV-I
    associated myelopathy (TSP/HAM)
  t. sprue
tropicalis
  Candida t.
tropicamide
tropism
tropoelastin
tropomodulin
troponin
  t. C
  cardiac t. T
  t. I
  t. I level
  t. T (TnT)
trough
  peak and t.
  t. tacrolimus level
Trousseau sign
trovafloxacin
Troyer syndrome
true
  t. histiocytic lymphoma
  t. macroglossia
  t. undescended testis
  t. vertigo

truncal
  t. acne
  t. asymmetry
  t. ataxia
  t. incurvation reflex
  t. obesity
  t. rash
truncus arteriosus
trunk
  t. control
  pulmonary arterial t.
  t. rotation
Truphylline
trust
  support t.
Tru-Trax
TruZone PFM
Trypanosoma
  T. brucei
  T. cruzi
trypanosomal chancre
trypanosome
trypanosomiasis
  African t.
  American t.
  cerebral t.
  Cruz t.
  Gambian t.
  Rhodesian t.
trypsin activation peptide (TAP)
trypsinization
trypsinogen
  immunoreactive t. (IRT)
tryptase
tryptophan
  t. ethylester
  t. malabsorption
TSB
  total serum bilirubin
TSC
  tuberous sclerosis complex
TSCC
  Trauma Symptom Checklist for Children
TSE
  transmissible spongiform encephalopathy
tsetse fly
TSF
  triceps skinfold thickness
TSH
  thyroid-stimulating hormone
    TSH surge
TSP
  tropical spastic paraparesis
TSP/HAM
  tropical spastic paraparesis/HTLV-I
    associated myelopathy

TSRH
   Texas Scottish Rite Hospital
      TSRH crosslink
TSS
   toxic shock syndrome
TSST-1
   toxic shock syndrome toxin-1
TST
   tuberculin skin test
T-Stat
tsutsugamushi
   t. fever
   Orientia t.
TT
   tetanus toxoid
   transfusion transmitted
      TT virus (TTV)
TTF-1
   thyroid transcription factor-1
tTG
   tissue transglutaminase
TTKG
   transtubular potassium concentration
      gradient
TTM
   transtelephonic monitoring
TTN
   transient tachypnea of newborn
TTP
   thrombotic thrombocytopenic purpura
TTR
   transthyretin
   Trauma Triage Rule
T-trophic
   T-cell trophic
T-tropic S1 strain
TTS
   transdermal therapeutic system
      Testoderm TTS
TTS-fentanyl
   therapeutic transdermal fentanyl
T-tube cholangiogram
t-tubules
TTV
   TT virus
tubal
   t. embryo stage transfer (TEST)
   t. embryo transfer (TET)
tube
   bilateral myringotomy t.'s
   bronchial t.
   chest t.

t. connector
cuffed endotracheal t.
cuffed ET t.
ear ventilation t.
endotracheal t.
EntriStar Skin Level T.
ET t.
eustachian t.
t. feed
feeding t.
Foley t.
gastrointestinal t.
gastrostomy t.
laser office ventilation of ears with
   insertion of t.'s (LOVE IT)
Linton t.
Malecot t.
myringotomy t.
nasogastric t. (NGT)
nasojejunal t.
neural t.
NG t.
NJ t.
OG t.
oral gastric t.
PE t.
Pedi PEG t.
PEG t.
percutaneous endoscopic
   gastrostomy t.
Pezzer t.
t. placement
polyethylene feeding t.
pressure equalization t. (PET)
Replogle sump t.
Rubin t.
Sengstaken-Blakemore t.
Shah permanent t.
t. thoracostomy
tracheal t.
tracheostomy t.
triple-lumen t.
tympanostomy t.
uncuffed endotracheal t.
ventilation t.
tuber
   cortical t.
   cryptic t.
tubercle
   choroid t.
   Ghon t.

NOTES

T

tubercle *(continued)*
  pubic t.
  tibial t.
tuberculid
  papulonecrotic t.
tuberculin
  t. skin test (TST)
  t. syringe
  t. test
tuberculoid
  borderline t. (BT)
  t. leprosy
tuberculoma
  infratentorial t.
tuberculoprotein
tuberculosis (TB)
  abdominal t.
  bovine t.
  cavitary t.
  congenital t.
  cutaneous t.
  disseminated t.
  endobronchial t.
  extrapulmonary t.
  extrathoracic t.
  gastrointestinal t.
  hematogenous primary t.
  infectious pulmonary t.
  intrathoracic t.
  miliary t.
  multidrug-resistant t. (MDR-TB)
  mycobacteria other than t. (MOTT)
  Mycobacterium t.
  orificial t.
  t. papulonecrotica
  pediatric t.
  primary pulmonary t.
  progressive primary pulmonary t.
  pulmonary t.
  reactivation t.
  renal t.
  spinal t.
  t. verrucosa cutis
  visceral t.
tuberculous
  t. abscess
  t. adenitis
  t. cervical lymphadenitis
  t. chancre
  t. colitis
  t. dactylitis
  t. enteritis
  t. gumma
  t. keratoconjunctivitis
  t. meningitis
  t. osteomyelitis
  t. peritonitis
  t. pleural effusion

  t. pneumonia
  t. spinal arachnoiditis
  t. spondylitis
tuberculum sella
tuberosity
  bicipital t.
tuberous
  t. breast abnormality
  t. sclerosis
  t. sclerosis complex (TSC)
  t. sclerosis syndrome
Tubigrip bandage
tubing
  blow-by through t.
  Mini-Med t.
tubocurarine chloride
tuboovarian abscess
tubular
  t. atrophy
  t. bone
  t. breathing
  t. disruption
  t. dysgenesis
  t. hypoplasia
  t. interstitial fibrosis
  t. necrosis
  t. proteinuria
tubularization
  in situ t.
tubularized incised plate (TIP)
tubule
  convoluted t.
  proximal convoluted t.
  renal t.
  seminiferous t.
tubuloglomerular feedback
tubulointerstitial
  t. lesion
  t. nephritis (TINU)
tubulopathy
  hypokalemic salt-losing t.
  t. of Lowe syndrome
  proximal t.
tuft
  digital t.
  distal t.
  epithelial t.
  glomerular t.
  t. of hair
  swollen glomerular t.
tugging at ears
tularemia
  glandular t.
  oculoglandular t.
  oropharyngeal t.
  pneumonic t.
  pulmonary t.
  t. (type A, B)

typhoidal t.
ulceroglandular t.
tularensis
   Francisella t.
tumbling E chart
tumescence
   physiologic t.
tumor
adrenal t.
aniridia-Wilms t.
Askin t.
atypical teratoid t.
atypical teratoid/rhabdoid t.
autonomic nerve t.
t. blush
brain t.
Brenner t.
t. burden
central primitive neuroectodermal t.
  (cPNET)
cervical cord t.
CNS t.
craniofacial t.
desmoplastic small round cell t.
  (DSRCT)
dumbbell t.
endodermal sinus t.
epithelial liver t.
Ewing t.
extragonadal germ cell t.
extrarenal rhabdoid t.
eyelid t.
Frantz t.
gastrointestinal autonomic nerve t.
  (GANT)
germ cell testicular t.
germinal cell t.
glomus t.
granulosa cell t.
granulosa-theca cell t.
hairlike t.
hormone-secreting t.
hypothalamic t.
infratentorial t.
insulin-secreting pancreatic t.
intraocular t.
intrinsic t.
islet cell t.
juvenile granulosa cell t. (JGCT)
juxtaglomerular cell t. (JGCT)
Koenen t.
Leydig cell t.

liver t.
t. lysis syndrome
malignant brain t.
malignant epithelial t.
malignant extrarenal rhabdoid t.
malignant germ cell t.
malignant mesodermal t.
malignant nerve sheath t.
mediastinal t.
mesodermal t.
metastatic t.
midline craniofacial t.
mulberry t.
t. necrosis
t. necrosis factor (TNF)
t. necrosis factor-alpha (TNF-alpha)
nerve sheath t.
neuroectodermal t.
t., node, metastases (TNM)
non-alpha cell t.
nonhematogenous t.
optic nerve t.
optic pathway t.
orbital t.
ovarian t.
pancreatic t.
paratesticular t.
pelvic t.
periaqueductal t.
peripheral neuroectodermal t.
peripheral primitive
  neuroectodermal t. (PPNET)
Phyllodes t.
piloid t.
pineal t.
pleomorphic spindle cell t.
posterior fossa t.
Pott puffy t.
prepubertal testicular t.
primary intraocular t.
primary tracheal t.
primitive neuroectodermal t.
  (PNET)
Purkinje cell t.
rhabdoid t.
round cell t.
sarcomatous t.
t. seeding
sex cord-stromal t.
single t.
sinus t.
solid t.

NOTES

tumor *(continued)*
    t. spillage
    spinal cord t.
    spindle cell t.
    sternomastoid t.
    stromal t.
    teratoid t.
    testicular t.
    testis t.
    theca cell t.
    Toronto t. (group I–IV)
    tracheal t.
    ventricular t.
    Wilms t. (stage I–V)
    yolk sac t.
tumorigenesis
tumor/medulloblastoma
    primitive neuroectodermal t./m.
      (PNET/MB)
Tums
tungiasis
tunica albuginea
tunnel
    intracardiac t.
    lateral atrial t. (LAT)
    subcutaneous t.
    t. vision
tunneled CVL
tunnel-view radiography
turbidity
Turbinaire
    Decadron T.
    Decadron Phosphate Nasal T.
turbinate
    t. bone
    nasal t.
turboinhaler
Turbuhaler
    budesonide T.
    Pulmicort T.
    Rhinocort T.
turbulence
turbulent airflow
turcica
    sella t.
Turco posteromedial release of clubfoot
Turcot syndrome
turgor
Turner
    T. mosaic
    T. mosaicism
    T. mosaic syndrome
    T. phenotype
    T. XO syndrome
turricephaly
Tusibron
Tusibron-DM
Tuss-DM

Tussin
    Clear T. 30
    Safe T. 30
Tussi-Organidin DM NR
Tusstat Syrup
TV
    tidal volume
TWAR
    Taiwan acute respiratory
TWAR agent
T-wave
    T-w. abnormality
    T-w. axis
    T-w. inversion
Tween 80
twenty-nail dystrophy
Twice-A-Day Nasal Solution
Twilite Oral
twill tape
twin
    conjoined t.
    diovular t.
    dissimilar t.
    dizygotic t.
    enzygotic t.
    equal conjoined t.
    fraternal t.
    heterologous t.
    heteroovular t.
    identical t.
    impacted t.
    incomplete conjoined t.
    monochorionic t.
    monovular t.
    monozygotic t.
    t. reversed arterial perfusion
     (TRAP)
    t. reversed arterial perfusion
     syndrome
    Siamese t.
    symmetrical conjoined t.
    unequal conjoined t.
    unlike t.
Twin-K
twinning
    cardiac t.
twin-to-twin
    t.-t.-t. transfusion
    t.-t.-t. transfusion reaction
    t.-t.-t. transfusion syndrome
twisted
    t. hair
    t. neck
twister cable
twitch
twitching
    arrhythmic t.
TwoCal HN formula

two-point discrimination
two-stage arterial switch operation
Tx
    thromboxane
Tycos aneroid sphygmomanometer
Tylenol
    T. and Codeine Elixir
    T. Cold, Children's
    T. Extra Strength
    T. With Codeine
    T. With Codeine No. 2, 3, 4
tylosis ciliaris
Tylox
tympani
    chorda t.
    scala t.
tympanic
    t. membrane
    t. membrane compliance
    t. membrane perforation
    t. temperature
tympanites
tympanitic abdomen
tympanocentesis (TPC)
tympanogram
tympanomastoid suture line
tympanometer
    Welch-Allyn MicroTymp
     impedance t.
tympanometric
    t. gradient
    t. width
tympanometry
    impedance t.
tympanosclerosis
tympanosquamous suture line
tympanostomy tube
tympanum
tympany
Ty-Pap
type
    acrofacial dysostosis (Nager t.)
    axonal t.
    Babesia WA1 t.
    Batten-Bielschowsky t.
    blood t.
    blood t. A, AB, B, O
    clinical t.
    dominantly hyperactive impulsive t.
    Finnish t.
    t. II pneumocyte
    t. IV RTA

    Landry t.
    low-grade B-cell lymphoma of
     MALT t.
    MALT t.
    normal female sex chromosome t.
     (XX)
    normal male sex chromosome t.
     (XY)
    peroneal muscular atrophy,
     axonal t.
    Pi t.
    protease inhibitor t.
    Spielmeyer-Vogt t.
typhi
    Rickettsia t.
    Salmonella t.
typhimurium
    Salmonella t.
typhlitis
typhoid
    t. fever
    t. vaccine
typhoidal tularemia
typhus
    flying squirrel t.
    t. group
    louse-borne t.
    murine t.
    North Asian tick t.
    Queensland tick t.
    recrudescent t.
    scrub t.
    sylvatic t.
    tick-borne t.
typical
    t. absence epilepsy
    t. measles
typing
    HLA t.
    newborn platelet antigen t.
    tissue t.
Tyrode's solution
tyrosinase-negative oculocutaneous albinism
tyrosinase-positive albinism
tyrosine
    t. kinase
    t. phosphatase
tyrosinemia
    hepatorenal t.
    hereditary t.
    oculocutaneous t.

NOTES

tyrosinemia *(continued)*
    transient t.
    t. (type I)

tyrosinosis
Tzanck smear

U-500
    Regular (Concentrated) Iletin II U-
        500
    Regular Iletin II U-500
UAC
    umbilical artery catheter
UALTE
    unexplained apparent life-threatening
        event
UAO
    urine acid output
UARS
    upper airway resistance syndrome
UBT
    urea breath test
U/C
    umbilical artery pulsatility index to
        middle cerebral artery pulsatility index
        ratio
        U/C ratio
Ucephan Oral
UCL
    ulnar collateral ligament
U-Cort Topical
UDCA
    ursodeoxycholic acid
UDP
    uridine diphosphate
UDP-galactose
UE
    upper extremity
uE3
    unconjugated estriol
UEP
    urinary excretion of protein
U/F
    Fulvicin U/F
Uhthoff
    U. sign
    U. symptom
UI
    uteroplacental insufficiency
U/L
    upper body segment to lower body
        segment ratio
        U/L ratio
ulcer
    aphthous oral u.
    chancroid u.
    chiclero u.
    collar button u.
    corneal u.
    Curling u.
    Cushing u.
    decubitus u.

duodenal u.
genital aphthous u.
herpetiform aphthous u.
herpetiform corneal u.
idiopathic u.
jejunal u.
oral u.
pterygoid u.
recurrent genital aphthous u.
shallow u.
stress-associated u.
ulcerans
    Mycobacterium u.
ulceration
    aphthous u.
    corneal u.
    digital u.
    esophageal u.
    genital u.
    nasal u.
    oral u.
    penile u.
    perianastomotic u.
    shallow u.
ulcerative
    u. blepharitis
    u. colitis
ulceroglandular
    u. disease
    u. tularemia
ULE
    unilateral laterothoracic exanthem
ulcgyria
ulinastatin
Ullrich
    U. disease
    U. syndrome
Ullrich-Feichtiger syndrome
Ullrich-Turner syndrome
ulna
ulnar
    u. clubhand
    u. collateral ligament (UCL)
    u. nerve block
    u. neuropathy
    u. palmar grasp
    u. styloid fracture
    u. tilt
ULR
    guaifenesin, phenylpropanolamine,
        phenylephrine
Ulrich-Turner stigmata
ultra
    U. Dream Ride car bed
    Grisactin U.

U

Ultracef
ultrafiltrate
Ultralente
    Humulin U U.
Ultralente U
Ultrase MT
ultrasensitive assay
ultrasonogram
ultrasonography
    Doppler u.
    graded compression u.
    intravascular u.
    transabdominal u.
    transvaginal u.
ultrasonologist
ultrasound
    abdominal u.
    cranial u.
    Doppler u.
    duplex u.
    u. fetometry
    head u.
    intracoronary u.
    intravascular u. (IVUS)
    noncontact u.
    pancreatic u.
    pelvic u.
    prenatal u.
    pulsed u.
    quantitative u. (QUS)
    renal u.
    u. scanning
    Sunlight Omnisense u.
    volumetric bladder u.
Ultravate
ultraviolet (UV)
    u. A, B
    u. light
umbilical
    u. anomaly
    u. arterial EDV
    u. arterial pH
    u. artery
    u. artery catheter (UAC)
    u. artery catheterization
    u. artery pulsatility index to
      middle cerebral artery pulsatility
      index ratio (U/C)
    u. blood sampling
    u. cord
    u. cord blood transplantation
    u. Doppler flow velocity
    u. granuloma
    u. hernia
    u. polyp
    u. stump
    u. swab
    u. vein

    u. vein catheter
    u. vein catheterization
    u. vein packed red blood cell
      transfusion
    u. vein platelet transfusion
    u. venous catheter (UVC)
    u. venous flow
    u. venous line (UVL)
    u. venous plasma amino acid
    u. vessel catheter
umbilicalis
    arteritis u.
umbilication of lesion
umbilicoplasty
umbilicus reconstruction
umbrella
    Bard PDA U.
    u. device
    u. sign
Unasyn
unbalanced AV canal defect
unbound iron
uncalcified
    u. bacterial plaque
    u. bone matrix
uncal herniation
uncinate fit
uncombable hair syndrome
uncompensated
    u. hydrocephalus
    u. shock
uncomplicated
    u. hernia
    u. measles
unconjugated
    u. bilirubin
    u. estriol (uE3)
    u. estriol level
    u. hyperbilirubinemia
uncuffed endotracheal tube
undecapeptide
undecylenic
    u. acid
    u. acid ointment
underdeveloped
    u. chin
    u. mandible
underdevelopment
    face u.
    middle one-third of face u.
underdose
underfeeding
underinflation
undernourished
undernutrition
understanding stage
undervascularity
    pulmonary u.

underwater weighing
Underwood disease
undescended
    u. testicle
    u. testis
undifferentiated rhabdomyosarcoma
Undoguent Topical
undulant fever
unemancipated
unequal
    u. aeration
    u. conjoined twin
    u. visual input
unexplained
    u. apparent life-threatening event
      (UALTE)
    u. fever
ungual
unguium
    tinea u.
UNHSP
    universal newborn hearing screening
    program
Uni-Ace
Uni-Bent Cough Syrup
unicameral bone cyst
unicentric
unicommisural
unidentified bright object
Uni-Dur
unifactorial disorder
unifocal clonic movement
unilambdoid synostosis
unilateral
    u. bar
    u. congenital ptosis
    u. cryptorchidism
    u. flank mass
    u. hearing impairment
    u. hemimegalencephaly
    u. hyperlucent lung
    u. hypoplastic pectoral muscle
    u. laterothoracic exanthem (ULE)
    u. lower lip paralysis
    u. megalencephaly
    u. mydriasis
    u. neonatal hydronephrosis
    u. occipital plagiocephaly
    u. optic neuritis
    u. optokinetic nystagmus
    u. renal agenesis

    u. stapling
    u. ureteral obstruction (UUO)
unilineal category
unilocular
uninhibited bladder
union
    delayed u.
uniparental disomy (UPD)
Unipen
    U. Injection
    U. Oral
Uniphyl
Uniplant
unipolar depression
Uni-Pro
Uniserts
    Bisacodyl U.
unit
    Bethesda u.
    colony-forming u. (CFU)
    dentoalveolar u.
    immunizing u. (IU)
    intensive special care u. (ISCU)
    International U. (IU)
    Kreiselman u.
    lipase u.
    Log-a-Rhythm Signal Acquisition u.
    neonatal intensive care u. (NICU)
    newborn intensive care u. (NBICU)
    newborn special care u. (NBSCU)
    Nytone enuretic control u.
    Orthotic Research and Locomotor
      Assessment U. (ORLAU)
    pediatric intensive care u. (PICU)
    pediatric sedation u. (PSU)
    plaque-forming u. (pfu)
    Wood u.
    Wrobleski u.
unitas
    oculus u. (both eyes) (o.u., OU)
United Network for Organ Sharing
  (UNOS)
units-erythroid
    burst-forming u.-e. (BFU-E)
Uni-tussin
    U.-t. DM
univariate
univentricular
universal
    u. bilirubin screen
    u. hearing screen

U

NOTES

universal *(continued)*
  u. newborn hearing screening program (UNHSP)
  u. nose of childhood
universalis
  alopecia u.
unlike twin
unmalleable
Unna-Thost syndrome
UNOS
  United Network for Organ Sharing
unoxygenated blood
unpasteurized
  u. milk product
unpredictable
unrecognized apnea
unregulated catabolism
unresponsive
  alertness, response to voice, response to pain, u. (AVPU)
unresponsiveness
  ACTH u.
unrestrictive ventricular septal defect
unroofed coronary sinus
unroofing
  endoscopic u.
  patch u.
unsaturated
  u. linolenic acid
  u. phosphatidylcholine
unspun urine
unstable
  u. bladder of childhood
  u. bladder syndrome
unusual hunger
Unverricht disease
Unverricht-Lundborg
  U.-L. disease
  U.-L. syndrome
up
  pinked u.
upbeat nystagmus
UPD
  uniparental disomy
UPJ
  ureteropelvic junction
  UPJ obstruction
upper
  u. airway noise
  u. airway resistance syndrome (UARS)
  u. airway sleep-disordered breathing
  u. body segment
  u. body segment to lower body segment ratio (U/L)
  u. extremity (UE)
  u. gastrointestinal
  u. gastrointestinal series

  u. GI lesion
  u. humeral epiphysis
  u. limb amelia
  u. limb deficiency
  u. motor neuron disease
  u. motor neuron sign
  u. motor neuron syndrome
  u. respiratory illness
  u. respiratory infection (URI)
  u. respiratory tract
  u. respiratory tract infection (URTI)
  u. urinary tract infection
UPPP
  uvulopalatopharyngoplasty
upregulation
upright
  u. abdominal radiograph
  u. chest film
  u. tilt-table testing
upsaliensis
  Campylobacter u.
upside-down ptosis
upslanting palpebral fissure
upstairs-downstairs heart
upstroke
uptake
  bone mineral u.
upward
  u. gaze
  u. gaze weakness
Urabeth
urachus
  patent u.
  persistent u.
urate
  u. nephropathy
  u. tophi
Urbach-Wiethe disease
urea
  u. breath test (UBT)
  u. cycle
  u. cycle disease
  u. cycle disorder
  u. cycle enzyme defect
  u. nitrogen
  u. plaster
urealyticum
  Ureaplasma u.
Ureaplasma urealyticum
Urecholine
ureidopenicillin
uremia
uremic
  u. encephalopathy
  u. state
  u. syndrome

ureter
    atretic u.
    duplicated u.
    ectopic u.
    ileal u.
    partially duplicated u.
    reimplantation of u.
    retrocaval u.
ureteral
    u. duplication
    u. ectopia
    u. obstruction
    u. rupture
    u. trigonal reimplantation
    u. valve
ureterocele
    ectopic u.
    prolapsed ectopic u.
    simple u.
ureterocystoplasty
    augmentation u.
ureteroneocystostomy
ureteropelvic
    u. junction (UPJ)
    u. junction obstruction
ureteropyelostomy
ureterosigmoidostomy
ureterostomy
    cutaneous u.
ureterovesical junction obstruction
urethra
    dilated posterior u.
    fusiform dilation of u.
    posterior u.
urethral
    u. atresia
    u. duplication
    u. elongation
    u. epithelium
    u. meatus
    u. plate
    u. plate division
    u. prolapse
    u. seam
    u. syndrome
    u. valve
urethritis
    chlamydial u.
    gonococcal u.
    nongonococcal u.
urethrocutaneous fistula
uretocalycostomy

Urex
urgency
URI
    upper respiratory infection
uric
    u. acid
    u. acid infarct
    u. acid lithiasis
    u. acid nephrolithiasis
    u. acid stone
uricosuria
uridine diphosphate (UDP)
uridyltransferase
    galactose-1-phosphate u. (GALT)
urinalysis
    bagged u.
    enhanced u.
urinary
    u. bladder
    u. catheter
    u. catheterization
    u. concentrating defect
    u. copper
    u. coproporphyrin
    u. coproporphyrin I
    u. excreted melatonin
    u. excretion
    u. excretion of protein (UEP)
    u. free cortisol
    u. glycosaminoglycan
    u. iodine
    u. mucopolysaccharide pattern
    u. obstruction
    u. orotic acid
    u. potassium wasting
    u. pterin
    u. sphincter
    u. stasis
    u. tract
    u. tract dilation
    u. tract dysplasia
    u. tract infection (UTI)
urine
    u. acid output (UAO)
    Coke-colored u.
    cola-colored u.
    concentrated u.
    u. culture
    dark u.
    dilute u.
    u. dipstick
    u. ferric chloride test

U

NOTES

urine *(continued)*
>   fetal u.
>   24-hour u. collection
>   u. ketoacid
>   u. ligase chain reaction
>   malodorous u.
>   maple syrup u.
>   u. mucopolysaccharide
>   u. organic acid
>   u. output
>   persistent alkaline u.
>   u. sample
>   u. sediment
>   suprapubic aspiration of u.
>   u. toxicology screen
>   unspun u.
>   u. vanillylmandelic acid
>   vin rose-colored u.

urine-reducing substance
uriniferous breath
urinoma
Uriscreen test
Urobak
urobilinogen excretion
urobilinogenuria
urobilinoid
urocanase deficiency
urocanic
>   u. acid
>   u. aciduria

Urocit-K
urocytogram
Urodine
urodynamic testing
uroflowmetry
urofollitropin
urogenital
>   u. sinus
>   u. tract

urogenitogram
Urogesic
urogram
>   excretory u.

urography
>   intravenous u. (IVU)

urokinase
urokinase-vancomycin lock
Uro-KP-Neutral
Urolene Blue Oral
urolithiasis
urologist
Uro-Mag
uropathogen
uropathy
>   obstructive u.

Uroplus
>   U. DS
>   U. SS

ursi
>   uva u.

Urso
ursodeoxycholic acid (UDCA)
ursodiol
URTI
>   upper respiratory tract infection

urticaria
>   acquired u.
>   acute u.
>   cholinergic u.
>   chronic idiopathic u.
>   cold u.
>   cutaneous u.
>   idiopathic u.
>   papular u.
>   u. pigmentosa
>   pressure u.
>   primary acquired u.
>   secondary solar u.
>   solar u.

urticarial raised lesion
urticate
urtication
use
>   compassionate u.
>   intravaginal foreign body u.
>   intravenous drug u. (IDU)

Usher syndrome (type 1)
uteri (*pl. of* uterus)
uterine
>   u. horn
>   u. outflow obstruction
>   u. tone

utero
>   in u. (IU)
>   u. sensitization

uteroplacental insufficiency (UI)
uterque
>   oculus u. (each eye) (o.u., OU)

uterus, pl. uteri
>   bicornuate u.
>   bifid u.
>   duplicate u.
>   hypoplastic u.

UTI
>   urinary tract infection
>   febrile UTI

Uticort Topical
utriculovaginal pouch
utterance
>   mean length of u. (MLU)

UUO
>   unilateral ureteral obstruction

UV
>   ultraviolet

Uval
uva ursi

UVC
    umbilical venous catheter
uveitis
        acute anterior u.
        posterior u.
uveokeratitis
uveomeningitic disease
uveomeningoencephalitic syndrome
uveoparotid
        u. fever
        u. fever syndrome

UVL
    umbilical venous line
uvula, pl. **uvuli**
      bifid u.
uvulitis
uvulopalatopharyngoplasty (UPPP)

NOTES

U

VA
  ventriculoatrial
    VA shunt
VAA
  verbal-auditory agnosia
VACA
  valvuloplasty and angioplasty of
    congenital anomalies
vaccinal thimerosal
vaccination (*See also* vaccine)
    bacille Calmette-Guérin v.
    rotavirus v.
    varicella v.
    yellow fever 17D v.
vaccinatum
    eczema v.
vaccine
    Acel-Imune v.
    acellular pertussis v.
    ActHIB v.
    V. Adverse Events Reporting
      System (VAERS)
    aP v.
    bacille Calmette-Guérin v.
    BCG v.
    Certiva v.
    chickenpox v.
    cholera v.
    cold-adapted influenza virus v.,
      trivalent (CAIV T)
    cold-attenuated intranasal
      influenza v. (CAIV)
    Comvax v.
    conjugate pneumococcal v.
    diphtheria, tetanus, acellular
      pertussis v.
    diphtheria, tetanus, pertussis v.
    diphtheria, tetanus toxoid, acellular
      pertussis v.
    diphtheria, tetanus (toxoids),
      accelerated pertussis v.
    diphtheria, tetanus toxoids, whole-
      cell pertussis v.
    DPT v.
    DTaP v.
    DTP v.
    Edmonston-Zagreb measles v.
    Engerix-B v.
    enhanced inactivated polio v.
      (eIPV)
    five-component v.
    GBS v.
    Haemophilus influenzae type b
      conjugate v.
    Havrix v.

    HB v.
    HBV v.
    hepatitis A v. (HAV)
    hepatitis B v.
    hepatitis B oligosaccharide-
      CRM197 v. (HbOC)
    Hib conjugate v.
    Hib polysaccharide v.
    HibTITER v.
    human diploid cell v.
    human diploid cell rabies v.
      (HDCV)
    inactivated polio v.
    inactivated poliomyelitis v.
    inactivated poliovirus v. (IPV)
    inactivated virus v.
    Infanrix v.
    influenza v.
    intranasal influenza v.
    IPOL poliovirus v.
    IPV v.
    killed virus v.
    live-attenuated virus v.
    live poliovirus v.
    Lyme disease v.
    measles, mumps, rubella v.
    MenCon v.
    meningococcal conjugate v.
    meningococcal polysaccharide v.
    MenPS v.
    mercury-free v.
    MMR v.
    M-M-R II v.
    nonvalent pneumococcal
      conjugate v. (PnCV)
    Oka strain varicella v.
    OmniHIB v.
    OPV v.
    oral attenuated *Salmonella typhi* v.
    oral polio v. (OPV)
    oral poliomyelitis v.
    oral poliovirus v. (OPV)
    Orimune poliovirus v.
    PCEC v.
    PedvaxHIB v.
    pentavalent v.
    PFP v.
    PncD v.
    PNCRM7 v.
    PncT v.
    pneumococcal conjugate v.
    pneumococcal polysaccharide v.
    pneumococcal protein conjugate v.
    pneumococcal 7-valent conjugate v.
      (PCV7)

vaccine *(continued)*
    poliovirus v.
    polyribose phosphate polysaccharide v.
    Prevnar pneumococcal v.
    ProHIBiT v.
    protein-conjugated v.
    purified chick embryo cell culture v.
    purified fusion protein v.
    rabies v.
    recombinant hepatitis B v.
    Recombivax v.
    Rhesus rotavirus tetravalent v.
    rOspA Lyme disease v.
    RotaShield rotavirus v.
    rotavirus v.
    RRV-TV v.
    Rv v.
    Sabin v.
    V. Safety Datalink (VSD)
    Salk v.
    split-virus v.
    swine-flu influenza v.
    TdaP v.
    TdaP-IPV v.
    Td-IPV v.
    Td toxoid v.
    tetanus and diphtheria toxoids v.
    tetanus toxoid and diphtheria v.
    thimerosal-free v.
    TriHIBit v.
    Tri-Immunol v.
    Tripedia v.
    typhoid v.
    7-valent pneumococcal conjugate v.
    Vaqta v.
    varicella virus v.
    varicella-zoster virus v. (VZVV)
    Varivax v.
    7VPnC v.
    VZV v.
    whole-cell diphtheria-tetanus-pertussis v.
    whole-cell DTP v.
    whole-virus v.
vaccine-acquired poliovirus
vaccine-associated
    v.-a. paralytic polio (VAPP)
    v.-a. paralytic poliomyelitis (VAPP)
    v.-a. pneumonia
vaccine-autism scare
vaccinia
    v. virus
    v. of vulva
vacciniforme
    hydroa v.
Vaccinium macrocarpon

VACTERL
    vertebral, anal, cardiac, tracheal, esophageal, renal, limb VACTERL syndrome
vacuo
    hydrocephalus ex v.
vacuolar myelopathy
vacuolation
vacuole
Vacutainer
    EDTA-anticoagulated V.
vacuum extraction
VAD
    vitamin A deficiency
VAERS
    Vaccine Adverse Events Reporting System
vagabond skin
vagal
    v. activity
    v. inhibition
    v. nerve stimulation
    v. tone
vagally mediated response
vagina
    atretic v.
    blind v.
    blind-ending v.
    distal v.
    duplicated v.
    exstrophic v.
    imperforate v.
    neutral pH of v.
    prepubescent v.
    rudimentary v.
    septate v.
    short v.
vaginal
    v. atresia
    v. candidosis
    v. discharge
    v. disinfection
    Gyne-Lotrimin V.
    v. introitus
    Monistat V.
    v. mucosa
    Mycelex-G V.
    v. plate
    v. pool
    v. sarcoma
    v. septum
    v. smear
    v. switch operation
    v. window
vaginalis
    Gardnerella v.
    obliterated processus v.
    persistent processus v.

processus v.
Trichomonas v.
vaginitis
nonspecific v.
Shigella v.
trichomonal v.
vaginography
vaginoplasty
vaginoscopy
vaginosis
bacterial v.
vagotomy
vagotonic
v. bradycardia
v. maneuver
vagus nerve
valacyclovir
7-valent
7-v. pneumococcal conjugate (7VPnC)
7-v. pneumococcal conjugate vaccine
valerate
hydrocortisone v.
Valergen
valerian
valga
coxa v.
valgum
genu v.
physiologic genu v.
valgus
forefoot v.
hallux v.
heel v.
hindfoot v.
obligatory heel v.
v. osteotomy
rearfoot v.
VALI
ventilatory-associated lung injury
validation
validity
valine
Valisone Topical
Valium
V. Injection
V. Oral
vallecula
Valley fever
valproate
valproic acid

Valsalva
V. maneuver
sinus of V.
V. sinus
Valtrex
value
Cronbach v.'s
EEG power v.
K v.'s
Tanner-Whitehouse bone age reference v.
valve
v. ablation
aortic v.
atrioventricular v.
Beall v.
bicuspid aortic v.
bleed-back v.
Delta V.
double-orifice mitral v.
Heimlich v.
Heyer-Schulte v.
Holter v.
Jatene v.
mitral v.
neoaortic v.
v. obstruction
one-way v.
parachute mitral v.
pop-off v.
porcine v.
posterior ureteral v.
posterior urethral v.
v. prolapse
pulmonary porcine v.
pulmonic v.
Ross pulmonary porcine v.
straddling atrioventricular v.
transurethral ablation of v.
tricuspid v.
trileaflet aortic v.
v.'s, unilateral reflux, dysplasia (VURD)
v.'s, unilateral reflux, dysplasia syndrome
ureteral v.
urethral v.
3-way Rudolph v.
valvectomy
valvotomy
aortic v.
balloon v.

V

NOTES

valvular
 v. insufficiency
 v. pulmonic stenosis
valvulitis
 murmur of v.
valvuloplasty
 v. and angioplasty of congenital
  anomalies (VACA)
 balloon pulmonary v.
 transcarotid balloon v.
Vamate Oral
Vaminolact
VAMP
 vincristine, actinomycin-D, methotrexate,
 prednisone
  VAMP chemotherapy
van
 v. Buchem syndrome
 v. den Bergh reaction
 v. der Hoeve syndrome
 v. der Woude syndrome
 V. Gehuchten lesion
 v. Ness procedure
vanadate
Vancenase
 V. AQ
 V. AQ Inhaler
 V. Nasal Inhaler
Vanceril
 V. Double Strength
 V. Oral Inhaler
Vancocin
 V. Injection
 V. Oral
Vancoled Injection
vancomycin
 v. hydrochloride
 v. intermediate resistant
  Staphylococcus aureus
vancomycin-resistant enterococcus (VRE)
Vanicream
vanillylmandelic acid (VMA)
vanished testes syndrome
vanishing
 v. bile duct
 v. testicle syndrome
Vanoxide
Vantin
VAP
 ventilator-associated pneumonia
vapocoolant
Vaponefrin
vaporizer
 cool-mist v.
 water v.
Vaporole
 Amyl Nitrate V.
vapor poisoning

VAPP
 vaccine-associated paralytic polio
 vaccine-associated paralytic poliomyelitis
Vaqta vaccine
vara
 adolescent tibia v.
 coxa v.
 idiopathic tibia v.
 infantile tibia v.
 juvenile tibia v.
 tibia v.
variabilis
 Dermacentor v.
 erythrokeratoderma v.
variability
 beat-to-beat v.
 heart rate v. (HRV)
 interobserver v.
variable deceleration
variance
Varian Spectra AA40
variant
 hyperammonemia v.
 hyperinsulinism with
  hyperammonemia v.
 Landau-Kleffner syndrome v.
 migraine v.
 Miller-Fisher v.
 papillary v.
 petit mal v.
varicella
 breakthrough v.
 v. bullosa
 bullous v.
 disseminated v.
 v. encephalitis
 v. gangrenosa
 v. immunization
 neonatal v.
 v. pneumonitis
 pustular v.
 v. pustulosa
 v. syndrome
 v. vaccination
 v. virus vaccine
varicella-zoster
 v.-z. encephalomyelitis
 v.-z. immune globulin (VZIG)
 v.-z. immunoglobulin (VZIG)
 v.-z. virus (VZV)
 v.-z. virus vaccine (VZVV)
varicelliform
varices (*pl. of* varix)
varicocele
varicocelectomy
variegata
 porphyria v.
variegate porphyria (VP)

varimax rotation
variola virus
varioliform
Varivax vaccine
varix, pl. varices
    endoscopic elastic band ligation
      of v.
    esophageal v. (EV)
varum
    developmental genu v.
    genu v.
    physiologic genu v.
    pseudo-genu v.
varus
    v. clubfoot
    congenital metatarsus v.
    cubitus v.
    dynamic pes v.
    forefoot v.
    metatarsus primus v.
    v. osteotomy
    rearfoot v.
VAS
    visual analog scale
vasa
    v. nervorum
    v. vasorum
vascular
    v. bed
    v. cell adhesion molecule (VCAM)
    v. clip applier
    v. congestion
    v. disease
    v. endothelial growth factor
      (VEGF)
    v. endothelium
    v. headache
    v. malformation
    v. myelopathy
    v. neoplasm
    v. nevus
    v. permeability
    v. permeability factor
    v. proliferative lesion
    v. resistance
    v. ring
    v. ring syndrome
    v. spider
    v. tone
vascularis
    strae v.
vascularized appendix

vasculature flow pattern
vasculitic
    v. erythema
    v. skin lesion
vasculitis
    asthma with v.
    Churg-Strauss v.
    cutaneous v.
    dermal v.
    disseminated granulomatous v.
    epididymal vessel v.
    fetal v.
    granulomatous v.
    gut v.
    hypersensitivity v.
    immune complex v.
    immune complex-mediated v.
    leukocytoclastic v.
    lymphocytic v.
    necrotizing granulomatous v.
    occlusive v.
    ovarian v.
    renal v.
    retinal v.
    v. syndrome
vasculogenesis
vasculopathy
    noncalcific v.
    proliferative v.
vas deferens
Vaseline-impregnated gauze
VasoClear Ophthalmic
Vasocon-A
Vasocon Regular Ophthalmic
vasoconstriction
    hypoxic v.
vasoconstrictor
vasodilation
    pulmonary v.
vasodilator cream
vasoepididymostomy
vasogenic edema
vasomotor rhinitis
vasoocclusion
vasoocclusive
    v. crisis
    v. episode
vasopathy
    calcifying v.
vasopressin
    v. analog
    arginine v. (AVP)

NOTES

V

vasopressin *(continued)*
  1-desamino-8-D-arginine v.
    (DDAVP)
vasopressor syncope
vasoregulation
vasorum
  vasa v.
vasospasm
  cerebral v.
  transient v.
Vasotec
  V. I.V.
  V. Oral
vasovagal
  v. faint
  v. syncope
vastus
  v. lateralis
  v. lateralis muscle
  v. medialis
VATER
  vertebral defects, anal atresia,
    tracheoesophageal fistula with
    esophageal atresia, radial and renal
    anomalies
  vertebral (defects), (imperforate) anus,
    tracheoesophageal (fistula), radial and
    renal (dysplasia)
    VATER syndrome
Vater
  ampulla of V.
  papilla of V.
VATS
  video-assisted thoracic surgery
  video-assisted thoracoscopic surgery
vault
  rectal v.
vaulting
VBM
  vertebral bone mass
vBMD
  volumetric bone mineral density
VC
  vital capacity
  Phenergan VC
VCA
  viral capsid antigen
VCAM
  vascular cell adhesion molecule
VCD
  vocal cord dysfunction
VCFS
  velocardiofacial syndrome
V-Cillin K
V code rational problems
VCUG
  voiding cystourethrogram

voiding cystourethrograph
voiding cystourethrography
VDRL
  Venereal Disease Research Laboratory
    CSF VDRL
vecuronium bromide
VEE
  Venezuelan equine encephalitis
Veetids
vegan
vegetable oil fat-based formula
vegetans
  pyoderma v.
vegetarian
vegetarianism
vegetation
  nonbacterial thrombotic v. (NBTV)
vegetative symptom
VEGF
  vascular endothelial growth factor
vehicle
  all-terrain v. (ATV)
Veillonella
  V. atypica
  V. dispar
  V. parvula
vein
  anomalous pulmonary v.
  antecubital v.
  axillary v.
  bridging v.
  cardinal v.
  cephalic v.
  dilated v.
  v. flap
  v. of Galen
  v. of Galen aneurysm
  v. of Galen malformation
  greater saphenous v.
  inferior mesenteric v.
  innominate v.
  internal jugular v.
  jugular v.
  left renal v.
  left vertical v.
  main renal v.
  mesenteric v.
  obliterated v.
  v. obstruction
  pulmonary v.
  renal v.
  saphenous v.
  splenic v.
  superior mesenteric v.
  umbilical v.
velamentous
  v. insertion
  v. placenta

Velban
vellus
    v. hair
    v. hypertrichosis
velocardiofacial syndrome (VCFS)
velocimetry
    Doppler v.
    fetal arterial v.
velocity, pl. velocities
    bone quantitative ultrasound v.
    cerebral blood flow v. (CBFV)
    end-diastolic v. (EDV)
    growth v. (GV)
    head growth v.
    height v. (HV)
    linear growth v.
    nerve conduction v. (NCV)
    peak growth v.
    sensory nerve conduction v.
    subnormal growth v.
    umbilical Doppler flow v.
velopharyngeal incompetence (VPI)
Velosef
Velosulin Human
Velpeau bandage
Velsar
Veltane Tablet
velum
vena cava
venenata
    dermatitis v.
venereal
    V. Disease Research Laboratory
      (VDRL)
    v. wart
venereum
    lymphogranuloma v. (LGV)
Venezuelan equine encephalitis (VEE)
Venilon human immunoglobulin
venipuncture
    external jugular v.
    v. site
venlafaxine hydrochloride
venodilation
Venoglobulin
Venoglobulin-I
Venoglobulin-S
venogram
venography
    contrast v.
    hepatic wedged v.

venom
    Hymenoptera v.
venoocclusive disease (VOD)
venosus
    ductus v.
    patent ductus v.
    sinus v.
venous
    v. angioma
    v. bleb
    v. blood sampling
    v. catheter
    v. engorgement
    v. flow
    v. hum
    v. lake
    v. line
    v. malformation (VM)
    v. obstruction
    v. occlusion plethysmography
    v. pH
    v. pooling
    v. pressure
    v. radical
    v. return
    v. sinus thrombophlebitis
    v. sinus thrombosis
    v. switch
    v. thromboembolism
venovenous (VV)
    v. ECMO
ventilation
    alveolar v.
    assisted v. (AV)
    bag-valve-mask v.
    endotracheal intubation and
      mechanical v. (EI/MV)
    high-frequency v. (HFV)
    high-frequency jet v. (HFJV)
    high-frequency oscillatory v.
      (HFOV)
    high-frequency positive-pressure v.
      (HFPPV)
    intermittent mandatory v. (IMV)
    intermittent mechanical v.
    intermittent positive-pressure v.
      (IPPV)
    intratracheal pulmonary v. (ITPV)
    inverse ratio v. (IRV)
    jet v.
    liquid v. (LV)

NOTES

V

ventilation *(continued)*
    liquid-assisted high-frequency
      oscillatory v. (LA-HFOV)
    mask and bag v.
    mechanical v.
    noninvasive motion v. (NIMV)
    oscillatory v.
    partial liquid v. (PLV)
    patient-triggered v.
    v. perfusion
    positive-pressure v. (PPV)
    pulmonary v.
    synchronized intermittent
      mandatory v. (SIMV)
    synchronized nasal intermittent
      positive-pressure v. (SNIPPV)
    tidal liquid v. (TLV)
    total liquid v. (TLV)
    transtracheal v.
    v. tube
    volume-controlled v.
ventilation-perfusion (V/Q)
    v. imbalance
    v. mismatch
    v. scan
ventilator
    Bennett PR-2 v.
    Bourns infant v.
    extrathoracic v.
    high-frequency v.
    high-oscillation v.
    Infant Star v.
    jet v.
    Newport Wave v.
    noninvasive extrathoracic v. (NEV)
    Porta-Lung noninvasive
      extrathoracic v.
    Pulmo-Aide v.
    Servo 900C v.
    Siemens Servo 300, 900C v.
    SLE 2000 v.
    Vix infant v.
    Wave v.
ventilator-associated pneumonia (VAP)
ventilator-induced lung injury (VILI)
ventilatory
    v. drive
    v. failure
    v. support
ventilatory-associated lung injury (VALI)
Ventolin
    V. Nebules
    V. Rotacaps
ventral
    v. mesentery
    v. pancreatic anlage
    v. suspension

ventricle
    v.'s to atrium
    common-inlet single right v.
    double-inlet left v.
    double-inlet right v.
    double-outlet v.
    double-outlet right v. (DORV)
    hyperdynamic v.
    hypoplastic left v.
    left v. (LV)
    v.'s to peritoneal cavity (VP)
    right v. (RV)
    single v.
ventricular
    v. afterload
    v. aneurysm
    v. assist device
    v. bypass
    v. catheter
    v. dysplasia
    v. dysrhythmia
    v. filling
    v. fluid
    v. hypertrophy
    v. inversion
    left v. (LV)
    v. outflow obstruction
    v. outflow tract reconstruction
    v. peritoneal (VP)
    v. preload
    v. premature contraction (VPC)
    v. premature depolarization
    v. puncture
    v. septal defect (VSD)
    v. septal defect patch closure
    v. septation
    v. septum
    v. shunt
    v. shunt procedure
    v. tachycardia
    v. tap
    v. tumor
ventriculitis
    gram-negative v.
ventriculoarterial
ventriculoatrial (VA)
    v. shunt
ventriculocisternostomy
ventriculoexternal shunt
ventriculography
    low-dose dobutamine stress
      radionuclide v.
    selective right v.
ventriculojugular shunt
ventriculomegaly
    cerebral v.

nonprogressive v.
posthemorrhagic v. (PHVM)
ventriculoperitoneal (VP)
occult trauma, postanoxia, v.
(OPV)
occult trauma, postictal v.
v. shunt (VPS)
v. shunting
ventriculopleural shunt
ventriculovascular shunt
ventrogluteal
venule
VEOS
very early onset schizophrenia
VEP
visual evoked potential
VEP acuity
flash VEP
VePesid
VER
visual evoked response
vera
polycythemia v.
verapamil
Verazinc
verbal
v. abuse
v. fluency
v. sequencing
verbal-auditory agnosia (VAA)
verbalize
verbally assaultive
Verelan
vergae
cavum v.
verge
anal v.
Vergogel Gel
Vergon
vermicularis
Enterobius v.
vermiform appendix
vermilion border of lip
vermis
agenesis of cerebellar v.
cerebellar v.
v. cerebelli
hypoplasia of v.
v. hypoplasia
hypoplastic superior cerebellar v.
partial agenesis of v.
selective aplasia of v.

Vermizine
Vermont-Oxford Neonatal Database
Vermox
vernal conjunctivitis
vernix caseosa
vero cytotoxin
verotoxin
verruca, pl. **verrucae**
mosaic v.
v. peruana
v. plana
v. plana juvenilis
v. plantaris
v. sock
v. vulgaris
verruciformis
epidermodysplasia v.
verrucous
v. endocarditis
v. papule
v. plaque
v. streaky epidermal nevus
Versed syrup
Versenate
Calcium Disodium V.
Versiclear
versicolor
pityriasis v.
tinea v.
version
California Verbal Learning Test-
Children's V.
Schedule for Affective Disorders
and Schizophrenia for School-Age
Children-Epidemiologic V. (K-
SADS-E)
tibial v.
versive seizure
vertebra, pl. **vertebrae**
apical v.
biconcave v.
block v.
butterfly v.
codfish v.
fishmouth v.
Goldenhar oculoauricular v.
v. plana
wedge v.
vertebral
v., anal, cardiac, tracheal,
esophageal, renal, limb
(VACTERL)

NOTES

V

629

vertebral *(continued)*
    v. arch defect
    v. artery compression
    v. body
    v. bone mass (VBM)
    v. column
    v. column defect
    v. defects, anal atresia, tracheoesophageal fistula with esophageal atresia, radial and renal anomalies (VATER)
    v. (defects), (imperforate) anus, tracheoesophageal (fistula), radial and renal (dysplasia) (VATER)
    v. laminar arch
    v. microfracture
    v. osteomyelitis
vertex presentation
vertical
    v. gaze palsy
    v. nystagmus
    v. striation
    v. talus
    v. transmission
vertically infected
verticillata
    cornea v.
vertiginous
    v. condition
    v. external anal sphincter
    v. seizure
    v. symptom
vertigo
    benign paroxysmal v. (BPV)
    epidemic v.
    Ménière v.
    paroxysmal v.
    true v.
Verukan Solution
verumontanum
very
    v. cold water near drowning
    v. early onset schizophrenia (VEOS)
    v. long chain acyl-CoA dehydrogenase (VLCAD)
    v. long chain fatty acid (VLCFA)
    v. low birth weight (VLBW)
    v. low birth weight child
    v. low birth weight infant
    v. low density lipoprotein (VLDL)
vesicle
    football-shaped v.
    skin v.
    tear-drop v.
vesicoamniotic shunt
vesicobullous
    v. disorder

    v. eruption
    v. skin lesion
vesicocutaneous fistula
vesicopustular lesion
vesicostomy
    cutaneous v.
vesicotomy
vesicoureteral reflux (grade I–V) (VUR)
vesicular
    v. breath sound
    v. exanthem
    v. palmar lesion
    v. skin lesion
    v. stomatitis virus (VSV)
vesiculation
    intraepidermal v.
vesiculopapular eruption
vesiculopustule
vesiculoulcerative
    v. lesion
    v. stomatitis
vessel
    afferent v.
    blood v.
    brachiocephalic v.
    complete transposition of great v.'s
    corkscrew conjunctival blood v.
    ghost v.
    great v.
    iris v.
    v. obliteration
    v. ostium
    palliation of great v.'s
    transposition of great v.'s (TGV)
vest
    E-Z-On V.
vestibular
    v. apparatus
    v. board
    v. damage
    v. fistula
    v. input
    v. nerve
    v. neuronitis
    v. nystagmus
    v. seizure
    v. stimulation
vestibulocochlear nerve
vestibulogenic
    v. epilepsy
    v. seizure
VFSS
    videofluoroscopic swallowing study
viable
Viard hypertrophy
Vibracare
Vibramycin
Vibra-Tabs

vibration sense
vibratory murmur
Vibrazole
Vibrio
    V. cholerae
    V. parahaemolyticus
    V. vulnificus
vibriocidal antibody
vibrotactile hearing aid
vicarious menstruation
Vicks
    V. Children's Chloraseptic
    V. Children's Nyquil Nighttime
      Cough/Cold
    V. Chloraseptic Sore Throat
    V. Formula 44
    V. Formula 44D
    V. Formula 44 Pediatric Formula
    V. Pediatric Formula 44E
    V. Sinex Nasal Solution
Vicodin ES, HP
Victa Ludorum by proxy
victimization
vidarabine
video
    v. camera
    v. electroencephalography
    v. game epilepsy
    v. monitoring
video-assisted
    v.-a. thoracic surgery (VATS)
    v.-a. thoracoscopic surgery (VATS)
videofluoroscopic swallowing study
  (VFSS)
videofluoroscopy
    modified barium swallow with v.
videoradiography
videosomnography
videourodynamic study
Videx Oral
vietnamiensis
    Burkholderia v.
view
    anteroposterior v.
    apical four-chamber v.
    calcaneal v.
    Caldwell v.
    comparison v.
    field of v.
    four-chamber v.
    frogleg v.
    Harris v.

    jughandle v.
    lateral v.
    long-axis v.
    Merchant v.
    mortise v.
    Neer v.
    oblique v.
    occipitomental v.
    open-mouth v.
    Panorex v.
    parasternal short-axis v.
    short-axis v.
    subcostal v.
    submentovertex v.
    sunrise v.
    suprasternal v.
    Waters v.
vigabatrin
vigilance
    generalized v.
vigorous infant
VILI
    ventilator-induced lung injury
villi (*pl. of* villus)
villonodular synovitis
villous
    v. atrophy
    v. atrophy of jejunum
    v. chorion
    v. edema
villus, pl. **villi**
    anchoring v.
    arachnoid v.
    flattened v.
vimentin
Vimule cap
vinblastine
Vincasar PFS
Vincent
    V. angina
    V. gingivitis
    V. infection
    V. stomatitis
vincristine
    v., actinomycin-D, methotrexate,
      prednisone (VAMP)
    v. and dexamethasone
Vineland
    V. Adaptive Behavior Scale
    V. Adaptive Behavior Scales,
      Survey Form

NOTES

V

Vineland *(continued)*
   V. Social Maturity Scale
   V. standard scores
vin rose-colored urine
vinyl chloride
Vioform hydrocortisone
Viokase
violaceous
   v. eruption
   v. erythema
   v. hue
   v. lesion
   v. polygonal papule
violence
   domestic v.
violent rage
violet
   gentian v.
viomycin
Vira-A
Viracept
viral
   v. arthritis
   v. capsid antigen (VCA)
   v. cerebellitis
   v. conjunctivitis
   v. culturing
   v. DNA polymerase
   v. encephalitis
   v. enteritis
   v. esophagitis
   v. exanthem
   v. hepatitis
   v. laryngitis
   v. laryngotracheobronchitis
   v. load
   v. meningitis
   v. meningoencephalitis
   v. myocarditis
   v. necrotizing bronchiolitis
   v. p24 antigen
   v. pharyngitis
   v. pneumonia
   v. prodrome
   v. shedding
   v. syndrome
   v. thymidine kinase
   v. upper respiratory tract infection
Viramune
Virazole
Virchow-Robin space
viremia
   plasma v.
   secondary v.
viremic phase
viridans
   v. enterococcus

Streptococcus v.
   v. streptococcus
virilization
   external v.
   strong v.
virion
virologic assay
virology
Viroptic Ophthalmic
virtual bronchoscopy
virulence
virulent
viruria
virus
   antibody to hepatitis A v. (anti-HAV)
   antirespiratory syncytial v. (anti-RSV)
   arthropod-borne v.
   Borna disease v.
   chickenpox v.
   chikungunya v.
   Congo v.
   cultivable v.
   dengue v.
   Dobrava v.
   ECHO 11 v.
   enteric cytopathogenic human orphan v.
   Epstein-Barr v. (EBV)
   fecal shedding of v.
   Hantaan v.
   hepatitis A v. (HAV)
   hepatitis B v. (HBV)
   hepatitis C v. (HCV, HVC)
   hepatitis D v. (HDV)
   hepatitis E v. (HEV)
   hepatitis F v. (HFV)
   hepatitis G v. (HGV)
   hepatotropic v.
   herpes v.
   herpes simplex v. (HSV)
   herpes simplex v. 1 (HSV1, HSV-1)
   herpes simplex v. 2 (HSV2, HSV-2)
   human immunodeficiency v. (HIV)
   human immunodeficiency v.-1 (HIV-1)
   human T-cell lymphotropic v. type I (HTLV-I)
   human T-cell lymphotropic v. type II (HTLV-II)
   human T-lymphotropic v. (type I, II)
   icosahedral triple-shelled v.
   influenza A v.
   Inoue-Melnick v.

Japanese B encephalitis v.
JC v.
Junin v.
La Crosse v.
Lassa v.
live-attenuated v.
lymphocytic choriomeningitis v. (LCMV)
Machupo v.
Marburg v.
Mayaro v.
measles v.
monkey polyoma v.
Montgomery County v.
murine leukemia v.
neonatal herpes simplex v.
non-A, non-B hepatotropic v.
Norwalk v.
Ockelbo v.
Omsk v.
o'nyong-nyong v.
parainfluenza v. (PIV)
parainfluenza v. type 1 (PF1)
parainfluenza v. type 2 (PF2)
parainfluenza v. type 3 (PF3)
parainfluenza v. type 4 (PF4)
Pogosta v.
recurrent Japanese encephalitis v.
respiratory syncytial v. (RSV)
Ross River v.
rubella v.
Sapporo v.
simian B v.
simplex v.
Sindbis v.
SinNombre v.
Snow Mountain v.
syphilis, toxoplasmosis, other agents, rubella, cytomegalovirus, herpes simplex v. (STORCH)
Theiler murine encephalomyelitis v.
tissue culture-grown attenuated v.
v. titer
toxoplasmosis, other agents, rubella, cytomegalovirus, herpes simplex v. (TORCH)
transfusion transmitted v.
TT v. (TTV)
vaccinia v.
varicella-zoster v. (VZV)
variola v.
vesicular stomatitis v. (VSV)

West Nile v.
wild v.
wild-type measles v.
virus-1
virus-induced epithelial damage
virus-neutralizing antibody (VNA)
viscera (*pl. of* viscus)
visceral
  v. abscess
  v. heterotaxy
  v. larva migrans
  v. leishmaniasis
  v. myopathy
  v. pain
  v. pericardiectomy
  v. protein status
  v. situs
  v. tuberculosis
visceroatrial
  v. situs
  v. situs inversus
visceromegaly
  v. syndrome
viscerosensory aura
viscid
viscosity
viscosus
  Actinomyces v.
viscous fluid
viscus, pl. **viscera**
  herniated viscera
  hollow viscera
  perforated v.
  in utero reduction of herniated viscera
visible peristalsis
Visine L.R. Ophthalmic
vision
  20/20 v.
  binocular v.
  blurred v.
  color v.
  cortical v.
  distance v.
  field of v.
  impaired v.
  low v.
  near v.
  peripheral v.
  residual v.
  v. therapist

V

NOTES

vision *(continued)*
    v. therapy
    tunnel v.
visna
Vistacon-50 Injection
Vistaquel Injection
Vistaril
    V. Injection
    V. Oral
Vistazine Injection
Vistide
visual
    v. acuity
    v. analog scale (VAS)
    v. aura
    v. cortex
    v. evoked potential (VEP)
    v. evoked response (VER)
    v. field
    v. field defect
    v. hallucination
    v. learner
    v. loss
    v. magnocellular system
    v. pathway
    v. phobic hallucination
    v. reflex epilepsy
    v. regard
    v. reinforcement audiometry (VRA)
    v. response audiometry (VRA)
    v. sequential memory
    v. spatial memory
    v. tracking
    v. tracking of red ring
    v. training exercise
visualization
    indirect v.
visual-motor
    v.-m. coordination
    v.-m. integration (VMI)
    v.-m. integration test
visual-perceptual test
visuomotor integration
visuoperceptual/simultaneous information processing
visuospatial
visuscope
Vita-C
Vitacarn
VitaGuard
    V. 1000 event recorder
    V. monitor
vital
    v. capacity (VC)
    V. HN formula
    v. signs
vitamin
    v. A

    v. A deficiency (VAD)
    v. A, D intoxication
    v. B_6
    v. B_{12}
    v. B_{12} absorption
    v. B_{12} deficiency
    v. B_6 dependence syndrome
    v. B_{12} level
    v. C deficiency
    V. C Drops
    v. D
    v. D deficiency
    v. D dependence
    v. D-dependent rickets
    v. D-resistant rickets
    v. E
    v. E deficiency
    v. K
    v. K deficiency
Vitaneed formula
Vita-Plus E
Vitec Topical
Vite E Creme
vitelline duct
vitiligo
    dermal v.
vitrectomy
vitreoretinopathy
    familial exudative v. (FEV)
vitreous
    v. band
    v. body
    v. chamber
    v. humor
    persistent hyperplastic primary v. (PHPV)
    v. seed
    v. seeding
vitro
    in v.
viuiria
vivax
    Plasmodium v.
Vivelle Transdermal
vivo
    in v.
Vivonex
    V. Pediatric
    V. Pediatric formula
    V. Plus formula
    V. Ten formula
Vix infant ventilator
VK
    Ledercillin VK
    Robicillin VK
V-Lax

VLBW
    very low birth weight
       VLBW infant
VLCAD
    very long chain acyl-CoA dehydrogenase
VLCFA
    very long chain fatty acid
VLDL
    very low density lipoprotein
VM
    venous malformation
VM-26
    teniposide
VMA
    vanillylmandelic acid
VMI
    visual-motor integration
VNA
    virus-neutralizing antibody
Vo_2
    oxygen consumption per minute
vocabulary
    Peabody Picture V.
    v. test
vocal
    v. cord
    v. cord dysfunction (VCD)
    v. cord paralysis
    v. fremitus
    v. nodule
    v. play
    v. tic
vocalization
    irregular stereotyped v.
vocalize
VOD
    venooclusive disease
Vogt
    V. cephalodactyly
    V. syndrome
Vogt-Koyanagi-Harada syndrome
Vogt-Koyanagi syndrome
Vogt-Spielmeyer disease
Vohwinkel syndrome
voice
    v. disorder
    high-pitched v.
    hoarse v.
    hot potato v.
    v. inflection
    nasal v.

    v. synthesizer
    too-soft v.
voiceless cry
voiceprint
void
    flow v.
voiding
    v. cystography
    v. cystourethrogram (VCUG)
    v. cystourethrograph (VCUG)
    v. cystourethrography (VCUG)
    v. dysfunction
    dysfunctional v.
    staccato v.
volar
    v. angulation
    v. ganglion
    v. hyperhidrosis
    v. splint
volitional movement
Volkmann
    V. deformity
    V. disease
    V. ischemic contracture
Volmax
Volpe method
voltage
Voltaren
    V. Ophthalmic
    V. Oral
Voltaren-XR Oral
volume
    blood v.
    cerebral blood v. (CBV)
    closing v. (CV)
    constant tidal v.
    v. contraction
    end-diastolic v. (EDV)
    end-expiratory lung v. (EELV)
    end-systolic v. (ESV)
    v. expander
    expiratory flow v.
    expiratory reserve v. (ERV)
    extracellular v. (ECV)
    forced expiratory v. (FEV)
    gastric residual v. (GRV)
    inspiratory reserve v. (IRV)
    intracranial v.
    intravascular v.
    v. load
    mean corpuscular v. (MCV)
    mean platelet v. (MPV)

NOTES

volume *(continued)*
    neonatal blood v.
    v. percent of cream in milk (CRCT)
    relaxation v.
    v. replacement
    residual v. (RV)
    testicular v.
    thoracic gas v. (TGV)
    tidal v. (TV, VT)
volume-controlled ventilation
volumetric
    v. bladder ultrasound
    v. bone mineral density (vBMD)
voluntary
    v. coughing
    v. urinary sphincter
volutrauma
volvulus
    gastric v.
    intestinal v.
    malrotation with midgut v.
    mesenteroaxial v.
    midgut v.
    neonatal v.
    v. neonatorum
    Onchocerca v.
    organoaxial v.
vomer
vomerian groove
vomiting
    bilious v.
    cyclic v.
    nonbilious v.
    pernicious v.
    projectile v.
    self-induced v.
vomitus
    bilious v.
von
    v. Gierke glycogen storage disease
    v. Graefe sign
    v. Hippel-Lindau disease
    v. Hippel-Lindau syndrome
    v. Meyenburg complex
    v. Recklinghausen disease
    v. Willebrand disease
    v. Willebrand factor (vWF)
    v. Willebrand factor antigen
    v. Willebrand panel
vowel sound
voyeurism
VP
    variegate porphyria
    ventricles to peritoneal cavity
    ventricular peritoneal
    ventriculoperitoneal

    VP shunt
    VP shunt tap
VP-16
    etoposide
VPC
    ventricular premature contraction
VPI
    velopharyngeal incompetence
7VPnC
    7-valent pneumococcal conjugate
        7VPnC vaccine
VPS
    ventriculoperitoneal shunt
V/Q
    ventilation-perfusion
        V/Q matching
        V/Q mismatch
VR
    Prostin VR
VRA
    visual reinforcement audiometry
    visual response audiometry
VRE
    vancomycin-resistant enterococcus
VSD
    Vaccine Safety Datalink
    ventricular septal defect
        perimembranous VSD
VSV
    vesicular stomatitis virus
VT
    tidal volume
vu
    déjà vu
    jamais vu
vue
vulgaris
    acne v.
    ichthyosis v.
    lupus v.
    neonatal pemphigus v.
    pemphigus v.
    psoriasis v.
    verruca v.
vulnerable child syndrome
vulnificus
    Vibrio v.
Vulpe Assessment Battery
vulva
    vaccinia of v.
vulvar
    v. condyloma
    v. congenital dysplastic angiopathy
    v. hidradenitis suppurativa
    v. hypopigmentation
    v. intercourse
    v. psoriasis
    v. wart

vulvitis
vulvovaginal
    v. candidiasis
    v. pouch
    v. pouch of Williams
vulvovaginitis
    contact v.
    irritative v.
    nonspecific v.
Vumon
VUR
    vesicoureteral reflux (grade I–V)
VURD
    valves, unilateral reflux, dysplasia
      VURD syndrome

VV
    venovenous
vWF
    von Willebrand factor
VX-478
    amprenavir
VZIG
    varicella-zoster immune globulin
    varicella-zoster immunoglobulin
VZV
    varicella-zoster virus
      VZV vaccine
VZV-specific IgM antibody
VZVV
    varicella-zoster virus vaccine

NOTES

V

W

W position of legs
W sign
W sitting position
Waardenburg-Klein syndrome
Waardenburg syndrome
Wada test
waddling gait
WADIC

Wing Autistic Disorder Interview
Checklist
wafer

Fiberall W.
WAGR

Wilms tumor, aniridia, genitourinary
malformations, mental retardation
WAGR syndrome
WAI

Weinberger Adjustment Inventory
waineri
waist

narrow mediastinal w.
waist-hip ratio (WHR)
waiter tip posture
waitlist control
Waldenström disease
Waldeyer ring
Wald test
walk

bear w.
walker

Maddacrawler w.
ORLAU swivel w.
swivel w.
Walker-Warburg syndrome
walking

idiopathic toe w. (ITW)
w. reflex
sideways w.
tandem w.
toe w.
wall

anterior thoracic w.
w. suction
wallaby

W. Phototherapy System
w. pouch
wallerian degeneration
walleye
walnut-shaped bladder
wandering atrial pacemaker
Warburg syndrome
ward

short-stay w. (SSW)
warfarin embryopathy

warm

w. antibody
w. shock
w. water near drowning
warmer

Ohio w.
radiant w.
warming stand
Warren shunt
wart

anogenital w.
brain w.
common w.
exophytic w.
filiform w.
flat w.
genital w.
laryngeal w.
mucous membrane w.
periungual w.
plantar w.
venereal w.
vulvar w.
Wartenberg sign
Warthin-Starry

W.-S. silver stain
W.-S. tissue Gram stain
warty dyskeratoma
WAS

Wiskott-Aldrich syndrome
wash

Benzac AC W.
Benzac W W.
Desquam-X W.
Dryox W.
gastric w.
hexachlorophene w.
nasal w.
nasopharyngeal w.
Oxy 10 W.
RSV nasal w.
Sastid Plain Therapeutic Shampoo
and Acne W.
Theroxide W.
washing

first-morning gastric w.
gastric w.
washout

antral w.
wasting

bicarbonate w.
cerebral salt w. (CSW)
phosphate w.
renal electrolyte w.
renal salt w.

wasting *(continued)*
 renal tubular bicarbonate w.
 salt w.
 sodium w.
 w. syndrome
 urinary potassium w.
water
 w. bottle appearance
 centimeters of w. (cm H_2O)
 w. enema
 extravascular lung w. (EVLW)
 w. intoxication
 w. lily sign
 w. loss
 w. on brain
 w. pacifier
 total body w. (TBW)
 w. vaporizer
waterhammer effect
Waterhouse-Friderichsen syndrome
water-perfused manometry catheter
watershed
 w. distribution
 w. lesion
 w. zone
water-soluble contrast enema
Waterston
 W. aortopulmonary anastomosis
 W. shunt
 W. shunt procedure
Waterston-Cooley procedure
Waters view
watery diarrhea
Watson-Alagille syndrome
Watson capsule
Watson-Crick double-helix DNA
Watson-Schwartz test
wave
 bifid P w.
 biphasic P w.
 brain w.
 broad P w.
 w. change
 delta w.
 fibrillatory w.
 flat T w.
 flattened T w.
 fluid w.
 flutter w.
 gastric peristaltic w.
 jugular venous A w.
 Mayer w.
 monophasic R w.
 notched P w.
 Osborne w.
 P w.
 peaked T w.
 peristaltic w.

 Q w.
 R w.
 sawtoothed flutter w.
 spiked P w.
 T w.
 tall P w.
 W. ventilator
waveform
4-Way Long Acting Nasal Solution
Wayson stain
WBC
 white blood cell
WBI
 whole-bowel irrigation
WBN
 well baby nursery
WCC
 well-child care
WCST
 Wisconsin Card Sorting Test
W-Ditching agent
WDL
 Wood-Downes-Lecks
 WDL asthma score
WE
 Wernicke encephalopathy
weak
 w. cry
 w. suck
weakness
 girdle w.
 homolateral w.
 hypotonic w.
 postictal w.
 proximal pattern w.
 upward gaze w.
wean-and-feed protocol
weaning brash
wearing position
Weaver syndrome
web
 esophageal w.
 gastric w.
 interdigital w.
 intraluminal w.
 laryngeal w.
 supraglottic w.
 windsock w.
webbed
 w. neck
 w. penis
webbing
Webb-McCall peak
Weber-Christian syndrome
Weber-Cockayne epidermolysis bullosa simplex
Weber test
Webril bandage

Wechsler
- W. Adult Intelligence Scale, 3rd edition
- W. Intelligence Scale for Children (WISC)
- W. Intelligence Scale for Children III (WISC-III)
- W. Intelligence Scale for Children, 3rd edition
- W. Intelligence Scale for Children-Revised (WISC-R)
- W. Memory Scale
- W. Preschool and Primary Scale of Intelligence (WPPSI)
- W. Preschool and Primary Scale of Intelligence-Revised (WPPSI-R)
- W. test

wedge
- w. osteotomy
- shoe w.
- w. vertebra

wedge-shaped platform

wedging

WEE
- western equine encephalitis

WeeFIM
- Functional Independence Measure for Children

weeping
- w. dermatitis
- w. lesion
- w. willow

Wegener granulomatosis (WG)

Weibel-Palade body

Weibull hazard

weighing
- underwater w.

weight
- birth w.
- dry w.
- extremely low birth w. (ELBW)
- w. gain
- low birth w. (LBW)
- low molecular w. (LMW)
- mean birth w.
- w. shifting
- very low birth w. (VLBW)
- w. z-score

weightbearing

weight/height (W/H)
- w./h. index

weight-lifter blackout

Weil-Felix
- W.-F. antibody testing
- W.-F. reaction

Weill-Marchesani syndrome

Weill sign

Weil syndrome

Weinberger Adjustment Inventory (WAI)

Weir equation

Welch
- W. Allyn AudioPath Platform hearing acuity instrument
- W. Allyn AudioScope
- W. Allyn SureSight eye chart

Welch-Allyn MicroTymp impedance tympanometer

welfare

well baby nursery (WBN)

Wellbutrin

well-child care (WCC)

Wellcovorin

well-hydrated baby

welt

Wenckebach
- W. heart block
- W. phenomena

Wender Utah Rating Scale (WURS)

Wepman Auditory Discrimination Test

Werdnig-Hoffmann
- W.-H. disease
- W.-H. disorder
- W.-H. paralysis
- W.-H. syndrome

werkmanii
- *Citrobacter w.*

werneckii
- *Exophiala w.*

Werner syndrome

Wernicke
- W. aphasia
- W. area
- W. disease
- W. encephalopathy (WE)
- W. syndrome

Wernicke-Korsakoff syndrome

Wessel colic

West
- W. Nile virus
- W. syndrome

Westcort Topical

westermani
- *Paragonimus w.*

NOTES

W

western
> W. blot
> W. blot test
> w. equine encephalitis (WEE)
> W. immunoblot

Westerner test
Westrim-I
Westrim-LA
wet
> w. brain syndrome
> w. burp
> w. drowning
> w. lung disease
> w. lung syndrome
> w. mount
> w. purpura

wetting defect of cornea
WG
> Wegener granulomatosis

W/H
> weight/height
> W/H index

Wharton jelly
wheal
> punctate w.

wheal-and-flare reaction
wheat
> spelt w.

Wheaton Pavlik harness
wheelchair sport
wheeze
> high-pitched w.
> monophonic w.
> nonmusical w.
> polyphonic w.

wheezer
> happy w.

wheezing
> high-pitched w.
> monophonic w.
> nonmusical w.
> polyphonic w.

wheezy bronchitis
whey
> hydrolyzed w.

whiff test
whiplash injury
Whipple
> W. disease
> W. procedure

whipworm
whispered pectoriloquy
Whitaker test
white
> w. blood cell (WBC)
> w. blood cell count
> w. blood cell lysosomal enzyme
> analysis

> w. coat effect
> w. dermographism
> w. forelock
> w. matter
> w. matter damage (WMD)
> w. matter degeneration
> w. matter lucency
> w. matter pallor
> w. papule
> w. plaque
> w. pseudomembranous material
> w. pupil
> w. pupillary reflex
> w. retinal infiltrate
> w. scleral hue
> w. strawberry tongue
> w. superficial onychomycosis
> w. tonsillitis

white-coat hypertension
whitehead
white-out
white-yellow plaque
Whitfield ointment
whitlow
> herpetic w.

Whitten media
Whittingham media
WHO
> World Health Organization
> WHO formula

whole-bowel irrigation (WBI)
whole-cell
> w.-c. diphtheria-tetanus-pertussis
> vaccine
> w.-c. DTP vaccine

whole-virus vaccine
whoop
> inspiratory w.

whooping cough
whorl
> hair w.

whorled macular hyperpigmentation
WHR
> waist-hip ratio

Wiberg
> center edge angle of W.

WIC
> women, infants, children
> Women, Infants, and Children Program
> WIC syndrome

Wickham stria
wide
> w. complex tachycardia
> w. cranial suture
> w. excision
> w. pulse pressure
> W. Range Achievement Test-
> Revised (WRAT-R)

w. range assessment of memory and learning (WRAML)

W. Range Assessment of Memory and Learning Test

wide-based shuffling gait

wide-field myringotomy

widely spaced eyes

widened

w. growth plate

w. metaphysis

w. symphysis pubis

widening

mediastinal w.

width

cardiac w.

chest w.

maximal cardiac w.

maximal chest w.

pulse w.

tympanometric w.

Wigraine

Wilcoxon

W. rank sum test

W. signed rank test

Wildervanck syndrome

wild-type measles virus

wild virus

Wilkie disease

Wilkins

W. disease

W. syndrome

Williams

W. syndrome (WS)

vulvovaginal pouch of W.

Williams-Beuren syndrome

Williams-Campbell syndrome

Willis

circle of W.

willow

weeping w.

Wilms

W. tumor, aniridia, genitourinary malformations, mental retardation (WAGR)

W. tumor (stage I–V)

Wilson disease

wilsonian

Wilson-Mikity syndrome

Wimberger

W. ring

W. sign

Winchester syndrome

Winckel disease

window

aortopulmonary w.

middle meatus nasal antral w.

nasal antral w.

w. operation

oval w.

transgastric w.

vaginal w.

windpipe

windsock web

windswept deformity

Wing Autistic Disorder Interview Checklist (WADIC)

wing-beating appearance

winging

scapular w.

wink

anal w.

Winks

WinRho SD, SDF

Winter

W. glans-cavernosal procedure

W. syndrome

wipe

disposable w.

wire

3F thermistor w.

Kirschner w.

lead w.

Teflon-coated w.

Wirsung

main duct of W.

Wirsungianus

ductus W.

WISC

Wechsler Intelligence Scale for Children

WISC-III

Wechsler Intelligence Scale for Children - Third Edition

WISC-III factor scores

Wisconsin Card Sorting Test (WCST)

WISC-R

Wechsler Intelligence Scale for Children-Revised

wisdom tooth

Wiskott-Aldrich syndrome (WAS)

wispy hair

witch's milk

withdrawal

w. bleeding

W

NOTES

withdrawal *(continued)*
  w. dyskinesia
  w. position
  social w.
withdrawn behavior
within-the-infant depressive disorder
WITS
  Women and Infants Transmission Study
WMD
  white matter damage
wolffi
wolffian duct
Wolf-Parkinson-White syndrome
Wolfram syndrome
Wolman disease
Wolraich questionnaire
womb
women
  w., infants, children (WIC)
  W., Infants, and Children Program
  (WIC)
  W., Infants, Children syndrome
  W. and Infants Transmission Study
  (WITS)
Wong-Baker Faces Pain Rating Scale
wood
  w. tick
  W. ultraviolet lamp
  W. unit
Woodcock-Johnson
  W.-J. Psychoeducational Battery
  W.-J. reading test
  W.-J. Tests of Achievement
Wood-Downes asthma score
Wood-Downes-Lecks (WDL)
  W.-D.-L. asthma score
woolly
  w. hair disease
  w. hair nevus
word
  W. catheter
  number of different w.'s (NDW)
work
  w. of breathing
  parent guidance w.
worker
  healthcare w. (HCW)
  social w.
workup
  malabsorption w.
  sepsis w.

world
  W. Association for Infant Mental
  Health
  W. Health Organization (WHO)
worm
  bag of w.'s
wormian bone
worried facial appearance
wound botulism
woven bone
WPPSI
  Wechsler Preschool and Primary Scale of
  Intelligence
WPPSI-R
  Wechsler Preschool and Primary Scale of
  Intelligence-Revised
WRAML
  wide range assessment of memory and
  learning
  WRAML test
wrap
  mummy w.
WRAT-R
  Wide Range Achievement Test-Revised
wrench
  E-tank w.
wrestling
Wright stain
Wright-stained smear
wringing
  hand w.
wrist
  gymnast's w.
  shaking w.
writer's cramp
writhing
Wrobleski unit
wry
  w. neck
  w. neck deformity
WS
  Williams syndrome
WURS
  Wender Utah Rating Scale
Wyamycin S
Wyburn-Mason syndrome
Wycillin
Wydase
Wygesic
Wymox

X
    X chromosome
Xa
xanthan/guar combination
xanthelasma
xanthine
xanthinuria, xanthiuria
xanthochromia therapy
xanthochromic
    x. CSF
    x. fluid
xanthogranuloma
    juvenile x. (JXG)
xanthogranulomatous
    x. infiltrate
    x. pyelonephritis
xanthoma
    Achilles tendon x.
    eruptive x.
    palmar x.
    x. striata palmaris
    tendon x.
xanthomatosis
    cerebrotendinous x.
    primary x.
Xanthomonas maltophilia
xanthopsia
xanthosis cutis
xanthous
xanthurenic
    x. acid
    x. aciduria
xenon
    x. arc
    x. clearance
    x. CT scan
xenopi
    Mycobacterium x.
xeroderma
    x. pigmentosa
    x. pigmentosum
xerophthalmia
xerosis
    x. conjunctiva
    x. cornea
xerostomia
xinafoate
    salmeterol x.
xiphisternum
XL
    Ditropan XL
    Procardia XL
XLA
    X-linked agammaglobulinemia

XLD
    X-linked dominant
XLHN
    X-linked hypercalciuric nephrolithiasis
XLHR
    X-linked hypophosphatemic rickets
X-linked
    X-l. adrenoleukodystrophy
    X-l. agammaglobulinemia (XLA)
    X-l. cardiomyopathy
    X-l. cardioskeletal myopathy
    X-l. cardioskeletal myopathy and
      neutropenia
    X-l. chronic granulomatous disease
    X-l. dominant (XLD)
    X-l. dominant disorder
    X-l. dyskeratosis congenita
    X-l. Ehlers-Danlos syndrome
    X-l. hydrocephalus
    X-l. hypercalciuric nephrolithiasis
      (XLHN)
    X-l. hypogammaglobulinemia
    X-l. hypophosphatemia
    X-l. hypophosphatemic rickets
      (XLHR)
    X-l. ichthyosis
    X-l. immunodeficiency with hyper
      IgM
    X-l. lymphoproliferative disease
    X-l. lymphoproliferative syndrome
    X-l. myotubular myopathy
    X-l. pyridoxine-responsive
      sideroblastic anemia
    X-l. recessive (XLR)
    X-l. recessive disorder
    X-l. recessive inheritance
    X-l. recessive nephrolithiasis
    X-l. recessive skeletal Ehlers-Danlos
      syndrome
    X-l. recessive-type diabetes
      insipidus
    X-l. retinoschisis
    X-l. severe combined
      immunodeficiency (X-SCID)
    X-l. severe combined
      immunodeficiency syndrome
    X-l. thrombocytopenia
XLR
    X-linked recessive
XO
    XO karyotype
    XO syndrome
XomaZyme-H65
Xopenex inhalation solution
Xp deletion

X

X-Prep Liquid
Xq
>isochromosome Xq

XR
>Dilacor XR

x-ray
>chest x-r. (CXR)
>dual-energy x-r.
>Lauenstein pelvic x-r.
>stand x-r.

X-SCID
>X-linked severe combined
>immunodeficiency

XX
>double strength
>normal female sex chromosome type

XXX
>mosaicism for XXX

XXY
>XXY karyotype
>XXY syndrome

XY
>normal male sex chromosome type
>46XY karyotype

xylitol
Xylocaine
>X. HCl I.V. Injection for Cardiac
>Arrhythmias
>X. Oral
>X. Topical Ointment
>X. Topical Solution
>X. Topical Spray
>X. With Epinephrine

xyloni
>*Solenopsis x.*

Xylo-Pfan
xylose lysine deaminase agar
xylosoxidans
>*Achromobacter x.*
>*Alcaligenes x.*

XYY syndrome

Y

Y chromosome
Y connector
Y shunt
Y shunting

Yale

Y. Global Tic Severity Scale
(YGTSS)
Y. Observation Scale

**Yale-Brown Obsessive Compulsive Scale
(YBOCS)**

Yankauer catheter

YAPA

young adult psychiatric assessment

yaws

dry crab y.

YBOCS

Yale-Brown Obsessive Compulsive Scale

year

y. of birth (YOB)
y. 7 conduct disorder

yeast

yellow

y. fever
y. fever 17D
y. fever 17D vaccination
y. jackets
y. nail
y. nail syndrome
y. OCA
y. retinal infiltrate
y. vernix syndrome

yellow-green pallor

Yersinia

Y. arthritis
Y. *enterocolitica*

Y. *pestis*
Y. pseudotuberculosis

yersinial infection

yersiniosis

YGTSS

Yale Global Tic Severity Scale

YOB

year of birth

Yodoxin

yohimbine

yolk

y. sac
y. sac tumor

young

y. adult psychiatric assessment
(YAPA)
Y. syndrome

youngae

Citrobacter y.

youth

gay, lesbian, bisexual y.'s
GLB y.'s
Great Smoky Mountains Study
of Y. (GSMS)
mature-onset diabetes of y.
maturity-onset diabetes of y.
(MODY)
y. risk behavioral survey (YRBS)
y. self-report (YSR)

YRBS

youth risk behavioral survey

YSR

youth self-report

Yunis Varon syndrome

Yuzpe method

Y

Z
Z band
Z foot
zafirlukast
zalcitabine (ddC)
zanamivir
Zancolli clawhand deformity repair
Zantac
Z. 75
zaprinast
Zarontin
Zaroxolyn
Zartan
ZDV
zidovudine
Zeasorb-AF
Zeasorb powder
zebra body
Zeis
pilosebaceous gland of Z.
Zellweger
Z. cerebrohepatorenal syndrome
Z. disease
Zemuron
Zenapax
Zenker solution
Zephrex LA
Zerit
zero
z. end-expiratory pressure
z. reject
Z. to Three diagnostic classification
zero-voltage baseline
Zestril
Zetar
Ziagen
zidovudine (ZDV)
Ziehen-Oppenheim syndrome
Ziehl-Neelsen
Z.-N. stain
Z.-N. test
Zilactin-B Medicated
zileuton
Zinacef Injection
zinc
z. deficiency
z. oxide
z. oxide ointment
z. oxide paste
z. protoporphyrin/heme (ZPP/H)
z. protoporphyrin/heme ratio
serum z.
z. stearate powder
z. sulfate
z. supplement

z. therapy
z. toxicity
Zinca-Pak
Zincate
zinc-free
z.-f. plastic bag
z.-f. plastic-lined diaper
z.-f. plastic specimen cup
Zinecard
Zinsser-Cole-Engman syndrome
Zinsser disease
ziprasidone
Zithromax
Zixoryn
Zofran ODT
zoledronate
Zolicef
Zollinger-Ellison syndrome
Zoloft
zolpidem
zona, pl. **zonae**
z. pellucida (ZP)
z. reticularis
zonal
z. aganglionosis
z. drilling
Zonalon Topical Cream
zone
chemoreceptor trigger z. (CTZ)
echo-free z.
extranodal marginal z.
germinal z.
growth z.
hypertrophic z. (HZ)
hypertrophic growth z.
marginal z.
z. of preparatory calcification (ZPC)
proliferative z. (PZ)
reserve z. (RZ)
toxicity z.
watershed z.
zonular cataract
zoonotic
zoster
herpes z.
z. myelitis
trigeminal herpes z.
zosteriform
z. lentiginous nevus
z. lesion
Zostrix
Zostrix-HP
Zosyn
Zovirax

Z

ZP
  zona pellucida
ZPC
  zone of preparatory calcification
ZPP/H
  zinc protoporphyrin/heme
  ZPP/H ratio
z-score
    height velocity z-s.
    weight z-s.
Z-shaped duodenum
ZstatFlu test
Zuckerkandl organ
Zydone
Zyflo
zygodactyly
zygoma
zygomatic
    z. arch

    z. bone
    z. head
    z. head of quadratus labiae
      superioris muscle
zygomaticofrontal region
zygomaticomaxillary fracture
zygomycosis
zygosity
zygosyndactyly
zygote
Zyklomat
Zyloprim
zymase
Zymenol
Zyprexa
Zyrtec syrup

Anatomical Illustrations

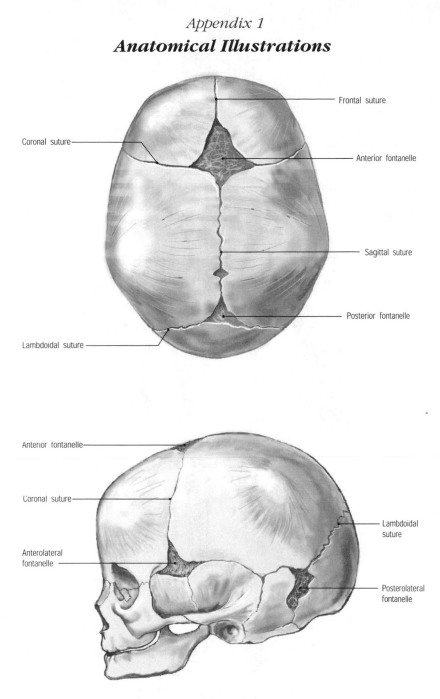

Figure 1. Newborn skull. Superior view (top). Lateral view (bottom).

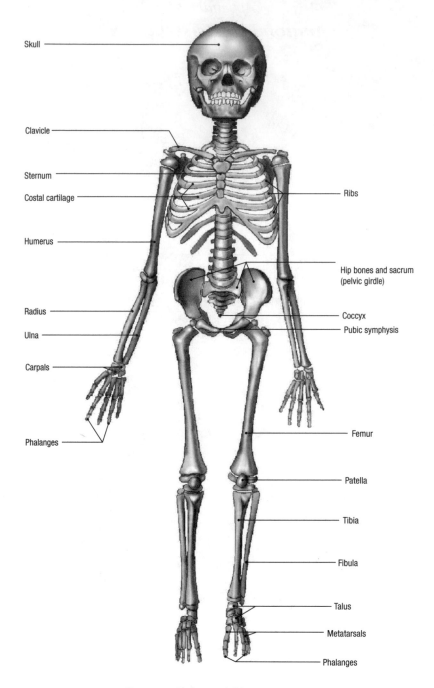

Figure 2. Skeleton, child. Anterior view.

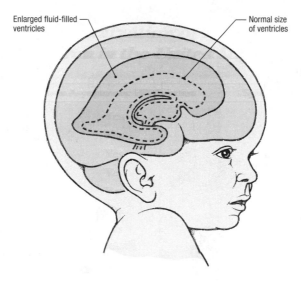

Enlarged fluid-filled
ventricles

Normal size
of ventricles

Figure 3. Hydrocephalus.

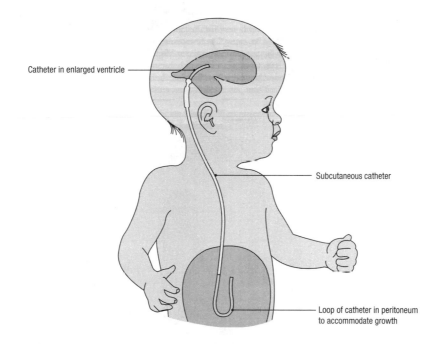

Catheter in enlarged ventricle

Subcutaneous catheter

Loop of catheter in peritoneum
to accommodate growth

Figure 4. Image of infant with ventriculoperitoneal shunt in place. The shunt removes excess cerebrospinal fluid from the ventricles and shunts it to the peritoneum. A one-way valve is present in the tubing behind the ear.

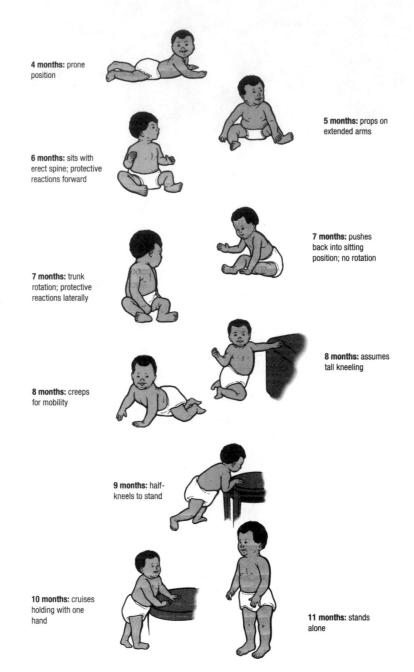

Figure 5. Developmental milestones. This image, created by Michael Schenk for *Stedman's Medical Dictionary, 27th Edition,* Baltimore, Lippincott Williams & Wilkins, 2000, p. 486, appears here with permission and courtesy of Lippincott Williams & Wilkins.

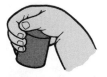

5 months: palmar grasp: fingers on top surface of object press it into center of palm; thumb abducted

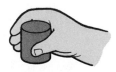

6 months: radial-palmar grasp: fingers on far side of object press it against opposed thumb and radial side of palm

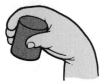

7 months: inferior-scissors grasp: raking into palm with abducted, totally flexed thumb and all flexed fingers, **or** raking object into palm with abducted, totally flexed thumb and 2 partly extended fingers

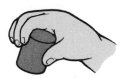

7 months: radial-palmar grasp: wrist straight

8 months: scissors grasp: between thumb and side of curled index finger, distal thumb joint slightly flexed; proximal thumb joint extended

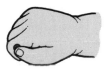

8 months: radial-digital grasp: object held with opposed thumb and fingertips, space visible between

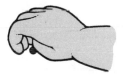

9 months: inferior-pincer grasp: between ventral surfaces of thumb and index finger, distal thumb joint extended; beginning thumb opposition

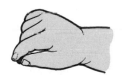

9 months: radial-digital grasp: wrist extended

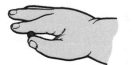

10 months: pincer grasp: between distal pads of thumb and index finger, distal thumb slightly flexed; thumb opposed

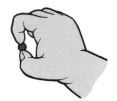

12 months: fine pincer grasp: between fingertips or fingernails; distal thumb joint flexed

Figure 6. Pinch and grasp patterns. This image, created by Michael Schenk for *Stedman's Medical Dictionary, 27th Edition,* Baltimore, Lippincott Williams & Wilkins, 2000, p. 1385, appears here with permission and courtesy of Lippincott Williams & Wilkins.

Appendix 1

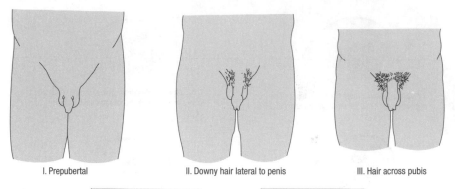

I. Prepubertal II. Downy hair lateral to penis III. Hair across pubis

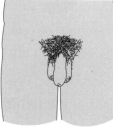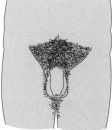

IV. Curled, adult distribution but
less abundant

V. Adult configuration

STAGE	GENITAL DEVELOPMENT	PUBIC HAIR
I	Prepubertal	Prepubertal
II	Enlargement of testes (> 4 mL volume) and scrotum with reddening of scrotal skin	Sparse, long, straight, slightly pigmented hair at base of penis
III	Growth of penis, primarily length, with further increase in size of testes and scrotum	Hair is darker and curlier with increased distribution on pubes
IV	Further increase in length and breadth of penis with development of glans, increase in testes and scrotum	Adult-type hair limited to pubes with no extension to medial thigh
V	Adult size and shape	Mature distribution with spread to medial thighs and lower abdomen

Figure 7. Tanner stages in the male. Rating I-V.

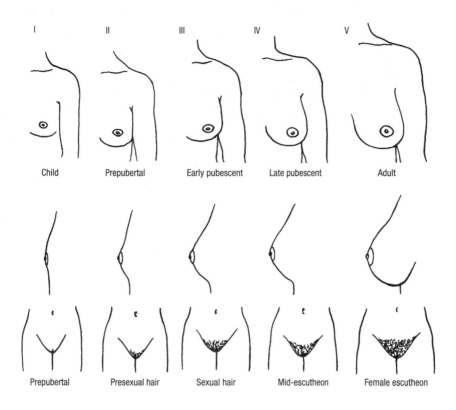

STAGE	BREAST	PUBIC HAIR
I	Prepubertal, elevation of papilla only	Prepubertal
II	Enlargement of areola, elevation of breast and papilla ("breast bud")	Sparse, long, straight, slight pigmented hair along labia
III	Further enlargement of breast and areola with no separation of contour	Hair is darker, curlier, and coarser with increased distribution on pubes
IV	Areola and papilla form a second mount above the breast	Adult-type hair limited to pubes with no extension to medial thigh
V	Mature breast	Mature distribution of inverse triangle with spread to medial thighs

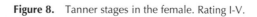

Figure 8. Tanner stages in the female. Rating I-V.

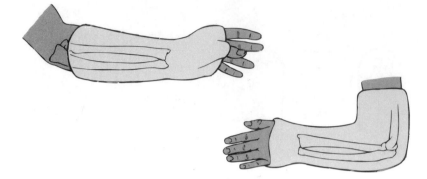

Figure 9. Gauntlet or thumb cast from the elbow down (left). Long arm cast from the biceps down (right). Radial styloid, ulnar styloid, and lateral epicondyle illustrated upon cast to show possible pressure area of cast.

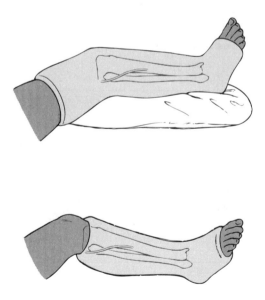

Figure 10. Long leg cast from the thigh to the foot and propped on a pillow (top). Short leg cast from the knee to the foot (bottom). Bones of lower leg and peroneal nerve shown to indicate possible pressure areas.

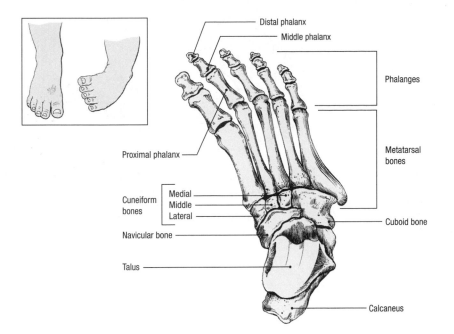

Figure 11. Clubfoot. Bones in a clubfoot deformity. Anterior view of a child's two feet, the left of which is clubbed (inset).

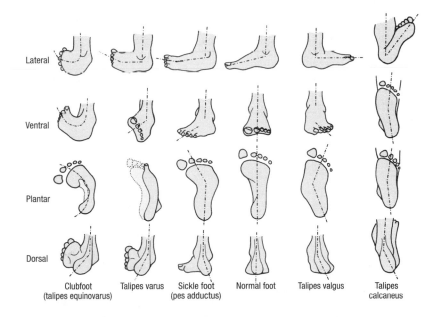

Figure 12. Foot deformities.

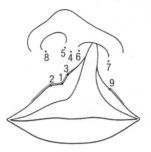

Figure 13. Anatomy of the normal and unrepaired unilateral cleft lip indicating key points used for planning repair: (1) lowest point in arch of Cupid's bow, midline of the lip; (2) peak of Cupid's bow on the noncleft side; (3) proposed peak of Cupid's bow; (4) midpoint of the columella; (5, 6) base of columella laterally; (7, 8) inset of alar base into nostril sill; (9) a point on the well-developed vermilion cutaneous roll of the lateral lip and the same horizontal plane as the peak of Cupid's bow on the noncleft side.

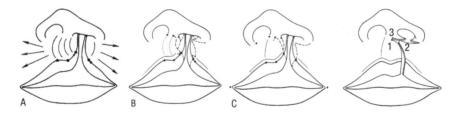

Figure 14. Cleft lip repair (A, B) and rotation advancement flap technique (C). (A) Unrepaired cleft lip stresses. (B) Incorporating stresses into repair. (1) Medial lip element. (2) Lateral lip element. (3) Small medial flap.

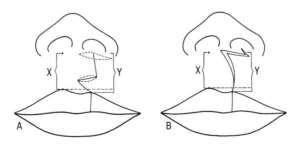

Figure 15. Cleft lip redo surgery. (A) Previous triangular or quadrangular repair flap. (B) Rotation advancement flap redo technique.

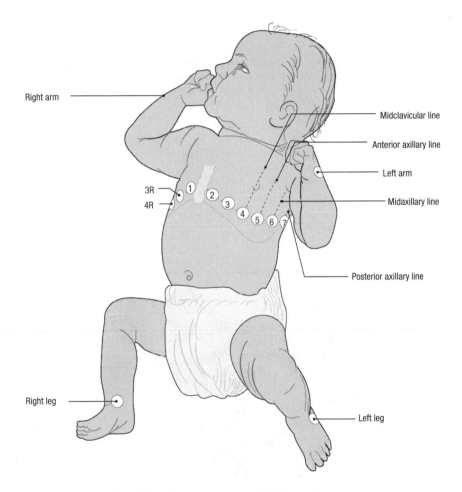

Right arm

Midclavicular line

Anterior axillary line

Left arm

3R

4R

1
2
3
4 5 6 7

Midaxillary line

Posterior axillary line

Right leg

Left leg

Figure 16. Electrocardiogram (ECG) lead placement.

Appendix 1

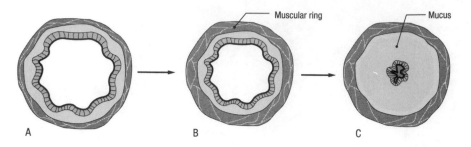

Figure 17. Pulmonary disorders, showing the effects asthma has on a bronchiole. (A) Normal bronchiole. (B) Muscular rings contract and thicken, decreasing lumen size. (C) Mucosal layers thicken, further closing lumen, which fills with thick mucus.

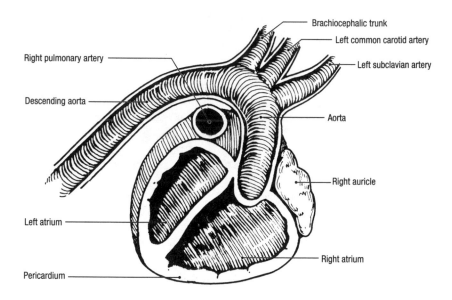

Figure 18. The aortic arch and descending aorta of a prone fetus in a vertex presentation.

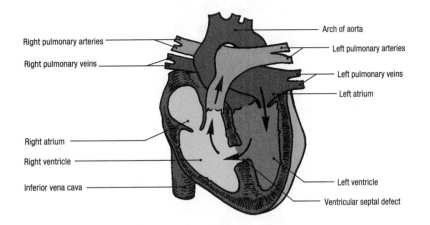

Right pulmonary arteries

Right pulmonary veins

Right atrium

Right ventricle

Inferior vena cava

Arch of aorta

Left pulmonary arteries

Left pulmonary veins

Left atrium

Left ventricle

Ventricular septal defect

Figure 19. Auscultation, ventricular septal defect (VSD). VSD is so large there is no pressure between the ventricles. Flow is dependent on systemic and pulmonary arterial resistance. If pulmonary vascular resistance (PVR) is less than systemic vascular resistance (SVR), a left-to-right shunt occurs.

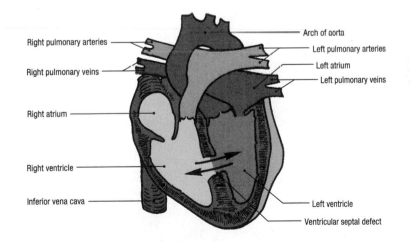

Right pulmonary arteries

Right pulmonary veins

Right atrium

Right ventricle

Inferior vena cava

Arch of aorta

Left pulmonary arteries

Left atrium

Left pulmonary veins

Left ventricle

Ventricular septal defect

Figure 20. Auscultation, ventricular septal defect (VSD). When pulmonary vascular resistance (PVR) is equal to or greater than systemic vascular resistance (SVR) in the presence of a large VSD, a murmur may not be detected due to low shunt volume. A loud single second sound is heard as aortic and pulmonary closures occur.

A13

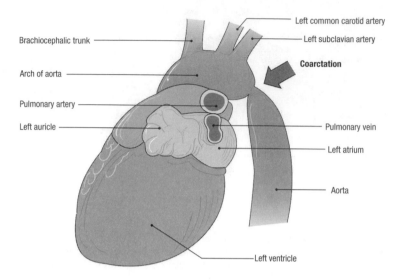

Left common carotid artery

Left subclavian artery

Brachiocephalic trunk

Coarctation

Arch of aorta

Pulmonary artery

Left auricle

Pulmonary vein

Left atrium

Aorta

Left ventricle

Figure 21. Coarctation of the aorta showing deformed descending aorta.

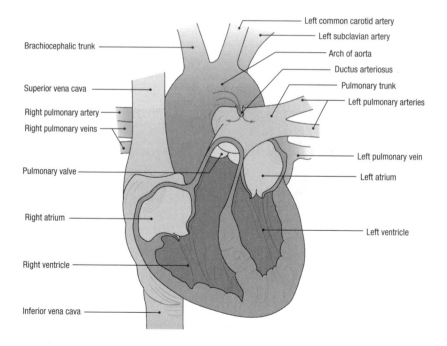

Left common carotid artery

Left subclavian artery

Brachiocephalic trunk

Arch of aorta

Ductus arteriosus

Superior vena cava

Pulmonary trunk

Right pulmonary artery

Left pulmonary arteries

Right pulmonary veins

Left pulmonary vein

Pulmonary valve

Left atrium

Right atrium

Left ventricle

Right ventricle

Inferior vena cava

Figure 22. Ductus arteriosus. Coronal view of heart with ductus arteriosus showing blood flow. Pulmonary trunk receives blood from aortic arch.

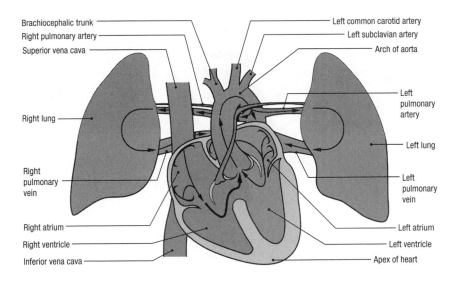

Figure 23. Coronal view of heart with pseudotruncus arteriosus. Altered blood circulation due to atresia of the pulmonic valve and absence of the main pulmonary artery is depicted.

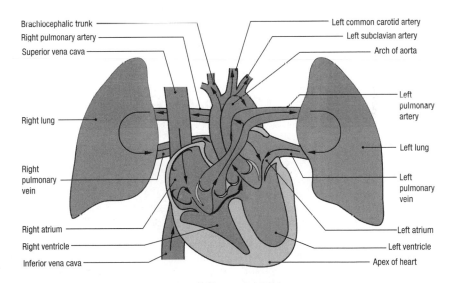

Figure 24. Coronal view of heart in tetralogy of Fallot. Characteristics include pulmonary trunk stenosis, right ventricular hypertrophy, dextroposition of the aorta, and ventricular septal defect (VSD). Blood flow is depicted.

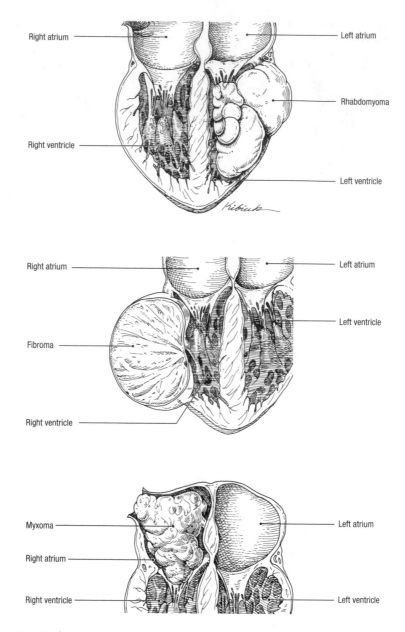

Figure 25. Cardiac tumors in children. Primary cardiac tumors in children appear to be associated with familial syndromes with autosomal dominant inheritance. Rhabdomyoma is the most common benign tumor and is derived from striated muscle elements. It is located within the wall of the myocardium (top). The fibroma is a solitary ventricular structure derived from fibrous connective tissue. It occurs in children under 10 years of age (middle). The myxoma arises from the lining of the atrium and resembles a polyp. It is a benign tumor (bottom).

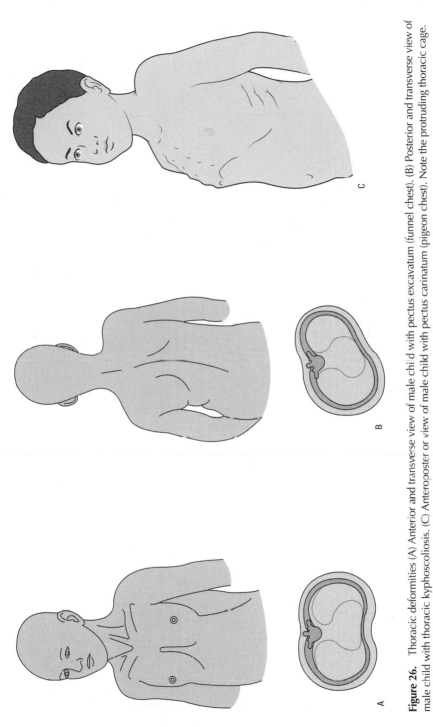

Figure 26. Thoracic deformities (A) Anterior and transverse view of male child with pectus excavatum (funnel chest). (B) Posterior and transverse view of male child with thoracic kyphoscoliosis. (C) Anteroposter or view of male child with pectus carinatum (pigeon chest). Note the protruding thoracic cage.

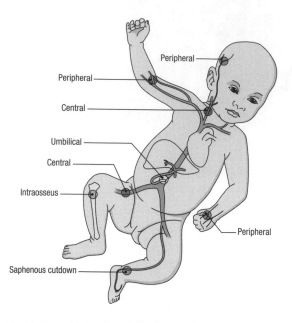

Figure 27. Pediatric IV sites: peripheral, umbilical, central, intraosseus, and saphenous cutdown.

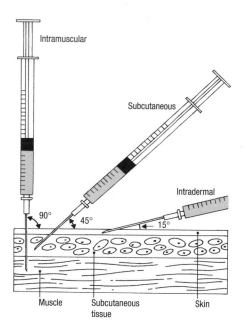

Figure 28. Angles of insertion of injection.

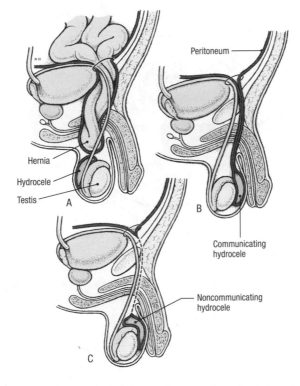

Figure 29. Types of hydroceles (peritoneum shown in dark gray).

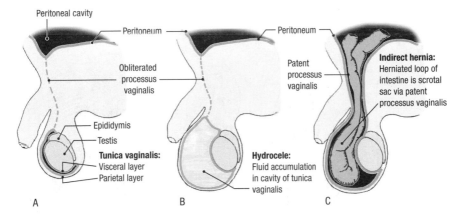

Figure 30. Processus vaginalis and tunica vaginalis. (A) Normal anatomy. (B) Hydrocele. (C) Indirect hernia.

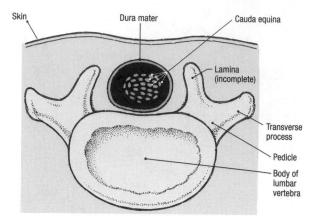

Figure 31. Spina bifida occulta.

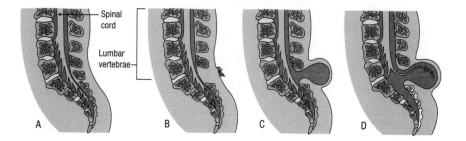

Figure 32. Four degrees of spinal cord anomalies. (A) Normal spinal cord. (B) Spina bifida occulta. (C) Meningocele. (D) Myelomeningocele.

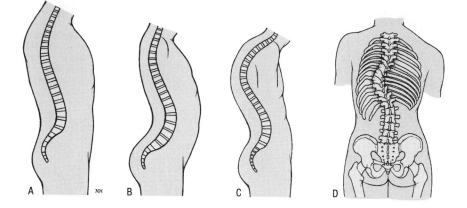

Figure 33. Spinal curvatures. (A) Normal. (B) Lordosis. (C) Kyphosis. (D) Scoliosis.

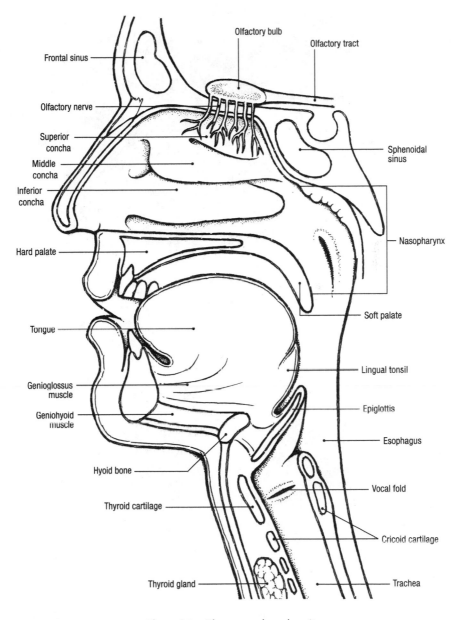

Figure 34. Pharynx and nasal cavity.

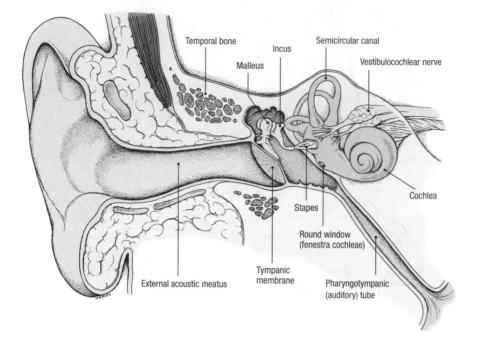

Figure 35. Ear.

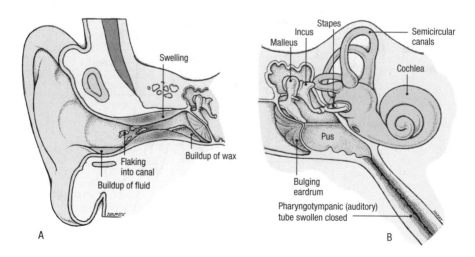

Figure 36. (A) Otitis externa. (B) Otitis media.

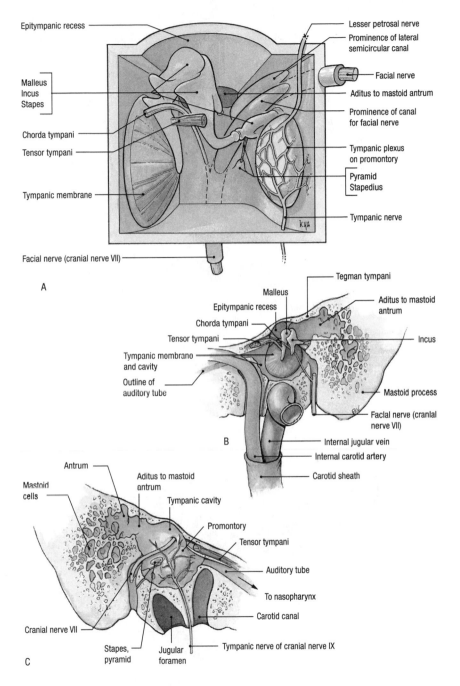

Epitympanic recess

Malleus
Incus
Stapes

Chorda tympani

Tensor tympani

Tympanic membrane

Facial nerve (cranial nerve VII)

A

Lesser petrosal nerve
Prominence of lateral
semicircular canal

Facial nerve

Aditus to mastoid antrum

Prominence of canal
for facial nerve

Tympanic plexus
on promontory

Pyramid
Stapedius

Tympanic nerve

Tegman tympani

Malleus

Epitympanic recess

Chorda tympani

Tensor tympani

Tympanic membrane
and cavity

Outline of
auditory tube

B

Aditus to mastoid
antrum

Incus

Mastoid process

Facial nerve (cranial
nerve VII)

Internal jugular vein

Internal carotid artery

Carotid sheath

Antrum

Mastoid
cells

Aditus to mastoid
antrum

Tympanic cavity

Promontory

Tensor tympani

Auditory tube

To nasopharynx

Carotid canal

Tympanic nerve of cranial nerve IX

Cranial nerve VII

Stapes,
pyramid

Jugular
foramen

C

Figure 37. Schematics of walls of tympanic cavity. (A) Anterior wall removed, anterior view. (B) Lateral wall, medial view. (C) Medial wall, lateral view.

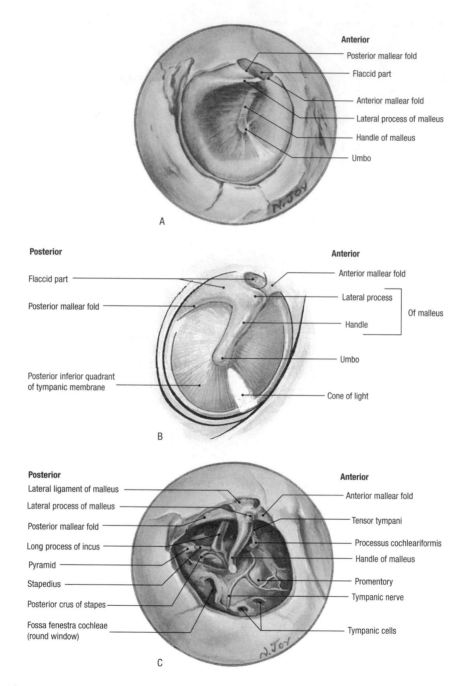

Figure 38. Tympanic membrane. (A) Lateral view. (B) Auriscopic view. (C) Tympanic membrane removed, inferolateral view.

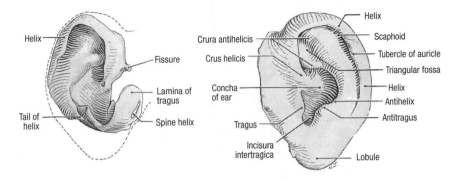

Helix

Crura antihelicis

Crus helicis

Concha of ear

Tragus

Incisura intertragica

Helix

Fissure

Lamina of tragus

Tail of helix

Spine helix

Helix

Scaphoid

Tubercle of auricle

Triangular fossa

Helix

Antihelix

Antitragus

Lobule

Figure 39. The auricle.

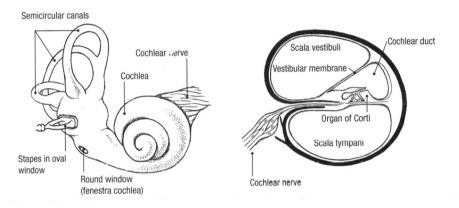

Semicircular canals

Cochlear nerve

Cochlea

Stapes in oval window

Round window (fenestra cochlea)

Scala vestibuli

Vestibular membrane

Cochlear duct

Organ of Corti

Scala tympani

Cochlear nerve

Figure 40. Cochlea, with cross-section.

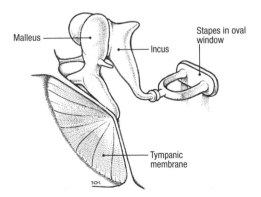

Malleus

Incus

Stapes in oval window

Tympanic membrane

Figure 41. Auditory ossicles.

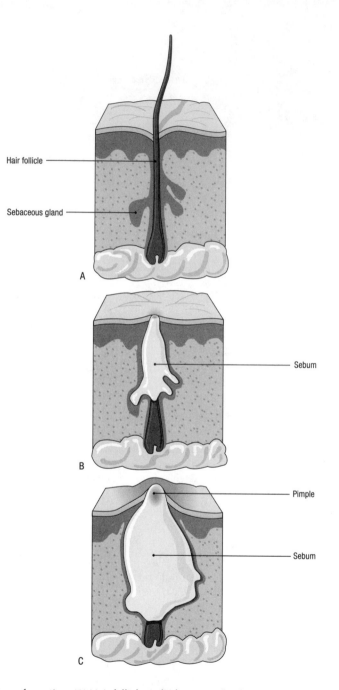

Figure 42. Acne formation. (A) Hair follicle and sebaceous gland. (B) First stage in acne development; follicle becomes blocked, sebum begins to fill follicle cavity. (C) Inflamed pustule and pimple; follicle is blocked, sebum has filled and expanded follicle cavity.

Normal Lab Values

Tests	Conventional Units	SI Units
acetone		
serum		
qualitative	negative	negative
quantitative	0.3–2.0 mg/dL	0.05–0.34 mmol/L
*alanine aminotransferase (ALT, SGPT), serum		
male	13–40 U/L (37°C)	0.22–0.68 μkat/L (37° C)
female	10–28 U/L (37°C)	0.17–0.48 μkat/L (37° C)
albumin		
serum		
adult	3.5–5.2 g/dL	35–52 g/L
urine		
qualitative	negative	negative
quantitative	50–80 mg/24 h	50–80 mg/24 h
CSF	10–30 mg/dL	100–300 mg/dL
ammonia		
plasma (Hep)	9–33 μmol/L	9–33 μmol/L
*amylase		
serum	27–131 U/L	0.46–2.23 μkat/L
*bilirubin		
serum		
neonates		
conjugated	0–0.6 mg/dL	0–10 μmol/L
unconjugated	0.6–10.5 mg/dL	10–180 μmol/L
total	1.5–12 mg/dL	1.7–180 μmol/L
calcium, serum	8.6–10.0 mg/dL (slightly higher in children)	2.15–2.50 mmol/L (slightly higher in children)
carbon dioxide (PCO_2), blood arterial	male 35–48 mmHg female 32–45 mmHg	4.66–6.38 kPa 4.26–5.99 kPa
carotene, serum	10–85 μg/dL	0.19–1.58 μmol/L
catecholamines, urine		
dopamine	65–400 μg/24 h	425–2610 nmol/24
epinephrine	0–20 μg/24 h	0–109 nmol/24
norepinephrine	15–80 μg/24 h	89–473 nmol/24
*cell counts, adult		
RBC male	$4.7–6.1 \times 10^6/\mu L$	$4.7–6.1 \times 10^{12}/L$
female	$4.2–5.4 \times 10^6/\mu L$	$4.2–5.4 \times 10^{12}/L$
leukocytes		
total	$4.8–10.8 \times 10^3/\mu L$	$4.8–10.8 \times 10^6/L$
platelets	$130–400 \times 10^3/\mu L$	$1340–400 \times 10^9/L$
reticulocytes	0.5–1.5% red cells	0.005–0.015 of RBC

continued

Tests	Conventional Units	SI Units
cells, CSF 0 RBC/ mm³	0–10 lymphocytes /mm³ 0 RBC/ mm³	0–10 lymphocytes /mm³
chloride serum or plasma	98–107 mmol/L	98–107 mmol/L

cholesterol, serum
    adult   desirable
            borderline
            high risk
    child (varies with age)
            age 1 to 4 years
            age 5 to 14 years
            age 15 to 20 years
	<200 mg/dL
	200–239 mg/dL
	≥240 mg/dL
	
	≤210 mg/dL
	≤220 mg/dL
	≤235 mg/dL
		<5.2 mmol/L
		5.2–6.2 mmol/L
		≥6.2 mmol/L
		
		≤5.4 mmol/L
		≤5.7 mmol/L
		≤6.1 mmol/L

coagulation tests
    antithrombin III
    (synthetic substrate)
    bleeding time (Duke)
    bleeding time (Ivy)
    bleeding time (template)
	80–120% of normal
	0–6 min
	1–6 min
	2.3–9.5 min
		0.8–1.2 of normal
		0–6 min
		1–6 min
		2.3–9.5 min

copper
    serum
        male
        female
	70–140 µg/dL
	80–155 µg/dL
		11–22µmol/L
		13–24µmol/L

cortisol, serum
    plasma (Hep, EDTA, Ox)
        8 a.m.
        4 p.m.
	5–23 µg/dL
	3–16 µg/dL
		138–635 nmol/L
		83–441 nmol/L

*creatinine
    serum or plasma, adult
        male
        female
	0.7–1.3 mg/dL
	0.6–1.1 mg/dL
		62–115 µmol/L
		53–97 µmol/L

ferritin, serum
    male
    female
	20–150 ng/mL
	10–120 ng/mL
		20–250 µg/L
		10–120 µg/L

*fibrinogen, plasma (NaCit)	200–400 mg/dL	2–4 g/L

glucose (fasting)
    blood
    plasma or serum
	65–95 mg/dL
	74–106 mg/dL
		3.5–5.3 mmol/L
		4.1–5.9 mmol/L

glucose, urine
    quantitative
    qualitative
	<500 mg/24 h
	negative
		<2.8 mmol/24 h
		negative

glucose, CSF	40–70 mg/dL	2.2–3.9 mmol/L

γ-glutamyltransferase
    (GGT), serum
    males
    females
	2–30 U/L (37°C)
	1–24 U/L (37°C)
		0.03–0.51 µkat/L (37°C)
		0.02–0.41 µkat/L (37°C)

continued

Tests	Conventional Units	SI Units
hematocrit		
newborns	53–65%	0.53–0.65
children (varies with age)	30–43%	0.30–0.43
hemoglobin (Hb)		
newborn	17.0–23.0 g/dL	2.64–3.57 mmol/L
children (varies with age)	11.2–16.5 g/dL	1.74–2.56 mmol/L
hemoglobin, fetal	≥1 y old: <2% of total Hb	≥1 y old: <0.02% of total Hb
hemoglobin electrophoresis whole blood (EDTA, Cit, or Hep)		
HbA	>95%	>0.95 Hb fraction
HbA$_2$	1.5–3.7%	0.015–0.37 Hb fraction
HbF	<2%	<0.02 Hb fraction
immunoglobulins, serum		
IgG	700–1600 mg/dL	7–16 g/L
IgA	70–400 mg/dL	0.7–4.0 g/L
IgM	40–230 mg/dL	0.42.3 g/L
IgD	0–8 mg/dL	0–80 mg/L
IgE	3–423 mg/dL	3–423kIU/L
*iron, serum		
males	65–175 µg/dL	11.6–31.3 µmol/L
females	50–170 µg/dL	9.0–30.4 µmol/L
*lactate dehydrogenase (LDH)		
newborn	290–775 U/L	4.9–13.2 µkat/L
neonate	545–2000 U/L	9.3–34 µkat/L
infant	180–430 U/L	3.1 7.3 µkat/L
child	110–295 U/L	1.9–5 µkat/L
lead, whole blood (Hep)	<25 µg/dL	<1.2 µmol/L
*lipase, serum	23–300 U/L (37°C)	0.39–5.1 µkat/L (37°C)
magnesium		
serum	1.3–2.1 mEq/L	0.65–1.07 mmol/L
	1.6–2.6 mg/dL	16–26 mg/L
osmolality		
urine	50–1200 mOsm/kg water	50–1200 mmol/kg water
oxygen, blood tension		
PO$_2$ arterial and capillary	83–108 mmHg	11.1–14.4 kPa
partial thromboplastin time activated (APTT)	<35 sec	<35 sec
pH		
blood, arterial	7.35–7.45	7.35–7.45
urine	4.6–8.0 (depends on diet)	same

continued

Tests	Conventional Units	SI Units
potassium		
serum		
premature		
cord	5.0–10.2 mmol/L	5.0–10.2 mmol/L
48 h	3.0–6.0 mmol/L	3.0–6.0 mmol/L
newborn cord	5.6–12.0 mmol/L	5.6–12.0 mmol/L
newborn	3.7–5.9 mmol/L	3.7–5.9 mmol/L
infant	4.1–5.3 mmol/L	4.1–5.3 mmol/L
child	3.4–4.7 mmol/L	3.4–4.7 mmol/L
*protein, serum		
total	6.4–8.3 g/dL	64–83 g/L
urine		
qualitative	negative	negative
quantitative	50–80 mg/24 h	50–80 mg/24 h
	(at rest)	(at rest)
CSF, total	8–32 mg/dL	80–320 mg/dL
*prothrombin time (PT)	12–14 sec	12–14 sec
sodium		
serum or plasma (Hep)		
premature		
cord	116–140mmol/L	116–140 mmol/L
48 h	128–148 mmol/L	128–148 mmol/L
newborn, cord	126–166 mmol/L	126–166 mmol/L
newborn	133–146 mmol/L	133–146 mmol/L
infant	139–146 mmol/L	139–146 mmol/L
child	138–145 mmol/L	138–145 mmol/L
specific gravity, urine	1.002–1.030	1.002–1.030
transferrin, serum		
newborn	130–275 mg/dL	1.30–2.75 g/L
triglycerides, serum, fasting		
desirable	<250 mg/dL	<2.83 mmol/L
urea nitrogen, serum	6–20 mg/dL	2.1–7.1 mmol Urea/L
*uric acid		
serum, enzymatic		
child	2.0–5.5 mg/dL	0.12–0.32 mmol/L

*Test values are method dependent.
Abbreviations: **CSF,** cerebrospinal fluid; **EDTA,** ethylenediaminetetraacetic acid; **Hep,** heparin; **Ox,** oxalate; **RBC,** red blood cell(s)

Apgar Score

After 60 seconds	Score	0	1	2
heart rate	—	absent	under 100	over 100
respiratory effort	—	absent	slow, irregular	good (screams)
muscle tone	—	limp	good in limbs	active movement
reaction to nasal catheter	—	none	makes grimaces	cough or sneezing
skin color	—	pale	rosy trunk, blue extremities	rosy
Score	—	(total points: 8–10 is normal)		

Developmental Milestones from Birth to 5 Years

Age (Months)	Adaptive/ Fine Motor	Language	Gross Motor	Personal-Social
1	Grasp reflex (hands fisted)	Facial response to sounds	Lifts head in prone position	Stares at face
2	Follows object with eyes past midline	Coos (vowel sounds)	Lifts head in prone position to 45°	Smiles in response to others
4	Hands open; brings objects to mouth	Laughs and squeals; turns toward voice	Sits; head steady; rolls to supine	Smiles spontaneously
6	Palmar grasp of objects	Babbles (consonant sounds)	Sits independently; stands, hands held	Reaches for toys; recognizes strangers
9	Pincer grasp	Says "mama," "dada" non-specifically; comprehends "no"	Pulls to stand	Feeds self; waves bye-bye
12	Helps turn pages of book	2–4 words; follows command with gesture	Stands independently; walks, one hand held	Points to indicate wants
15	Scribbles	4–6 words; follows command no gesture	Walks independently	Drinks from cup, imitates activities
18	Turns pages of book	10–20 words; points to 4 body parts	Walks up steps	Feeds self with spoon
24	Solves single-piece puzzles	Combines 2–3 words; uses "I" and "you"	Jumps; kicks ball	Removes coat; verbalizes wants
30	Imitates horizontal and vertical lines	Names all body parts	Rides tricycle using pedals	Pulls up pants; washes and dries hands
36	Copies circle; draws person with 3 parts	Gives full name, age, and sex; names 2 colors	Throws ball overhand; walks up stairs (alternating feet)	Toilet trained; puts on shirt, knows front from back
42	Copies cross	Understands "cold," "tired," "hungry"	Stands on one foot for 2–3 seconds	Engages in associative play

Age (Months)	Adaptive/ Fine Motor	Language	Gross Motor	Personal-Social
48	Counts 4 objects; identifies some numbers and letters	Understands prepositions (under, on, behind, in front of); asks "how" and "why"	Hops on one foot	Dresses with little assistance; shoes on correct feet
54	Copies square; draws person with 6 parts	Understands opposites	Broad-jumps 24 inches	Bosses and criticizes; shows off
60	Prints first name; counts 10 objects	Asks meaning of words	Skips (alternating feet)	Ties shoes

Appendix 5
Recommended Immunizations

Immunization	Recommended Age
Hepatitis B virus vaccine (Hep B)	# 1: Birth to 2 months # 2: 1 month to 4 months # 3: 6 months to 18 months
Diphtheria, Tetanus, Pertussis (DTaP)	2 months 4 months 6 months 15 months to 18 months 4 years to 6 years
Td	11 years to 16 years Every 10 years throughout life
Haemophilus influenzae type b (Hib)	2 months 4 months 6 months 12 months to 15 months
Inactivated Polio (IPV)	2 months 4 months 6 months to 18 months 4 years to 6 years
Pneumococcal Conjugate (PCV)	2 months 4 months 6 months 12 to 18 months
Measles, Mumps, Rubella (MMR)	12 months to 15 months 4 years to 6 years 11 years to 12 years
Varicella (Var)	12 months to 18 months 11 years to 12 years
Hepatitis A (Hep A)	24 months to 12 years (in selected areas)

For additional information, please visit the Centers for Disease Control and Prevention (CDC) National Immunization Program (NIP) web site at *http://www.cdc.gov/nip/*.

Appendix 6

Routine Immunization of HIV-Infected Children in the United States

Vaccine	Known Asymptomatic HIV Infection	Symptomatic HIV Infection
Hepatitis B	Yes	Yes
DTaP (or DTP)	Yes	Yes
IPV*	Yes	Yes
MMR	Yes	Yes[†]
HiB	Yes	Yes
Pneumococcal[‡]	Yes	Yes
Influenza[§]	Yes	Yes
Varicella[‖]	No	No

(Adapted from the American Academy of Pediatrics. In Peter G, ed. *1997 Red Book: Report of the Committee on Infectious Diseases.* 24th ed. Elk Grove Village, IL: American Academy of Pediatrics, 1997.)
DTP = diphtheria and tetanus toxoids and pertussis vaccine; DTaP = diphtheria and tetanus toxoids acellular pertussis vaccine; IPV = inactivated poliovirus vaccine; MMR = live-virus measles, mumps, and rubella; Hib = *Haemophilus influenzae* type b conjugate.
*Only IPV should be used for HIV-infected children, HIV-exposed infants who status is indeterminate, and household contacts of HIV-infected patients.
[†]Severely immunocompromised HIV-infected children should not receive MMR vaccine.
[‡]Pneumococcal vaccine should be administered at 2 years of age to all HIV-infected children. Children who are older than 2 years of age should receive pneumococcal vaccine at the time of diagnosis. Revaccination after 3 to 5 years is recommended in either circumstance.
[§]Influenza vaccine should be provided each fall and repeated annually for HIV-exposed infants 6 months of age and older, HIV-infected children and adolescents, and for house-hold contacts of HIV-infected patients.
[‖]Varicella vaccine is not currently indicated for HIV-exposed or HIV-infected patients, but studies are in progress to determine safety and possible indication.

Appendix 7
Oral Rehydration Fluids and Infant Formulas

Commercially Available Oral Rehydration Formulas

Lytren

Pedialyte

Rehydralyte

WHO Formula

Infant Formulas

Cow's milk-based standard formulas	Soy-based standard formulas	Preterm formulas	Special formulas #
Enfamil (Mead Johnson); with/without iron	Isomil (Ross)	Similac Special Care (Ross)	Nutramigen (Mead Johnson)
Similac (Ross); with/without iron	Prosobee (Mead Johnson)	Enfamil Premature (Mead Johnson); with/without iron	Pregestimil (Mead Johnson)
PM 60/40 (Ross)†		Similac Neocare (Ross)‖	Portagen (Mead Johnson)
Gerber; with/without iron (Gerber)			Alimentum (Ross)‖
Good Start (Carnation)†			Lactofree (Mead Johnson)
			Neocate (Scientific Hospital Supplies, Inc.)

†Formula with a low renal solute load. ‖Available only as ready-to-feed.

#Indications for Special Formulas:

Name	Indications
Nutramigen	Cow's milk allergy, severe or multiple food allergies, severe or persistent diarrhea, galactosemia
Pregestimil	Malabsorption, intestinal resection, severe or persistent diarrhea, food allergies
Portagen	Steatorrhea secondary to cystic fibrosis, intestinal reactions, pancreatic insufficiency, biliary atresia, lymphatic anomalies, celiac disease
Alimentum	Problems with digestion or absorption, severe or prolonged diarrhea, cystic fibrosis, steatorrhea, food allergies, intestinal resection
Lactofree	Lactose intolerance without cow's mild protein intolerance
Neocate	Cow's milk allergy, soy and protein hydrolysate intolerance, multiple food protein intolerance

Appendix 8

Poisonous Plants

Azalea
Buttercup
Calla Lily
Creeping Charlie (Ground Ivy)
Daffodil
Delphinium
Elderberry
Holly berries
Hyacinth bulbs
Hydrangea
Iris
Ivy (Boston and English)
Jimson Weed
Larkspur
Laurel
Lily-of-the-Valley
Mistletoe
Morning Glory
Nightshade
Periwinkle
Philodendron
Poison Ivy
Poison Oak
Rhododendron
Sweet Pea
Tomato vines
Tulip
Wisteria
Yew

Appendix 9

Sample Reports

ASTHMA: DISCHARGE SUMMARY

ADMISSION DIAGNOSIS: Status asthmaticus, hypoxia, and sinus arrhythmia.

HISTORY OF PRESENT ILLNESS: The patient is an 8-year-old male who presented to the emergency room with a history of wheezing. He is a known asthmatic. He presented with two days of shortness of breath and cough. Home management has consisted of Claritin, Singulair, and p.r.n. albuterol nebulization. Normal peak flows reported in the 250s. He has had no recent fever or viral illnesses.

ALLERGIES: Peanuts, soy, and eggs.

PHYSICAL EXAMINATION
GENERAL: On admission, the patient was a well-developed, well-nourished child in mild distress, well hydrated.
VITAL SIGNS: Pulse 124, respiratory rate 24, blood pressure 107/60 and temperature 98 orally.
SKIN: The skin was warm and dry with no rashes.
LYMPHATICS: No lymphadenopathy.
HEENT: There was fluid behind the left TM, but it was mobile. Otherwise, unremarkable.
NECK: Supple. Full range of movement.
CHEST: Regular rate and rhythm without murmurs. Good cap refill.
LUNGS: Bilateral inspiratory and expiratory wheezes present with subcostal and intercostal retractions. Fair aeration throughout.
ABDOMEN: Soft and nontender. Nondistended. Bowel sounds present. No hepatosplenomegaly or masses.
MUSCULOSKELETAL: Warm and well perfused. Moves all extremities.
NEUROLOGIC: Nonfocal. Alert and oriented, cooperative and talking.

HOSPITAL COURSE: The patient was initially evaluated in the emergency room and admitted to the pediatric ICU on continuous albuterol nebulization at 10 mg an hour, which he received for 30 hours and was then weaned to 2.5 mg nebs q.2h., which lengthened to q.4h. the same day. He was also treated with Solu-Medrol 4 mg/kg/d and discharged on steroids. He was treated with Atrovent nebs 0.5 mg q.4h. and chest PT q.4h. On admission to the PICU, he was maintained on IV fluids of D5 1/3 normal saline with 20 mEq of KCl/L at maintenance which was hep locked when he was tolerating a regular diet.

Another problem was hypoxia. On presentation to the emergency room, his saturations were 95% to 98%. On the night after admission to the PICU he did develop an oxygen requirement. On room air, saturations fell into the high 80s. The patient was on maximum of 2 liters a minute nasal cannula and was weaned to room air for approximately 18 hours prior to discharge.

Sinus arrhythmia: During admission, irregular heartbeat was noted on monitor. An EKG was obtained and read by cardiology as a sinus arrhythmia with no followup recommended. The patient was otherwise asymptomatic during hospitalization.

The patient was discharged to the care of his mother. Medications given were prednisone 20 mg p.o. b.i.d. times three days, albuterol nebs 2.5 mg q.4h., Singulair 5 mg p.o. daily, and Flovent MDI 44 mcg two puffs b.i.d. He is to follow up in one week.

CIRCUMCISION

PREOPERATIVE DIAGNOSIS: Congenital phimosis.

POSTOPERATIVE DIAGNOSIS: Congenital phimosis.

ANESTHESIA: None.

ESTIMATED BLOOD LOSS: Nil.

DESCRIPTION: This newborn infant was taken to the OB procedure room, prepped, and draped in the usual manner. After cleansing with chlorhexidine, the foreskin was grasped at the 2 and 10 o'clock position. Dorsal crush injury was created, and a dorsal slit was made. The foreskin was bluntly dissected away from the glans. It was taken down all of the way to the corona. A 1.1 Gomco bell was placed. The clamp was applied. The foreskin was sharply dissected away. The clamp was left on for a full five minutes. The clamp was removed. There was no evidence of congenital hypospadias. The infant tolerated the procedure and was taken back to his mother in good condition.

EPILEPSY IN A DEVELOPMENTALLY DELAYED CHILD: DISCHARGE SUMMARY

DISCHARGE DIAGNOSES
1. Status epilepticus.
2. Lissencephaly.
3. Scoliosis.
4. Hip contracture.
5. Gastrostomy tube.

CONSULTATION: Pediatric neurology.

HISTORY OF PRESENT ILLNESS: The patient is an 11-year-old female with lissencephaly and seizures who presented with status epilepticus. The patient's seizures have not been well controlled, and she had been on a maximum dose of vigabatrin. The neurologist had been attempting to wean off the vigabatrin and place the patient on zonisamide. The last dose adjustment was one week prior to admission. The patient routinely does well for several weeks, then has a "bad day" with breakthrough seizures which are treated with G tube nitrazepam. She has not required inpatient care for seizures in several years. She did have an increase in her seizure activity five days prior to admission and was managed at home. She had been back to her baseline status and then developed problems approximately 9:30 at school on the day of admission. She developed generalized tonic-clonic seizures which lasted longer than 30 minutes, so she was brought to the emergency department by EMS. There was no noted airway compromise. She was treated in the emergency department with a total of 7 mg of IV Ativan with a slowing in her seizure frequency but not a complete resolution. She was admitted to the pediatric intensive care unit for further management of her seizures.

PAST MEDICAL HISTORY: Lissencephaly diagnosed at four months of age. The patient does see, hear, and vocalizes, but she does not speak. She has a significant seizure disorder. Her seizures usually consist of myoclonic jerks and raising of her head. She also has the orthopedic problems previously mentioned of scoliosis and hip contractures. She had a history of a ruptured tympanic membrane one year ago and has a gastrostomy tube, although has no Nissen and no history of aspiration pneumonia.

FAMILY HISTORY: Noncontributory.

SOCIAL HISTORY: She lives with her parents and two siblings. She is in a special school during the day.

CURRENT MEDICATIONS
1. Vigabatrin 500 mg per G tube in the morning and 750 mg in the evening.

2. Topamax 67.5 mg via G tube b.i.d.
3. Zonisamide 25 mg via G tube in the morning and 100 mg in the evening.

ALLERGIES: There are no allergies.

REVIEW OF SYSTEMS: There has been no recent fever, illness, or ill contacts.

ADMITTING PHYSICAL EXAMINATION
GENERAL: She was sleeping and shivering. She was noted to be severely developmentally delayed, although she was somewhat responsive and in no significant distress.
VITAL SIGNS: Her blood pressure was 90/60, heart rate 150s, respiratory rate in the 20s, with a temperature of 100.3 after her seizure activity.
SKIN: Skin was warm and dry without rashes.
LYMPHATICS: No adenopathy.
HEENT: She was noted to have significant microcephaly with normal TMs and oropharynx.
NECK: Supple.
CHEST: Her lungs were clear with intermittent snoring. She did have good aeration and was apparently handling her secretions well.
CARDIAC: She had regular rate and rhythm without murmur, rub, or gallop. She was warm and well perfused distally.
ABDOMEN: Soft and nontender. G tube site clean, no hepatosplenomegaly.
MUSCULOSKELETAL: There was significant scoliosis and hip contractures.
NEUROLOGICAL: She was noted to have increased tone throughout. She was responsive and had spontaneous eye opening at times. She had frequent episodes of increased myoclonic tone in her neck and back tone. She did have a gag on admission.

HOSPITAL COURSE: The patient was admitted to the pediatric ICU and her hospital course was as follows:

NEUROLOGIC: The patient continued to have frequent myoclonic jerks throughout her first several hours of hospitalization. She had been given one dose of nitrazepam at home of 2.5 mg, and this was repeated several hours after her arrival in the PICU. At that time, her seizure activity seemed to wane, although she did become quite a bit more somnolent. She did, however, maintain good airway protective responses at all times. The patient remained somnolent for several hours and then awoke after about 10 hours in the PICU. At that point, she regained her baseline neurologic status. At the time of discharge, she was alert with eyes open and responsive and smiling at mom. She had had only two mild events overnight with no airway compromise. Her medications were discussed with her normal neurologist, and it was decided that her vigabatrin would be increased to 750 mg b.i.d. and her zonisamide increased to 50 mg in the morning and 100 mg in the evening. The Topamax would remain as it was previously prescribed.

RESPIRATORY SYSTEM: The patient maintained good saturations on room air throughout. She never appeared to aspirate and had no respiratory distress. She had clear lungs at the time of discharge.

CARDIOVASCULAR SYSTEM: She remained stable throughout with heart rates in the 120s and blood pressure in the 120s/60s.

FLUIDS, ELECTROLYTES, AND NUTRITION: The patient was started on Ensure feeds on the night after her admission, and she tolerated these very well through her G tube. She was transitioned to p.o. feeds on the morning of discharge and had no problems. Her abdomen was soft and nontender throughout, and her admitting electrolytes were unremarkable. Also, a calcium was normal at 9.0. Her glucose was slightly elevated at 231 after her seizure, and this was repeated the following morning and was 91. Her LFTs were within normal limits.

HEMATOLOGIC: She had a hematocrit on admission that was 34.5, platelet count 301, white count 10.6, with 68 polys, 26 lymphs, 5 monocytes, and 2 eosinophils.

INFECTIOUS DISEASE: She remained afebrile throughout her hospitalization and was started on no antibiotics as there was no evidence of bacterial infection.

The patient was discharged to home to the care of her mother. The mother stated that she was comfortable managing her at this point, and the patient had been stable overnight. She was instructed to go home on the following medications:
1. Vigabatrin 750 mg through the G tube b.i.d.
2. Topamax 67.5 mg through the G tube b.i.d.
3. Zonisamide 50 mg through the G tube q.a.m., 100 mg through the G tube q.h.s.
4. Nitrazepam 2.5 mg via G tube p.r.n. for increasing seizure activity as previously prescribed by her neurologist.

The mother was given instructions to call her neurologist or bring the patient back to the emergency department if her seizures became more frequent or if she had any respiratory compromise with them. She was instructed to make an appointment with the neurologist approximately one week after discharge. Her private medical doctor was called and agreed with the plan.

HYPERBILIRUBINEMIA: DISCHARGE SUMMARY

DISCHARGE DIAGNOSES
1. Live newborn female infant.
2. ABO incompatibility.
3. Hyperbilirubinemia.

PROCEDURE: Phototherapy.

HISTORY OF PRESENT ILLNESS: The baby is the 7-pound 8-ounce product of a 41-week gestation, born via spontaneous vaginal delivery to a 38-year-old, G2, P2 female. Apgar scores were 8 and 9.

PHYSICAL EXAMINATION: Physical exam upon admission to the newborn nursery revealed a normal infant who was noted to be slightly jaundiced at the time of the first physical exam. The rest of the exam at that point had been normal.

HOSPITAL COURSE: A bilirubin level drawn at approximately 14 hours of life revealed a total bilirubin of 1.06 with a direct of 0.1. The baby was started on phototherapy as well as a Bili-Blanket. The bilirubin level at 22 hours of life was 10.6. It was then repeated at 32 hours of life and was noted to be 10.9. At that point, the baby was transferred to the pediatric floor and phototherapy was continued. The baby's blood type was noted to be B positive, Coombs positive. The baby was breastfed, supplemented with formula, and improved.

The day after admission, the phototherapy was discontinued. A repeat bilirubin was checked and was noted to be 9.5. The baby was subsequently discharged to home with the mother to follow up in the office.

LUMBAR PUNCTURE

INDICATIONS: Rule out meningitis.

PROCEDURE SUMMARY: The patient was placed on a warmer and was held in a left lateral decubitus position. The spine was bent and after preparing the area with Betadine and draping in a sterile fashion, a 1½-inch long 22-gauge spinal needle with a stylet was introduced at the level of L4-L5. There was a small amount of clear CSF, which was collected in one tube. There was no further dripping of CSF for which another spinal needle was introduced at the level of L3-L4 with good CSF dripping back, which was collected in the first tube plus into other tubes. Total amount of CSF was about 3 cc, which was clear with some red blood cells noted in it. After collection of the tubes, the spinal needle was removed.

After cleaning with alcohol, the puncture wound was covered with a Band-Aid. The patient tolerated the procedure well with no complications. There was a drop of blood at the puncture wounds.

CSF will be sent in three separate tubes. Tube one will be for Gram stain, culture, and Bactigen panel. Tube two will be for chemistries, glucose, and protein. Tube three will be for cell count with differential.

MYRINGOTOMY

PREOPERATIVE DIAGNOSIS: Chronic otitis media.

POSTOPERATIVE DIAGNOSIS: Chronic otitis media.

ANESTHESIA: General.

COMPLICATIONS: None.

DESCRIPTION: The patient was brought to the operating room where general mask anesthesia was induced. With the use of an operating microscope, an anterior inferior myringotomy was performed on the left tympanic membrane, and through it no effusion was suctioned. An Armstrong tube was placed and ear drops following into the canal. With the use of an operating microscope, an anterior inferior myringotomy was performed on the right tympanic membrane, and through it no effusion was suctioned. An Armstrong tube was placed and ear drops following into the canal. The patient was awakened and taken to the recovery room in satisfactory condition.

NASAL PHARYNGOSCOPY AND BILATERAL TYMPANOSTOMY

PREOPERATIVE DIAGNOSIS: Bilateral recurrent otitis media with effusion.

POSTOPERATIVE DIAGNOSIS: Bilateral recurrent otitis media with effusion.

ANESTHESIA: Ultane, nitrous oxide, and oxygen.

NARRATIVE SUMMARY: In the supine position and under the above adequate general mask anesthesia, the patient was prepped and draped in the usual aseptic manner consistent for this procedure. Using the Zeiss operating microscope, the left tympanic membrane was visualized. The canal was cleaned of cerumen. A radial incision was made in the anteroinferior quadrant. "Glue" was found behind this ear, and this was suctioned. A 0.40 Shepard tube was put into place. Cortisporin Otic suspension drops were instilled, and a cotton ball was placed at the meatus. The right tympanic membrane was then visualized using the same Zeiss operating microscope. The canal was cleaned of cerumen. A radial incision was made in the anteroinferior quadrant.

The patient was then placed in a Rose position, and under apnea conditions, the McIvor mouthgag was quickly placed in the mouth. A red rubber catheter was placed in the right nostril and brought out through the mouth, thus retracting the palate. Using the laryngeal mirror, the adenoid tissue was found to be moderately enlarged. No adenoid tissue was removed. The red rubber catheter and McIvor mouthgag were quickly removed. The patient was then awakened and removed to the recovery room in apparent good condition.

NEONATOLOGY HISTORY AND PHYSICAL

HISTORY OF PRESENT ILLNESS: I was asked to see this child in the newborn nursery as a consultation because of tachypnea. Briefly, the patient is a full-term baby approximately 18 hours old. He was born to a 25-year-old, gravida 1, para 1 by normal spontaneous vaginal delivery. Apgar scores were 9, 9, and 9 at one, five, and ten minutes respectively. Birth weight was 9 pounds 4 ounces. There was no prolonged rupture of membranes or maternal temperature. The child's temperature was 101.4 rectally at delivery. The mother was rubella nonimmune, A positive, antibody negative, HIV negative, RPR nonreactive, alpha fetoprotein negative, and hepatitis B negative with a normal glucose tolerance test. She was also group B *Streptococcus* negative.

At 12 hours of age, the patient was noted by his primary pediatrician to have an increased respiratory rate. Chest x-ray was obtained and found to have a normal cardiothymic silhouette with primary pulmonary markings without infiltrate or pneumothorax. The patient remained tachypneic yet saturated 100% in room air. No cyanosis was noted. On observation in special-care nursery, the child desaturated twice into the 80s, continued to have respiratory rates in the 80s, and is now admitted to the special-care nursery for transient tachypnea of the newborn versus rule out sepsis.

PHYSICAL EXAMINATION
VITAL SIGNS: On admission, temperature is 98.3, heart rate 126 to 150, respirations 62 to 80, oxygen saturation 100% on room air, blood pressure 62/42.
HEENT: Examination reveals an abrasion on the scalp. Anterior fontanel is open and soft. Mucous membranes are moist. There is no cleft palate. Extraocular movements are intact. Pupils are equally round and reactive to light. The oropharynx is clear. There is no nasal flaring.
CHEST: Clear to auscultation bilaterally without retractions.
CARDIAC: Examination reveals a regular rate and rhythm without murmur.
ABDOMEN: Soft and not tender, not distended, with positive bowel sounds. No hepatosplenomegaly.
EXTREMITIES: Show no cyanosis, clubbing, or edema.
GENITOURINARY: Reveals a normal male with testes descended bilaterally.
NEUROLOGIC: Examination reveals a positive suck, Moro, and grasp with movements of all four extremities.

LABORATORIES: Includes an initial white count of 29.0 with a differential of 56 neutrophils, 14 bands, 24 lymphocytes, and 4 monocytes. Hemoglobin is 18.2, hematocrit 53.5 with 289 platelets. Blood culture is pending. Glucose results by Dextrostix are 59 and 62.

PLAN

1. Admit the child to the special-care nursery.
2. Maintain the child n.p.o. and on intravenous fluids for now.
3. Place the child on ampicillin and gentamicin while blood cultures are followed in the laboratory.

PREMATURE INFANT DISCHARGE SUMMARY

DISCHARGE DIAGNOSES

1. Premature male infant, 24 to 25 weeks' gestation, appropriate for gestational age.
2. Respiratory failure.
3. Severe respiratory distress syndrome/pulmonary interstitial emphysema.
4. Intraventricular hemorrhage, grade 4.
5. Hypotension.
6. Patent ductus arteriosus, treated with Indocin.
7. Anemia.
8. Hyperbilirubinemia.
9. Suspected sepsis.
10. Pneumoperitoneum and probable necrotizing enterocolitis.

ADMITTING HISTORY

The baby is 728 grams birth weight at admission, extremely premature male infant, delivered by emergency cesarean section for footling breech presentation and vaginal bleeding with preterm labor. The infant was 25-5/7 weeks' gestation by dates, but by examination the infant's maturity was 24–25 weeks AGA.

Mother had prenatal care. Mother is married, gravida 3, para 0-1-1-0. Mother's blood type O, Rh positive, rubella immune, RPR nonreactive, hepatitis B surface antigen negative. She had a previous 24-week gestation premature baby, who expired with grade 4 intraventricular hemorrhage and necrotizing enterocolitis.

The infant's Apgar scores were 4 at one minute, 5 at five minutes, and 5 at ten minutes. The infant was intubated at birth and given positive pressure ventilation. Umbilical venous catheterization was done. First dose of Survanta was given by the transport team. Antibiotics were started. The infant was transported on a ventilator.

PHYSICAL EXAMINATION AT ADMISSION

GENERAL: Examination on admission revealed an extremely premature male infant. The skin was shiny and transparent. There were several areas of bruising noted over all extremities, and bruising was noted on the scalp and over the back. The skin over the feet was breaking down. Extremities were cool to touch. The infant's color was pale pink, with no external congenital anomalies noted.

VITAL SIGNS: Temperature 36°C rectally. Heart rate 178 per minute. Respiratory rate 60 per minute, which was same as intermittent mandatory ventilation. Blood pressure 24/14 mmHg. Weight 728g, head circumference 23 cm, length 33 cm.

HEAD: Anterior fontanel open and soft, sutures approximated.

EYES: Revealed tightly fused eyelids.

EARS: Normally placed. Pinnae were flat and folded easily.

NOSE: Nares patent.

MOUTH: Palate intact.

NECK: No masses.

CHEST/HEART: Moderate chest retractions. Bilateral breath sounds were equal, with rales. There was no heart murmur heard. Normal sinus rhythm. Precordium was quiet. Pulses were palpable. Capillary filling time was about 3 seconds.

ABDOMEN: Soft, no distention. No organomegaly noted.

ANUS: Patent. The infant passed stools.

GENITALIA: Scrotum was very small. Left testicle was palpable in the inguinal canal. Right testicle was not palpable.

EXTREMITIES: Full range of motion.

BACK AND SPINE: Intact.

NEUROLOGIC: The infant was not very active but was responding to stimulation. Spontaneous respirations were present. Suck was absent. Grasp was weak. No seizures. Muscle tone was hypotonic but appropriate for gestation.

HOSPITAL COURSE

RESPIRATORY FAILURE/RESPIRATORY DISTRESS SYNDROME/PULMONARY INTERSTITIAL EMPHYSEMA:

The infant's admission chest x-ray revealed severe respiratory distress syndrome. The infant was placed on conventional ventilator with initial settings of SIMV 60, PIP 18, PEEP +4, FIO_2 1.0. Umbilical arterial catheterization was done under sterile conditions for blood gas monitoring. The previous umbilical venous catheter was replaced due to malposition. Arterial blood gases were followed. The infant was given second and third doses of Survanta at 12-hour intervals. There was some improvement, with decrease in oxygen requirement for some time; but again, the infant's oxygen requirement went up to 100%, and there was respiratory acidosis on arterial blood gases. Therefore, ventilator was changed to a high-frequency oscillatory ventilator on day ___. The infant was on high-frequency oscillatory ventilator from day ___ until day ___, when the respirator was changed to a conventional ventilator due to low ventilator settings. The infant had to be placed back on a high-frequency oscillatory ventilator the next day on day ___. Ventilators were switched a few times between high-frequency oscillatory ventilator and conventional ventilator. Due to the development of severe cystic BPD and pulmonary interstitial emphysema, especially in the left lung with hyperinflation of the left lung, the infant was placed on his left side for a few days. Also, the endotracheal tube was advanced to the right main stem bronchus to ventilate only the right lung and to achieve atelectasis of the left lung, which was successful. There was a lot of improvement in the lung fields of both right and left lungs. The infant's respiratory settings could be reduced. The infant was given intravenous hydrocortisone starting on day ___. Hydrocortisone was discontinued and Decadron was started on day ___, for bronchopulmonary dysplasia. Aminophylline was started on day ___. Arterial blood gases were followed as needed. On day ___, the infant's ventilator settings were SIMV 30, PIP 16, PEEP +4 and oxygen requirement was about 30%.

INTRAVENTRICULAR HEMORRHAGE, GRADE 4: Head ultrasound test, done on day ___, reported a large intraventricular hemorrhage in the left frontal horn, extending into the adjacent left frontal lobe. Blood was also seen attached to the atria of both lateral ventricles, right greater than left. Blood was seen layering the occipital horns bilaterally. The lateral ventricles were dilated, right greater than left. No other parenchymal hemorrhage was seen. Head ultrasound, repeated on day ___, reported ventricular dilatation, right greater than left, similar to the prior study, interval partial resorption of bilateral intraventricular as well as left periventricular hemorrhage. No new hemorrhage was seen. The infant was started on phenobarbital prophylactically soon after admission. There were no clinical seizures noted. The infant's anterior fontanel was soft and was not bulging. Sagittal sutures were approximated.

HYPOTENSION: The infant's admission blood pressure was low, 24/14 mmHg. The infant was started on intravenous dopamine infusion at 5 mcg/kg/min. Also, packed red blood cell transfusion was given due to low hematocrit of 35%. This helped to improve blood pressure. Dopamine was discontinued on the third day, since the infant's blood pressure had improved.

PATENT DUCTUS ARTERIOSUS, TREATED WITH INDOCIN: On the third day of life, echocardiogram was done to rule out patent ductus arteriosus. No heart murmur was heard clinically. The echocardiogram reported patent ductus arteriosus with at least mild to moderate amount of left-to-right shunt, some dilatation of the right ventricle with slight tricuspid regurgitation, and estimated right ventricular systolic pressure of approximately 30 mmHg, which was approximately two-thirds of the systemic blood pressure. The infant was treated with one course of indomethacin. Echocardiogram was repeated on day ___. The test reported that ductus arteriosus was no longer detected at this time. Right atrium and right ventricle were not dilated. Slight tricuspid regurgitation was present with an estimated right ventricular systolic pressure of 35 mmHg, which was approximately 62% of systemic pressure. Some degree of right ventricular hypertension, therefore, appeared to still be present. Echocardiogram was repeated again on day ___ for reevaluation and to rule out any evidence for hypertrophic cardiomyopathy secondary to Decadron use. The echocardiogram reported normal study. There was no evidence of patent ductus arteriosus. There was no evidence of septal hypertrophy.

ANEMIA: The infant's admission hematocrit was 35%. He was transfused with 10 cc/kg of packed red blood cells due to anemia and hypotension. The infant required two packed red blood cell transfusions during the first three days of life, which was probably secondary to intraventricular hemorrhage. During the infant's hospital stay a total of at least six red blood cell transfusions were given for low hematocrit, due to the infant's extreme prematurity and respiratory support needed.

HYPERBILIRUBINEMIA: The mother's blood type is O Rh positive. The infant's blood type is A Rh negative. Mother's antibody screen was negative. Direct Coombs IgG was negative. The infant was started on prophylactic phototherapy soon after admission due to severe bruising over the scalp and over the extremities, as well as bruising over the trunk. Bilirubin levels were followed. Phototherapy was discontinued on day ___. Peak bilirubin level was 5.1 total and indirect bilirubin 4.4.

SUSPECTED SEPSIS: The infant's initial CBC was within normal limits, with white blood cell count of 19,200 and normal differential count. Platelet count was 229,000. The infant was started on intravenous ampicillin and gentamicin prior to transport. Admission blood culture was negative. Nose and rectal cultures were negative. On day ___, gentamicin was discontinued and cefotaxime was started due to oliguria. Ampicillin and cefotaxime were discontinued on day five of life since both admission blood cultures were negative. On day ___, during the night, there was a small area of bluish-green discoloration noted over the lower abdomen, on the left side, which had spread over the lower abdomen and peripherally over the upper abdominal skin. The abdomen was not distended. The abdomen was very soft. On removing the tape of the bridge for umbilical artery catheter and umbilical venous catheter, it was noted that there was an area of skin break down and an abrasion 3 x 0.4 cm with oozing of serous fluid. Culture from this abdominal wound area was sent for bacterial cultures and fungal culture. Also, blood cultures were drawn from a peripheral site, from the umbilical artery catheter, and from the umbilical venous catheter for both bacterial cultures and fungal cultures. The infant's CBC on day ___ was abnormal with elevated white blood cell count to 41,700, with shift to the left on differential count. Platelet count was low at 69,000. A pediatric infectious disease specialist was consulted. As per the specialist's recommendation, cultures for bacteria and fungi were sent, as mentioned above. The infant was started on intravenous antibiotic therapy with intravenous Zosyn, which had piperacillin plus tazobactam. The infant was also started on intravenous tobramycin. Intravenous Zosyn and tobramycin were started for gram-positive as well as gram-negative coverage, including *Pseudomonas aeruginosa*. Due to presence of hyphal elements seen on Gram stain of the abdominal wound site, the infant was started on intravenous amphotericin B. Also, topical amphotericin B ointment was started for the abdominal skin wound. There was no hepatomegaly. The urine output was decent. The abdomen was soft and nondistended. All three blood cultures were negative. The tip of the umbilical venous catheter culture was also negative. The abdominal site culture reported moderate *Staphylococcus epidermidis,* a few *Aspergillus, Fumigatus,* and fungal culture from the left knee area site reported growing a few *Candida parapsilosis.* The infant was given a test dose of amphotericin B on day ___, and then amphotericin B was given daily intravenously over four to six hours. The discoloration over the abdomen seemed to be resolving, and the abdominal wound of abrasion area began to heal. Intravenous Zosyn and Tobramycin were discontinued on day ___. Intravenous amphotericin B and topical amphotericin B were continued. Followup CBC showed improvement with white blood cell count of 17,400 on day ___, with normal differential count and platelet count of 333,000. The infant was transfused with volume-depleted platelet transfusion once on day ___.

PNEUMOPERITONEUM AND PROBABLE NECROTIZING ENTEROCOLITIS:
This infant has never been fed and was given intravenous total parenteral nutrition during his hospital course. There was no organomegaly or palpable abdominal mass noted at any time. Several abdominal x-rays were followed. There was paucity of bowel gas seen when sepsis was suspected on day ___, but followup x-ray showed bowel gas which was mainly seen over the left side of the abdomen. There was no intramural air or pneumatosis intestinalis noted on abdominal x-rays. There was no significant bowel dilatation. Since ___, the infant's respiratory status had much improved with improvement seen in the lung fields on chest x-ray; the infant's ventilator settings could be lowered considerably. Unfortunately, on the morning of day ___, the infant's abdomen was soft and slightly distended, and on x-rays of the abdomen a large pneumoperitoneum was seen. Due to probable bowel perforation and necrotizing enterocolitis, the infant was started on intravenous clindamycin and gentamicin. Also, fresh frozen plasma 10 cc/kg was given. Arrangements were made for transport to ___ Hospital for surgical evaluation and further necessary treatment.

The infant's parents were informed, and they came to visit the infant in the neonatal intensive care unit prior to transport of the infant to ___ Hospital. The parents were made aware that this is a very serious problem and that the infant's prognosis is guarded.

RIGHT HERNIORRHAPHY WITH HYDROCELECTOMY

PROCEDURE: The patient was identified in the preop holding area and taken to the operating room where he was placed in supine position. General anesthesia was induced and the abdomen prepped with Betadine and draped out in sterile fashion. This included the genital and perineal area. A scalpel incision was made in the right groin overlying the inguinal canal in line with the skin crease. This was carried down with blunt dissection to Scarpa fascia, which was divided sharply and further blunt dissection carried down to the aponeurosis. Inferior aspect of the aponeurosis was identified and followed down to the external ring. The external ring was identified and a hemostat inserted through this before dividing the most distal aspect of the aponeurosis at the ring. Cremasteric fibers were then lifted and divided sharply, identifying the underlying cord structures. Hydrocele sac was identified in the anteromedial aspect, and the cord structures including the vas and vascular structures were identified and dissected free from this with gentle blunt dissection. A vascular loop was used for retraction of these structures away from the hydrocele sac. As it was dissected free, its distal end stopped midcord, not extending down in the scrotum. The proximal aspect was followed all the way up to the internal ring where its border was identified until retraction showed preperitoneal fat. Here it was suture ligated and simple ligated with 3–0 PDS before dividing 0.5 cm distal to the ties. This was passed off as a specimen. Inspection was undertaken and showed good hemostasis. The external aponeurosis was closed down to the external ring with a running suture. Scarpa and subcutaneous tissues were reapproximated with simple interrupted absorbable sutures. Monocryl 5–0 was used to reapproximate the skin edges in running subcuticular fashion. Mastisol and Steri-Strips were applied, and the procedure was terminated. The patient tolerated the procedure well and was transferred to the recovery room in stable condition.

SICKLE CELL DISEASE: DISCHARGE SUMMARY

PRIMARY DIAGNOSIS: Sickle thalassemia disease.

SECONDARY DIAGNOSES
1. Pain crisis.
2. Sympathetic left knee effusion.

HISTORY OF PRESENT ILLNESS: The patient is a 15-year-old African-American male who presented to the emergency room on the morning of admission with a history of knee pain and bilateral ankle pain. The patient had no fever at the time but was in severe pain. He gave a scale of 10/10 for the pain. The patient was seen in the emergency room and started on intravenous fluids and narcotic medication. The patient received several doses of narcotics, including morphine and Dilaudid, and had intermittent relief. Over the course of the day, the patient had persistent pain, and I was called by the emergency room staff to evaluate this patient for admission.

On arrival to the emergency room, the patient was found to be in acute distress. His temperature at that time had been elevated to 101, and he was lying in bed crying with the report of pain in his left knee and both ankles. At the time, the physical exam was benign. He had tenderness over the left patella region with no evidence of swelling. The patient also had slight tachycardia at the time. Oxygen saturations were 95% on room air, and he had no respiratory distress. His laboratory studies in the emergency room showed normal white count and acceptable hemoglobin level. After discussion with the hematologist, the decision was made to admit him for management of his pain and assessment of his fever.

HOSPITAL COURSE: The patient was admitted to the pediatric floor and was started on intravenous ceftriaxone and patient-controlled analgesic. His pump was set at 3.5 mg morphine per hour. This was weaned gradually over the course of the next few days, and after 48 hours, the patient was switched to oral pain medicine with good control. Also during the course of the illness, the patient developed swelling of his left knee joint. This was evaluated by orthopedics who diagnosed sympathetic knee effusion in that joint. His ankles remained painful, but he had no objective lesions present. In evaluating the left knee swelling, a bone scan was done to rule out osteomyelitis, and this came back negative. Also during the course of admission, the patient hemolyzed his hemoglobin from 8.4 down to 6.4 gm/dl, and he received two units of compatible packed red cells. The repeat hemoglobin after this was 8.8 gm/dl.

During the course of the patient's admission, he had a chest x-ray which showed increase in his cardiac silhouette for which he had a cardiac consult and an echocardiogram which showed some left ventricular hypertrophy but without any pericardial involvement and no symptomatology.

On the physical examination on admission, the patient was found to be in acute distress in the emergency room. His temperature at that time was 101 axillary. His pulse was 94. Respiratory rate was 20. On exam, his neck was supple. His tympanic membranes were clear. His throat was without exudate or erythema. He had equal and reactive pupils. He had no jaundice at this point. The jaundice developed on the second day of admission in his sclerae, and this cleared prior to discharge. On cardiovascular exam, the patient had regular tachycardia and had a 2/6 systolic ejection murmur over the left sternal border and base of the heart consistent with a flow murmur secondary to chronic hemolytic process (anemia). His lungs were clear bilaterally. He had no chest pain and no respiratory distress. The abdomen was benign, soft, and nontender. No organomegaly was noted. Neurologically he was intact, and extremities were positive for left knee pain, especially around the anterior lower aspect of the knee joint, and positive soft tissue swelling on the second day of admission, with a difference of 3 cm between his left and right knees. There was no skin erythema or rash seen.

LABORATORY STUDIES DURING ADMISSION: The patient was admitted with a hemoglobin of 8.3 gm/dl, and this went down to 6.4 gm/dl. On the second day of admission, he received two packed red blood cell units to correct his anemia, and this was brought back up to 8.8 gm/dl on discharge home. The patient had a very mildly elevated white count on admission with a normal differential. He had not much bandemia, and on discharge his leukocytosis had resolved.

Other relevant laboratory studies and workup during admission: The patient had an HIV and CMV, which were negative. He had chemistries and liver function tests, which were within normal limits. He also had blood cultures, which were negative. Urine was within normal limits. Bone scan was normal. Hip film of his left hip to rule out avascular necrosis was normal. The chest x-ray was unremarkable for any focal infiltrate.

DISPOSITION ON DISCHARGE: After five days of intravenous hydration, IV antibiotics and pain control, the patient had recovery from his pain crisis and hemolytic crisis. He went home on the following medications: Percocet one to two tablets every four to six hours as needed for pain, Colace for constipation, and he was to continue his regular prophylactic penicillin and folic acid for his sickle cell disease.

On discharge home, the patient was without much pain in his knee. He had grade 2/10 pain in his left knee, and he was to use hot packs as needed for symptomatic treatment of his left knee effusion. Followup with his pediatrician in one week and followup with the orthopedist in one week also.

TONSILLECTOMY AND ADENOIDECTOMY: CHRONIC ADENOID TONSILLITIS

PREOPERATIVE DIAGNOSIS: Chronic adenoid tonsillitis.

POSTOPERATIVE DIAGNOSIS: Chronic adenoid tonsillitis.

ANESTHESIA: General.

COMPLICATIONS: None.

DESCRIPTION: The patient was brought to the operating room where general anesthesia was induced and maintained through an endotracheal tube. A Crowe-Davis mouthgag was inserted and red rubber Robinson passed through the nose and retrieved through the oropharynx for retraction of the palate. An adenoid curette was used to remove the adenoid tissue from the nasopharynx. Hemostasis was obtained with electrocautery. The left tonsil was grasped, and using electrocautery it was dissected from the fossa and transected at the base. The right tonsil was removed in a similar manner. The patient was awakened, extubated, and then taken to the recovery room in satisfactory condition.

TONSILLECTOMY AND ADENOIDECTOMY: OBSTRUCTIVE SLEEP APNEA SECONDARY TO TONSILLAR AND ADENOID HYPERTROPHY

PREOPERATIVE DIAGNOSIS: Obstructive sleep apnea secondary to tonsillar and adenoid hypertrophy.

POSTOPERATIVE DIAGNOSIS: Obstructive sleep apnea secondary to tonsillar and adenoid hypertrophy.

ANESTHESIA: Ultane, nitrous oxide, and oxygen with 0.25% Marcaine with 1:100,000 units of epinephrine local.

NARRATIVE SUMMARY: In the supine position and under the above adequate general endotracheal anesthetic, the patient was prepped and draped in the usual aseptic manner consistent with this procedure.

With the patient in the Rose position, the McIvor mouthgag was placed in the mouth, thus retracting the tongue. A red rubber catheter was placed in the right nostril and brought out through the mouth, thus restricting the palate. It was difficult getting this through the nose. Using the laryngeal mirror, the adenoid tissue was found to be very enlarged and totally obstructing the back of the nose. Using midline and lateral sweeps of the adenoid curette, the vast majority of the adenoid tissue was removed and sent to pathology for diagnosis. Hemostasis was secured with electrocautery and adenoid pack. It must be noted a rim of adenoidal tissue was left inferiorly for closure of the palate.

The right tonsil was clamped with a curved Allis clamp. An incision was made in the anterior, superior, and posterior pillar mucosa. The capsule was delineated, and capsule and tonsillar tissue was dissected free of the underlying muscle. Using the electrocautery, the tonsil was amputated at its base and sent to pathology for diagnosis. Using the electrocautery, hemostasis was secured.

The left tonsil was then clamped with a curved Allis clamp. Significant cryptitis was present. The purulent material that was extruded was cultured and sent to pathology for culture and sensitivity. An incision was made in the anterior, superior, and posterior pillar mucosa. The capsule was delineated, and capsule and tonsillar tissue were dissected free of the underlying muscle. Using the electrocautery, the tonsil was amputated at its base and sent to pathology for diagnosis. Hemostasis was secured with electrocautery.

A solution of 0.25% Marcaine with 1:100,000 units of epinephrine was injected into the tonsillar fossas for pain control. The uvula was slit posteriorly with a #12 blade in the usual manner. The mouth then was irrigated and suctioned.

The red rubber catheter was removed. The McIvor mouthgag was removed.

The patient was then awakened and removed to the recovery room in apparent good condition.

UMBILICAL VEIN CATHETERIZATION, UMBILICAL ARTERY CATHETERIZATION

UMBILICAL VEIN CATHETERIZATION INDICATION: Need for IV fluids.

The patient was placed on the warmer. After restraining the extremities, the umbilical area was prepared with Betadine while the umbilical stump was held by a nurse. The base of the umbilical stump was tied with a piece of tape. The umbilical stump was then cut with a #11 blade at about 0.5 cm to the skin. After identifying the umbilical vein, a 5.0 single-lumen catheter was introduced and fixed at 11 cm. Followup x-ray showed a loop of the catheter almost at the level of the point of entry in the umbilical stump. The tip of the catheter was at the level of the liver not passing the level of the diaphragm. This catheter was removed, and another 5.0 single-lumen catheter was introduced. Followup x-ray showed the tip in the right ventricle for which the catheter was withdrawn a few centimeters and again fixed at about 11 cm showing the tip of the catheter in good position. The patient tolerated the procedure well and with no complications. There was a small amount of bleeding.

UMBILICAL ARTERY CATHETERIZATION INDICATION: Respiratory distress, need to monitor blood gases.

The patient was prepared and draped as above. After having placed the umbilical vein catheter, one of the umbilical arteries was identified and its lumen was dilated using forceps. A 3.5 single-lumen catheter was then introduced and fixed at 10 cm using 3–0 silk. Followup x-ray shows the tip of the catheter in good position at the level of L4. The patient tolerated the procedure well and with no complications. There was no bleeding.

Common Terms by Procedure

Asthma: Discharge Summary
aeration
albuterol nebulization
Atrovent
cap refill
chest PT
Claritin
continuous albuterol nebulization
D5 1/3 normal saline
EKG
electrocardiogram (EKG)
Flovent metered dose inhaler (MDI)
hepatosplenomegaly
hypoxia
intercostal retraction
irregular heartbeat
KCl
mcg
mEq
microgram (mcg)
milliequivalent (mEq)
nasal cannula
normal peak flow
pediatric intensive care unit (PICU)
PICU
potassium chloride (KCl)
prednisone
room air
saturation
shortness of breath
Singulair
sinus arrhythmia
Solu-Medrol
status asthmaticus
steroid
subcostal retraction
wheezing

Circumcision
chlorhexidine

congenital epispadias
congenital hypospadias
congenital phimosis
corona
dorsal crush injury
dorsal slit
foreskin
glans
Gomco bell

Epilepsy in a Developmentally Delayed Child: Discharge Summary
airway protection response
aspirate
aspiration pneumonia
Ativan
electrolyte
Ensure
eosinophil
G tube
gastrostomy tube
generalized tonic-clonic seizure
hepatosplenomegaly
hip contracture
lissencephaly
liver function test (LFT)
LFT
lymph
microcephaly
monocyte
myoclonic jerk
Nissen
pediatric intensive care unit (PICU)
PICU
polymorphonuclear leukocyte (poly)
scoliosis
seizure
somnolent
status epilepticus
Topamax

vigabatrin
zonisamide

Hyperbilirubinemia: Discharge Summary

Apgar score
Bili-Blanket
bilirubin level
blood group system (ABO) incompatibility
blood type B positive
breastfed
Coombs test
G2, P2
gestation
hyperbilirubinemia
jaundice
phototherapy
spontaneous vaginal delivery

Lumbar Puncture

Bactigen panel
Band-Aid
Betadine
CSF
cell count
cerebrospinal fluid (CSF)
chemistries
differential
22-gauge spinal needle
glucose
Gram stain
left lateral decubitus
meningitis
puncture wound
stylet
warmer

Myringotomy

anterior inferior myringotomy
Armstrong tube
chronic otitis media
effusion
general mask anesthesia

operating microscope
tympanic membrane

Nasal Pharyngoscopy and Bilateral Tympanostomies

adenoid tissue
anteroinferior quadrant
apnea
cerumen
Cortisporin Otic suspension drops
cotton ball
general mask anesthesia
laryngeal mirror
McIvor mouthgag
meatus
nasal pharyngoscopy
nitrous oxide
nostril
oxygen
palate
radial incision
red rubber catheter
Rose position
supine position
Ultane
Zeiss operating microscope

Neonatology History and Physical

alpha fetoprotein
ampicillin
anterior fontanel
Apgar score
band
birth weight
blood culture
cardiothymic silhouette
cleft palate
cyanosis
Dextrostix
gentamicin
gestational age
glucose tolerance test

gravida 1, para 1
group B *Streptococcus*
hematocrit
hemoglobin
hepatitis B
HIV
human immunodeficiency virus (HIV)
lymphocyte
monocyte
Moro (reflex)
nasal flaring
neutrophil
normal spontaneous vaginal delivery
oxygen saturation 100% on room air
platelet
positive suck
RPR nonreactive
rubella nonimmune
rupture of membrane
sepsis
special-care nursery
tachypnea

Premature Infant Discharge Summary
AGA
aminophylline
amphotericin B
ampicillin
anemia
anterior fontanel
appropriate for gestational age (AGA)
approximated
arterial blood gas
Aspergillus
atelectasis
bacterial culture
bilateral breath sound
bilateral intraventricular hemorrhage
bilirubin
blood gas monitoring
blood type A
blood type O

bowel dilatation
bowel perforation
bronchopulmonary dysplasia
Candida parapsilosis
capillary filling time
CBC
cefotaxime
chest x-ray
clindamycin
clinical seizure
complete blood (cell) count (CBC)
conventional ventilator
cystic bronchopulmonary dysplasia (BPD)
Decadron
differential count
dilated
direct Coombs test
dopamine
echocardiogram
emergency cesarean section
endotracheal tube
external congenital anomaly
FIO_2
footling breech presentation
fresh frozen plasma
Fumigatus
fungal culture
fused eyelid
gentamicin
gestation
gestational age
Gram stain
gram-negative coverage
gram-positive coverage
grasp
gravida 3, para 0-1-1-0
head circumference
head ultrasound test
heart murmur
hematocrit
hepatitis B surface antigen negative
hepatomegaly

high-frequency oscillatory ventilator
hydrocortisone
hyperbilirubinemia
hyperinflation
Hyphal element
hypotension
hypotonic
IgG
immunoglobulin G (IgG)
indirect bilirubin
Indocin
indomethacin
inguinal canal
intermittent mandatory ventilation
interval partial resorption
intramural air
intravenous total parental nutrition
intraventricular hemorrhage
left frontal horn
left frontal lobe
left-to-right shunt
mainstem bronchus
malposition
millimeters of mercury (mmHg)
mmHg
moderate chest retraction
muscle tone
nares patent
necrotizing enterocolitis
normal sinus rhythm
occipital horn
organomegaly
packed red blood cell transfusion
parenchymal hemorrhage
patent ductus arteriosus
paucity
peak end-expiratory pressure (PEEP)
peak inspiratory pressure (PIP)
PEEP
periventricular hemorrhage
phenobarbital
pinna
PIP

piperacillin
platelet count
platelet transfusion
pneumatosis intestinalis
pneumoperitoneum
positive pressure ventilation
precordium
preterm labor
prophylactic phototherapy
prophylactically
Pseudomonas aeruginosa
pulmonary interstitial emphysema
rale
respirator
respiratory acidosis
respiratory distress syndrome
respiratory failure
Rh negative
Rh positive
right atrium
right ventricle
right ventricular hypertension
right ventricular systolic pressure
RPR nonreactive
rubella immune
sagittal suture
scrotum
seizure
sepsis
septal hypertrophy
serous fluid
severe respiratory distress syndrome
SIMV 30
SIMV 60
spontaneous intermittent mandatory
  ventilation (SIMV) 30
spontaneous intermittent mandatory
  ventilation (SIMV) 60
spontaneous respiration
Staphylococcus epidermidis
sterile condition
suck
Survanta

sutures approximated
tazobactam
tightly fused eyelid
tobramycin
total bilirubin
transport team
tricuspid regurgitation
umbilical arterial catheterization
umbilical venous catheter
umbilical venous catheterization
vaginal bleeding
ventilator
ventricular dilation
white blood cell count
Zosyn

Right Herniorrhaphy With Hydrocelectomy

3–0 PDS
anteromedial aspect
aponeurosis
Betadine
blunt dissection
cord structure
cremasteric fiber
divided sharply
draped in sterile fashion
external ring
general anesthesia
groin
hemostasis
hydrocele sac
hydrocele scar
inguinal canal
internal ring
Mastisol
midcord
Monocryl 5–0
preperitoneal fat
running subcuticular fashion
Scarpa fascia
scrotum
simple ligated
skin crease

Steri-Strip
subcutaneous tissue
supine position
suture ligated
vas deferens
vascular loop
vascular structure

Sickle Cell Disease: Discharge Summary

2/6 systolic ejection murmur
acute distress
anemia
avascular necrosis focal infiltrate
bandemia
bone scan
cardiac silhouette
ceftriaxone
chest x-ray
chronic hemolytic process
CMV
cytomegalovirus (CMV)
Colace
Dilaudid
echocardiogram
erythema
exudate
flow murmur
folic acid
hemolytic crisis
hemolyzed
HIV
human immunodeficiency virus (HIV)
hot pack
jaundice
left sternal border
leukocytosis
morphine
organomegaly
osteomyelitis
oxygen saturation
packed red blood cell
packed red cell
pain scale 10/10

patella region
patient-controlled analgesic
penicillin
Percocet
room air
sclera
sickle cell disease
sickle thalassemia disease
sympathetic left knee effusion
symptomatic treatment
symptomatology
tachycardia
ventricular hypertrophy

Tonsillectomy and Adenoidectomy: Chronic Adenoid Tonsillitis

adenoid curet
adenoid tonsillitis
Crowe-Davis mouthgag
dissected
electrocautery
endotracheal tube
extubated
fossa
general anesthesia
hemostasis
nasopharynx
oropharynx
red rubber Robinson
transected

Tonsillectomy and Adenoidectomy: Obstructive Sleep Apnea Secondary to Tonsillar and Adenoid Hypertrophy

adenoid hypertrophy
adenoid pack
adenoidectomy
amputated
aseptic manner
#12 blade
capsule

cryptitis
culture and sensitivity
curved Allis clamp
delineated
electrocautery
epinephrine local
general endotracheal anesthetic
hemostasis
laryngeal mirror
lateral sweep
Marcaine
McIvor mouthgag
midline sweep
nitrous oxide
obstructive sleep apnea
palate
pillar mucosa
red rubber catheter
Rose position
supine position
tonsillar fossa
tonsillar hypertrophy
tonsillar tissue
tonsillectomy
Ultane
uvula

Umbilical Vein Cathetcrization, Umbilical Artery Catheterization

Betadine
#11 blade
diaphragm
dilated
forceps
IV fluid
monitor blood gases
respiratory distress
3–0 silk
single-lumen catheter
umbilical stump
ventricle
warmer

Appendix 11
Drugs by Therapeutic Category and Key Word

ACNE PRODUCT
benzoyl peroxide
clindamycin
isotretinoin
tetracycline
tretinoin

ADJUVANT THERAPY, PENICILLIN LEVEL PROLONGATION
probenecid

ADRENAL CORTICOSTEROID AGENT
beclomethasone
betamethasone
budesonide
corticotropin
cortisone
cosyntropin
dexamethasone
fludrocortisone
flunisolide
fluocinolone
fluocinonide
fluorometholone
fluticasone
hydrocortisone
methylprednisolone
prednisolone
prednisone
triamcinolone

ADRENERGIC AGONIST AGENT
Ophthalmic
dipivefrin
naphazoline
phenylephrine
Miscellaneous

albuterol
bitolterol
clonidine
dobutamine
dopamine
epinephrine
isoetharine
isoproterenol
metaproterenol
norepinephrine
oxymetazoline
phenylephrine
phenylpropanolamine
pseudoephedrine
salmeterol
terbutaline

ALCOHOL FREE AGENT
acetaminophen and codeine
albuterol
amiodarone
citrate and citric acid
fluoride
lorazepam
theophylline

ALKALINIZING AGENT
Oral
citrate and citric acid
sodium bicarbonate
Parenteral
sodium acetate
sodium bicarbonate
tromethamine

ALPHA-ADRENERGIC AGENT
Agonist
clonidine
norepinephrine
phenylephrine

Blocking Agent, Oral
  ergotamine
  phenoxybenzamine
  prazosin
Blocking Agent, Parenteral
  phentolamine
  tolazoline
  trimethaphan camsylate
Inhibitors, Central
  methyldopa

ALPHA-/BETA-ADRENERGIC BLOCKER
  labetalol

AMEBICIDE
  chloroquine
  iodoquinol
  metronidazole
  paromomycin

5-AMINOSALICYLIC ACID DERIVATIVE
  mesalamine
  olsalazine
  sulfasalazine

AMMONIUM DETOXICANT
  lactulose
  neomycin
  sodium benzoate
  sodium phenylacetate and sodium
    benzoate
  sodium phenylbutyrate

AMPHETAMINE
  dextroamphetamine

ANALGESIC
Narcotic
  acetaminophen and codeine
  alfentanil
  codeine
  droperidol and fentanyl
  fentanyl

  hydrocodone and acetaminophen
  hydromorphone
  meperidine
  methadone
  morphine sulfate
  nalbuphine
  opium tincture
  oxycodone and acetaminophen
  oxycodone and aspirin
  paregoric
  pentazocine
  propoxyphene
  propoxyphene and acetaminophen
  sufentanil
Non-Narcotic
  acetaminophen
  aspirin
  choline magnesium trisalicylate
  diclofenac
  flurbiprofen
  ibuprofen
  indomethacin
  ketorolac
  naproxen
  piroxicam
  sulindac
  tolmetin
Non-Narcotic (Epidural)
  clonidine
Topical
  benzocaine
  capsaicin
  cocaine
  dibucaine
  lidocaine
  lidocaine and prilocaine
  tetracaine
Urinary
  phenazopyridine

ANDROGEN
  fluoxymesterone
  testosterone

ANGIOTENSIN-CONVERTING ENZYME (ACE) INHIBITOR
captopril
enalapril/enalaprilat
lisinopril

ANOREXIANT
dextroamphetamine
phenylpropanolamine

ANTACID
antacid preparations
calcium supplements
magnesium supplements
sodium bicarbonate

ANTHELMINTIC AGENT
mebendazole
niclosamide
piperazine
praziquantel
pyrantel pamoate
thiabendazole

ANTIANGINAL AGENT
atenolol
diltiazem
nadolol
nifedipine
nitroglycerin
propranolol
verapamil

ANTIANXIETY AGENT
alprazolam
buspirone
diazepam
doxepin
hydroxyzine
lorazepam

ANTIARRHYTHMIC AGENT
Class I-A
disopyramide
procainamide
quinidine
Class I-B
lidocaine
mexiletine
phenytoin
Class I-C
flecainide
Class II
esmolol
nadolol
propranolol
Class III
amiodarone
bretylium
Class IV
verapamil
Miscellaneous
adenosine
digoxin

ANTIASTHMATIC AGENT
albuterol
aminophylline
atropine
beclomethasone
bitolterol
budesonide
cromolyn
dexamethasone
epinephrine
flunisolide
fluticasone
hydrocortisone
ipratropium
isoetharine
isoproterenol
metaproterenol
methylprednisolone
montelukast
nedocromil
prednisolone
prednisone

salmeterol
terbutaline
theophylline
triamcinolone
zafirlukast
zileuton

ANTIBIOTIC
Aminoglycoside
  amikacin
  gentamicin
  neomycin
  streptomycin
  tobramycin
Anaerobic
  clindamycin
  metronidazole
Beta-lactam and Beta-lactamase
    Combination
  amoxicillin and clavulanic acid
  ampicillin and sulbactam
  piperacillin and tazobactam
  ticarcillin and clavulanate potassium
Carbacephem
  loracarbef
Carbapenem
  imipenem and cilastatin
Cephalosporin (First Generation)
  cefazolin
  cephalexin
  cephalothin
  cephapirin
  cephradine
Cephalosporin (Second Generation)
  cefaclor
  cefotetan
  ccfoxitin
  cefpodoxime
  cefprozil
  cefuroxime
Cephalosporin (Third Generation)
  cefixime
  cefoperazone

cefotaxime
ceftazidime
ceftizoxime
ceftriaxone
Cephalosporin (Fourth Generation)
  cefepime
Macrolide
  azithromycin
  clarithromycin
  erythromycin
  erythromycin and sulfisoxazole
  troleandomycin
Ophthalmic
  bacitracin
  bacitracin and polymyxin B
  chloramphenicol
  ciprofloxacin
  dexamethasone, neomycin, and
    polymyxin B
  gentamicin
  neomycin, (bacitracin) polymyxin B,
    and hydrocortisone
  neomycin, polymyxin B, and
    bacitracin
  neomycin, polymyxin B, and
    prednisolone
  polymyxin B
  prednisolone and gentamicin
  sulfacetamide
  tetracycline
  tobramycin
Oral Rinse
  chlorhexidine gluconate
  hydrogen peroxide
Otic
  chloramphenicol
  hydrogen peroxide
  neomycin, (bacitracin) polymyxin B,
    and hydrocortisone
Penicillin
  amoxicillin
  amoxicillin and clavulanic acid
  ampicillin

ampicillin and sulbactam
penicillin G benzathine
penicillin G, parenteral, aqueous
penicillin G procaine
penicillin V potassium
Penicillin (Antipseudomonal)
  carbenicillin
  mezlocillin
  piperacillin
  piperacillin and tazobactam
  ticarcillin
  ticarcillin and clavulanate potassium
Penicillin (Antistaphylococcal)
  cloxacillin
  dicloxacillin
  methicillin
  nafcillin
  oxacillin
Quinolone
  ciprofloxacin
  nalidixic acid
Sulfonamide Derivative
  co-trimoxazole
  erythromycin and sulfisoxazole
  sulfacetamide
  sulfadiazine
  sulfamethoxazole
  sulfisoxazole
Sulfone
  dapsone
Tetracycline Derivative
  demeclocycline
  doxycycline
  tetracycline
Topical
  bacitracin
  bacitracin and polymyxin B
  chlorhexidine gluconate
  gentamicin
  gentian violet
  hexachlorophene
  hydrogen peroxide
  mafenide

metronidazole
mupirocin
neomycin
neomycin and polymyxin B
neomycin, (bacitracin) polymyxin B,
  and hydrocortisone
neomycin, polymyxin B, and
  bacitracin
silver sulfadiazine
tetracycline
Urinary Irrigation
  neomycin and polymyxin B
  polymyxin B
Miscellaneous
  aztreonam
  bacitracin
  chloramphenicol
  clindamycin
  clofazimine
  cycloserine
  furazolidone
  methenamine
  nitrofurantoin
  pentamidine
  polymyxin B
  rifabutin
  rifampin
  trimethoprim
  vancomycin

ANTICHOLINERGIC AGENT

Ophthalmic
  atropine
  cyclopentolate
  homatropine
  scopolamine
Transdermal
  scopolamine
Miscellaneous
  atropine
  benztropine
  dicyclomine

glycopyrrolate
hyoscyamine
hyoscyamine, atropine, scopolamine,
  and phenobarbital
ipratropium
propantheline
scopolamine
trihexyphenidyl
trimethaphan camsylate

ANTICOAGULANT AGENT
enoxaparin
heparin
warfarin

ANTICONVULSANT AGENT
Barbiturate
  mephobarbital
  pentobarbital
  phenobarbital
  primidone
  thiopental
Benzodiazepine
  clonazepam
  clorazepate
  diazepam
  lorazepam
  midazolam
Hydantoin
  fosphenytoin
  mephenytoin
  phenytoin
Succinimide
  ethosuximide
  methsuximide
Miscellaneous
  acctazolamide
  carbamazepine
  felbamate
  gabapentin
  lamotrigine
  magnesium supplements
  paraldehyde

tiagabine
topiramate
valproic acid and derivatives

ANTIDEPRESSANT AGENT
Serotonin Reuptake Inhibitor
  fluoxetine
  paroxetine
Tricyclic
  amitriptyline
  desipramine
  doxepin
  imipramine
  nortriptyline
Miscellaneous
  trazodone

ANTIDIABETIC AGENT
insulin preparations

ANTIDIARRHEAL AGENT
attapulgite
bismuth subsalicylate
charcoal
diphenoxylate and atropine
kaolin and pectin
lactobacillus acidophilus and
  lactobacillus bulgaricus
loperamide
octreotidc acctatc
opium tincture
paregoric

ANTIDIURETIC HORMONE ANALOG
vasopressin

ANTIDOTE
Acetaminophen
  acetylcysteine
Absorbent
  charcoal
Aluminum Toxicity
  deferoxamine

Anticholinergic Agent
  physostigmine
Anticholinesterase
  pralidoxime
Arsenic Toxicity
  dimercaprol
Benzodiazepine
  flumazenil
Cisplatin
  amifostine
  sodium thiosulfate
Copper Toxicity
  penicillamine
Cyanide
  amyl nitrite
  methylene blue
  sodium thiosulfate
Cyclophosphamide-Induced
  Hemorrhagic Cystitis
  mesna
Cycloserine Toxicity
  pyridoxine
Digoxin
  digoxin immune fab
Drug-Induced Dystonic Reactions
  benztropine
  diphenhydramine
  trihexyphenidyl
Drug-Induced Methemoglobinemia
  methylene blue
Emetic
  ipecac syrup
Extravasation
  hyaluronidase
  phentolamine
  sodium thiosulfate
Gold Toxicity
  dimercaprol
Heparin
  protamine
Hydralazine Toxicity
  pyridoxine
Hypercalcemia
  calcitonin

edetate disodium
etidronate disodium
pamidronate
plicamycin
Hyperkalemia
  sodium polystyrene sulfonate
Hypersensitivity Reactions
  diphenhydramine
  epinephrine
Ifosfamide-Induced Hemorrhagic
  Cystitis
  mesna
Iron Toxicity
  deferoxamine
Isoniazid Toxicity
  dimercaprol
  edetate calcium disodium
  penicillamine
  succimer
Malignant Hyperthermia
  dantrolene
Mercury Toxicity
  dimercaprol
Methotrexate
  leucovorin
Narcotic Agonists
  naloxone
Neuromuscular Blocking Agent
  edrophonium
  neostigmine
  pyridostigmine
Organophosphate Poisoning
  atropine
  pralidoxime

ANTIEMETIC AGENT

chlorpromazine
dexamethasone
dimenhydrinate
dolasetron
dronabinol
granisetron
hydroxyzine
lorazepam

meclizine
metoclopramide
ondansetron
prochlorperazine
promethazine
thiethylperazine
trimethobenzamide

ANTIFLATULENT AGENT
charcoal
simethicone

ANTIFUNGAL AGENT
Oral Nonabsorbed
clotrimazole
nystatin
Systemic
amphotericin B
amphotericin B lipid complex
amphotericin B liposome
fluconazole
flucytosine
griseofulvin
itraconazole
ketoconazole
miconazole
Topical
amphotericin B
clioquinol
clotrimazole
econazole
gentian violet
haloprogin
ketoconazole
miconazole
nystatin
sodium thiosulfate
tolnaftate
undecylenic acid and derivatives
Vaginal
clotrimazole
miconazole
nystatin

ANTIGOUT AGENT
allopurinol
colchicine
probenecid

ANTIHEMOPHILIC AGENT
antihemophilic factor (human)
desmopressin
factor IX complex (human)
tranexamic acid

ANTIHISTAMINE
Antihistamine/Decongestant
  Combination
  brompheniramine and
    phenylpropanolamine
  carbinoxamine and pseudoephedrine
  promethazine and phenylephrine
  promethazine, phenylephrine, and
    codeine
  triprolidine and pseudoephedrine
Nasal
  azelastine
Miscellaneous
  astemizole
  brompheniramine
  cetirizine
  chlorpheniramine
  clemastine
  cyproheptadine
  dimenhydrinate
  hydroxyzine
  loratadine
  meclizine
  terfenadine

ANTIHYPERTENSIVE AGENT
Combination
  hydrochlorothiazide and
    spironolactone
Miscellaneous
  atenolol
  bumetanide

A69

captopril
chlorothiazide
clonidine
diazoxide
diltiazem
enalapril/enalaprilat
esmolol
ethacrynic acid
furosemide
hydralazine
hydrochlorothiazide
labetalol
lisinopril
methyldopa
metolazone
minoxidil
nadolol
nifedipine
nitroglycerin
nitroprusside
phenoxybenzamine
phentolamine
prazosin
propranolol
spironolactone
timolol
tolazoline
torsemide
triamterene
trimethaphan camsylate
verapamil

ANTIHYPOGLYCEMIC AGENT
diazoxide
glucagon

ANTIINFLAMMATORY AGENT
Ophthalmic
  dexamethasone
  fluorometholone
  flurbiprofen

medrysone
prednisolone
Rectal
  hydrocortisone
  mesalamine
Miscellaneous
  aspirin
  beclomethasone
  betamethasone
  budesonide
  choline magnesium trisalicylate
  colchicine
  cortisone
  dexamethasone
  diclofenac
  flunisolide
  fluocinolone
  flurbiprofen
  hydrocortisone
  ibuprofen
  indomethacin
  ketorolac
  mesalamine
  methylprednisolone
  naproxen
  olsalazine
  piroxicam
  prednisolone
  sulfasalazine
  sulindac
  triamcinolone

ANTILIPEMIC AGENT
cholestyramine resin
niacin

ANTIMALARIAL AGENT
chloroquine
hydroxychloroquine
primaquine
pyrimethamine
quinine
sulfadoxine and pyrimethamine

ANTIMANIC AGENT
lithium

ANTIMIGRAINE AGENT
amitriptyline
ergotamine
nadolol
papaverine
propranolol
sumatriptan
timolol

ANTINEOPLASTIC AGENT
Adjuvant
  azathioprine
Alkylating Agent
  busulfan
  carboplatin
  cisplatin
  ifosfamide
  thiotepa
Alkylating Agent (Nitrogen Mustard)
  chlorambucil
  cyclophosphamide
  mechlorethamine
  melphalan
Alkylating Agent (Nitrosourea)
  carmustine
  lomustine
Anthracycline
  daunorubicin
  doxorubicin
  idarubicin
  mitoxantrone
Antibiotic
  bleomycin
  dactinomycin
  daunorubicin
  doxorubicin
  idarubicin
  mitomycin
  mitoxantrone
  plicamycin

Antimetabolite
  cytarabine
  fludarabine
  fluorouracil
  mercaptopurine
  methotrexate
  thioguanine
Antimetabolite (Purine)
  cladribine
Antimicrotubular
  paclitaxel
Hormone (Gonadotropin Hormone-
    Releasing Antigen)
  leuprolide
Miotic Inhibitor
  etoposide
  vinblastine
  vincristine
Purine
  mercaptopurine
Miscellaneous
  asparaginase
  dacarbazine
  dexrazoxane
  hydroxyurea
  interferon alfa-2a
  interferon alfa-2b
  pegaspargase
  procarbazine

ANTIPARASITIC AGENT, TOPICAL
lindane
permethrin

ANTI-PARKINSONS AGENT
amantadine
benztropine
levodopa
trihexyphenidyl

ANTIPLATELET AGENT
aspirin
dipyridamole

ANTIPROTOZOAL AGENT
atovaquone
furazolidone
metronidazole
pentamidine

ANTIPRURITIC AGENT, TOPICAL
lidocaine and prilocaine

ANTIPSORIATIC AGENT, TOPICAL
coal tar

ANTIPSYCHOTIC AGENT
chlorpromazine
droperidol
haloperidol
prochlorperazine
thioridazine
thiothixene

ANTIPYRETIC AGENT
acetaminophen
aspirin
ibuprofen
indomethacin
ketorolac
naproxen

ANTIRETROVIRAL AGENT
abacavir
didanosine
efavirenz
indinavir
lamivudine
nelfinavir
nevirapine
ritonavir
saquinavir
stavudine
zalcitabine
zidovudine

ANTISEBORRHEIC AGENT, TOPICAL
coal tar
selenium sulfide
sulfur and salicylic acid

ANTISECRETORY AGENT
octreotide acetate

ANTISPASMODIC AGENT
Gastrointestinal
atropine
dicyclomine
glycopyrrolate
hyoscyamine
hyoscyamine, atropine, scopolamine, and phenobarbital
propantheline
Urinary
oxybutynin
propantheline

ANTITUBERCULAR AGENT
cycloserine
ethambutol
ethionamide
isoniazid
pyrazinamide
rifabutin
rifampin
streptomycin

ANTITUSSIVE AGENT
codeine
dextromethorphan
guaifenesin and codeine
guaifenesin and dextromethorphan
hydrocodone and acetaminophen
hydromorphone
promethazine and codeine
promethazine, phenylephrine, and codeine

ANTIVENIN AGENT
antivenin (crotalidae) polyvalent

ANTIVIRAL AGENT
Inhalation Therapy
  ribavirin
Ophthalmic
  idoxuridine
  trifluridine
  vidarabine
Oral
  acyclovir
  amantadine
  famciclovir
  rimantadine
Parenteral
  acyclovir
  foscarnet
  ganciclovir
Topical
  acyclovir

BARBITURATE
  mephobarbital
  methohexital
  pentobarbital
  phenobarbital
  primidone
  secobarbital
  thiopental

BENZODIAZEPINE
  alprazolam
  clonazepam
  clorazepate
  diazepam
  flurazepam
  midazolam
  triazolam

BETA-ADRENERGIC BLOCKER
Ophthalmic
  levobunolol
  timolol
Miscellaneous
  atenolol

  esmolol
  nadolol
  propranolol
  timolol

BETA$_1$ & BETA$_2$-ADRENERGIC AGONIST AGENT
  albuterol
  bitolterol
  metaproterenol
  salmeterol
  terbutaline

BIOLOGICAL RESPONSE MODULATOR
  interferon alfa-2a
  interferon alfa-2b

BIOTINIDASE DEFICIENCY, TREATMENT AGENT
  biotin

BISPHOSPHONATE DERIVATIVE
  etidronate disodium
  pamidronate

BLOOD PRODUCT DERIVATIVE
  albumin
  antihemophilic factor (human)
  factor IX complex (human)

BLOOD VISCOSITY REDUCER AGENT
  pentoxifylline

BRONCHODILATOR
  albuterol
  aminophylline
  atropine
  bitolterol

epinephrine
ipratropium
isoetharine
isoproterenol
metaproterenol
salmeterol
terbutaline
theophylline

CALCIUM CHANNEL BLOCKER

diltiazem
nifedipine
verapamil

CALCIUM SALT

calcium supplements

CALORIC AGENT

fat emulsion
medium chain triglycerides

CARBONIC ANHYDRASE INHIBITOR

acetazolamide

CARDIAC GLYCOSIDE

digoxin

CARDIOPROTECTIVE AGENT

dexrazoxane

CENTRAL NERVOUS SYSTEM STIMULANT

Amphetamine
dextroamphetamine
Nonamphetamine
caffeine, citrated
doxapram
methylphenidate
pemoline

CHELATING AGENT

Oral

penicillamine
succimer
Parenteral
deferoxamine
dimercaprol
edetate calcium disodium
edetate disodium
Miscellaneous
dexrazoxane

CHOLINERGIC AGENT

Ophthalmic
acetylcholine
physostigmine
pilocarpine
Miscellaneous
bethanechol
edrophonium
neostigmine
physostigmine
pilocarpine
pyridostigmine

COLONY STIMULATING FACTOR

epoetin alfa
filgrastim
sargramostim

CONTRACEPTIVE AGENT

Oral
norethindrone
Progestin Only
medroxyprogesterone
norethindrone

CONTROLLED SUBSTANCE

II
alfentanil
cocaine
codeine
dextroamphetamine
dronabinol
droperidol and fentanyl

fentanyl
hydromorphone
meperidine
methadone
methylphenidate
morphine sulfate
opium tincture
oxycodone and acetaminophen
oxycodone and aspirin
pentobarbital
secobarbital
sufentanil
III
acetaminophen and codeine
fluoxymesterone
hydrocodone and acetaminophen
ketamine
paregoric
pentobarbital
testosterone
thiopental
IV
alprazolam
chloral hydrate
clonazepam
clorazepate
diazepam
flurazepam
lorazepam
mephobarbital
methohexital
midazolam
paraldehyde
pemoline
pentazocine
phenobarbital
propoxyphene
propoxyphene and acetaminophen
triazolam
V
acetaminophen and codeine
diphenoxylate and atropine
guaifenesin and codeine

promethazine and codeine
promethazine, phenylephrine, and
codeine

CORTICOSTEROID

Inhalant (Oral)
beclomethasone
budesonide
dexamethasone
flunisolide
fluticasone
triamcinolone
Intranasal
beclomethasone
budesonide
dexamethasone
flunisolide
fluticasone
triamcinolone
Ophthalmic
dexamethasone
dexamethasone, neomycin, and
polymyxin B
fluorometholone
medrysone
neomycin, (bacitracin) polymyxin B,
and hydrocortisone
neomycin, polymyxin B, and
prednisolone
prednisolone
prednisolone and gentamicin
Otic
neomycin, (bacitracin) polymyxin B,
and hydrocortisone
Rectal
hydrocortisone
Systemic
betamethasone
cortisone
dexamethasone
fludrocortisone
hydrocortisone
methylprednisolone

prednisolone
prednisone
triamcinolone
Topical
  betamethasone
  dexamethasone
  fluocinolone
  fluocinonide
  fluticasone
  hydrocortisone
  neomycin, (bacitracin) polymyxin B,
    and hydrocortisone

COUGH PREPARATION
codeine
dextromethorphan
guaifenesin and codeine
guaifenesin and dextromethorphan
hydrocodone and acetaminophen
hydromorphone
promethazine and codeine
promethazine, phenylephrine, and
  codeine

CYSTINOSIS, TREATMENT AGENT
cysteamine

CYTOPROTECTIVE AGENT
amifostine

DECONGESTANT
Nasal
  naphazoline
  oxymetazoline
Miscellaneous
  brompheniramine and
    phenylpropanolamine
  guaifenesin, phenylpropanolamine,
    and phenylephrine
  phenylpropanolamine
  pseudoephedrine

DIAGNOSTIC AGENT
Adrenocortical Insufficiency
  corticotropin
  cosyntropin
Gonadotrophic Hormone
  gonadorelin
Growth Hormone Function
  arginine
  levodopa
Hypothalamic-Pituitary ACTH
    Function
  metyrapone
Intestinal Absorption
  d-Xylose
Myasthenia Gravis
  edrophonium
  neostigmine
Pancreatic Exocrine Insufficiency
  secretin
Penicillin Allergy Skin Test
  benzylpenicilloyl-polylysine
Pheochromocytoma
  phentolamine
Thyroid Function
  protirelin
Zollinger-Ellison Syndrome and
    Pancreatic Exocrine Disease
  secretin

DIURETIC AGENT
Carbonic Anhydrase Inhibitor
  acetazolamide
Combination
  hydrochlorothiazide and
    spironolactone
Loop
  bumetanide
  ethacrynic acid
  furosemide
  torsemide
Osmotic
  mannitol

Potassium Sparing
  spironolactone
  triamterene
Thiazide
  chlorothiazide
  hydrochlorothiazide
Miscellaneous
  metolazone

DYE FREE AGENT
  lorazepam
  theophylline

ELECTROLYTE SUPPLEMENT
Oral
  calcium supplements
  magnesium supplements
  phosphate supplements
  potassium supplements
  sodium bicarbonate
  sodium chloride
Parenteral
  calcium supplements
  magnesium supplements
  phosphate supplements
  sodium acetate
  sodium bicarbonate
  sodium chloride

ENZYME
Glucocerebrosidase
  alglucerase
Inhalant
  dornase alfa
Pancreatic
  pancreatin
  pancrelipase
Topical Debridement
  sutilains

ERGOT ALKALOID AND DERIVATIVE
  ergotamine

ESTROGEN DERIVATIVE, VAGINAL
  estradiol
  estrogens, conjugated

EXPECTORANT
  guaifenesin
  guaifenesin and codeine
  guaifenesin and dextromethorphan
  guaifenesin, phenylpropanolamine,
    and phenylephrine
  potassium iodide

FOLIC ACID DERIVATIVE
  leucovorin

GALLSTONE DISSOLUTION AGENT
  ursodiol

GANGLIONIC BLOCKING AGENT
  trimethaphan camsylate

GASTRIC ACID SECRETION INHIBITOR
  lansoprazole
  omeprazole

GASTROINTESTINAL AGENT
Gastric or Duodenal Ulcer Treatment
  antacid preparations
  bismuth subsalicylate
  cimetidine
  famotidine
  lansoprazole
  misoprostol
  nizatidine
  omeprazole

ranitidine
sucralfate
Prokinetic
cisapride
metoclopramide

GENERAL ANESTHETIC
alfentanil
fentanyl
ketamine
methohexital
pentobarbital
propofol
sufentanil
thiopental

GENITOURINARY IRRIGANT
neomycin and polymyxin B

GLUCOCORTICOID
beclomethasone
betamethasone
budesonide
cortisone
dexamethasone
fludrocortisone
flunisolide
fluocinolone
fluocinonide
fluticasone
hydrocortisone
methylprednisolone
prednisolone
prednisone
triamcinolone

GOLD COMPOUND
auranofin
aurothioglucose
gold sodium thiomalate

GONADOTROPIN
chorionic gonadotropin
gonadorelin

GONADOTROPIN RELEASING HORMONE ANALOG
histrelin

GROWTH HORMONE
human growth hormone

HEMOSTATIC AGENT
aminocaproic acid
aprotinin
desmopressin
thrombin, topical

HISTAMINE H$_2$ ANTAGONIST
cimetidine
famotidine
nizatidine
ranitidine

HIV AGENT (ANTI-HIV AGENT)
abacavir
didanosine
efavirenz
indinavir
lamivudine
nelfinavir
nevirapine
ritonavir
saquinavir
stavudine
zalcitabine
zidovudine

HOMOCYSTINURIA, TREATMENT AGENT
betaine anhydrous

HORMONE, POSTERIOR PITUITARY
vasopressin

HYPERAMMONEMIA AGENT

lactulose
neomycin
sodium benzoate
sodium phenylacetate and sodium
benzoate
sodium phenylbutyrate

HYPERTHERMIA, TREATMENT

dantrolene

HYPNOTIC AGENT

chloral hydrate
diazepam
flurazepam
lorazepam
midazolam
paraldehyde
pentobarbital
phenobarbital
secobarbital
thiopental
triazolam

IMMUNE GLOBULIN

immune globulin, intravenous
respiratory syncytial virus immune
globulin (intravenous)
rh$_o$(D) immune globulin
rh$_o$(D) immune globulin, intravenous

IMMUNOSUPPRESSANT AGENT

azathioprine
cyclosporine
dacliximab
lymphocyte immune globulin
muromonab-CD3
mycophenolate
tacrolimus

INFANTILE SPASM, TREATMENT

corticotropin
valproic acid and derivatives

INHALATION, MISCELLANEOUS

cromolyn
nedocromil

INTERFERON

interferon alfa-2a
interferon alfa-2b

INTRAVENOUS NUTRITIONAL THERAPY

fat emulsion

IRON SALT

iron dextran complex
iron supplements

KERATOLYTIC AGENT

podophyllum resin
salicylic acid

LAXATIVE

Bowel Evacuant
polyethylene glycol-electrolyte
solution
Bulk-Producing
malt soup extract
psyllium
Hyperosmolar
sorbitol
Lubricant
mineral oil
Osmotic
glycerin
magnesium supplements
polyethylene glycol-electrolyte
solution
sorbitol

A79

Saline
  phosphate supplements
Stimulant
  bisacodyl
  cascara sagrada
  castor oil
  docusate and casanthranol
  senna
Surfactant
  docusate
  docusate and casanthranol
Miscellaneous
  lactulose

LEPROSTATIC AGENT
  clofazimine
  dapsone

LEUKOTRIENE RECEPTOR ANTAGONIST
  montelukast
  zafirlukast
  zileuton

LOCAL ANESTHETIC AGENT
Injectable
  bupivacaine
  lidocaine
  lidocaine and epinephrine
  tetracaine
Ophthalmic
  proparacaine
  tetracaine
Oral
  benzocaine
  dyclonine
  tetracaine
Topical
  benzocaine
  cocaine
  dibucaine
  lidocaine
  lidocaine and prilocaine

  tetracaine
Urinary
  phenazopyridine

LUBRICANT, OCULAR
  ocular lubricant
  sodium chloride

LOW MOLECULAR WEIGHT HEPARIN
  enoxaparin

LUNG SURFACTANT
  beractant
  calfactant
  colfosceril

LUTEINIZING HORMONE-RELEASING HORMONE ANALOG
  leuprolide

MAGNESIUM SALT
  magnesium supplements

METABOLIC ALKALOSIS AGENT
  ammonium chloride
  arginine

MINERAL
Oral
  fluoride
  iron supplements
  zinc supplements
Oral Topical
  fluoride
Parenteral
  iron dextran complex
  trace metals
  zinc supplements

MINERALOCORTICOID
  fludrocortisone

MONOCLONAL ANTIBODY
palivizumab

MUCOLYTIC AGENT
acetylcysteine
dornase alfa

NASAL AGENT, VASOCONSTRICTOR
naphazoline
oxymetazoline
phenylephrine

NEUROMUSCULAR BLOCKER AGENT
Depolarizing
succinylcholine
Nondepolarizing
atracurium
cisatracurium
doxacurium
mivacurium
pancuronium
rocuronium
tubocurarine
vecuronium

NITRATE
nitroglycerin

NONNUCLEOSIDE REVERSE TRANSCRIPTASE INHIBITOR (NNRTI)
efavirenz
nevirapine

NONSTEROIDAL ANTIINFLAMMATORY DRUG (NSAID)
Ophthalmic
diclofenac
flurbiprofen
ketorolac
Oral
aspirin
choline magnesium trisalicylate
diclofenac
ibuprofen
indomethacin
ketorolac
naproxen
piroxicam
sulindac
tolmetin
Parenteral
indomethacin
ketorolac

NUCLEOSIDE ANALOG REVERSE TRANSCRIPTASE INHIBITOR (NRTI)
abacavir
didanosine
lamivudine
stavudine
zalcitabine
zidovudine

NUTRITIONAL SUPPLEMENT
ascorbic acid
biotin
carnitine
cyanocobalamin
cysteine
dihydrotachysterol
ergocalciferol
folic acid
medium chain triglycerides
niacin
phytonadione
pyridoxine
riboflavin
thiamine
vitamin A
vitamin E

OPHTHALMIC AGENT
Miotic
  acetylcholine
  pilocarpine
Mydriatic
  atropine
  cyclopentolate
  homatropine
  phenylephrine
  scopolamine
  tropicamide
Vasoconstrictor
  dipivefrin
  naphazoline
Miscellaneous
  ocular lubricant
  silver nitrate

OPIATE PARTIAL AGONIST
  nalbuphine
  pentazocine

OTIC AGENT
Analgesic
  antipyrine and benzocaine
Ceruminolytic
  antipyrine and benzocaine
  carbamide peroxide
  triethanolamine polypeptide oleate-
    condensate

OVULATION STIMULATOR
  chorionic gonadotropin

PANCREATIC ENZYME
  pancreatin
  pancrelipase

PEDICULICIDE
  lindane
  permethrin

PHENOTHIAZINE DERIVATIVE
  chlorpromazine
  haloperidol
  prochlorperazine
  promethazine
  promethazine and codeine
  thiethylperazine
  thioridazine
  thiothixene

PHOSPHATE SALT
  phosphate supplements

PHOSPHODIESTERASE ENZYME INHIBITOR
  amrinone
  milrinone

PLASMA VOLUME EXPANDER
  albumin
  dextran
  hetastarch

POTASSIUM SALT
  phosphate supplements
  potassium supplements

PRESERVATIVE FREE AGENT
  adenosine
  alfentanil
  atracurium
  bupivacaine
  clonidine
  cytarabine
  doxorubicin
  enoxaparin
  epoetin alfa
  fentanyl
  filgrastim
  gentamicin
  heparin
  lidocaine
  mesna
  metaproterenol

methotrexate
morphine sulfate
pegaspargase
ranitidine
respiratory syncytial virus immune
    globulin (intravenous)
timolol
tobramycin
urokinase

PROGESTIN
medroxyprogesterone
norethindrone

PROSTAGLANDIN
alprostadil
misoprostol

PROTEASE INHIBITOR
indinavir
nelfinavir
ritonavir
saquinavir

RECOMBINANT HUMAN ERYTHROPOIETIN
epoetin alfa

RESPIRATORY STIMULANT
aminophylline
caffeine, citrated
doxapram
theophylline

RETINOIC ACID DERIVATIVE
isotretinoin
tretinoin

SALICYLATE
aspirin
choline magnesium trisalicylate

SCABICIDAL AGENT
crotamiton
lindane
permethrin

SEDATIVE
chloral hydrate
clorazepate
diazepam
diphenhydramine
flurazepam
hydroxyzine
lorazepam
mephobarbital
methohexital
midazolam
paraldehyde
pentazocine
pentobarbital
phenobarbital
promethazine
secobarbital
thiopental
triazolam

SHAMPOO
lindane
selenium sulfide

SKELETAL MUSCLE RELAXANT
Nonparalytic
baclofen
chlorzoxazone
cyclobenzaprine
dantrolene
methocarbamol
Paralytic
atracurium
cisatracurium
doxacurium
mivacurium
pancuronium
rocuronium

succinylcholine
tubocurarine
vecuronium
Miscellaneous
quinine

SOAP
hexachlorophene

SODIUM SALT
phosphate supplements
sodium acetate
sodium bicarbonate
sodium chloride

SOMATOSTATIN ANALOG
octreotide acetate

STOOL SOFTENER
docusate
docusate and casanthranol

SUCRASE DEFICIENCY, TREATMENT AGENT
sacrosidase

SUGAR FREE AGENT
albuterol
calcium supplements
citrate and citric acid
fluoride
metoclopramide
psyllium
theophylline

SYMPATHOMIMETIC AGENT
albuterol
bitolterol
dobutamine
dopamine
epinephrine
isoetharine
isoproterenol
metaproterenol
norepinephrine
phenylephrine
phenylpropanolamine
pseudoephedrine
terbutaline
triprolidine and pseudoephedrine

THEOPHYLLINE DERIVATIVE
aminophylline
theophylline

THROMBOLYTIC AGENT
streptokinase
urokinase

THYROID PRODUCT
levothyroxine
liothyronine

TOCOLYTIC AGENT
terbutaline

TOPICAL SKIN PRODUCT
aluminum acetate
benzoyl peroxide
calamine lotion
capsaicin
hemorrhoidal preparations
iodine
silver nitrate
zinc oxide

TRACE ELEMENT, PARENTERAL
trace metals

UREA CYCLE DISORDER (UCD) TREATMENT AGENT
sodium benzoate
sodium phenylacetate and sodium
  benzoate
sodium phenylbutyrate

URIC ACID LOWERING AGENT
allopurinol
probenecid

URICOSURIC AGENT
probenecid

URINARY ACIDIFYING AGENT
ammonium chloride
ascorbic acid
phosphate supplements

VACCINE
Inactivated Bacteria
pneumococcal vaccine
Live Virus
rotavirus vaccine

VASOCONSTRICTOR
Nasal
oxymetazoline
Ophthalmic
oxymetazoline

VASODILATOR
Coronary
amyl nitrite
dipyridamole
nitroglycerin
Miscellaneous
diazoxide
hydralazine
minoxidil
nitroglycerin
nitroprusside
papaverine

phenoxybenzamine
phentolamine
prazosin
tolazoline

VASOPRESSIN ANALOG, SYNTHETIC
desmopressin

VITAMIN A DERIVATIVE
isotretinoin

VITAMIN D ANALOG
calcitriol
dihydrotachysterol
ergocalciferol

VITAMIN
Fat Soluble
calcitriol
dihydrotachysterol
ergocalciferol
phytonadione
vitamin A
vitamin E
Topical
tretinoin
vitamin E
Water Soluble
ascorbic acid
biotin
cyanocobalamin
folic acid
niacin
pyridoxine
riboflavin
thiamine

NOTES

NOTES

NOTES

NOTES

NOTES

NOTES

NOTES

NOTES

NOTES

NOTES

NOTES

NOTES

NOTES

NOTES

NOTES